AN OFFICIAL REPORT OF THE AMERICAN PUBLIC HEALTH ASSOCIATION

CONTROL OF
COMMUNICABLE
DISEASES
MANUAL   20th Edition

David L. Heymann, MD, Editor

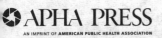

APHA PRESS
AN IMPRINT OF AMERICAN PUBLIC HEALTH ASSOCIATION

American Public Health Association
800 I Street, NW
Washington, DC 20001-3710
www.apha.org

DISCLAIMER: The views expressed in the publications of the
American Public Health Association are those of the author
and do not necessarily reflect the views of the American Public
Health Association, or its staff, advisory panels, officers, or
members of the Association's Executive Board.

Georges C. Benjamin, MD, FACP, FACEP(E), FNAPA,
FRSPH(Hon), FFPH(Hon), Executive Director
Ashell R. Alston, Interim Director of Publications
Brian Selzer, Interim Deputy Director of Publications
Maya Ribault, Book Production Editor

Printed and bound in the United States of America
Typesetting: The Charlesworth Group
Cover Design: Alan Giarcanella
Printing and Binding: United Book Press, Inc.

ISBN 978-0-87553-018-5 softcover

iii

Paul E. M. Fine, VMD, PhD
London School of Hygiene & Tropical Medicine
United Kingdom

Johan Giesecke, MD
Karolinska Institute
Sweden

Donato Greco, MD
Italy

Duane J. Gubler, ScD, MS
Duke-NUS Graduate Medical School
Singapore

Paul R. Gully, MB, ChB, FRCPC, FFPH
University of British Columbia School of Population and Public Health
Canada

Pengiran Hishamuddin Badaruddin, BMBS, MPH
Ministry of Health
Singapore

James M. Hughes, MD
Emory University School of Medicine
United States

Martyn Jeggo, BVetMed, MSc, PhD, FAICD, FTSE, MRCVS
Geelong Centre for Emerging Infectious Diseases
Australia

T. Jacob John, MBBS, FRCP, PhD, DSc
Child Health Foundation
India

I. Nyoman Kandun, MD
Field Epidemiology Training Programme
Indonesia

Rima F. Khabbaz, MD
Centers for Diseases Control and Prevention
United States

Omar A. Khan, MD, MHS
Christiana Care Health System
United States

Ann Marie Kimball, MD, MPH
Bill and Melinda Gates Foundation
United States

Sait Kit (Ken) Lam
University of Malaya
Malaysia

James W. LeDuc, PhD
University of Texas Medical Branch
United States

Marlo Libel, MD, MPH
Brazil

Prof. David Mabey
London School of Hygiene & Tropical Medicine
United Kingdom

John S. Mackenzie, PhD
Curtin University
Australia

Jaouad Mahjour
World Health Organization
Regional Office for the Eastern Mediterranean
Egypt

Helene Mambu-ma-Disu, MD, MPH
Sabin Vaccine Institute
Democratic Republic of the Congo,
Republic of the Congo, Madagascar

Ziad A. Memish, MD, FRCP(Can), FRCP(Edin), FRCP(Lond)
Alfaisal University
Kingdom of Saudi Arabia

Jai P. Narain, MBBS, MD, MPH
National Centre for Disease Control
India

Angus Nicoll, MD
European Centre for Disease Prevention and Control
Sweden

Jean-Marie Okwo-Bele, MD, MPH
World Health Organization
Switzerland

Marguerite Pappaioanou, DVM, MPVM, DACVPM, PhD
Centers for Disease Control and Prevention
United States

Didier Pittet, MD, MS, CBE
The University of Geneva Hospitals and Faculty of Medicine
Switzerland

Guénaël Rodier, MD
World Health Organization
Regional Office for Europe
Denmark

Bijan Sadrizadeh, MD
Academy of Medical Sciences
Iran

Jørgen Schlundt, DVM, PhD
Technical University of Denmark
Denmark

Oyewale Tomori, DVM, PhD
Redeemer's University
Nigeria

Suwit Wibulpolprasert, MD
Thailand Ministry of Public Health
Thailand

Burton W. Wilcke, Jr, PhD
University of Vermont
United States

REVIEWERS

Dr. Rosemawati Ariffin
ASEAN/FETN
Malaysia

Shaharom Nor Azian, CMDin, MD, MPH, EIP Malaysia
Ministry of Health
Malaysia

Dr. Sopon Iamsirithavorn
ASEAN/FETN
Thailand

Dr. Chuleeporn Jiraphongsa
ASEAN/FETN
Thailand

Dr. Muhammad Amir Kamaludin
ASEAN/FETN
United Kingdom

Dr. Fadzilah Kamaludin
ASEAN/FETN
Malaysia

Andrew Kiyu, MBBS, DrPH, MPH
Sarawak Health Department
Malaysia

Saraswathi Bina Rai, MBBS, MPH
Ministry of Health
Malaysia

Kumnuan Ungchusak
Ministry of Public Health
Thailand

Dr. Ahmad Faudzi Yusof
ASEAN/FETN
Malaysia

Dr. Mohamed Paid Bin Yusof
ASEAN/FETN
Malaysia

Oliverio Welsh, MD, DrSc
University Hospital Monterrey
Mexico

Ed E. Zijlstra, FRCP, FRCPath, PhD
Rotterdam Centre for Tropical Medicine
The Netherlands

Ahmed Fahal, FRCS
University of Khartoum
Sudan

CHAPTER AUTHORS

Centers for Disease Control and Prevention
1600 Clifton Road, Atlanta, GA 30329, USA
http://www.cdc.gov

Anderson A. D.
Barskey A.
Barton Behravesh C.
Beach M.
Beard C. B.
Belay E.
Bertherat E.
Bialek S. R.
Blaney D.
Bowen A.
Bower W.
Brandt M.
Brunkard J. M.
Cantey P.
Clark T.
Cleveland A. A.
Cohn A.
Dasch G.
Deming M.
Doker T.
Dunne E. F.
Eberhard M.
Fischer M.
Fox L.
Franka R.
Gage K.
Galloway R.
Gorwitz R.
Gould L. H.
Griffin P. M.
Guerra M.
Hall A.
Hall R.
Harris J.
Herwaldt B. L.
Hicks L.
Hills S. L.
Hoffmaster A.

Hunsperger E.
Introcaso C. E.
Iwane M.
Jackson K. A.
Jones J.
Kato C.
Kersh G. J.
Kidd S.
Knust B.
Lammie P.
Lanzieri T. M.
Lasker B.
Litvintseva A.
Lockhart S.
Lopman B.
Mahon B.
Margolis H.
Marin M.
Martin D.
McQuiston J.
Mead P.
Meites E.
Meslin F.
Mintz E.
Mody R. K.
Montgomery S.
Moore M.
Muñoz J.
Ndowa F.
Neblett Fanfair R.
Nelson C.
Nichol S.
Nicholson W.
Nielsen H. V.
O'Reilly C.
Papp J.
Patel M.
Patrick M.

Peterman T.
Pillay A.
Powers A.
Purfield A. E.
Rabe I.
Rao A. K.
Reef S.
Regan J.
Reynolds M.
Rollin P. E.
Routh J.
Roy M.
Roy S.
Schillinger J. A.
Schneider E.
Schriefer M.

Shadomy S.
Silk B.
Slayton R.
Smith R.
Spradling P. R.
Staples E.
Taylor M. M.
Tiwari T. S. P.
Tomashek K.
Torrone E.
Van Beneden C.
Visvesvara G.
Walters M.
Yendell S.
Yoder J.

World Health Organization

Avenue Appia 20, 1211 Geneva 27, Switzerland
http://www.who.int

Abela-Ridder B.
Arrowood M.
Aylward R. B.
Ball A.
Barbeschi M.
Besselaar T.
Bridges C. B.
Dagne D. A.
Fitzner J.
Franco J. R.
Gabrielli A.
Gayer M.
Getahun H.
Hardiman M.
Ichimori K.
Jannin J.
Kern P.
Magnino S.

Mariotti S. P.
Meslin F.
Montresor A.
Mounts A.
Newman R. D.
Perry R.
Previsani N.
Raviglione M.
Rietveld A. E. C.
Roth C.
Savioli L.
Schantz P.
Shindo N.
Simarro P.
Solomon A.
Tam J. S.
Vandemaele K.

WHO Disclaimer: since 2008, all WHO recommendations are derived through a rigorous process to ensure that they are evidence-based; further, the evidence is assessed for quality and relevance using the GRADE analysis. The application of these standards is overseen by a WHO Guidelines Review Committee (GRC). Chapters prepared by WHO authors which have recommendations in accord with guidelines approved by the GRC since 2008, and therefore meet these standards, are identified next, while the remaining chapters written by WHO authors have recommendations derived from expert opinion, other accepted standards, and reviews of the recent literature.

WHO-authored chapters consistent with GRC-standard guidelines are as follows: "Communicable Disease Control in Humanitarian Emergencies," "Malaria," "Measles," "Poliomyelitis," and "Tuberculosis and Other Mycobacterial Diseases."

Other Organizations

Badaruddin H.
Bermingham A.
Cardosa M. J.
Cook L. B. M.
Enwonwu C. O.
Harbarth S.
Heymann D. L.
Ho M.
John T. J.
King L. J.
Kiyu A.
Lee V. J.

Maznieda M.
Ong F. G. L.
Ooi M. H.
Pebody R.
Perera D.
Pittet D.
Schlundt J.
Smith D.
Stewardson A.
Watson J. M.
Wilcke B.
Yeoh E. K.

TABLE OF CONTENTS

FOREWORD

Since 2008 we have seen an explosion in infectious diseases of international concern. In 2009 we had the H1N1 pandemic. In 2012 a new, highly fatal coronavirus named Middle East Respiratory Syndrome (MERS) was first reported out of Saudi Arabia. And as we go to press, an old foe—Ebola—is creating the largest epidemic of Ebola virus disease (EVD) in human history. All 3 of these cases reinforce the need for health practitioners to have an expert guide in the use of sound infection control practices. This new version of *Control of Communicable Diseases Manual (CCDM)*, the 20th revision of this 96-year-old favorite of the health community, is now available to address these important concerns.

The text was initially written in the early 20th century, as a pamphlet for New England health officials, by Dr. Francis Curtis, then the health officer of Newton, Massachusetts. Later, Dr. Robert Hoyt, a health officer from Manchester, New Hampshire, recognized its importance and convinced the American Public Health Association (APHA) at our annual meeting in Cincinnati, Ohio, to review, edit, and adopt the text as our own. In 1917, it was published in *Public Health Reports* (32:41:1706-1733) by the US Public Health Service. Its 30 pages contained disease control measures for the 38 communicable diseases that were then reportable in the United States. It was available from the Government Printing Office for a modest 5 cents. This manual is now the classic by which all other infectious disease manuals are measured. *CCDM* has undergone several rewrites over the years. Even the last word in the title was changed from "Man" to "Manual" to remove the perception of gender bias. This text remains a global treasure and continues to be translated into multiple languages. We continue to embrace change; this edition will also be available as a downloadable E-book, enhancing access and portability, and allowing for more frequent updates to keep pace with a changing environment and advancing knowledge.

The 5 people who have served as editors for *CCDM* over the years are to be saluted for their efforts:

Haven Emerson: 1st–7th editions
John Gordon: 8th–10th editions
Abram S. Benenson: 11th–16th editions
James Chin: 17th edition
David L. Heymann: 18th–20th editions

This updated edition of *CCDM* strengthens the value of this text as a global resource. Dr. David L. Heymann and his team of experts from around the world continue to uphold the highest standards of quality and expertise, and I thank them for their work. I also want to thank the many men and women who work silently behind the scenes and on occasion have given their lives to contain the threat of infectious disease.

Georges C. Benjamin, MD, FACP, FACEP(E), FNAPA,
FRSPH(Hon), FFPH(Hon)
Executive Director
American Public Health Association

PREFACE TO THE 20TH EDITION

At a time in mid-2014 when the Ebola virus is spreading in major urban areas in West Africa, when the Middle East Respiratory Syndrome coronavirus (MERS-CoV) remains a risk in countries where hospital infection control is not up to standard, when endemic infectious diseases remain a major cause of mortality in the least developed countries, and when antimicrobial resistance is decreasing the effectiveness of treatment for many of these endemic infections, *Control of Communicable Diseases Manual* (*CCDM*) remains as relevant today as when it was first edited by Dr. Haven Emerson just over 100 years ago.

This 20th edition of the manual has been reformatted and decreased in size to ensure that the printed version remains convenient to carry to the field as a quick reference for information such as clinical signs and symptoms, modes of transmission, incubation periods, and measures for prevention and control. It has been updated by a diversity of world-leading experts, and once updated each chapter has been peer-reviewed by at least 2 members of the editorial board as well as the editor. Chapter authors have signed off on each chapter and have signed a conflict of interest statement that is kept by the American Public Health Association (APHA).

This process has led to a reliable and fit-for-purpose printed manual as the APHA works on a Web-based interactive and searchable version of the same format, due out in early 2015. The Web-based manual will permit more timely and frequent chapter updates, making *CCDM* more relevant in a world where rapid changes are occurring in communicable disease epidemiology and new communicable diseases.

During the process of editing *CCDM20*, some of the subsections of previous editions have become new stand-alone chapters because of their increasing relevance. These include "Japanese Encephalitis," "West Nile Virus Disease," "Rift Valley Fever," "Rotavirus Infection," "Norovirus Infection," and "SARS, MERS, and Other Coronavirus Infections." Other chapters have been merged, reorganized, or renamed, and cancers linked to communicable diseases have now been included in the chapter with the relevant infection. Finally, 2 new chapters have been added to *CCDM20*—one on noma, the other on communicable diseases at the animal/human interface. The latter describes the interconnectedness of infections of humans and animals and the role of the environment in the emergence and spread of communicable diseases that has led to the One Health movement.

It has been a privilege to work with the world's experts in communicable diseases and public health who have volunteered their time and knowledge to update this 20th edition of the *CCDM* and to serve as members of the editorial board. But it was with great sadness that we learned of the death of Prof. Peter Ndumbe, who was a member of the editorial board, and a true friend and colleague to public health workers around the world. His death represents a great loss to his native country Cameroon and to the global health community of which he was an active and devoted member. This edition of *CCDM* bears testament to the lasting value of Prof. Ndumbe's life and work.

David L. Heymann, MD

READER'S GUIDE TO *CCDM20*

Each disease chapter in *Control of Communicable Diseases Manual*, 20th edition, (*CCDM20*) is presented in a standardized format that includes the following information:

Disease name: each disease is identified by the numeric code assigned by the WHO's *International Classification of Diseases, 10th Revision (ICD-10)*. Common names are also listed and can be matched to the *ICD* names using the index in the back of the manual.

1. **Clinical features:** presents the main signs and symptoms of the disease and differentiates the disease from others that may have a similar clinical picture. Case-fatality rates may also be included.

2. **Causative agent(s):** identifies the specific agent or agents that cause the disease; classifies the agent(s); describes variations, subtypes, and strains; and may indicate important characteristics.

3. **Diagnosis:** describes methods most commonly used to diagnose the disease and provides information on how results should be interpreted.

4. **Occurrence:** provides information on where the disease is known to occur and the magnitude of its burden. Information on past and current outbreaks may also be included.

5. **Reservoir(s):** describes any person, animal, arthropod, plant, or substance—or combination of these—in which an infectious agent normally lives and reproduces itself in such a manner that it can be transmitted to a susceptible host. Intermediate hosts and animal populations at risk are described in this section.

6. **Incubation period:** describes the time interval between infection and the first appearance of symptoms associated with the infection.

7. **Transmission:** provides information on the mechanisms by which the infectious agent is spread to or among humans; the period of time during which it may be transferred to humans from an infected human, reservoir, or vector; and the factors that influence transmissibility.

8. **Risk groups:** describes human population groups at increased risk of infection or development of disease or that are resistant to either infection or disease. Information on immunity subsequent to infection may also be given.

9. **Prevention:** describes measures that can be used to prevent infection of individuals and/or groups.

10. **Management of patient:** gives an overview of best clinical practice (including accepted treatment) and other measures necessary in patient management to reduce morbidity and mortality, minimize the period of communicability, and prevent spread to others. This manual is not intended to be a therapeutic guide. Readers must be aware of contra-indications and side effects of any treatment recommended in the manual and determine the risk-benefit profile, including for the use of antimicrobials in pregnant women and young children. For example, because tetracyclines, including doxycycline, could pose a small, dose-dependent risk of staining teeth that are under development in young children, the risk of dental staining from their use in children younger than 8 years should be weighed against the potential benefit of its use for treatment. Specific dosages and clinical management are described primarily for those diseases for which delay in instituting therapy might jeopardize the patient's life.

11. **Management of contacts and the immediate environment:** describes procedures recommended for managing contacts and the immediate environment that are designed to limit the spread of the disease. General information can be found in themed chapters "Communicable Disease Alert and Response During Mass Gatherings" and "Response to an Outbreak."

12. **Special considerations:** describes any special considerations relevant for the disease. For instance, when applicable, it notes reporting requirements, whether free drugs are available through WHO or CDC, and what measures are recommended for public health workers in case of deliberate use of biological agents to cause harm. Disaster implications or special epidemic measures are also described, if applicable. General information can be found in themed chapters "Reporting of Communicable Diseases Under the International Health Regulations," "Communicable Disease Control in Humanitarian Emergencies," and "Outbreak Response in Case of Deliberate Use of Biological Agents to Cause Harm."

REPORTING OF COMMUNICABLE DISEASES UNDER THE INTERNATIONAL HEALTH REGULATIONS

Background

The principal global agreement for addressing the risks of the international spread of infectious disease is the International Health Regulations (IHR), issued under the WHO constitution and adopted by its member states. The first version (then called the International Sanitary Regulations) was agreed in 1951, and since then there have been a number of revisions, the most recent of which entered into force as a binding legal agreement in 2007. The current IHR (2005), hereafter referred to as IHR in this manual, has a much broader scope of application than that of earlier versions, which had focused on 3 infectious diseases after smallpox had been eradicated: cholera, plague, and yellow fever. In addition, the IHR was updated to take account of the new challenges presented by an increasingly globalized world and advances in information and communication technology. At time of writing in early 2013, the IHR has entered into force for 195 of the world's countries, including all the WHO member states.

The IHR provides broad new mandates and obligations both for participating countries and for WHO, with the following goal:

> To prevent, protect against, control, and provide a public health response to the international spread of disease in ways that are commensurate with, and restricted to, public health risks, and which avoid unnecessary interference with international traffic and trade. (IHR)

The IHR depends heavily on global surveillance, alert, and response activities, which aim to support countries and the international community in identifying and responding to emerging public health risks. In this respect, the IHR now recognizes and mandates the use of information from a variety of sources, and not only the information officially reported by the country in which the health event may be occurring.

The IHR aims to avoid the stigmatization of particular diseases or of the countries in which they are occurring—factors that proved significant barriers to compliance with the previous regulations. In addition to the provisions dealing with the detection and response to emergency events, the IHR also mandates certain routine measures related to preventing the international spread of diseases (e.g., the use of the International Certificate of Vaccination or Prophylaxis in travelers from areas at risk of yellow fever transmission; see International Measures in Special Considerations in "Yellow Fever").

A1

A new component of the IHR is commitments by the States Parties to strengthen or reestablish the public health infrastructures designed to facilitate early recognition of, and rapid response to, emerging disease threats—which, for a variety of reasons, have either never been established or have declined in effectiveness in some parts of the world over recent decades.

The text of IHR consists of 66 articles and 9 annexes. This section addresses only those articles and annexes most directly relevant to the detection of, international reporting or notification of, and response to communicable disease outbreaks.

Surveillance Under IHR

The process of global surveillance involves the systematic collection of information from many different sources, its assessment, and taking prompt public health action based on the conclusion. When an event is assessed as a *potential* public health emergency of international concern (PHEIC), it shall then be notified to WHO while verification and further information are sought from the affected country. On the basis of the information thus obtained, events may be discarded from consideration or may undergo repeated risk assessment to monitor ongoing need for further information or response activities. The surveillance-related provisions of the IHR provide a firm institutional mandate and legal framework for key elements of this process within WHO.

The provisions of the IHR do not of themselves create the basis for any international system of surveillance for specific diseases. Instead, the regulatory requirements—including those for notification to WHO and obligations to respond to WHO requests for verification—aim to identify any public health event that may constitute a public health emergency of international concern, or PHEIC (see Public Health Emergencies of International Concern section in this chapter), as determined through a standard decision protocol.

National IHR focal points and WHO IHR contact points

Under the IHR, urgent communications, including those concerning country reporting, are transmitted to WHO through specific National IHR Focal Points. Each of the 6 WHO regional offices has established an IHR Contact Point for the countries within its respective region; and as of early 2013, almost all WHO member states have identified national IHR Focal Points.

Notification

A central reporting obligation under the IHR is the mandatory duty for countries to carry out an assessment of public health events occurring within their territories, in accordance with the decision protocols and criteria found in Annex 2 of the regulations, and then to notify WHO of all qualifying events within 24 hours of the assessment. The events that are to be notified are effectively defined by 4 criteria in the decision protocol:

1) Whether the event has a serious public health impact.
2) Whether the event is unusual or unexpected.
3) Whether the event risks spreading internationally.
4) Whether the event risks resulting in restrictions on international trade and/or travel.

If an event within a country fulfills 2 of the 4 listed criteria, it qualifies as an event that *may* constitute an international emergency and so must be notified by that country to WHO through the National IHR Focal Point. In addition to these criteria, there are a number of subquestions and indicative examples of factual contexts to guide use of the decision protocol.

Consistent with the broad scope of the IHR, the decision protocol—and hence notification—does not require that the event involve a particular disease or type of causative agent (i.e., biological, chemical, or nuclear). The decision protocol was designed to allow the assessment of events where the nature of any disease or agent is still undefined at the time of assessment and does not exclude events based upon whether they are or may be accidental, natural, or intentional in nature.

While the decision protocol and Annex 2 of IHR require that all events remain subject to assessment as indicated, they also specifically require that certain events, involving a limited number of specific diseases that have demonstrated the ability to cause serious public health impact and to spread rapidly internationally, must always be analyzed utilizing the decision protocol. These must be notified if the analysis indicates that they fulfill 2 of the 4 criteria.

The diseases in this category are:

- Cholera
- Pneumonic plague
- Yellow fever
- Viral hemorrhagic fevers (e.g., dengue hemorrhagic fever, Ebola, Marburg)
- West Nile fever
- Other diseases of special national or regional concern (e.g., dengue fever, Rift Valley fever, and meningococcal disease)

Finally, the IHR identifies 4 specific disease entities that are always considered unusual or unexpected, and which may have serious public health impact, and hence which always may constitute a public health emergency of international concern. Accordingly, even 1 case of these diseases must be notified to WHO.

These diseases are as follows:

- Smallpox
- Poliomyelitis due to wild-type poliovirus
- Human influenza caused by a new subtype (e.g., H5N1 in humans)
- Severe acute respiratory syndrome (SARS)

WHO maintains the case definitions for the notification of cases of these diseases.

Other types of reporting under IHR

As a complement to the obligation to notify, the IHR provides an option for countries to keep WHO informed, on a confidential basis, about events within their territories that are not notifiable as discussed earlier and to consult with WHO on the appropriate responsive health measures. This provision focuses in particular on those events for which there is insufficient available information to complete the decision protocol.

Countries are also required to inform WHO within 24 hours of receipt of evidence of a public health risk identified outside their territory that may cause international disease spread, as manifested by exported or imported:

1) Human cases
2) Vectors carrying infection or contamination
3) Goods that are contaminated

The IHR does not include any provision referring explicitly to reporting suspected intentional or deliberate releases of harmful agents. However, the IHR stipulates that where a country has evidence of an unexpected or unusual public health event within its territory—irrespective of origin or source—that may constitute a public health emergency of international concern, the country must provide to WHO all relevant public health information.

Response Under IHR

The IHR requires WHO to collaborate with countries in the risk assessment and response to public health events whenever they request WHO to do so. Such collaboration can include the provision of technical guidance, assessment of the effectiveness of control measures, and mobilization of international teams either for risk assessment or for control purposes.

The WHO event detection and verification activities provide risk assessment support needed by member states to protect the health of their populations during certain public health events. This support can take the form of different types of assistance to countries already affected by the event, as well as the provision of information regarding the event to countries as yet unaffected. This is so that the latter can take action to prevent their populations from becoming affected or prepare themselves to take effective response actions should they become affected.

WHO ensures that countries have rapid access to the most appropriate experts and resources for risk assessment and outbreak response, through the Global Outbreak Alert and Response Network of institutions able to provide support and expertise. The Global Outbreak Alert and Response Network partnership was formalized in April 2000 to improve the coordination of international outbreak responses, and to provide an operational framework to focus the delivery of support to countries. The network's primary aims are as follows:

- To support countries with disease control efforts by ensuring rapid and appropriate technical expertise to affected populations.
- To investigate and characterize events and assess risks of rapidly emerging epidemic disease threats.
- To support national outbreak preparedness by ensuring that responses contribute to sustained containment of epidemic threats.

More information can be found at: http://www.who.int/csr/outbreaknetwork/en.

Provision of information

Providing authoritative information on public health events that have particular international significance is an important part of an effective public health response. WHO manages the information provided by an affected country in ways that both protect that country from unjustified overreaction by other countries and ensures that other countries are provided with the information they need to protect their populations—including citizens who travel to the affected country/countries.

As part of an incentive to State Parties to notify and report events to WHO, the IHR guarantees that information in notifications, reports, and consultations under the IHR is not made generally available to other countries unless circumstances arise that justify dissemination in order to address the risk of international spread. The contexts that justify communication of the information to other State Parties are clearly specified and include situations where the Director-General has declared a public health emergency of international concern (see PHEIC section, discussed next), where international spread has been confirmed, where control measures are not likely to succeed, and/or where implementation of international control measures is required immediately.

When WHO intends to make such information available to other countries, it has an obligation to consult with the country experiencing the event. WHO may also make information available in the public domain, if other information about the event is already public and if a need exists for public availability of information that is authoritative and independent.

Public Health Emergencies of International Concern (PHEIC)

The experience gained during the international collaboration to respond to the emergence of severe acute respiratory syndrome (SARS) led to the inclusion within the IHR of specific provisions governing actions in response to rare and serious events, which are called PHEIC. The responsibility of determining whether a potential PHEIC falls into this category lies with the Director-General of WHO, acting on the advice of the WHO Secretariat, and requires the convening of a committee of health experts (the IHR Emergency Committee). If the Director-General determines that the event constitutes a PHEIC, the IHR Emergency Committee advises WHO Director-General on appropriate Temporary Recommendations of health measures to be implemented by States Parties. The Emergency Committee continues to advise the Director-General throughout the period of the PHEIC, including advising on necessary changes to the recommended measures for control and on the termination of the PHEIC.

Development and Maintenance of Core Surveillance Capacities

One of the most important elements of the IHR is the requirement for all participating countries to develop and maintain core public health capacities for surveillance and response, in accordance with the functions described in Annex 1 of the IHR. These core public health capacities had to be developed within 5 years of entry into force of the IHR for each country, but most countries have requested a 2-year extension in June 2012, and some countries may require 2 more years, until June 2015, to develop the minimum core capacities.

Through these requirements, the IHR seeks to ensure that all countries have the basic infrastructure, human resources, and procedures needed in order to undertake the timely identification and risk assessment of, and response to, outbreaks of disease and other public health events when and where they occur. This is key to avoid or minimize the international spread of such public health risks.

Note

This chapter concentrates on those elements of the IHR that are of relevance to the control of communicable disease, and particularly the recognition of and response to public health events such as disease outbreaks. The IHR also contains provisions for the routine application of health measures in the context of international travel and transportation in the absence of such events. Where these measures have relevance to a specific communicable disease (e.g., those pertaining to the international certificate of vaccination), they are mentioned in the relevant chapter of this book.

The main Web page for the IHR can be found at: http://www.who.int/csr/ihr/en.

National Reporting of Communicable Diseases

Surveillance is the cornerstone for effective disease prevention and control efforts, and disease reporting is one of the 3 legs of the surveillance platform, the others being timely and appropriate analysis followed by the provision of the information needed to guide intervention. While the reporting of individual and aggregated data on disease occurrence are not the only inputs to the surveillance process, they are the most common and form the bedrock on which public health surveillance is built.

The practice of, and the recommendations and requirements for, disease reporting vary widely between countries as a consequence of differences in epidemiological contexts, health care provision, role of national legislation, administrative structures, and available resources. The planned use to be made of the derived information will also influence the type of reporting needed; for example reporting against very specific and detailed case definitions may be needed for clinical research purposes, while much broader and simpler definitions may suffice for the monitoring of health facility utilization. An increasing number of countries are supplementing case-based disease data reported from health information systems with event-based data from media reports or other informal sources to assist in the early detection of public health events requiring an urgent response.

Disease reporting usually takes the form of either a case report or infection reports (some countries only require aggregate reporting), or an outbreak or event report.

1) Case reports: case reporting provides diagnosis, age, sex, and date of onset for each person with the disease. Sometimes it includes identifying information, such as the name and address of the person with the disease. Additional information, such as treatment provided and its duration, are required for certain case reports.

   National legislation or guidelines often indicate which diseases must be reported, who is responsible for reporting, the format for reporting, and how case reports are to be entered into and forwarded within the national system. If there is a requirement for international case reporting (see next section), national governments report to WHO.

2) Outbreak or event reports: outbreak reporting provides information about an increase in the number of cases above a certain threshold. However, the specific disease causing an outbreak may not be included in the list of diseases officially reportable, or it may be of unknown etiology if it is newly recognized or emerging. It would then lead to the report of an event of unknown etiology.

National legislation or guidelines may indicate which types of outbreak or event must be reported, who is responsible for reporting, the format for reporting, and how case reports are to be entered into and forwarded within the national system. In general, outbreak reporting is required by the most rapid means of communication available. When there is a requirement for outbreak or event reporting internationally (see next section), national governments report to WHO. General advice on the reporting of diseases listed in *CCDM20* is provided under the Special Considerations section for each disease. While the international legal requirement for disease reporting is described in the section on the International Health Regulations, it is important to note that, in addition to this, WHO has a number of diseases under routine international surveillance including:

- Louse-borne typhus fever
- Relapsing fever
- Meningococcal meningitis
- Paralytic poliomyelitis
- Malaria
- Tuberculosis
- HIV/AIDS
- Influenza
- SARS

[M. Hardiman]

RESPONSE TO AN OUTBREAK

The response to a report of an outbreak must include the management of those infected and the containment or mitigation of the outbreak by interrupting or reducing transmission of the suspected infectious agent. Steps in an outbreak response should be systematic and based on epidemiological evidence.

Public and political reaction, urgency, and the need for immediate pre-cautionary measures may, however, present challenges to this routine approach. The following is a minimal list of the steps essential for responding to outbreaks. Often they can be undertaken concurrently.

1) Confirming the outbreak.
2) Establishing a task force and designate an outbreak control team.
3) Establishing and maintaining regular communications.
4) Managing sick persons.
5) Conducting an outbreak investigation:

- Identifying additional persons with infection by active surveillance.
- Identifying possible source(s) of infection and means of transmission.
- Defining the population at risk.

6) Preventing further transmission.
7) Monitoring the response.

Confirming the Outbreak

To confirm an outbreak, laboratory specimens must be obtained from the initial cases reported and from successive cases if initial cases are no longer available. Specimens should be provided to a laboratory with the capacity to screen for numerous pathogens and should be clearly labeled with clinical information that describes the illness. If the outbreak is life-threatening, it may be necessary to recommend immediate precautionary measures of prevention based on knowledge about infections that are clinically similar. Once laboratory diagnosis is available, precautionary measures must be reassessed and altered if new evidence makes changes possible (discussed later).

Establishing a Task Force and Designating an Outbreak Control Team

Once an outbreak has been confirmed, a task force should be established to serve as the command-and-control center for the outbreak response. Task force members should have technical and political understanding from the various sectors involved in the outbreak and should meet regularly, with minutes of meetings recorded. In its role as command center, the task force should designate an outbreak control leader and team to conduct the outbreak investigation, establish and maintain regular communications, analyze the data, determine evidence-based control measures, and contain or mitigate the outbreak by applying the control measures. The task force should meet regularly and formally until the outbreak has been contained or mitigated, should provide a final report that includes recommendations to prevent recurrence, and consider a formal scientific report for peer review and publication in a medical journal or epidemiological bulletin. The complexity of the outbreak control team will depend on the population(s) affected.

Establishing and Maintaining Regular Communications

Regular communications about the outbreak and the risk of infection is one of the most important parts of an outbreak response and serves to reassure the population that a response is underway, avoid undue panic or concern, create an environment where additional cases can be identified, and help individuals and communities understand how transmission can be stopped. Time spent explaining the evidence and control measures with responsible journalists—whether they are from newspaper, radio, television, or other outlets—will facilitate the outbreak response by creating an environment of understanding. Regular simple information (outbreak facts such as case numbers, case definition, studies underway, and suspected incubation period) should be provided at intervals. Social media are also important means of communication and must be a part of the outbreak response as well, as reports from reliable sources may be necessary to counteract less reliable communication. To ensure credibility with the general public, it is usually preferable to nominate a specific press communications person.

Managing Sick Persons

Priority must be given to those who are sick. Their symptoms must be treated (e.g., antipyretics for fever, antiemetics for vomiting, oral or parenteral fluids for dehydration), and if the etiology is suspected but not confirmed, the sick persons must be treated presumptively with anti-infective medications. Signs, symptoms, and other information must be recorded, and information about management procedures that appear to be effective provided to other health care workers wherever the outbreak is occurring. Once a laboratory diagnosis has been established, evidence-based changes in patient management must be made if necessary. An attempt should also be made to identify any possible sources of infection by questioning patients or their families. Information such as contact with other sick persons or wild animals, ingestion of unusual foods, travel, or other suspicious contact situations is necessary to fully conduct an outbreak investigation.

Patients must be isolated while they are being treated, and health workers must be protected so that the disease is not spread to other patients, to health workers, and to their families. Health workers are often at great risk of infection, especially from an emerging infection that has not yet been recognized as part of an outbreak or from a disease that is easily spread by respiratory and other body secretions. In such instances, all medical staff in contact with patients should use personal protection equipment.

Information collected from each patient should be recorded on specially prepared line lists, which should then be used to construct the epidemic curve. From the epidemic curve, attempts should be made to determine the incubation period and glean other information to establish the epidemiological characteristics of the patients and the outbreak.

Conducting an Outbreak Investigation

Identifying additional persons with infection by active surveillance

A surveillance case definition must be established using information collected from the line list of patients. A surveillance case definition describes the signs and symptoms of a person who is a part of the outbreak, and sometimes provides other information, such as the age or sex of those at risk or geographic areas where the outbreak is known to be occurring. Case definitions should be highly sensitive (for a possible and/or a probable—sometimes called presumptive—case), and once the etiology is known, highly specific (a laboratory-confirmed case). Some infections may be asymptomatic or have atypical symptoms, and they should be identified during the course of an outbreak investigation by contact tracing once the etiology is understood.

Surveillance teams should be organized and active, and a systematic search for persons who fit the case definition should be conducted in the geographic area of the outbreak. All persons identified by active surveillance as fitting the possible, probable, or confirmed case definition should be placed under observation and managed in a hospital setting using isolation procedures, avoiding contact with other patients, including those who fit the confirmed case definition.

Contacts—persons who have had contact with those people fitting the case definition during the presumptive incubation period—should be identified, located, and asked to report to a health worker should they develop any symptoms. In some settings they might be asked to self-isolate at home or to present to a facility designated for quarantine. If a contact develops symptoms, he or she should be placed under health facility isolation and observation but not in contact with known patients until they can be confirmed.

Identifying possible source(s) of infection and means of transmission

At times the possible source of infection and means of transmission will be highly suspect based on patient history (e.g., eating a certain food, contact with an animal, or some factor in the environment) while at other times further questioning of patients or their families will be necessary to identify possible sources. Once a possible source or sources have been identified, a hypothesis about the means of transmission should be developed, and a case-control study conducted to attempt to better describe the transmission risks.

Defining the population at risk

The population at risk of infection must be identified, and this provides the denominator required and ensures that active surveillance and prevention measures can be ensured in a broad enough geographic area. Overall or specific attack rates (age-specific, village-specific) should be calculated and may lead to new hypotheses requiring further investigation and additional study designs.

Once the population at risk is defined, screening and additional laboratory testing may be required (e.g., collection of nasal swab specimens for laboratory investigation of nasal carriage, microbiological typing, genomic sequencing, and susceptibility to antimicrobials) that can then provide evidence for additional prevention and control measures.

Preventing Further Transmission

Early in an outbreak investigation it may not be possible to confirm the etiology, source, or means of transmission and, based on experience and evidence from similar outbreaks in the past, it may be necessary to apply precautionary measures in an attempt to stop transmission. A large respiratory outbreak, for example, may require social distancing measures such as closing schools before the outbreak is fully understood, avoidance of certain foods, or culling of animals thought to be a source of infection. Such measures are often costly and must be managed accordingly, with modification if required as soon as evidence from the present outbreak investigation becomes available.

As soon as recommendations for prevention and control have been made they must be provided to health workers, updated as new evidence becomes available, and fully implemented by public health teams and the public in order to fully contain or mitigate the outbreak. At times recommendations must be made for home management and/or burial practices as well (see "Ebola-Marburg Viral Diseases").

Monitoring the Response
Continued active surveillance is necessary until the outbreak has been contained. Regular supervision of health workers as they manage patients, of the response team as it conducts surveillance and implements control, and of any other partners is required. Monitoring of the outbreak response team should be ensured by the task force and line supervisors. An outbreak can generally be considered contained if active surveillance has been maintained and has identified no new cases during a period twice as long as the presumed incubation period of the infection. Other sectors involved in the outbreak (e.g., animal or food sectors) should thereafter maintain any measures necessary to remove or isolate the source of infection and maintain eventual upstream preventive measures undertaken (see "One Health: Communicable Diseases at the Human/Animal Interface").

The key to an effective outbreak response is coordination by the outbreak control team of those they represent, including clinicians, epidemiologists, microbiologists, health educators, the public health authority, and the local community that is overseen by an appropriately constructed task force.

Outbreaks with characteristics considered as possible public health events of international concern (PHEIC), based on comparison to the decision tree of the International Health Regulations (see "Reporting Of Communicable Diseases Under the International Health Regulations"), should be reported to WHO as soon as possible through the national focal point.

[Editorial Board]

COMMUNICABLE DISEASE ALERT AND RESPONSE DURING MASS GATHERINGS

Introduction

Mass gatherings are events in which large numbers of people come together for a common goal or purpose. A communicable disease outbreak at a mass gathering has the potential to overwhelm the public health system of the community or country in which the mass gathering is occurring. Even when public health and other support services are adequate to detect and respond to communicable disease outbreaks in the community, they may not be able to provide adequate support when there is an influx of large numbers of people (national and/or international). Planning for mass gatherings should therefore include a risk assessment for communicable disease outbreaks and for the management of those risks.

Risk Assessment

Gatherings of people from within the same country may increase the risk of outbreaks from communicable diseases caused by indigenous pathogens. However, gatherings that draw visitors from different nations, regions, and cultures have the potential for importation of communicable disease pathogens that are not present in the host community and which may require public health expertise not normally available. In addition, responses to such outbreaks may require accommodating the needs of populations with differing languages, social norms, and customs. Because there is the potential that those affected may have already returned to their home countries, processes for contact tracing overseas should be considered.

Systematic risk assessment prior to the gathering helps identify potential outbreak risks and guides the establishment of realistic risk management goals. Sporting events or rock concerts, for example, may have risks associated with alcohol and/or drug abuse including bloodborne infections from unsafe injecting practices or sexually transmitted infections from unprotected sex. The risk management goal in such instances is to ensure that active health promotion activities are in place and that prevention measures and counseling services are made available.

Religious and/or faith healing gatherings might attract a significant number of the ill and infirm who have increased susceptibility to communicable diseases. Additional risks include hypothermia from sleeping outside or from inclement weather conditions and hyperthermia if temperatures are high. Likewise, gatherings of senior citizens may have an increased risk of serious respiratory or other communicable diseases. Risk management goals at such events would be to provide facility-based health care services along with preventive measures such as isolation of those who are ill.

Of particular concern during a mass gathering event are food supplies that could contain contaminated food, unsafe water, and substandard hygiene and sanitation. Risk management goals to address these concerns must be appropriately designed and implemented well before the gathering occurs.

Finally, systematic risk assessment will also help identify vulnerabilities that could increase the risk of deliberately caused outbreaks, requiring interaction with security and other government agencies (for further information, see "Outbreak Response in Case of Deliberate Use of Biological Agents to Cause Harm").

The risk assessment framework and methodology for communicable disease outbreaks are provided in "Response to an Outbreak." Some of the specific information required for successful risk analysis in advance of a mass gathering could take the form of a checklist, including the following considerations.

General features of the gathering:

- Age and sex of those likely to participate.
- Likely number of participants and countries of provenance.
- Season in which the gathering will occur.
- Potential insect and animal vectors present.
- Quality of water and sanitation services.
- Likely food vendors, if any.
- Characteristics of the hosting location (e.g., geographic/regional features, climate and weather, language(s), and customs/traditions of inhabitants, including ethnic groups).
- Accommodation and potential for overcrowding/overflow.
- Political, security, or other vulnerabilities that could fail to prevent deliberately caused communicable disease outbreaks.

Specific communicable disease information:

- Indigenous infectious agents circulating in local populations and animals, as well as in populations likely to participate.
- Infectious agents circulating where participants originate.
- Health intelligence obtained from previous mass gatherings.
- Vaccine coverage/immunity levels in hosting communities and in participants.

Diseases that are important causes of outbreaks at mass gatherings include those that are highly infectious and have modes of transmission likely to be enhanced by close person-to-person contact, unsafe water supply and sanitation, and/or unsafe food supplies. They should be considered a high priority during risk assessment, remembering that such incidents cause considerable political and media concern.

If risk assessment suggests political or other vulnerabilities that could facilitate deliberate attempts to cause outbreaks, links should be planned and operationally tested with agencies dealing with criminality (for further information, see the list of agents with potential for deliberate use in "Outbreak Response in Case of Deliberate Use of Biological Agents to Cause Harm").

Risk Management and Planning

Effective risk management for communicable diseases in mass gatherings requires advance planning in order to ensure that the necessary services and resources are available. It is complicated by high event visibility, and political and media pressure may make it necessary to apply precautionary measures for control before evidence is available.

Planning for mass gatherings should therefore ensure the following:

- Surveillance and outbreak alert systems to identify risks and/or outbreaks, established at least a year before the mass gathering in order to collect baseline data. Systems should be based on an enhanced business-as-usual approach.
- Health services adequately equipped to offer preventive services and to control an outbreak, linked with other services responsible for personal security, food safety, sanitation, and water.
- Contact tracing/quarantine measures.
- Provisions for management of dead bodies (see "Communicable Disease Control in Humanitarian Emergencies").
- Communications and counseling capacity to cope with projected needs (see "Response to an Outbreak"), with a lead for public health messaging agreed to in advance in order to ensure rapid and clear communication.
- Standard operating procedures that ensure that all involved in outbreak management understand their roles and responsibilities, with robust advance testing and exercising.
- Early stakeholder engagement to ensure understanding of roles, responsibilities, and reporting/working requirements.
- Post–mass gathering systems to provide support to the sick after the event and risk information to other countries and to transport hubs that take attendees home.

A budget should be prepared and obtained for any necessary reinforcement in infrastructure or health manpower, and training should be provided to health staff and others as required to ensure adequate detection, investigation, and response capacity for potential outbreaks.

Legacy of Planning

Care should be taken to ensure that planning maximizes the public health legacy: while some investments made during the planning phase may be beneficial only for the duration of the mass gathering, others will provide permanent benefit to public health infrastructure.

Since the investments may be costly, decision-makers should clearly understand which lasting benefits will result and that investment in advance will prevent greater, unnecessary cost should an outbreak occur.

Surveillance and Outbreak Alert

The communicable disease surveillance and notification system for mass gatherings should build on the preexisting routine system. It should be in place at least 12 months before the gathering in order to provide seasonal baseline data with case definitions for indigenous and/or potential imported disease risks available; it should also ensure detection of unexpected events should they occur. The system should be proactive and based on an electronic platform for rapid communication. If reporting in the routine system is not daily, consideration should be given to increasing the level to daily reporting just before and during the mass gathering.

An event management system is required that provides the electronic platform, electronic tools, and procedures to manage reports of communicable diseases in a format that permits verification and risk assessment in a seamless and reproducible process. Daily event management is required, including preplanned protection of information and secure distribution.

Public health laboratory support should be in place and able to identify known pathogens, especially those that preexist before the gathering and others that could enter with participants who arrive from other geographic and climatic areas. They should make provisions for rapid and safe transport and storage of specimens, with a capacity that exceeds normal demand, and maintain internal and external quality control.

In the absence of suitable national laboratories, an international laboratory should be identified that can provide the relevant training and/or services, and guidelines should be established for the transfer of specimens between laboratories.

The relevant domestic and international detection and reporting required under IHR serve as a means of ensuring essential national reporting and apply to international participants as well (see "Reporting of Communicable Diseases Under the International Health Regulations").

Health Services

Prevention and patient management require robust health services that can be assessed with the following checklist:

- Frontline prevention and patient management services, including counseling.
- Emergency medical staff.
- Geographical proximity to the mass gathering site.
- Surge capacity.
- Transport to other medical facilities.
- Supplies for prevention, including vaccines.

- Medicines that correspond to potential risks.
- Reliable diagnostic laboratory support.
- Safe medical facility water, sanitation, and food supplies.
- Sustainability for a prolonged period of heightened alert and response.
- Language interpreters/cultural experts if the gathering includes international participants.
- Means for rapid mobilization of additional equipment.
- Fact sheets with prepared prevention and control messages (these may need translation).
- Distribution system able to safely and securely handle large quantities of supplies (e.g., blankets, food, and clothing).

Patient management and outbreak containment are described more fully in other chapters. Infection control, contact tracing, quarantine, management of dead bodies, and outbreak communication may, however, be of a greater magnitude and complexity in a mass gathering. The following section describes these functions more fully in the context of mass gatherings.

Infection Control

Infection control procedures and capacities must be robust enough to accommodate increased numbers of people seeking medical care (see "Infection Prevention and Control"). It is therefore important to identify, in advance, other medical facilities where large-scale isolation of patients may be assured if there is an outbreak of infectious disease and secure transport systems so that contacts do not become infected.

The language and culture of participants should also be considered so that infection control guidance can be understood.

Contact Tracing/Quarantine

Contact tracing and quarantine measures, including fever surveillance (daily temperature checking among contacts), require close links with:

- Air and other types of public transport systems, and their hubs.
- Hotels, hostels, boarding houses, and camping grounds.
- Diplomatic missions and embassies of countries from which participants come.
- Law enforcement authorities and others to help locate and identify contacts.
- Border control.
- Any systems that detail participant movements.

These links should occur as part of the planning process and well in advance for their mutual operation in the event of an outbreak. Special scenario exercises should be considered to better understand how these linkages will work together should it be required.

In some instances, mass drug or vaccine prophylaxis may be required, and plans and supplies should also be in place (see "Mass Vaccination and Public Health").

Management of Dead Bodies

Dead bodies should be handled safely, respecting the rites and customs of the religions or cultures of participants (see Management of Dead Bodies section in "Communicable Disease Control in Humanitarian Emergencies"). Religious or other leaders should be identified during the planning process, as should potential emergency mortuary facilities with forensic pathologists if bodies are not readily recognizable. Planning should also include the necessary agreements for repatriation of dead bodies that involve cross-border/international transport.

Outbreak Communication

Outbreak communication follows the procedures described in the Establishing and Maintaining Regular Communications section of "Response to an Outbreak." Multiple language capabilities may be required and should be planned for in advance. Communication may be especially important in assuring participants that risks are being dealt with effectively. Predetermined routine risk management-related information should be agreed in advance so that it is clear and consistent. Relevant information should be provided to the press once or twice daily during the gathering.

Counseling

A disease outbreak or other health emergency may increase the demand for psychological counseling and support services for those who are affected, as well as those who fear they are at risk. Counseling is particularly important if the event is widespread, has severe health impact, or is the result of a deliberate act. Counseling services must be planned in advance and must ensure appropriate emotional and/or psychological support at the mass gathering site and also make allowance for counseling of friends and family at home.

Religious leaders, counselors, and social workers who provide counseling may need to respond by telephone and may require assistance from organizations such as the International Federation of Red Cross and Red Crescent Societies.

Standard Operating Procedures

Planning for the activities discussed earlier should include the development of a coordination mechanism with standard operating procedures. Several different operational units may need to operate simultaneously and may require decision-making at a level above them with their supervising authority. Preagreed primacy, roles, and responsibilities and single points of contact must therefore be clearly defined.

Carefully prepared and tested standard operating procedures that clearly outline the role of each of the required services are a good way of assuring coordination. An operations center should be established in advance to provide the necessary coordination and command/control required. Liaison officers in each operational unit must also be identified in advance to form a network through which information to and from the operations center is communicated. To prevent confusion, standard operating procedures must be well practiced in scenario exercises during the planning phase.

Further information and guidance can be found at: http://www.who.int/csr/mass_gathering/en/index.html.

[M. Barbeschi]

OUTBREAK RESPONSE IN CASE OF DELIBERATE USE OF BIOLOGICAL AGENTS TO CAUSE HARM

The deliberate or intentional release of biological agents is an unpredictable threat and a public health event of potential national and international importance when it occurs. This was clearly demonstrated in 2001 when anthrax spores were deliberately disseminated in envelopes addressed to several prominent personalities throughout the USA, causing 22 infections and 5 deaths. The public health response included identifying all those at risk of infection through the postal system and prescribing antibiotics to more than 32,000 persons identified as potentially in contact with envelopes contaminated with anthrax spores. It also involved emergency and law enforcement services in the USA and in other countries where numerous false alarms occurred simultaneously, causing unprecedented demands on public health laboratory services.

The sociopolitical implications of deliberate events require national health agencies to collaborate with security and other sectors for the response. This in turn may change the context in which public health services are delivered because of widespread fear, the potential for multiple closely grouped events, high visibility, and coinvestigation with law enforcement. The capacity for managing the health risks of potential outbreaks involving the deliberate use of pathogens or biological toxins depends on the capacity of the emergency and facility-based health care systems to accommodate a surge in patients and on the knowledge and skills of health workers in dealing with infectious disease outbreaks. The security and other sectors should be included in planning for the response to deliberately caused outbreaks. Strengthening detection systems for naturally occurring outbreaks will also increase their capacity to detect outbreaks that may be deliberately caused.

Strengthening the core public health capacities under the revised IHR is deemed to be the best method of ensuring detection and a public health response where and when an outbreak occurs, whether it is naturally occurring or deliberately caused.

Key Issues to Consider
Key considerations related to the health risks of deliberate use of pathogens or toxins include:

- The alert and response mechanism for dealing with suspected or confirmed deliberate events is the same as for detecting naturally occurring events (e.g., severe acute respiratory syndrome [SARS], avian influenza).
- Epidemiological and laboratory capacities may need to be enhanced in order to cope with both the public health response and coordination with security/investigative agencies (e.g., carrying out forensic epidemiology, ensuring chain of custody and chronological documentation, safeguarding confidentiality, carrying out sample collection, preserving evidence).

A deliberately caused outbreak at a mass gathering is especially important as it has the potential to overwhelm the public health system (see "Communicable Disease Alert and Response During Mass Gatherings"). If the biological agent in question is widely dispersed and/or easily transmissible, surge capacity requirements may be greater than anticipated, and flexible systems must be available for the rapid mobilization and distribution of medicines or vaccines. In certain types of outbreaks, alternative models of response must be considered. For example, should an event with a highly communicable disease occur in a stadium, it may be necessary to bring clinical capacity to the location of the outbreak rather than transporting contaminated and infectious people and substances to health care facilities through urban public transport systems, the capacity of which could thus be compromised or overwhelmed. An inappropriate response runs the risk of amplifying transmission rather than stopping it.

In the event that the agent is transmissible, additional capacity is required for contact tracing and active surveillance. Incubation period, period of communicability, and susceptibility are agent-specific. Some of the infectious agents of concern include bacteria and rickettsia (anthrax, brucellosis, melioidosis, plague, Q fever, tularemia, and typhus), fungi (coccidioidomycosis) and viruses (arboviruses, hemorrhagic fever viruses, and variola virus). International threat analysis considers that deliberate use of biological agents to cause harm is a real threat that can occur at any time.

Such risk analysis is not, however, generally considered a public health function. A more complete illustrative list of agents with potential for deliberate use follows later in this chapter.

The prevention of the deliberate use of biological agents presupposes accurate and up-to-date intelligence about deliberate users and their activities. The agents may be manufactured using equipment necessary for the routine manufacture of drugs and vaccines, and the possibility of dual use of these facilities adds to the complexity of prevention. This has led many analysts to regard a strong public health infrastructure, with rapid and effective detection and response mechanisms for naturally occurring infectious diseases of outbreak potential, as an essential part of a society's response to the threat of deliberately caused outbreaks of infectious disease.

The deliberate release of a biological agent may occur overtly or covertly. If the release of a biological agent is perpetrated overtly in the setting of an "announced event," it may result in immediate mass hysteria. Such an occurrence, whether related to a real event, to a hoax, or to a perceived event, could quickly overwhelm and incapacitate an entire health care system if not managed quickly and appropriately.

The first indication of a covert biological attack could be the inexplicable and rapid onset of respiratory distress and incapacitation of victims. Early response should also take into account the possibility of an accidental release of a toxic agent. Symptoms may be masked in the first instance if the release is accompanied by an explosion and attendant trauma and panic. Alternatively, if the biological agent has been administered to food or beverage supplies at a mass gathering, the first symptoms will be more typical of rapid onset food poisoning that might not become manifest before the attendees depart, with symptoms developing up to 1 or 2 days after the population has disseminated. If the symptoms are atypical, they may need to be supported by hospital laboratory diagnosis and/or epidemiological surveillance.

Standard Operating Procedures

Organizations that respond to deliberately caused outbreaks should consider developing, testing, and implementing standard operating procedures in advance through desktop or field exercises. These exercises should help to identify roles and responsibilities and should set out the key tasks to be undertaken by specific staff in the first 48 hours following the onset of an emergency. Aspects of the response that need to be clarified, and their operation rehearsed in simulation exercises, include:

- Multiagency working protocols and procedures to establish the roles of the medical services in preparedness and response in the event of a covert or overt deliberately caused outbreak, including command, control, and coordination procedures at strategic, tactical, and operational venues/levels.

- Means of informing the local and national public and media, of interacting with local and national governments, and of informing and/ or seeking assistance from key regional and international organizations (e.g., WHO, World Organization for Animal Health in the case of biological agents that could affect or be transmitted by animals).

- Infection control because of the risk of the deliberate release of chemical/biological/radiological/nuclear agents that could affect medical personnel if infection control procedures are incomplete or inadequate (e.g., those regarding the use of specialized personal protective equipment and decontamination) or are not followed rigorously.

Routine national and global surveillance systems for naturally occurring outbreak-prone and emerging infectious diseases provide the capacity to detect and respond to deliberately caused infectious diseases because the public health detection and response mechanisms are similar. Adequate background information on the natural behavior of infectious diseases will facilitate recognition of an unusual event and help to determine whether suspicions of deliberate use should be investigated.

Planning for naturally occurring outbreaks should include elements to cope with suspected or confirmed deliberate release as well as indications of actions to be taken should such a release be suspected.

Most health workers have little or no experience in managing illness arising from some of the infectious agents with the greatest potential for deliberate use to cause harm; training in clinical recognition and initial management may therefore be needed for first responders. This training should include methods for infection control, safe handling of diagnostic specimens and body fluids, and decontamination procedures. One of the most difficult issues for the public health system is to decide whether preparedness should include stockpiling of drugs, vaccines, and equipment.

Outbreaks of international importance, whether naturally occurring or thought to have been deliberately caused, should be reported electronically by national governments to: outbreak@who.int. For further information on reporting obligations, see "Reporting of Communicable Diseases Under the International Health Regulations."

Further information on preparedness for deliberate outbreaks can be found on the relevant WHO website at: http://www.who.int/csr/en.

Illustrative List of Agents with Potential for Deliberate Use

With current movement toward an all-hazard, all-pathogens approach to both naturally occurring and deliberately caused communicable disease outbreaks, proscriptive lists are losing meaning. There are a number of lists of infectious agents that are more or less suited to different contexts and threat assessments, and meaningful preparedness for deliberate use must fully take into account the specific nation/space/time for which it is considered.

Generalized lists (e.g., those generated by CDC, the EU, or Association of Southeast Asian Nations [ASEAN]) while useful for budgeting and planning are by no means all-inclusive. They should be considered as illustrative lists, the relevance of which is affected by changing targets, pathogens (natural or genetically modified), the means/path of delivery, and other factors. In addition, such lists change quickly over time as more is understood about the agents in question and their potential for use in a deliberate attack.

The following is an illustrative list of a number of pathogens (thought potentially suitable for deliberate attacks) that have been or are thought to be under development in biological offensive programs, or that have been deliberately used in the past to cause outbreaks.

Bacteria, such as:

- Anthrax (*Bacillus anthracis*)
- Brucellosis (*Brucella abortus*, *Brucella suis*, and *Brucella melitensis*)
- Glanders (*Burkholderia mallei*)
- Melioidosis (*Burkholderia pseudommallei*)
- Tularemia (*Francisella tularensis*)
- Plague (*Yersinia pestis*)
- Q Fever (*Coxiella burnetii*)
- Typhus Fever (*Rickettsia prowazeki*)

Fungi, such as:

- Coccidioidomycosis (*Coccidiodes immitis*)

Viruses, such as:

- SARS
- Ebola, Marburg, and other viral hemorrhagic fevers
- Venezuelan equine encephalomyelitis
- Smallpox (*Variola* virus)

Bacterial toxins, such as:

- Staphylococcal enterotoxins
- Botulinal neurotoxins

For more information and illustrative examples of more comprehensive lists, see the following lists from CDC and WHO at:

- http://www.bt.cdc.gov/agent/agentlist.asp
- http://www.who.int/csr/delibepidemics/annex3.pdf

Illustrative List of Indicators That an Outbreak/Incident Is Potentially a Deliberate Event

The following criteria constitute an illustrative list of potential indicators for deliberate events, based on pathogens/toxins that have been or are thought to be under development in biological offensive programs, or that have been deliberately used in the past to cause outbreaks (to be considered also in relation to Annex 2 of the IHR reporting mechanisms, if appropriate):

- Large or multiple simultaneous outbreaks of an infectious disease.
- Recognition of infectious diseases that are not endemic to an area.
- Presentation of multiple patients with infectious diseases that may be endemic to an area but that rarely infect humans.
- A cluster of 2 or more cases, related in time and space, of the following syndromes (single cases of severe illness in a previously well person may also be considered):

  - Neurological syndrome—meningitis, encephalitis, encephalopathy, or neurological disturbance.
  - Respiratory syndrome—pneumonia, infiltrates, pneumonitis, acute respiratory distress syndrome (ARDS).
  - Acute fulminating septicemia or shock.
  - Fulminant hepatitis or hepatic failure.

Illustrative List of Alert and Surveillance Signals

To be integrated into routine surveillance and alert systems:

- Overt threat of deliberate use.
- All rumors and reports of smallpox-like illness.
- All rumors and reports of disease with test results confirming a specific agent with potential for deliberate use in a nonendemic area (e.g., pulmonary anthrax, tularemia, or plague).
- Previously well persons presenting with severe unexplained disease or syndrome, or death.
- Disease of known etiology occurring in an unusual setting, population or season, or with an atypical clinical presentation/higher morbidity and mortality.
- Multicentric outbreaks—same syndrome or confirmed disease in noncontiguous areas.
- Illness or deaths among animals that precede or accompany illness or death in humans.
- Suspected or known deliberate or accidental release in another country.
- Illness affecting a key sector of the community (e.g., political, financial) or a mass gathering event.

Illustrative List of Indicators Based on Clinical and Epidemiological Findings

- Failure of a common disease to respond to usual therapy/prophylaxis.
- Unusually short median/mean incubation period for a known disease.
- Previously unknown modes and/or routes of transmission.
- Infectivity (the number of people infected by a single person, or a high value) significantly higher than expected (increased transmissibility).
- Case-fatality rate significantly higher than expected (increased virulence).
- Dose response, for example, lower attack rates among people who had been indoors, especially in areas with filtered air or closed ventilation systems, compared with people who had been outdoors.
- An unusual increase in the number of people seeking health care, especially if presenting with fever, respiratory, neurological, or gastrointestinal symptoms.

Suggestive Laboratory Findings

- Confirmed atypical, genetically engineered, or antiquated strain of an agent.
- Laboratory confirmed case/cluster of specific agent with no known risk factors for a natural infection.
- Indistinguishable molecular and genetic characteristics of agents detected in temporally or spatially distinct sources.

The WHO Strategy for Global Health Security can be found in the WHO World Health Report 2007 on Global Health Security at: http://www.who.int/whr/2007/en.

[M. Barbeschi]

ONE HEALTH: COMMUNICABLE DISEASES AT THE HUMAN-ANIMAL INTERFACE

Introduction

Humans, animals, and the environment are inextricably linked and connected in a world with more than 7 billion people. The human-animal interface is expanding, and the global environment, ecosystems, and habitats have been permanently altered, creating a changing ecological milieu that is leading to an increase in emergence and reemergence of infectious diseases.

During the last 3 decades there has been a significant increase in outbreaks, including hantavirus, plague, new variant Creutzfeldt-Jakob disease (CJD), Nipah virus, West Nile, Rift Valley fever, anthrax, severe acute respiratory syndrome (SARS), Marburg hemorrhagic fever, Ebola, *Escherichia coli*, 0157:H7, *Salmonella* Saintpaul, Q fever, H5N1 and H1N1 influenza A viruses, and numerous antimicrobial-resistant pathogens. Approximately 75% of these have been zoonotic, and the challenge is to create and implement an integrated approach to address human health, with an emphasis on prevention of emerging and reemerging infectious diseases at their origin, rather than continuing a reactionary response that often causes a negative economic impact in addition to human suffering and death. This integrated and holistic approach is the essence of the concept of One Health.

One Health is the collaborative effort of multiple disciplines to attain optimal health for humans and animals while protecting the environment. Factors that must be considered in One Health include adaptation of microbes, global travel and trade, host susceptibility, deliberate intent to do harm, climate change, economic development and land use, human demographics and behavior, and a breakdown of both public and animal health infrastructures linked to poverty and social inequality.

Most of these factors are man-made and have produced "the 21st century global mixing bowl" in which microbes have many opportunities to create new niches, cross species boundaries, and rapidly travel worldwide to cause infection and outbreaks in humans and animals. These factors are likely to accelerate in intensity and complexity and are important for understanding of One Health and communicable diseases.

Humans

The world population has a growth rate of 1.2% per year and the next century will represent a period of exponential growth. Approximately 90% of this growth is occurring in developing countries. Almost 1 billion people live in periurban or slum settings in the developing world's largest cities, and these sites are where the most rapid growth in human populations is projected. Communicable diseases are spread not only by travel but also by immigration, translocation, and other movement of people worldwide. And there are a significant and increasing number of immunocompromised individuals who are especially susceptible to infections, including foodborne and waterborne illnesses.

Animals

As per capita incomes rise, people consume more calories and eat different products, increasing demand for meat and protein from animal sources. With relative increases in wealth and technological advances in livestock and poultry production, global increases and consumption of livestock products is a certainty. The Food and Agriculture Organization (FAO) estimates that there will be a 50% increase in demand for animal protein in the next 1–2 decades, and as the entire global food system becomes more intensive, it will progressively shift to developing countries, where veterinary and public health infrastructures are minimal. The number of companion animals and pets is also rapidly increasing, and wildlife is increasingly sought for food—thereby carrying and transmitting zoonotic infections that cause diseases such as rabies, West Nile virus, Lyme disease, and infections with other viruses such as Nipah, Hendra, and hantavirus. Bats are thought to be hosts for a variety of infectious agents including Nipah, Ebola, and Marburg. Influenza A viruses are also found across a number of bird and animal species and often evolve, adapt, and move through avian and porcine hosts prior to human adaptation.

Environment and Climate Change

The environment continues to undergo change, mostly to the detriment of the ecosystem. Habitat disruption and altering land use may, for example, have an impact on carrier populations such as rodents. Climate change also has the potential to alter the environment and geographic range of insect vectors. During the past decade there has been an increase in the incidence of tickborne diseases such as Crimean Congo hemorrhagic fever, Lyme disease, and Rocky Mountain spotted fever.

The global threat from dengue is thought to have occurred in part because of a shift in geographic range of mosquitoes that is associated with temperature and humidity change. The Rift Valley fever virus has caused animal and human epidemics in Africa after flooding and the associated increased number of mosquito breeding sites. The recent increase in the incidence of coccidioidomycosis in the southwestern USA is likely due to a combination of hot and dry conditions and disruption of the land from new construction that aerosolizes this microbe.

Working Successfully at the Human-Animal Interface: One Health

Currently, global alert and effective response are the major means of protecting against emerging infections. One Health shifts the response farther upstream closer to the origins of emergence caused by risk factors in animals and the environment. Canine rabies, for example, has been eliminated in many countries by national programs to vaccinate canine populations. The cost savings to health care and the benefits to human health have been significant. New and emerging infections—for which there are no vaccines—must be prevented and controlled by action on vectors, habitats, and other aspects of the ecosystem, and disease surveillance must be expanded to include animals and risk factors in order to accumulate the evidence base that will permit the development of interventions to prevent and control emerging infections at their source.

Food safety and the adoption of a Hazard Analysis Critical Control Points strategy is based on One Health and aims to reduce or eliminate pathogen loads in animals, animal products, and food processes to prevent human exposures. National animal disease control campaigns for brucellosis, tuberculosis, rabies, bovine spongiform encephalitis (BSE), psittacosis, and equine encephalitis have all greatly reduced morbidity and mortality in animals and have concurrently reduced human exposures and disease. The elimination and reduction of influenza in poultry and swine populations is a critical strategy to reduce human risk.

Use of Rift Valley virus vaccines in livestock can prevent human exposure to infected ruminant animals, and vector control, such as mosquito abatement, reduces potential exposures to mosquito-borne infections. Limiting human exposure at live-animal markets is a proven means of preventing emerging infection events such as SARS in China, and preventing exposure of animals and humans to bats is thought to be a further means of decreasing the risk of Nipah, Ebola, and Marburg viruses.

Global interdependence and growing convergence of animals, animal products, and humans will continue to provide possibilities for emergence and international spread of infectious diseases in humans and to create economic losses in goods, services, travel, and trade in addition to human sickness and death. Infectious diseases are therefore no longer only a concern to the health sector. Their prevention and control requires the work of epidemiologists, clinicians, ecologists, veterinarians, entomologists, climatologists, engineers, and many more experts coming together to provide new insights and perspectives, using new scientific and technological tools. Together they must expand and integrate surveillance of humans, animals, and the ecosystem and create a workforce with the skills and knowledge to work across sectors to prevent emergence of infectious diseases at the human-animal interface.

[L. J. King]

INFECTION PREVENTION AND CONTROL

I. HEALTH CARE FACILITIES

Health care–associated infections occur as a result of health care in facilities, or in the community. Infections can take place in all types of facilities, independent of resources, and are a major cause of death and increased morbidity in hospitalized patients worldwide. The most severe health care–associated infections are found where very ill patients are being treated.

At any one time, over 1.4 million people worldwide suffer from infectious complications of health care. In developed countries, about 5%–10% of patients admitted to acute care hospitals acquire an infection; in resource-poor countries, the burden of health care–associated infections is even greater.

Health care workers may also become infected, and therefore prevention and control measures increase safety for them as well as for patients. Special measures may be required to reduce the risk of infection for visitors to health care facilities.

Health care settings can act as amplifiers of infection, resulting in outbreaks, with an impact on both hospital and community health. For example, nosocomial transmission varied from hospital to hospital and accounted for 20%–57% of recorded probable cases of severe acute respiratory syndrome (SARS). In outbreaks of Ebola and Marburg viral hemorrhagic fevers in Africa, health care workers have accounted for up to 10% of all cases and have served as sources of infection in their families and communities.

Epidemiology

The modes of transmission of infections in health care settings, and in the community, are alike, but processes in health care settings may serve to amplify and facilitate the spread of infections. Microorganisms causing health care–associated infections can be considered to arise from endogenous or exogenous sources. The former refers to the patient's own flora, which can be transferred during health care from a site that is routinely colonized (e.g., skin or gastrointestinal tract) to a normally sterile site (e.g., blood or cerebrospinal fluid). Exogenous sources are external to the patient, such as health care workers, other patients, or the environment. In health care facilities, opportunities for contact between infected and susceptible patients are increased, particularly when health care workers manipulate infectious materials and then touch susceptible patients without proper hand hygiene or when they reuse improperly cleaned equipment involved in patient care. Invasive devices can also facilitate transmission and bypass natural barriers to infection.

Infectious agents causing health care–associated infections may vary greatly from one facility to another, depending on the type of patient (e.g., adults or children), the scope of health services provided, the predominant sites of infection, and the incidence of infections in the community. Most health care–associated infections are caused by bacteria from the normal or transitory flora of the skin, the intestine, the upper respiratory tract, and the upper digestive tract. Viral agents are less frequent and are mostly associated with infections in children, such as acute respiratory or intestinal infections; the exceptions are bloodborne viral infections, such as hepatitis B and C viruses, HIV, and norovirus, which is responsible for large outbreaks among the elderly and in long-term care facilities. The evolution of diagnostic laboratory techniques will no doubt reveal nosocomial viral infections in the future that are unrecognized at present. Fungi are infrequent pathogens in hospital-acquired infections, with the exception of *Candida* spp., which can cause bloodstream infections in patients with central venous catheters or parenteral nutrition; and *Aspergillus* spp., which is present in pulmonary infections of immunocompromised hosts.

The majority of health care–associated infections are sporadic, but a small proportion is associated with outbreaks. Outbreaks can originate from community-infected patients (e.g., acute respiratory infections [ARIs] with adenovirus), from the contamination of a common source within the facility (e.g., contamination of antiseptic solutions or intravenous medications), or as a result of systematic breakdown of aseptic technique for a given procedure.

Host risk factors, such as age and severity of underlying disease, are a major influence on the incidence of most types of health care–associated infections. Some practices, such as use and manipulation of invasive devices (e.g., urinary and central vascular catheters, naso-orotracheal tubes, and mechanical ventilation) and procedures (e.g., surgery) are also associated with infections, and high rates can be observed when there is inadequate infection prevention and control. Contamination of air, water, or equipment surfaces plays a minor role in most health care–associated infections.

While host factors cannot easily be modified, health care practices and procedures can be successfully modified using various preventive strategies. Environmental risk factors can be modified, but the impact of such interventions may be limited to reduction of risk of only certain very specific infections (e.g., airborne viruses, *Aspergillus* spp., *Legionella* spp., and vancomycin-resistant enterococcus).

Health care workers with infections or who are colonized with transmissible microbial agents—particularly those workers treating patients— are a risk for patients. Their infections may be minor (e.g., skin infections, conjunctivitis, and upper respiratory tract infections) but can severely affect certain patients, such as the immunocompromised. At times, health care workers must be treated and/or removed from certain direct patient-care procedures until the infection is cleared and the risk of transmission is over.

Health care workers are frequently exposed to injuries and infectious agents through occupational activities, particularly infections that are bloodborne (e.g., hepatitis B virus) and airborne (e.g., *M. tuberculosis*). Health care workers must therefore be evaluated periodically for infections and for the risk of infection, as must the procedures they perform. Preventive measures such as vaccination of staff against hepatitis B, use of personal protective equipment, and effective postexposure management or treatment must be practiced in all health care facilities. Health care workers should also be vaccinated against seasonal infections that could be carried into the health care setting and infect patients (e.g., seasonal influenza).

Prevention and Control

The most frequent prevention and control measures are intended to reduce the presence of microbiological agents in a health care facility through the use of Standard Precautions during patient care, in order to prevent cross infection, and to ensure prompt and effective treatment of infected patients.

Standard Precautions are a series of procedures that must be performed when dealing with all patients, independent of their infectious status. The key elements of Standard Precautions are:

- **Hand hygiene** before touching a patient, before clean/aseptic tasks, after body fluid exposure, after touching a patient, and after touching a patient's surroundings. For standard precautions, the preferred product is an alcohol-based hand rub, unless hands are visibly soiled, when soap and water should be used. Glove use is not a substitute for appropriate hand hygiene.
- Use of **personal protective equipment** (e.g., gloves, gowns, masks, and eye protection) based on the risk assessment of the procedure (see table at the end of this section).
- **Safe injection practices**, ensuring that only disposable needles and syringes are used, and never reused. Sharp equipment and materials should be handled in such a way as to prevent injuries to the handler or others, particularly if the equipment has been in contact with blood or any body fluid, secretion, or excretion.
- **Environmental cleaning** (both routine and following specific exposure risks), disinfection of reusable equipment, and appropriate disposal of waste.
- **Respiratory hygiene**, by covering the nose and mouth with a tissue when coughing or sneezing, disposing of the tissue after use, and performing hand hygiene afterwards.
- Use of **aseptic technique** whenever natural host barriers are breached (e.g., any incision or puncture) or during manipulation of a port of entry, such as hubs of intravenous lines or the site of catheter insertions.

Adherence to infection control measures should be monitored, with feedback of results to health care workers and supervisors, and there should be formal liaison with public health services, especially when infections involve the community.

Transmission-based precautions are implemented in specific circumstances of increased risk to prevent pathogen spread by direct contact, by respiratory droplets, or by the airborne route. They include: contact precautions (e.g., hand hygiene, gown, gloves, and patient-dedicated equipment), droplet precautions (e.g., surgical mask and separation of ≥ 1 m), and airborne precautions (e.g., approved respirator and negative pressure room).

Treatment is sometimes complicated by the presence of infectious agents, mainly bacteria, that are resistant to anti-infective drugs. Health-facility–associated infections with anti-infective drug resistant organisms are more frequently observed in intensive care units and other settings containing severely ill patients or among those hospitalized for the long-term. Antimicrobial resistance and antimicrobial stewardship are dealt with more fully in Antimicrobial Resistance section in this chapter.

The dissemination of resistant strains throughout a health care facility is by the same routes as with any other infectious agent. Asymptomatic carriers—both patients and health care workers—are of special importance in the dissemination of resistant strains, since they may not be recognized, and preventive measures may therefore not be in place.

For effective control, it may be necessary to place infected or colonized patients with the same known pathogen in the same designated unit (in the same space and with the same staff working on the unit), to which patients without the infection cannot be admitted. This is sometimes referred to as "cohorting."

Infection Control Programs

Infection control programs must comply with Standard Precautions and ensure prompt patient management. The effectiveness of good infection prevention and control programs in reducing the risk of infection in hospitals has been clearly demonstrated, and hospitals with an ongoing culture of safe practices are better prepared to control sporadic infections and to avoid outbreaks. Successful models of infection control in health care facilities include:

- Specialized infection control staff, with appropriate training.
- Policies and guidelines for health care practices.
- Supervision of clinical procedures.
- Surveillance of infections and of process and other outcome measures, with feedback to health care staff.

Infection control programs require trained medical and nursing professionals with time allocated to perform the necessary functions and an infection control committee that sets policies and monitors the impact of infection control activities. To be effective, senior management of a facility must support the committee by ensuring that infection control activities are routinely integrated into hospital policies, training strategies, and supervision of patient-care practices.

Surveillance is required to provide data to describe the incidence, trends, risk factors, and etiology of health care–associated infections; to identify high-risk patients; to detect outbreaks early; and to assess the impact of interventions.

There are several surveillance models, and all require standard case definitions and systematic active case finding procedures. Surveillance must be designed in such as way as to satisfy information needs, while allowing health care workers the necessary time to implement prevention and control measures. Process and outcome indicators are also monitored and fed back to health care staff and organization management to motivate change and improvement.

Health care workers themselves will often be the first to notice the emergence of an infection, or of changes in the epidemiology of an existing infection in the community (i.e., changes in incidence and/or prevalence, mode of transmission, disease severity and/or susceptibility to treatment). Timely reporting to community-based public health services is required. Likewise, community outbreaks or other communicable disease emergencies should be reported directly to health care facilities by community public health services in order to ensure best possible outbreak management and to prevent spread to other patients, visitors, and health care workers.

Over the past decades, the field of infection control has accumulated a large body of evidence-based recommendations to prevent health care–associated infections, but significant gaps still exist between knowledge and implementation.

II. ANTIMICROBIAL RESISTANCE

Introduction

Antimicrobial resistance reduces the options and effectiveness of anti-infective therapy in all infectious disease areas: bacterial, viral, fungal, and parasitic. The emergence of antimicrobial resistance is a natural phenomenon, but can be promoted by the use of anti-infective drugs. In certain circumstances, the evolution of antimicrobial resistance is greatly accelerated when anti-infective drugs are used inappropriately.

Antimicrobial resistance costs money and human lives. It leads to increased morbidity and mortality and the need for prolonged treatment, sometimes with more expensive and toxic combination therapies. It also prolongs the periods during which patients are infectious and can spread disease.

Evolution of Antimicrobial Drug Resistance

The emergence of antimicrobial resistance is the result of constant evolutionary selection in infectious diseases: bacterial, viral, fungal, and parasitic. Microbes reproduce rapidly, mutate frequently, are able readily and freely to exchange genetic material, and therefore easily develop or acquire resistance to anti-infective therapy. Anti-infective drugs eliminate susceptible pathogens while selecting resistant ones, providing them with an evolutionary advantage. Resistance genes encode various mechanisms that allow microorganisms to resist specific anti-infective drug therapy. These mechanisms offer resistance to other antimicrobials of the same class and sometimes to several different antimicrobial classes. The prevalence of resistance varies between geographical regions, and over time, but it has become clear that, sooner or later, resistance will emerge to almost every antimicrobial drug.

Several issues apply specifically to the emergence of antimicrobial resistance in developing countries: inadequate or inconsistent access to antimicrobials leading to truncated treatment courses; the availability of antimicrobial agents without prescription or health care advice; and the sale of counterfeit, often substandard drugs. Among 46 recent reports of counterfeit drugs from 20 countries, 32% of the drugs in question contained no active ingredient, and the rest contained either incorrect quantities of active ingredients or impurities. Substandard doses of antimicrobials place selection pressure on resistant organisms and lead to more rapid evolution of resistance.

In high-income countries, overprescribing of anti-infective treatment by health care workers, and excessive demand by the general population, contribute to increased selection pressure on resistant organisms. Other issues include the empiric prescription of antimicrobials in the absence of laboratory confirmation of infection and the use of excessively broad-spectrum antimicrobials.

A significant portion of the global use of antimicrobial agents occurs amongst animals, particularly the food-production industry. Antimicrobial drugs have been used not only for the treatment of infections in animals, but have also been added to animal feed as prophylaxis against infections, or as growth promoters, mainly in the mass production of poultry, pigs, and fish. Antimicrobials used in this context have included those classed as important in human medicine, raising concern about the role of the food-production industry in the emergence of clinically significant antimicrobial resistance, and its subsequent dissemination to humans through direct contact, environmental contamination, and the food chain. Furthermore, anti-infective drugs are used as pesticides in agriculture products. It is thought that the development and transfer of drug resistance to other organisms may be caused by such agricultural use, but the mechanisms are not well-understood.

Reduced investment in research and development of new classes of anti-infective drugs contributes to the seriousness of antimicrobial resistance and its impact on public health.

Measures to contain antimicrobial resistance

To reduce the selective pressure of antimicrobial drugs, all aspects of drug use in humans, animals, and agriculture must be addressed. The components of a broad strategy include the following:

- Targeted education of all stakeholders (the general population, prescribers, policy-makers, and members of the food-production industry) about the appropriate use of antimicrobials and methods to prevent pathogen transmission and infection.
- Enabling appropriate use of antimicrobials in humans by development of clinical treatment guidelines and decision support, improvements in diagnostics, and auditing and feedback of prescriber practices.
- Aiming to require a prescription in order to access antimicrobial agents.
- Using infection control and prevention strategies to reduce the emergence and transfer of antimicrobial resistance in health care settings, including the control of antimicrobial use (antimicrobial stewardship).
- Legislation to regulate sale of, and where appropriate, enforce the banning of, certain anti-infective drugs such as their use as growth-promoters in livestock.
- Surveillance of antimicrobial use and antimicrobial resistance in human and veterinary settings.
- Vigilance against counterfeit drugs.

Global Trends in Antimicrobial Drug Resistance Development—Some Examples

Tuberculosis

Approximately 3.7% of all new patients with tuberculosis and 20% of those having previously received antituberculous treatment, have multidrug resistant tuberculosis (MDR-TB), representing approximately 440,000 cases and 150,000 deaths each year.

For more information on TB, see "Tuberculosis and Other Mycobacterial Diseases."

MRSA

Infections with methicillin-resistant *Staphylococcus aureus* (MRSA) have long been associated with health care facilities, causing adverse patient outcomes and increased health care costs. Since the 1980s, the frequency of isolates of MRSA among *S. aureus* has increased to almost 70% in health care facilities in Japan and the Republic of Korea, and around 40% in facilities in the USA and Europe. Decreased vancomycin susceptibility has also emerged within most MRSA lineages. MRSA is also of concern outside of health care facilities, with the rate of invasive community-acquired MRSA approaching 10% in some countries. Most often, it causes skin and soft tissue infections, as well as also invasive infections, such as necrotizing pneumonia. Community-acquired MRSA strains are genetically different from hospital-associated strains, and in contrast to most health care–associated MRSA, are usually susceptible to a wider range of antibiotics, such as clindamycin, trimethoprim/sulfamethoxazole, and gentamicin.

Gram-negative bacilli

Since 2000, treatment of infections due to Gram-negative bacilli has been complicated by a rapid emergence and global dissemination of cephalosporin-resistance, mediated by extended-spectrum beta-lactamase (ESBL) enzymes. Of particular note is the community-based spread of the pandemic ESBL-producing *Escherichia coli* ST131 strain. Frequent coresistance to aminoglycosides and fluoroquinolones compromises the effectiveness of traditional first-line agents. In Europe, 3%–36% of *E. coli* isolates were resistant to third generation cephalosporins in 2011. Carbapenem-resistant *Enterobactericeae* represent an emerging crisis, with such strains being susceptible only to limited antibiotics or pan-resistant. Examples include *Klebsiella pneumoniae* carbapenamase, originally identified in the USA in 1996, and New Delhi metallo-beta-lactamase 1, which was first described in 2009 in a Swedish traveler to India. Both enzyme types have subsequently spread globally.

Influenza

Various seasonal influenza-causing strains (e.g., A/H3N2) have been found to show high levels of resistance to both amantadine and rimantadine, 2 drugs regularly used in the past to treat seasonal influenza. Resistance of seasonal influenza viruses has also recently developed to oseltamivir. In the 2008–2009 influenza season, 99.4% of seasonal influenza A (H1N1) viruses tested by the US Centers for Disease Control and Prevention were resistant to oseltamivir, though this fell in subsequent years. In Thailand, resistance to oseltamivir has been shown in H5N1 human infections—causing concern should H5N1 develop into a human pandemic influenza strain. For more information on influenza, see "Influenza."

HIV

HIV is a highly mutant virus that easily develops drug resistance. In high-income countries, where antiretroviral therapy (ART) has been widely accessible for over a decade, an estimated 10%–17% of persons diagnosed with HIV are infected with virus resistant to at least one class of ART drugs. In low- and middle-income countries, where ART is based on an effective three-drug regimen, transmitted antiviral resistance was lower but is increasing with increasing exposure to antiretroviral therapy. For more information on HIV, see "HIV Infection and AIDS."

Malaria

Chloroquine resistance of *Plasmodium falciparum* malaria is now prevalent worldwide. Mortality estimates from public health records in Africa indicate a two- to eleven-fold increase in malaria-associated mortality among children when drug resistance develops, with hospital attendance showing similar increasing trends. Following the global occurrence and spread of high-level resistance against 2 second-line antimalarials, sulfadoxine-pyrimethamine and mefloquine, the recommended treatment of malaria relies on combination therapy with artemisinin and its derivatives as 1 component. Currently, resistance is developing to antimalarial drugs with increasing rapidity, and it is recommended that multidrug combinations be used exclusively, in an effort to slow the development of resistance and to better preserve the effectiveness of existing antimalarial drugs. However, artemisinin-resistance has recently emerged in western Cambodia and in the Thailand-Myanmar border region.

Clostridium difficile

Clostridium difficile are gram-positive spore-forming bacteria that are part of the normal intestinal flora. In those treated with broad spectrum antibiotics that decrease the normal bacterial flora in the gut and interfere with bacterial competition that maintains their balance, *C. difficile* can proliferate and cause severe intestinal disease with watery diarrhea (≤ 15 movements/day), severe abdominal pain, loss of appetite, fever, blood or pus in stool with weight loss and death. *C. difficile* is one of the major hospital-acquired infections in many parts of the world and is the cause of severe illness in the elderly and those who are immunosuppressed or otherwise debilitated.

[A. Stewardson, D. Pittet]

Table: Summary of infection control precautions
Individual barriers: Standard, Contact, Droplet, and Airborne Precautions

Measures	Occasion for use	Hand hygiene	Gloves	Gown	Medical mask	Filtering face piece*	Eye wear
Standard precautions	Before and after patient contact, and after contact with contaminated environmental surfaces or equipment	Always					
	In cases of direct contact with patient blood and body fluids, secretions, excretions, mucous membranes or nonintact skin	Based on risk assessment	✓				
	If there is a risk of spills of infectious material onto the health care worker's body and face	Based on risk assessment		✓	✓	✓	✓
Contact precautions	Always,** on entering patient room***	✓	✓	✓			
Droplet precautions	Always,** on entering patient room***	✓			✓		
Airborne precautions	Always,** on entering patient room***	✓				✓	

*Filtering face pieces for use in health care are particulate respirators with high filtration efficiency (e.g., EU FFP2, US NIOSH-certified N95)

**Whenever entering the patient room or whenever providing care for the patient

***Single room facilitates the application of specific contact and droplet precautions and is obligatory for the application of airborne precautions. In addition, the room for airborne precautions should be adequately ventilated.

MASS VACCINATION IN PUBLIC HEALTH

Mass vaccination campaigns, conducted over short time periods, continue to play an important role in the control of vaccine-preventable diseases, in both industrialized and developing country settings. Mass vaccination is particularly important for:

- Preventing or containing emerging outbreaks of vaccine-preventable diseases.
- Optimizing the impact of a new vaccine.
- Achieving very high herd immunity levels to attain disease control goals.

Mass vaccination and routine immunization are a necessary alliance for attaining both national and international goals in the control of vaccine-preventable diseases.

Preventing or Containing Infectious Disease Outbreaks

The most widely accepted reason for using mass vaccination is to increase population (herd) immunity rapidly in the setting of an existing or potential communicable disease outbreak, thereby limiting the morbidity and mortality that might result. The rationale for using a mass vaccination approach is particularly strong when the incidence of an epidemic-prone disease is beginning to rise; when it is suspected that community immunity is suboptimal; and/or when there has been no routine vaccination because vaccines are unsuitable for routine use or because populations have been displaced and routine immunization services disrupted.

Even with well-managed immunization programs, numbers of susceptible individuals can slowly accumulate to the point where there are enough to sustain outbreaks and ongoing transmission. This phenomenon can be accelerated by primary vaccine courses waning in effectiveness in older children, influxes of unvaccinated migrants, and temporary or sustained vaccination scares affecting groups of children, often in age cohorts. Such situations can be verified by seroepidemiology or administrative surveys indicating that there are growing numbers of susceptible individuals; modeling is then applied to indicate the risk of outbreaks, and mass vaccination "catch-up" campaigns are used to head off resurgence, targeting susceptible groups or whole populations. Some examples of mass vaccination to prevent or contain infectious disease outbreaks follow.

Meningitis

Meningococcal meningitis is one of a number of diseases for which mass vaccination is a standard, proven element of epidemic control. Although meningococcal meningitis occurs throughout the world, the largest epidemics occur in the semiarid areas of 12 sub-Saharan African countries, designated the "African meningitis belt." Most countries within the meningitis belt experience increased transmission each year during the dry season, with large epidemics occurring every 8-12 years during the past 50 years, particularly in regions with extensive communication and mixing of populations.

Meningitis epidemics in sub-Saharan Africa are generally caused by serogroup A organisms, though W135 serogroups have also recently played an important role. Meningococcal vaccines based on capsular polysaccharide antigens are often then deployed. Polysaccharide meningitis vaccines are not routinely used in early childhood because of their general lack of efficacy in infants and young children, those at greatest risk of infection and disease. A conjugate meningitis A vaccine that overcomes this problem is now available and being integrated into routine immunization programs (discussed later).

When increased transmission of meningitis occurs in sub-Saharan Africa, epidemiological surveillance is important in order to determine when the threshold of transmission that leads to epidemics has been reached. Once that threshold is reached (currently 5 confirmed cases/100,000 population/week in rural areas, and 2 confirmed cases/week in urban areas), mass vaccination should be started, targeted at an age group of 1-29 years, and sometimes at the whole population. Rapidly organized and conducted mass vaccination campaigns effectively protect susceptibles and can often interrupt epidemic transmission within 2 or 3 weeks. Mass vaccinations are usually provided by mobile vaccination teams or by fixed vaccination stations at health centers or other community facilities. A meningococcus A conjugate vaccine that is protective in infants and young children is now being introduced in a strategy to vaccinate 1-29 year-olds in an effort to eliminate serogroup A epidemic meningitis. This conjugate vaccine is also being included in national immunization programs in areas at high risk of meningococcal disease, thus compensating for the lack of efficacy of the polysaccharide vaccine in this age group.

Influenza

The need to alter vaccine antigenic composition each year makes it necessary to rapidly vaccinate populations at risk during the winter months in both the northern and southern hemisphere, before the seasonal influenza epidemics begin. The influenza virus is highly unstable and constantly mutates through a process called antigenic drift. At times, when there is an influenza pandemic, a major antigenic shift occurs as a new influenza virus enters human populations. Because antigenic drift and shift decrease the efficacy of influenza vaccine, the recommended antigenic composition of the vaccine is altered annually, based on prevalent virus strains—once in February for the Northern Hemisphere influenza season that will begin roughly 11 months later, and again in August for the influenza season in the Southern Hemisphere.

WHO estimates that up to 500,000 persons die each year from seasonal influenza, mainly those older than 60 years or with other underlying medical conditions. As soon as new vaccines become available each year, they are provided to these populations at risk (usually the elderly, and in some countries to health care workers as well), through mass vaccination at fixed health facilities. Some countries recommend vaccination of populations of all ages with influenza vaccine based on analysis of its cost-benefit. Although it is known that seasonal influenza epidemics occur in developing countries, further study is needed to understand the target populations and vaccination strategy required to optimize the impact of mass vaccination in these settings.

Yellow fever

The yellow fever vaccine is integrated into routine immunization programs in some countries at risk, but not all (see "Yellow Fever"). A severe epidemic of human-to-human transmission is most likely to occur when conditions allow the density of mosquito vector populations to increase substantially, as often happens during the rainy season. Epidemiological surveillance is a key strategy for limiting yellow fever epidemics by rapidly identifying human infections when they occur. Mosquito control is also an effective supplemental prevention strategy. However, the most effective means of preventing yellow fever epidemics is through vaccination at 9 months of age, using the vaccine as part of routine immunization programs.

If routine immunization at 9 months old does not reach the level needed for herd immunity among the general population, epidemic transmission is a risk, and mass vaccination is required to fill the immunity gap. The target population for mass vaccination, once yellow fever has been identified in human populations, is the entire population living or working in the area from which the infection has been identified.

When financial resources or vaccine supply are limited, the primary target population for mass vaccination is usually children aged between 9 months and 14 years. Vaccinations are generally provided through house-to-house campaigns, during which there is active questioning to determine whether additional human infections are occurring. As with any epidemic, planning and implementation of mass vaccination must begin as soon as possible after an outbreak is confirmed, and emergency supplies of 17D yellow fever vaccine must be ordered immediately.

Outbreaks among displaced persons

Sudden and large or massive influxes into a single area of people with varied backgrounds and immunization status can occur during civil disturbance, war, and natural disasters. In such situations, routine immunization activities are often not available. Where displaced populations live in close proximity, and where sanitation and water supplies may be compromised, an environment is created that is particularly conducive to epidemics of vaccine-preventable diseases.

Major vaccines used in mass campaigns among displaced persons are those for measles, meningococcal meningitis, and yellow fever. Mass vaccination for measles is usually conducted immediately after displaced persons congregate, particularly if vaccine coverage rates are estimated to be less than 80%. The target population is often extended to a lower age limit of 6 months and an upper limit of 14 years, with revaccination of infants when they reach 12 months of age. Mass vaccination for meningitis and yellow fever is conducted if risk factors for epidemics are present, while studies of the applicability of the new typhoid and cholera vaccines in displaced populations are under way at time of writing in several geographic areas to evaluate their usefulness in mass campaigns among displaced persons.

Deliberately caused outbreaks

There are a variety of circumstances under which public health authorities gauge the risk of a deliberately caused epidemic or biologic threat. Mass vaccination campaigns are then sometimes conducted as a deterrent and to prevent or limit a deliberately caused outbreak should one occur. Some countries perceive a particular threat from disease, such as smallpox and/or anthrax, and have begun to stockpile vaccines against these perceived threats that would be used for mass vaccination of entire populations should such a threat be realized.

Strategies for the use of these vaccines vary, but most countries state as the first priority mass vaccination of primary responders, followed by mass vaccination of the general population if the deliberately used infectious agent has the potential to spread from person to person. The strategies for mass vaccination may, however, be much more complex than for other indications due to the deterrent nature and the need to be as safe as possible. For example, because infection with HIV has been associated with generalized vaccinia and death after vaccination with traditional smallpox vaccines, strategies of preventive mass vaccination using these vaccines need to incorporate the ability to avoid vaccination of HIV-infected persons and to provide them with protection by other means, such as passive immunization with vaccinia immune globulin.

For more information on planning for, and reaction to, the deliberate use of infectious agents, see "Outbreak Response in Case of Deliberate Use of Biological Agents to Cause Harm."

Optimizing the impact of a new vaccine

A second important use of mass vaccination strategies is to rapidly increase coverage with a new vaccine at the time of its introduction into routine immunization programs. During the past 60 years, more than 20 new vaccines have become available. Mass vaccination is a key element of new vaccine introduction, the goal being to quickly reduce the proportion of susceptible persons at risk at the time the new vaccine is introduced into the routine immunization program. The impact of the mass campaign is to equalize population immunity levels, thus preventing a potential exacerbation of the targeted disease due to a sudden change in its transmission patterns or other epidemiological characteristics, which might occur as a result of vaccinating only a portion of the susceptible population through routine immunization programs. At the time of new vaccine introduction, persons considered at risk of infection are vaccinated in mass vaccination campaigns to "mop up" or protect all those who are susceptible. Mass vaccination is then ended, and the vaccines remain incorporated in routine immunization programs to vaccinate susceptible persons as they enter the cohort of susceptibility (usually at, or shortly after birth). A first clear example of this strategy occurred in the 1950s, when the Salk inactivated polio vaccine was first licensed. Initially it was offered in mass campaigns to all populations considered at risk of polio, and then it was incorporated into routine childhood immunization programs to ensure that children entering the birth cohort were fully protected.

Although routine childhood immunization against rubella is now a standard component of vaccination programs in industrialized countries, the vaccine has until recently seen limited uptake in developing countries. Decision-making on whether or not to introduce rubella vaccine has been complicated by concern that routine childhood immunization against the disease can shift the average age of infection to older girls, inadvertently increasing, at least transiently, the risk of disease in pregnant women, and thus the incidence of congenital rubella syndrome. Consequently, the introduction of routine childhood immunization against rubella is sometimes accompanied by a one-time mass campaign, targeting all girls younger than 15 years, and in some countries targeting all women of childbearing age.

It is likewise recommended standard practice to accompany the introduction of yellow fever and meningococcal A conjugate vaccine into routine childhood immunization programs with a one-time mass vaccination campaign. In these campaigns, children aged younger than 15 years are targeted in order to prevent yellow fever epidemics, and adults and children younger than 30 years are targeted to prevent meningitis epidemics which could continue to occur because of the immunization gap that would exist until immunized childhood cohorts reach adulthood.

Achieving Very High Herd Immunity Levels to Attain Disease Control Goals

Mass vaccination is also used to attain the herd immunity levels required to accelerate prevention and mortality reduction, and in some instances for eradication. Since the late 1980s, international and national accelerated disease control targets have been established for eradication, for mortality reduction, and for heightened control (sometimes called elimination) of infectious diseases. Reaching these targets requires rapidly increasing population immunity, usually with the goal of interrupting human-to-human transmission of the causative infectious agent. Mass vaccination campaigns are a particularly important element of these efforts as the vaccination coverage levels required to achieve herd immunity, especially in densely populated areas, often exceed the coverage rates from routine immunization programs.

Polio eradication

Polio vaccination has been included in routine immunization programs since the licensing of the Salk and Sabin vaccines. In 1988, when the goal of eradicating polio was set, an increasing number of countries had already interrupted human-to-human transmission of wild poliovirus by using oral poliovirus vaccine (OPV) or inactivated polio vaccines (IPV) in routine immunization programs. In many countries in Latin America, where routine immunization programs had not ever achieved high-level control, it was demonstrated that by supplementing routine immunization with mass vaccination, these tropical and semitropical developing countries could rapidly increase herd immunity and interrupt transmission.

The mass vaccination strategy currently used in polio eradication targets all children younger than 5 years during National Immunization Days or Weeks in which OPV is administered to children through fixed sites, with house-to-house mop-up campaigns that sometimes target a broader age group—if required—to interrupt the final chains of transmission. In some densely populated areas, interrupting poliovirus transmission has required well over 90% coverage in multiple mass vaccination campaigns each year. Areas with low standards of sanitation and high-population densities have required the greatest number of campaigns.

Prior to conducting mass vaccination, district-level microplanning is used to identify areas where children younger than 5 years may be living and to prepare maps that are used by social mobilizers and vaccinators as they pass from community to community and house to house. The oral route of OPV administration allows the widespread use of health care workers, school-teachers, and community volunteers trained in short courses to administer polio vaccine during the campaigns. Mass vaccination is done in countries that remain polio-endemic, countries that have reestablished polio transmission due to imported virus, countries where it is necessary to prevent and/or control outbreaks following polio importation, and countries that are considered to be at high risk of wild poliovirus importation.

Despite the impact of the global polio eradication initiative to date, the use of mass vaccination strategies with the endpoint of eradication remains in uneasy alliance with routine immunization programs, largely due to the massive marginal and opportunity costs associated with eliminating the final chains of human-to-human transmission. This debate has led to the establishment of careful and comprehensive criteria for considering future eradication programs, particularly the need for explicit and appropriate cost-benefit analysis in advance, and the establishment of capacity to sustain sufficient societal and political support throughout the process.

Measles mortality reduction

Although measles vaccine is universally included in routine immunization programs in developing countries (see "Measles"), there is frequent failure of children to seroconvert to measles vaccine because of the presence of maternal antibody to measles. Once maternal antibody disappears, the window of opportunity to vaccinate children effectively before natural infection is short and operationally difficult to exploit. Mass vaccination campaigns are a frequently used strategy for overcoming this problem.

Based on the age profile of measles susceptibility (and therefore mean duration of protection from maternal antibody), a one-time nationwide catch-up campaign is conducted in Latin America and some parts of sub-Saharan Africa each year to reduce population susceptibility to measles and interrupt transmission. Usually all children younger than 15 years are targeted, regardless of prior measles immunization status. Follow-up mass vaccination campaigns, targeting children aged 9 months to 4 years are then conducted every 3–4 years thereafter, giving those who have not previously seroconverted a second opportunity, thus preventing outbreaks in older children. Countries achieving very high coverage through routine immunization programs generally provide this second opportunity prior to school entry.

Prevention of maternal and neonatal tetanus

To prevent maternal and neonatal tetanus, mass vaccination campaigns are conducted in high-risk areas delineated using surveillance data and data on the prevalence of safe and clean birth and delivery practices. In most countries with the explicit goal of eliminating maternal and neonatal tetanus, districts are now ranked from highest to lowest risk of these diseases. Multiple rounds of mass vaccination, targeting young girls and women of childbearing age, are often required for rapid boosting of immunity against tetanus.

[D. L. Heymann]

COMMUNICABLE DISEASE CONTROL IN HUMANITARIAN EMERGENCIES

Communicable Disease Risk in Humanitarian Emergencies

Communicable diseases are a potential major cause of mortality and morbidity in humanitarian emergencies, and they can occur at any time after the initial injuries and death (mainly trauma and drowning) related to the emergency itself.

Humanitarian emergencies include natural disasters such as floods, earthquakes, and drought, as well as conflict situations such as war or civil strife leading to large-scale population displacement. In this chapter, the generic term "emergency" encompasses all situations in which populations are displaced and in need of humanitarian assistance.

People who are displaced across national borders are termed "refugees," whereas those who have been displaced within their country are called "internally displaced persons." There are an estimated 10.4 million refugees and 26.4 million internally displaced persons worldwide, and in 2014 there were more than 60 emergency-affected countries requiring humanitarian assistance, the majority of which were in sub-Saharan Africa and the Middle East.

The communicable disease risk after an emergency is influenced by the type of emergency, its geographic location, and the following risk factors:

1) Prior baseline health of the displaced population, including prevalence of malnutrition and immune status.
2) Size and other characteristics (e.g., age) of the displaced population.
3) Access to appropriate and adequate shelter, food, water, and sanitation after the emergency has occurred.
4) Level of overcrowding in host communities, temporary settlements, or camps.
5) Access to basic health services including primary and referral health care and to public health services including immunizations.

Natural disasters are sometimes associated with large-scale communicable disease outbreaks, especially if there is significant population displacement with a decrease in living standards and provision for basic needs.

But it is conflict and postconflict settings that are most often at risk of epidemics, often compounded by poor baseline population health and prior long-term disruption to essential services and disease control programs.

Children in these settings are at particular risk, and diarrheal diseases, acute respiratory infections (ARIs), measles, and malaria can be major causes of mortality. Other communicable diseases, such as epidemic meningococcal disease, relapsing fever, and typhus are also a risk. It is also important to address diseases such as tuberculosis and HIV in these situations.

Emergencies occur in both industrialized and developing countries. But the impact is often much greater in the latter where essential services may not be available and where inadequate shelter, lack of safe water and sanitation facilities, overcrowding, and substandard immunization services prior to the emergency all contribute to the high risk of communicable disease transmission. It is important to remember that nondisplaced and other populations living in conflict-affected countries can also be at increased risk of communicable diseases.

Major Pathogens

Water-related diseases

Diarrheal diseases are a major cause of mortality and morbidity in emergencies. They result mainly from inadequate quality and quantity of water, substandard and insufficient sanitation facilities, overcrowding, poor hygiene, and scarcity of soap. In camp settings, diarrheal diseases have accounted for more than 40% of deaths in the acute phase of an emergency, with more than 80% of these deaths occurring in children younger than 2 years. The common sources of diarrheal disease outbreaks include pollution of water sources (by fecal contamination of surface water entering incompletely sealed wells), contamination of water during transport and storage (through contact with hands or containers soiled by feces), unsanitary sharing of water containers and cooking pots, scarcity of soap, and contamination of foods.

Developing countries have an especially high risk of diarrheal disease outbreaks following an emergency. After the influx of 800,000 Rwandan refugees into North Kivu, Democratic Republic of the Congo (DRC), in 1994, for example, 85% of the 50,000 deaths that were recorded in the first month were caused by diarrheal diseases, of which 60% were cholera and 40% shigellosis. Cholera outbreaks have been recurrent in DRC throughout the last decade, particularly in conflict-affected eastern DRC. In Aceh Province, Indonesia, a rapid health assessment in the town of Calang 2 weeks after the tsunami in December 2004 found that 100% of the survivors drank from unprotected wells and that 85% of the town's population had reported diarrhea in the previous 2 weeks.

An outbreak of diarrheal disease after flooding in Bangladesh in 2004 led to more than 17,000 cases: *Vibrio cholerae* (O1 Ogawa and O1 Inaba) and enterotoxigenic *Escherichia coli* were isolated. A large cholera epidemic (O1 Ogawa) with over 16,000 cases occurred in West Bengal in 1998 following floods. Cholera was confirmed in Pakistan in the aftermath of the South Asia earthquake in 2005, as well as after the nationwide flooding disaster in 2010. A major cholera outbreak started 9 months after the earthquake in Haiti in 2010, thought from an imported strain and subsequent rapid transmission. Cholera was also confirmed in several countries after drought in the Horn of Africa in 2011 and after food insecurity and floods in the Sahel in 2012.

Hepatitis A and E, also transmitted by the fecal-oral route, in association with lack of access to safe water and sanitation, are also a risk. Hepatitis A is endemic in most developing countries, and most children are exposed and develop immunity at an early age. As a result, the risk for large outbreaks is usually low in emergency settings. In hepatitis E endemic areas, outbreaks frequently follow heavy rains and floods; the illness is generally mild and self-limited, but for pregnant women case-fatality rates can reach 25%. After the 2005 earthquake in Pakistan, sporadic hepatitis E cases and clusters were common in areas with poor access to safe water. Prolonged outbreaks of Hepatitis E occurred in conflict-affected Darfur, Sudan, and eastern Chad in 2004, as well as in refugee camps in South Sudan during 2012 and 2013.

Leptospirosis is an epidemic-prone zoonotic bacterial disease that can be transmitted by direct contact with water contaminated with the urine of rodents and other animal carriers. Flooding and heavy rainfall facilitates spread of the organism because of the proliferation of rodents and the proximity of rodents to humans on shared high ground. Outbreaks of leptospirosis have occurred in numerous countries worldwide related to disasters. In Central America, leptospirosis outbreaks have been reported in most countries and especially in Nicaragua—the highest case numbers coinciding with a tropical storm in 2007 and hurricane in 2010. Other major outbreaks have occurred in Taiwan (associated with Typhoon Nali) in 2001 and after flooding in Mumbai in 2000, in Argentina in 1998, and in the Krasnodar region of Russia in 1997. After flooding in Brazil in 1996, incidence rates of leptospirosis doubled in the flood-prone areas of Rio de Janeiro. Water and/or trauma-related infections (e.g., Vibrio, *Aeromonas* and *Pseudomonas* spp.) are frequent after flooding or tsunamis.

It is not only developing countries that are at risk; there are reports of diarrheal disease outbreaks after disasters in industrialized countries as well. In the USA, for example, outbreaks of diarrheal illness was noted after Hurricane Allison in 1995 and Hurricane Katrina in 2005. After Katrina, norovirus *Salmonella* and toxigenic and nontoxigenic *V. cholerae* were confirmed among displaced populations, and a norovirus outbreak also occurred after an earthquake in Japan in 2011. In contrast, in developed parts of Europe, diarrheal diseases are less often a feature of natural disasters.

Diseases associated with overcrowding

Overcrowding is common in populations displaced by natural disaster or conflict situations and can facilitate the transmission of communicable diseases.

Measles risk in an emergency is dependent on baseline immunization coverage among the affected population and, in particular, among children aged younger than 15 years. Overcrowding is associated with increased reproductive ratio of measles requiring very high vaccination coverage levels to prevent outbreaks. Case-fatality rates are estimated at 3%–5% in developing countries, but may be as high as 10%–30% in displaced populations, particularly where the prevalence of malnutrition is high; in eastern Sudan and Somalia in 1995, measles accounted for 53% and 42% of deaths in refugees, respectively. The large-scale epidemics reported in the 1980s and 1990s are not presently reported as frequently, probably due to the prompt implementation of mass measles immunization campaigns in emergencies as part of humanitarian responses, and to global measles control efforts that have markedly increased vaccination coverage and protection. However, protracted emergencies disrupt vaccination programs over the long-term and can leave large populations and older age groups vulnerable to measles outbreaks. In such settings, while 60% of cases still occur in children younger than 5 years, 20% of cases occur in the 5–15 year age group.

ARIs are a major cause of illness and death among displaced populations, particularly in children less than five years of age. Systematic review has shown ARIs cause between 20% and 35% of deaths, with case-fatality rates (CFRs) up to 30%–35% in emergency settings. Lack of access to health services and to antimicrobial agents for treatment further increases the risk of death from ARIs. Risk factors among displaced persons include crowding, exposure to indoor cooking using open flames, inadequate shelter, lack of blankets (especially in cold climates), and poor nutrition.

Meningitis is transmitted from person to person, particularly in situations of crowding. Large outbreaks of meningococcal meningitis are well documented in populations displaced by conflict, but have not been recently reported following natural disasters. Serogroup A *Neisseria meningitidis* is the main cause of epidemic meningococcal meningitis (80%–85%), although serogroup W135 has become increasingly prevalent in sub-Saharan Africa. Epidemics are also occurring beyond the traditional meningitis belt to include east, southern, and central Africa (e.g., Burundi, Rwanda, and Tanzania; June–October 2002). Cases and deaths from meningitis among displaced people in Aceh and Pakistan have also been documented. With the introduction of the new meningococcal A conjugate vaccine in late 2010, outbreaks of meningococcal A meningitis are being eliminated.

Vector-borne diseases

Natural disasters, particularly cyclones, hurricanes, and flooding, can affect vector breeding sites and vector-borne disease transmission. While initial flooding may wash away existing mosquito breeding sites, standing water caused by heavy rainfall or overflow of rivers can create new breeding sites. This situation can result (typically with some weeks delay) in an increase of the vector population and potential for disease transmission, depending on the local mosquito vector species and its preferred habitat. The crowding of infected and susceptible hosts, inadequate access to health services preventing early and appropriate treatment, a weakened public health infrastructure, and interruptions of ongoing control programs all increase vectorborne disease transmission.

Malaria outbreaks in the wake of disasters are a well-known phenomenon. For example, an earthquake in Costa Rica's Atlantic Region in 1991 was associated with changes in habitat that were beneficial for mosquito breeding and preceded an extreme rise in malaria cases. Additionally, periodic flooding linked to *El Niño*/Southern Oscillation has been associated with malaria epidemics in the dry coastal region of northern Peru.

Populations moving from areas of low endemicity (including nonimmune people) to hyperendemic areas are exposed to high malarial transmission. A large malaria epidemic occurred in Burundi between October 2000 and March 2001 affecting 7 of 17 provinces and causing over 2.8 million cases in a country with a population of 7 million. Other vectorborne diseases of concern in emergency settings are Rift Valley fever, dengue, yellow fever, Japanese encephalitis (mosquito-borne), epidemic typhus, and relapsing fever (louse-borne). Rift Valley fever outbreaks affected Kenya (CFR 23%), Somalia (CFR 45%), and the United Republic of Tanzania (CFR 41%) after flooding in late 2006–2007 and, while endemic, there were upsurges in both Crimean-Congo hemorrhagic fever (CCHF) and dengue related to floods in Pakistan in 2010. A yellow fever outbreak occurred in Darfur, Sudan, in late 2012 (CFR 20%).

Other diseases associated with emergencies
Tetanus is caused by a toxin released by the anerobic tetanus bacillus *Clostridium tetani*. Contaminated wounds, particularly in populations where vaccination coverage levels are low, are associated with illness and death from tetanus. A cluster of 106 cases of tetanus, including 20 deaths, occurred in Aceh in 2004, peaking two and a half weeks after the tsunami. Cases were also reported in Pakistan following the 2005 earthquake.

Methods of Control in Emergency Response
A systematic approach to the control of communicable diseases is a key component of humanitarian emergency response, and is crucial to protecting the health of affected populations.

The main methods of control are as follows:

A. Preparedness measures
Many emergencies, while not predictable, are more likely to occur in areas predisposed to natural phenomena—such as earthquake zones or regions liable to flooding or seasonal severe weather events—and preparedness is therefore a possibility. Even in the case of war or conflict, there is often a long period in advance of hostilities where preparations can be made to ensure a more functional and rapid response. Activities include risk analysis and mapping, contingency planning, stockpiling, training, development of surge capacity in health facilities, improving the physical resilience of health facilities, and undertaking simulation exercises. Such disaster or emergency planning is vital to ensure a smooth, multisectoral response that will reduce deaths and disease. Steps required are:

1) Identify and analyze emergency risks, population vulnerabilities, and likely impact/consequences.
2) Engage in multisectoral contingency planning for prevention, detection, and control of potential priority communicable diseases, and conduct desktop simulation exercises.
3) Implement relevant preparedness measures such as immunization, heightened vector control, stockpiling, and staff training.

B. Rapid risk assessment after emergency onset

After an emergency, rapid risk assessment is required to determine the baseline health status of the emergency-affected population; identify the communicable disease threats, including those with epidemic potential; and determine priority interventions. Steps required are:

1) Identify the lead health agency or authority.
2) Identify and determine the capacity of international and local health partners.
3) Establish health coordination mechanisms.
4) Obtain health data on the host country and countries of origin of displaced persons, as well as on the areas through which they may have passed.
5) Identify main disease threats, including potential epidemic diseases and their geographic distribution.
6) Assess the staffing and capacity of health facilities, including laboratories.
7) Determine priority public health interventions.

C. Preventive measures

Prevent communicable disease by maintaining a healthy physical environment and good general living conditions. Required activities are:

1) Select and plan shelter sites to minimize overcrowding and maximize ventilation.
2) Ensure adequate supply of safe water and water storage containers that can be closed or tapped.
3) Ensure adequate sanitation and hygiene facilities and waste management.
4) Ensure availability of food and cooking facilities.
5) Provide essential clinical services.
6) Control insect vectors and infection reservoirs.
7) Implement mass immunization campaigns (e.g., measles) and other interventions, based on the risk assessment.
8) Provide community education on hygiene and other preventive measures.

D. Control of patient and contacts

The use of standard diagnostic algorithms and treatment protocols in health facilities with agreed upon first-line drugs is crucial in order to ensure effective diagnosis and treatment. Simplified drug regimens are particularly important in emergencies. Infection control and appropriate waste management in health facilities can help prevent nosocomial transmission.

1) Review disease risks identified by risk assessment.
2) Develop simple treatment protocols (e.g., for cholera, meningitis, ARIs, malaria).

3) Train health care workers in management of major diseases and those of outbreak potential.

4) Ensure regular supply of medicines and other supplies, including point of care and other rapid diagnostic tests.

5) Develop clear systems of referral for management of patients with severe disease.

6) Educate the community on health risks and early health care seeking.

7) Implement infection prevention and control practices in health care facilities in line with globally accepted Standard Precautions.

E. Surveillance/early warning system

Set up or strengthen a disease surveillance system with an early warning mechanism to ensure the early reporting of cases, to monitor disease trends, and to facilitate prompt detection and response to outbreaks.

1) Identify target diseases/syndromes for surveillance based on risk assessment.

2) Develop simple case definitions for reporting by participating health facilities.

3) Establish simple and robust, regular reporting mechanisms (including a rapid alert system).

4) Ensure adequate laboratory confirmation services.

5) Monitor disease trends and carry out continuous risk assessment.

6) Feed information back to participating facilities and health sector partners.

F. Epidemic measures

Ensure outbreaks are rapidly controlled using preparedness measures (i.e., stockpiles of medical supplies, treatment protocols, and staff training) and rapid response (i.e., rapid verification, investigation, confirmation, and implementation of control measures).

1) Constitute multisectoral outbreak control committee for outbreak management.

2) Identify and train epidemic response teams.

3) Ensure adequate supplies of vaccines, drugs, and equipment.

4) Establish standard operating procedures for alert or trend verification, investigation and confirmation, and implementation of control measures.

5) Ensure appropriate risk communication with the community, partners, government, and media.

Management of Dead Bodies

Deaths associated with natural disasters are most often caused by blunt trauma, crush-related injuries, or drowning. Violence in a conflict situation can also lead to large numbers of deaths due to deliberate injury. The sudden presence of large numbers of dead bodies (corpses) in an emergency-affected area can fuel fears of outbreaks.

There is no evidence that dead bodies pose a risk of epidemics following natural disasters or acute conflict situations where deaths are due to violence, though they may cause personal communicable disease risks to relief workers who have direct and routine contact. The source of any infection is more likely to be survivors than those killed by the natural disaster or acute conflict. At the time of death, most victims of disasters are unlikely to have a concurrent epidemic-causing disease. Even when deaths are due to communicable diseases, most pathogenic organisms do not survive longer than 48 hours in the human body following death (with the exception of HIV, which can survive in the body ≤6 days after death).

Corpses from those from persons who died from cholera, shigellosis, or hemorrhagic fevers require special attention, especially if burial practices involve touching the corpse. Despite such exceptions, the risk of outbreaks from corpses after natural disasters and acute conflict is frequently exaggerated by both health officials and the media.

Those who do not touch dead bodies have a negligible risk of infection. On the other hand, health workers and emergency relief workers who routinely handle corpses may be at risk of contracting tuberculosis, bloodborne viruses (e.g., hemorrhagic fevers, hepatitis B, hepatitis C, HIV), and gastrointestinal infections (e.g., rotavirus diarrhea, salmonellosis, *Escherichia coli*, typhoid/paratyphoid fevers, hepatitis A, shigellosis, cholera).

- Tuberculosis can be acquired if the bacillus is aerosolized (via exhalation of residual air in lungs, or fluid from lungs spurted up through nose/mouth during handling of the corpse).
- Bloodborne infections can occur from direct contact with blood or body fluid of the corpse through skin lesions, by injury from bone fragments and other sharp body protrusions, or from exposure of the mucus membranes, especially if there is splashing of blood or body fluids.
- Gastrointestinal infections can occur when dead bodies leak feces. Transmission occurs via the fecal-oral route through direct contact with the body and soiled clothes or contaminated vehicles or equipment. Dead bodies may contaminate the water supply through leaking of feces, which could cause gastrointestinal infections, however this has never been documented.

The management of dead bodies is often a concern because of the false belief that they represent an epidemic hazard if they are not buried or burned immediately. Immediate burial or cremation, however, does not constitute an essential public health measure and may violate important social norms.

When managing dead bodies in a humanitarian emergency, best practices are the following:

1) Burial is preferable to cremation in mass casualty situations.
2) Every effort should be made to identify all corpses.
3) Mass burials should be avoided if at all possible.
4) Families should have the opportunity to conduct culturally appropriate funerals and burials according to social custom with the understanding that any practices that could transmit disease from the corpse to the family members, such as cleaning the mouth or coming in contact with body secretions, should be avoided.
5) Where customs vary, separate areas should be available for each social group to exercise their own funerary traditions with dignity.
6) Where existing facilities such as graveyards or crematoria are inadequate, alternative locations or facilities should be provided.
7) The affected community should also have access to materials to meet their needs for culturally acceptable funeral pyres and other funeral rites.

Additional procedures/guidelines for emergency relief workers who routinely handle dead bodies:

8) Ensure Standard Precautions for blood and body fluids.
9) Ensure use and correct disposal of gloves and boots (face masks are not necessary).
10) Use body bags if available.
11) Wash hands with soap and water or rub hands with an alcohol-based hand-rub after handling bodies and before eating.
12) Wash and disinfect vehicles and equipment used in transport of dead bodies.
13) Disinfect bodies before burial only in exceptional cases (e.g., deaths due to cholera, shigellosis, or hemorrhagic fever).
14) Ensure that the bottom of any grave is at least 1.5 m above the water table, with a 0.7 m unsaturated zone.
15) Ensure sufficient time for ventilation (due to toxic gases) before recovery of body if it has been confined in an unventilated space for several days.

Conclusion

Much of the excess mortality and morbidity due to communicable diseases that occur in emergency-affected populations is avoidable through appropriate risk analysis, planning, and preparedness. Effective interventions are usually available, and if rapidly implemented along with preventive measures as part of the humanitarian response, can significantly reduce the impact of these diseases on the population. Coordination between governments, UN agencies, and nongovernmental agencies working at local, national, and international levels, and collaboration between all sectors providing emergency relief—health, food, nutrition, shelter, water, and sanitation—is crucial in order to protect the health of emergency-affected populations.

[M. Gayer]

HANDLING OF INFECTIOUS MATERIALS

Biorisk Management/Biosafety/Laboratory Biosecurity
Laboratory biorisk management includes both laboratory biosafety (the containment principles, technologies, and practices implemented to prevent unintentional exposure to pathogens and toxins, or their accidental release) and laboratory biosecurity (the protection, control, and accountability for valuable biological material within laboratories, in order to prevent unauthorized access, loss, theft, misuse, diversion, or intentional release). Valuable biological materials are biological materials that require—according to their owners, users, custodians, caretakers, or regulators—administrative oversight, control, accountability, and specific protective and monitoring measures in laboratories to protect their economic and historical (archival) value, and/or the population from their potential to cause harm.

Biorisk management describes the use of a risk-based management system approach to work associated with biological agents and toxins, as well as the structures and processes that are essential in controlling biorisk in an organization, regardless of the complexity and the hazards encountered. To ensure work is conducted safely and securely, a comprehensive and effective laboratory biorisk management system will address the following elements: management and organization; risk assessment; pathogen and toxin inventory; general safety; competent personnel; good microbiological technique; clothing and personal protective equipment; human factors; health care; emergency response and contingency plans; accident/incident investigation procedures; facility physical requirements; equipment, maintenance, and calibration; disinfection and decontamination; transport procedures; and security.

Transport and Transfer of Infectious Substances
Specimens collected from humans and/or animals must be transported safely and efficiently, packaged in such a way as to protect those engaged in their transportation from the risk of infection from any pathogen present.

Shipping of infectious substances is highly regulated to ensure appropriateness and consistency and to make sure that materials are accompanied with adequate information.

Specimens that potentially contain infectious substances are divided into 2 categories. Category A specimens potentially contain pathogens capable of causing permanent disability, life-threatening or fatal disease in otherwise healthy humans or animals. Category B specimens are those infectious substances that do not meet the criteria for inclusion in Category A.

For Category A specimens, UN-approved triple-packaging must be used consisting of the following 3 layers:

1) Watertight and leakproof primary receptacle containing the specimen that is wrapped in cushioning and sufficient absorbent material to absorb all fluid in case of leakage.
2) Secondary durable, watertight, leakproof packaging to enclose and protect the primary receptacle(s). Several primary receptacles may be placed in the same secondary packaging, as long as applicable volume and weight limitations are respected.
3) Outer packaging bearing the UN specification marking, thus confirming it has passed the performance tests to the satisfaction of the competent authority.

Less stringent requirements apply for the shipment of Category B specimens, for which 3 layers of packaging are also required.

Specific labeling requirements apply for Category A and Category B shipments, and both categories require additional labeling when other dangerous goods (e.g., dry ice, liquid nitrogen) are used to keep the samples frozen.

Shipping documents accompanying the consignments must include appropriate import/export permits if required. A shipper's Declaration for Dangerous Goods is required for shipments of Category A substances. It is the responsibility and full liability of the shipper to ensure the correct classification, packaging, labeling, and documentation of all potentially infectious substances destined for transport. Noncompliance can lead to civil penalties and/or prosecution as well as delays in delivery.

Transfer

Shipments of specimens across borders require import/export permits from the countries of departure, transit, and destination. The details of the required documentation are dictated by the characteristics of the agents being transported. Generally, transfer issues are addressed by national health, agriculture, and/or customs authorities.

Efficient transport and transfer require coordination between the shipper, the carrier, and the receiver in order to ensure they are transported safely, they arrive on time, and they are in good condition. Such coordination depends upon well-established communication and the existence of a good working relationship between all 3 parties. It is recommended that such a working relationship be assured in advance of shipping.

Shippers, carriers, and receivers have specific responsibilities in ensuring successful transportation. Compliance with applicable regulations in the execution of these responsibilities will reduce the likelihood that packages are damaged and leak, thereby reducing human exposure and possible infection and improving the efficiency of package delivery.

Countries that do not have specific transport regulations in place are encouraged to adopt the UN system for the transport of infectious substances. Only through focused efforts to address any issues that are an impediment to transport will suitable conditions be developed and maintained that ensure the efficient, timely, legal, and worldwide transport and transfer of infectious substances.

Further substantive information on transport of infectious substances, including guidelines, diagrams, and checklists for packaging, international regulations, and spill clean-up procedure can be found at: http://www.who.int/ihr/publications/who_hse_ihr_2012.12/en.

[N. Previsani]

ACTINOMYCOSIS

DISEASE	ICD-10 CODE
ACTINOMYCOSIS	ICD-10 A42

1. Clinical features—A chronic bacterial disease, most frequently localized in the orocervicofacial (55%), thoracic (15%), or abdominopelvic (20%) regions. The lesions, firmly indurated areas of purulence and fibrosis, spread slowly to contiguous tissues. Eventually, draining sinuses may appear and surface on the skin. In infected tissue, the organism grows in clusters, called "sulfur granules."

2. Causative agents—*Actinomyces israelii* is the usual human pathogen. However, many other *Actinomyces* spp. have been associated with disease; the most common are *Actinomyces gerencseriae*, *Actinomyces naeslundii*, *Actinomyces meyeri*, *Actinomyces odontolyticus*, *Actinomyces turicensis*, and *Actinomyces viscosus*. *Propionibacterium propionicus* is also reported to cause actinomycosis. All species are Gram-positive, non-acid-fast, anaerobic to microaerophilic higher bacteria that may be part of normal oral flora. Most, if not all, actinomycosis results from polymicrobial infection with other commensal organisms.

3. Diagnosis—A high index of suspicion is required for initial diagnosis as actinomycosis often mimics other conditions, such as malignancy or tuberculosis. Demonstration in tissue or pus of slim, non-spore-forming, Gram-positive bacilli, with or without branching, or evidence of "sulfur granules." Also by isolating microorganisms from samples of appropriate clinical materials not contaminated with normal flora during collection. Clinical findings and culture allow distinction between actinomycosis and actinomycetoma (for further information, see "Mycetoma and Nocardiosis").

4. Occurrence—Infrequent, occurring sporadically worldwide. Men and women of all races and age groups may be affected, but frequency is maximal between 20 and 60 years. The male:female ratio is approximately 3:1.

5. Reservoir—Humans are the natural reservoir of *A. israelii* and other agents. In the normal oral cavity, the organisms grow in dental plaque and in tonsillar crypts, without apparent penetration or cellular response in adjacent tissues. Surveys in Sweden, the USA, and other countries have demonstrated *A. israelii* microscopically in 40% of extirpated tonsillar crypts and by anaerobic culture in up to 48% of specimens of saliva or material from carious teeth. *A. israelii* has been found in vaginal secretions of approximately 10% of women using intrauterine devices. No external environmental reservoir has been demonstrated.

6. Incubation period—Irregular; probably many years after colonization in the oral tissues and days or months after a precipitating event causing disruption of the mucosal barrier.

7. Transmission—Oral cavity colonization with Actinomyces is nearly 100% by 2 years of age. However, except for rare instances of human bite, there is no evidence for human-to-human disease transmission. The source of clinical disease is endogenous. From the oral cavity, the organism may be aspirated into the lung or introduced into jaw tissues through injury, extraction of teeth, or mucosal abrasion. Abdominal disease also results from introduction through breaks in the mucosal barrier. Pelvic disease is most often associated with the presence of an intrauterine device (IUD).

8. Risk groups—Those with mucosal barrier disruption caused by trauma, surgery or irradiation and immunocompromising conditions (e.g., diabetes, steroid use, HIV), and females with prolonged IUD use. Immunity following infection has not been demonstrated.

9. Prevention—Maintenance of oral hygiene, particularly removal of accumulating dental plaque, will reduce the risk of oral infection.

10. Management of patient—Treatment: no spontaneous recovery. Prolonged administration of penicillin in high doses is usually effective; tetracycline, erythromycin, clindamycin, and cephalosporins are alternatives. Surgical drainage of abscesses or removal of IUD is often necessary.

11. Management of contacts and immediate environment—It is not beneficial to investigate contacts and seek the source of infection.

12. Special considerations—None.

[W. Bower]

❖

AMEBIC INFECTIONS

DISEASE	ICD-10 CODE
AMEBIASIS	ICD-10 A06
INFECTIONS WITH FREE-LIVING AMEBA	ICD-10 B60.2, B60.1

I. AMEBIASIS (amoebiasis)

1. Clinical features—Most infections are asymptomatic and commensal, but some may be invasive and give rise to intestinal or extra-intestinal disease. Intestinal disease varies from acute or fulminating dysentery with fever, chills, and bloody or mucoid diarrhea (amebic dysentery), to mild abdominal discomfort with diarrhea containing blood or mucus, alternating with periods of constipation or remission. Amebic granulomata (ameboma), sometimes mistaken for carcinoma, may occur in the wall of the large intestine in patients with intermittent dysentery or colitis of long duration. Dissemination through the bloodstream may occur and produce abscesses of the liver, and less commonly of the lung or brain. Painful ulceration of the skin is a rare manifestation that can occur anywhere, but most commonly in the perianal and genital regions, usually in association with amebic dysentery. Penile lesions may result from anal intercourse. Amebae reach the skin either directly through contact with contaminated feces or indirectly through hematogenous spread; amebic colitis is often confused with forms of inflammatory bowel disease, such as ulcerative colitis; care should be taken to distinguish the two, since corticosteroids may exacerbate amebic colitis. Amebiasis can also mimic numerous noninfectious and infectious diseases. Conversely, the presence of amebae may be misinterpreted as the cause of diarrhea in a person whose primary enteric illness is the result of another condition.

2. Causative agent—*Entamoeba histolytica*, a parasitic organism. Other similar organisms are *Entamoeba hartmanni*, *Entamoeba dispar*, *Entamoeba moshkovskii*, *Entamoeba bangladeshi*, *Escherichia coli*, or other intestinal protozoa. Not all *E. histolytica* strains are equally virulent. Additionally, the morphologically identical *E. dispar*, present in many asymptomatic cyst passers and once thought to be nonpathogenic, has recently been associated with cases of amebic colitis and amebic liver abscess, putting into question its avirulent status. Immunological differences, isoenzyme patterns, and polymerase chain reaction (PCR) permit differentiation of *E. histolytica* from *E. dispar*.

3. Diagnosis—By microscopic demonstration of trophozoites or cysts in fresh or suitably preserved fecal specimens, smears of aspirates, scrapings obtained by proctoscopy, or aspirates of abscesses or sections of tissue. The presence of trophozoites containing red blood cells is indicative of invasive amebiasis. Examination should be done on fresh fecal specimens by a trained microscopist, as the organism must be differentiated from macrophages. However, even trained microscopists cannot differentiate *E. histolytica* from the morphologically identical *E. dispar* and *E. moshkovskii*. In patients with intestinal disease, examination of at least 3 specimens collected on 3 separate days will increase the yield of organisms from approximately 50% in a single specimen to 75%-95%, but the yield in stool from patients with amebic liver abscesses is only 8%-44%, even with repeated stool examinations. Only one commercially available stool antigen-detection test distinguishes *E. histolytica* from *E. dispar*. Other available assays specific for *E. histolytica*, such as enzyme immunoassay (EIA) and PCR, may require reference laboratory services. Serological tests, particularly immunodiffusion and enzyme-linked immunosorbent assay (ELISA), are very useful in diagnosis of invasive disease in persons living in nonendemic areas. Scintillography, ultrasonography, and computerized axial tomography (CAT) scanning are helpful in revealing the presence and location of an amebic liver abscess and can be considered diagnostic when associated with a specific antibody response to *E. histolytica* in persons from a nonendemic area.

4. Occurrence—Amebiasis is ubiquitous. Persons of all ages are susceptible, but infection is less common in infants and young children. Females and males are equally likely to be infected, but invasive disease is more common in males. For example, liver abscesses occur predominantly in adult males. Asymptomatic carriers are common in endemic areas. The proportion of cyst passers who have clinical disease is usually low. Published prevalence rates of cyst passage, usually based on cyst morphology, vary from place to place, with rates generally higher in areas with poor sanitation and crowding, in mental institutions, and among sexually promiscuous male homosexuals. In areas with good sanitation, amebic infections tend to cluster in households and institutions.

5. Reservoir—Humans, usually a chronically ill or asymptomatic cyst passer.

6. Incubation period—Variable, from a few days to several months or years; commonly 2-4 weeks.

7. Transmission—Either person-to-person or through ingestion of fecally contaminated food or water containing amebic cysts, which are relatively chlorine-resistant. Cysts can survive in moist environmental conditions for weeks to months. Transmission may occur sexually by oral-anal contact with a chronically ill or asymptomatic cyst passer. The period of communicability lasts as long as cysts are passed, which may be for months or years. Patients with acute amebic dysentery probably pose only limited danger to others because of the absence of cysts in dysenteric stools and the fragility of trophozoites.

8. Risk groups—Those at greatest risk live in areas of poor sanitation, crowding, and unsafe drinking water or where unsafe water or human fecal fertilizer ("night soil") is used in agriculture. Other risk groups include immigrants from or travelers to endemic areas and persons partaking in oral-anal sexual activity.

9. **Prevention**—

1) Educate the general public and asymptomatic carriers in personal hygiene, particularly the sanitary disposal of feces and hand-washing after defecation, and before preparing or eating food. Disseminate information regarding the risks involved in eating unwashed (with potable water) or uncooked fruits and vegetables and in drinking water of questionable purity.

2) Dispose of human feces in a sanitary manner and do not use as fertilizer.

3) Protect public water supplies from fecal contamination. Sand filters and diatomaceous earth filters remove nearly all cysts from water. Water of undetermined quality can be made safe by boiling for 1 minute (at altitudes >6,562 ft or 2,000 m, water should be boiled for ≥3 minutes). Chlorination of water as generally practiced in municipal water treatment does not always kill cysts; small quantities of water are better treated with prescribed concentrations of iodine, either liquid or crystalline, or in water purification tablets (tetraglycine hydroperiodide), allowing for at least 30 minutes of contact time and longer for colder water. The most effective treatment of small quantities of water is achieved through the use of portable filters with an absolute pore size of 1.0 μm or less.

4) Treat asymptomatic carriers with a luminal amebicide in order to reduce the risk of transmission and protect the patient from symptomatic amebiasis. Common luminal amebicides are paromomycin and iodoquinol.

5) Educate high-risk groups to avoid sexual practices that facilitate fecal-oral transmission.

6) Health agencies should regulate the sanitary practices of people who prepare and serve food in public eating places and the general cleanliness of the premises involved. Routine examination of food handlers as a control measure is impractical.

7) Disinfectant dips for fruits and vegetables are of unproven value in preventing transmission of *E. histolytica*. Thorough washing with potable water and keeping fruits and vegetables dry might help; cysts are killed by desiccation, by temperatures above 50°C (122°F), and by irradiation.

8) Chemoprophylaxis is not advised.

10. **Management of patient—**

1) Isolation: for hospitalized patients, enteric precautions in the handling of feces, contaminated clothing, and bed linen. Exclusion of individuals infected with *E. histolytica* from food handling and from direct care of hospitalized and institutionalized patients; release to return to work when chemotherapy is completed.

2) Sanitary disposal of feces.

3) Treatment: symptomatic amebiasis should be treated with a systemically active compound, such as metronidazole, tinidazole, ornidazole, or secnidazole, followed by a luminal amebicide to eliminate any surviving organisms in the colon. Follow-up stool examination is recommended after completion of therapy to rule out cyst carriage. If a patient with a liver abscess remains febrile after 5–7 days of metronidazole treatment, nonsurgical aspiration might be indicated. Chloroquine is sometimes added to metronidazole for treating a refractory liver abscess. Abscesses may require surgical aspiration if there is a risk of rupture or if the abscess continues to enlarge despite treatment. Metronidazole is not recommended for use during the first trimester of pregnancy; however, it may be a life-saving drug in case of fulminating amebiasis in late pregnancy, and there has been no proof of teratogenicity in humans.

11. Management of contacts and immediate environment— Household members and other suspected contacts should have adequate microscopic examination of feces and be treated if results are positive for *E. histolytica*. Adequate handwashing after defecation, sanitary disposal of feces, and treatment of drinking water will control the spread of infection. If a common vehicle is indicated, such as water or food, appropriate measures should be taken to correct the situation. The use of condoms and avoidance of sexual practices that permit fecal-oral contact can control sexual transmission. Persons diagnosed with amebiasis should refrain from using recreational water venues until treatment with a luminal drug is completed and any diarrhea has resolved.

12. Special considerations—Disruption of normal sanitary facilities and food management will favor an outbreak of amebiasis, especially in populations that include large numbers of cyst passers.

II. INFECTIONS WITH FREE-LIVING AMEBA (naegleriasis, acanthamoebiasis, balamuthiasis)

1. Clinical features—Naegleriasis causes a typical syndrome of fulminating pyogenic meningoencephalitis (primary amebic meningoencephalitis,

[PAM]) with severe frontal headache, occasional olfactory hallucinations, nausea, vomiting, high fever, nuchal rigidity and somnolence, and death within an average of 5.3 days (range 1–12 days) of symptom onset. The mortality rate of PAM in the USA is greater than 99%. Acanthamoebiasis causes a granulomatous disease (granulomatous amebic encephalitis [GAE]) of insidious onset and lasting from weeks to several months. Balamuthiasis also causes GAE. The mortality rate of GAE in the USA is greater than 90%. In addition to causing GAE, several species of *Acanthamoeba* (*A. polyphaga*, *A. castellanii*, *A. hatchetti*) have been associated with chronic granulomatous lesions of the skin, with or without secondary invasion of the central nervous system (CNS). *Balamuthia mandrillaris* has also been associated with skin lesions preceding CNS infections in some cases. Infections of the cornea (keratoconjunctivitis due to *Acanthamoeba*) have resulted in blindness.

2. **Causative agents**—*Naegleria fowleri*, several species of *Acanthamoeba* (*A. culbertsoni*, *A. polyphaga*, *A. castellanii*, *A. astronyxis*, *A. hatchetti*, *A. rhysodes*, and *A. lenticulata*), and *Balamuthia mandrillaris*.

3. **Diagnosis**—Although free-living amebae (*N. fowleri*, *Acanthamoeba* species, and *Balamuthia*) have sometimes been misidentified as macrophages or *Entamoeba histolytica*, they can be differentiated morphologically and through immunohistochemical staining and PCR testing of brain tissue in PAM and GAE cases. As well, *N. fowleri* and *Acanthamoeba* species can be cultured on nonnutrient agar seeded with *Escherichia coli*, *Enterobacter aerogenes*, or other suitable *Enterobacter* species; *Balamuthia* require mammalian cell cultures for isolation. These techniques can also be used with skin scrapings, swabs, and aspirates in suspected *Acanthamoeba* and *Balamuthia* infections involving the skin. Likewise, suspected *Acanthameoba* eye infections can be diagnosed by histology, PCR, or culture of corneal scrapings; confocal microscopy can also be used. In addition, PAM can be diagnosed through microscopic examination of wet mount preparations of fresh cerebrospinal fluid (CSF) showing motile amebae and of stained smears of CSF.

4. **Occurrence**—The organisms are distributed globally in the environment. Cases have been diagnosed in many countries on all continents except Antarctica, including more than 160 cases of PAM in healthy people, more than 100 cases of GAE in immunodeficient patients (including those with AIDS), and more than 1,000 cases of keratitis, primarily in wearers of contact lenses.

5. **Reservoirs**—*Acanthamoeba* and *Naegleria* are free-living in aquatic and soil habitats. Little is known about the reservoir of *Balamuthia*, although it has recently been isolated from soil and dust and its deoxyribonucleic acid [DNA] has been identified in water and soil.

6. **Incubation period**—From 1-7 days (mean 5 days) in documented US cases of *Naegleria* infection; usually longer in infections with *Acanthamoeba* and *Balamuthia*.

7. **Transmission**—Naegleriasis occurs through exposure of the nasal passages to contaminated water, most commonly by diving or swimming in warm freshwater, especially ponds or lakes in warm climate areas or during late summer, thermal springs or bodies of water warmed by the effluent of industrial plants, or inadequately maintained swimming pools. Naegleriasis has also occurred following direct nasal irrigation with contaminated water or with solutions made from contaminated water. After entering the sinuses, *Naegleria* trophozoites invade brain and meninges by extension along the olfactory nerves. *Acanthamoeba* and *Balamuthia* trophozoites reach the CNS through hematogenous spread, probably from a skin lesion or other sites of primary colonization, such as the respiratory tract. Acanthamoebiasis frequently occurs in chronically ill or immunosuppressed patients with no history of swimming or known source of infection. Balamuthiasis also occurs in such patients but develops in immunocompetent patients as well. Additionally, transmission of *Balamuthia* through solid organ transplantation has been documented in the USA on 3 separate occasions since 2009. Contact lens use, homemade saline used as a cleaning or wetting solution, a brand of multipurpose contact lens solution no longer on the market, and contact lens exposure to water have been implicated as risk factors for corneal *Acanthamoeba* infection. Other than solid organ transplant transmission, no person-to-person transmission has been observed with any of the free-living amebae.

8. **Risk groups**—Naegleriasis occurs mainly in active immunocompetent children and young men and women who have had recent contact with warm, fresh water.

Immunodeficient individuals have increased susceptibility to infection with *Acanthamoeba* and probably *Balamuthia*, although balamuthiasis occurs in immunocompetent persons as well and appears to occur more frequently in persons of Hispanic ethnicity. Eye infections associated with *Acanthamoeba* have occurred primarily in contact lens wearers.

9. **Prevention**—

1) PAM and swimming: the only sure way to prevent swimming-associated PAM is to refrain from swimming and other water-related activities in warm fresh water. Infections may be reduced by educating the public about the risks of swimming in lakes and ponds during periods of warm water temperatures (particularly where infection is known or presumed to have been acquired) and of allowing such water to go up the nose through diving or underwater swimming. Protect the nasopharynx from exposure to

water likely to contain *N. fowleri* (e.g., through the use of nose clips). In practice, this is difficult, since the amebae may occur in a wide variety of aquatic bodies, including inadequately treated swimming pools. Swimming pools containing residual free chlorine of 1-2 ppm are considered safe. No infection is known to have been acquired in a well-maintained chlorinated swimming pool.

2) PAM and sinus irrigation: solutions used for nasal irrigation should be made with boiled, distilled, or sterile water.

3) *Acanthamoeba* keratitis: contact lens wearers should not wear lenses while bathing, showering, or swimming or while using hot tubs and should follow strictly the wear and care procedures recommended by lens manufacturers and health care professionals.

10. Management of patient—Despite the sensitivity of the organisms to antibiotics in laboratory studies, effective treatment for PAM and GAE has not been established and recoveries have been rare. Recovery from PAM occurred in two case patients (one each from the USA and Mexico) following intravenous (with and without intrathecal) administration of amphotericin B at various dosages, oral rifampicin, and an intravenous azole (miconazole or fluconazole), along with dexamethasone to treat cerebral edema. *N. fowleri* is also sensitive to azithromycin, which could be added to the other medications. GAE recoveries have occurred with varying combinations of pentamidine, sulfadiazine, flucytosine, fluconazole, and miltefosine. Like *N. fowleri*, *Balamuthia* is sensitive to azithromycin, which has also been successfully added to the drug cocktail. For eye infections due to *Acanthamoeba*, topical chlorhexidine and/or polyhexamethylene biguanide have been used successfully, often with the addition of the diamidines propamidine, or hexamidine.

11. Management of contacts and the immediate environment—A history of swimming or introducing water into the nose (e.g., sinus irrigation) within 1 week prior to the onset of PAM symptoms may suggest the source of infection. Sources of *Acanthamoeba* and *Balamuthia* infection are less well understood but a history of soil exposure (either recreationally or occupationally) is sometimes elicited from GAE patients; freshwater exposure might also be a source of infection.

12. Special considerations—Any grouping of cases warrants prompt epidemiological investigation. If GAE occurs in a recent transplant patient, investigation of the donor and other organ recipients from the same donor should be initiated.

[S. Roy, J. Yoder, M. Beach, G. Visvesvara]

ANGIOSTRONGYLIASIS

DISEASE	ICD-10 CODE
ANGIOSTRONGYLIASIS	ICD-10 B83.2
INTESTINAL ANGIOSTRONGYLIASIS	ICD-10 B81.3

I. ANGIOSTRONGYLIASIS (eosinophilic meningoencephalitis, eosinophilic meningitis)

1. Clinical features—Angiostrongyliasis affecting the central nervous system (CNS), also known as eosinophilic meningitis, may be asymptomatic or symptomatic; it is commonly characterized by severe headache, neck and back stiffness, and paresthesias. Temporary facial paralysis occurs in 5% of patients. Low-grade fever may be present. Illness is usually self-limiting and may last a few days to several months. Deaths have rarely been reported. Differential diagnosis includes cerebral cysticercosis, paragonimiasis, echinococcosis, gnathostomiasis, tuberculous, coccidioidal or aseptic meningitis, and neurosyphilis.

2. Causative agents—*Parastrongylus* (*Angiostrongylus*) *cantonensis*, a zoonotic nematode (lungworm of rats). The third-stage larvae in the intermediate host (terrestrial or marine mollusks) are infective for humans.

3. Diagnosis—The worm has been found in the cerebrospinal fluid (CSF) and lung, and, rarely, in the eye. CSF usually exhibits pleocytosis with over 10% eosinophils; blood eosinophilia is not always present but can be quite elevated. Presence of eosinophils in the CSF and a history of eating raw mollusks or eating raw foods that may be contaminated by snails or slugs suggest the diagnosis, especially in endemic areas. Immunodiagnostic tests are presumptive; demonstration of worms in CSF or at autopsy is confirmatory. Some research laboratories have developed polymerase chain reaction (PCR) tests for use with CSF and tissue.

4. Occurrence—Widely distributed, reported as far north as Japan; as far south as Brisbane, Australia; in Africa as far West as Côte d'Ivoire; and also in Egypt, Madagascar, the USA, and Puerto Rico. Most cases of infection are diagnosed in China (including Taiwan), Cuba, Indonesia, Malaysia, the Philippines, Thailand, Viet Nam, Pacific islands including Hawaii and Tahiti, and much of the Caribbean.

5. Reservoirs—The rat (*Rattus* and *Bandicota* spp.).

6. Incubation period—Usually 1-3 weeks.

7. Transmission—Ingestion of raw or insufficiently cooked mollusks (snails, slugs, or land planarians), which are intermediate or transport hosts harboring infective larvae. The mollusks are infected by first-stage larvae excreted by an infected rodent; when third-stage larvae have developed in the mollusks, rodents (and people) ingesting the mollusks are infected. Prawns, fish, and land crabs that have ingested snails or slugs may also transport infective larvae. Lettuce and other leafy vegetables contaminated by small mollusks may serve as a source of infection.

In the rat, larvae migrate to the brain and mature to the adult stage; young adults migrate to the surface of the brain and through the venous system to reach their final site in the pulmonary arteries, where they become sexually mature and mate. After mating, the female worm deposits eggs that hatch in terminal branches of the pulmonary arteries; first-stage larvae enter the bronchial system, pass up the trachea, are swallowed, and are passed in the feces. In humans, young adult worms are not able to leave the brain, do not reach maturity, and do not complete the life cycle. This explains the typical neurological symptomatology, which is mainly attributable to the death of young adult worms in the CNS. Angiostrongyliasis is not transmitted from person to person, and humans are a final host.

8. Risk groups—Malnutrition and debilitating diseases may contribute to an increase in severity, and even (rarely), in the case of the central nervous system disease, to a fatal outcome.

9. Prevention—

1) Avoid eating raw or undercooked snails, slugs, and other possible hosts.
2) Control rats.
3) Boil or cook snails, slugs, prawns, fish, and crabs for 3–5 minutes, or freeze at $-15°C$ ($5°F$) for 24 hours; this effectively kills the larvae.
4) Avoid eating raw foods that may be contaminated by snails or slugs; thoroughly cleaning lettuce and other greens does not always eliminate infective larvae.
5) Wear gloves (and wash hands) if snails or slugs are handled.

10. Management of patient—Treatment is usually supportive with the use of analgesics for pain and corticosteroids to limit the inflammatory reaction. Careful removal of CSF at frequent intervals can help to relieve headache in patients with elevated intracranial pressure. Anthelminthic treatment is controversial; no anthelminthic drug is proven effective, and some patients have worsened with therapy. Mebendazole or albendazole may shorten the course of infection. The usefulness of any treatment is debated because the infection is usually self-limiting and because the pathology is attributable to dead worms rather than to live ones.

11. Management of contacts and immediate environment— Identify source of food involved and investigate its preparation.

12. Special considerations—Any grouping of cases in a particular geographic area or institution warrants prompt epidemiological investigation and appropriate control measures.

II. INTESTINAL ANGIOSTRONGYLIASIS

1. Clinical features—Common findings of the intestinal form of angiostrongyliasis include abdominal pain and tenderness in the right iliac fossa and flank, fever, anorexia, vomiting, abdominal rigidity, a tumor-like mass in the right lower quadrant, and pain on rectal examination. Fever, anorexia, vomiting, constipation, or diarrhea are frequent in children. Leukocytosis is usually present, with eosinophils ranging from 20%–60%. Adult worms and eggs in the mesenteric arteries damage the endothelium, causing inflammation, thrombosis, and necrosis. On surgery, the whole wall of the intestine is thickened and hardened, with yellow granulations in the subserosa of the intestinal wall; adult worms are found in the small arteries, generally in the ileocecal area, while eggs and larvae are found in lymph nodes, intestinal wall, and omentum. Intestinal obstruction and perforation can occur. Differential diagnosis includes malignant tumors, appendicitis, Crohn's disease, and Meckel's diverticulum.

2. Causative agents—_Parastrongylus_ (_Angiostrongylus_) _costaricensis_, a nematode worm. The third-stage larvae in the intermediate host (slugs) are infective for humans.

3. Diagnosis—High eosinophilia suggests the diagnosis, especially in children living in endemic areas. Clinical diagnosis may be aided by X-ray. Serological diagnostic techniques are also available. Parasitological diagnosis by biopsy or resective surgery is confirmative. In humans, eggs are not found in feces.

4. Occurrence—Reported in Argentina, Brazil, Colombia, Costa Rica, Dominican Republic, Ecuador, El Salvador, Guadeloupe, Guatemala, Honduras, Martinique, Nicaragua, Panama, Peru, USA, and Venezuela. It is not understood whether transmission occurs outside the Caribbean and Americas.

5. Reservoirs—The cotton rat _(Sigmodon hispidus)_. Several species of other rodents and mammals, such as marmosets, dogs, and coatimundis, can be final hosts, like humans.

6. Incubation period—Usually 2-4 weeks, although can be months.

7. Transmission—Ingestion of raw or insufficiently cooked slugs, which are intermediate or transport hosts harboring infective larvae; also ingestion of slug's slime (mucus) on lettuce and other leafy vegetables, or following playing with slugs (in children). Slugs are infected when they ingest first-stage larvae excreted with feces by an infected rodent; when third-stage larvae have developed in the slugs, rodents (and humans) ingesting the slugs are infected. In the cotton rat, larvae penetrate the intestinal wall and migrate to the lymphatics of the intestinal wall and mesentery. After molting into young adults, they migrate to the mesenteric arteries, where they mature and release eggs that hatch and are excreted with feces by 24 days after infection. In humans, adult worms release eggs into the intestinal tissues. The eggs and larvae degenerate and cause intense local inflammatory reactions and do not appear to be shed in the stool.

8. Risk groups—Risk groups are not well established but are likely to include those who ingest infected slugs or raw vegetables contaminated with slugs or their slime, which contain larvae. Some reports have shown higher case rates in children 6-12 years and in males.

9. Prevention—

1) Avoid eating raw or undercooked snails, slugs, and other possible hosts.
2) Control rats.
3) Boil snails and slugs for 3-5 minutes, or freeze at −15°C (5°F) for 24 hours; this effectively kills the larvae.
4) Avoid eating raw foods that may be contaminated by snails or slugs; thoroughly cleaning lettuce and other greens does not always eliminate infective larvae.
5) Wear gloves (and wash hands) if snails or slugs are handled.

10. Management of patient—Thiabendazole, albendazole, and diethylcarbamazine have shown some effect, but there are no clinical trials demonstrating efficacy. The usefulness of any medical treatment is debated, however, because the infection is usually self-limiting in a few weeks to many months. Death of adult worms following chemotherapy causes acute inflammation in the surrounding tissues, and surviving worms might wander erratically and cause further lesions. In advanced stages of disease, surgery is a common form of treatment; in light infections only the appendix might be involved, but in heavy infections the terminal ileum, cecum, and ascending colon might require excision.

11. Management of contacts and immediate environment—Identify source of food involved and investigate its preparation.

12. Special considerations—Any grouping of cases in a particular geographic area or institution warrants prompt epidemiological investigation and appropriate control measures.

[L. Fox]

ANISAKIASIS

DISEASE	ICD-10 CODE
ANISAKIASIS	ICD-10 B81.0

1. Clinical features—Symptoms vary according to the site of *Anisakis* larval invasion into gastrointestinal mucosa. After eating uncooked/undercooked seafood, abdominal pain, nausea and vomiting, and occasionally hematemesis, starting within several hours, result from invasion in gastric mucosa (gastric Anisakiasis). Subsequently, or alternatively, abdominal pain, distension, diarrhea often with blood/mucus and mild fever, may occur about 1-2 weeks after eating seafood, and persist (granulomatous enteritis called enteric Anisakiasis). In heavy infestation, larvae may lodge in the esophagus, causing esophagitis with pain and difficulty in swallowing. In some, allergic symptoms like skin rash including urticaria, itching, and rarely, anaphylaxis, may develop. Occasionally, only the allergic manifestations occur without larval infestation. Rarely, submucosal granulomas can cause intestinal obstruction; intestinal perforation may also occur, leading to peritonitis.

2. Causative agents—Human Anisakiasis is caused by tissue invasion by the third stage larvae of *Anisakis simplex* (and other *Anisakis* species) or *Pseudoterranova decipiens*, nematode parasites of marine mammals. Although the adult worms are in marine mammals, the third stage larvae are found in fish and squid. Larvae do not develop further in humans. The larvae are 2-5 cm long and remain coiled on the mucosal surface, or embedded in tissue, both in fish and in humans.

3. Diagnosis—Requires clinical suspicion based on history of eating seafood. Endoscopic detection of larvae confirms diagnosis. Embedded dead larvae within granulomas are identified by histopathology of resected tissue. A skin-prick test with *A. simplex* antigen and a serological test for immunoglobulin class E (IgE) antibody against *A. simplex* are available, and both are helpful in diagnosis.

4. Occurrence—The disease occurs in individuals who eat uncooked, undercooked, and inadequately treated (refrigerated, frozen for brief period, salted, marinated, or smoked) saltwater fish or squid. Most cases have been recognized in Japan, where thousands of cases have been described (after eating sushi and sashimi). Cases have also been detected in Scandinavian countries (eating gravlax); on the Pacific coast of Latin America (ceviche); in the Netherlands (herring), and Spain (anchovies). With increasing consumption of raw fish, cases are seen with increasing frequency.

5. Reservoir—*Anisakis* species are widely distributed in all oceans and many sea mammals. The natural life cycle involves transmission of larvae through predation from small crustaceans to squid, or fish, then to sea mammals, the definitive hosts. In fish and squid, the third stage larvae migrate to fleshy body tissues, from which humans get infected as they are eaten. As accidental and dead end hosts, humans do not contribute to the nematode's life cycle.

6. Incubation period—Gastric symptoms may develop within a few hours of ingestion. Symptoms referable to the small intestines occur within a few days or weeks, depending on the number of ingested larvae. Allergic reactions may occur within hours, or take more time—days to weeks. Even dead larvae in raw or undercooked fish could elicit allergic reactions without larval infestation.

7. Transmission—Through ingestion of uncooked, undercooked, or inadequately treated marine fish and squid containing nematode larvae. The larvae may remain in the gastrointestinal tract of the fish and migrate into the internal organs or flesh (muscles) even after the fish dies. When ingested by humans and liberated through digestion in the stomach, they may penetrate the gastric or intestinal mucosa. There is no human-to-human transmission.

8. Risk groups—Persons eating uncooked, undercooked, or inadequately treated marine fish and squid.

9. Prevention—

1) Avoid ingestion of inadequately cooked marine fish and squid. Larvae are killed by heating to 60°C (140°F) for 10 minutes; blast-freezing to −35°C (−31°F) or below for 15 hours; or freezing by regular means at −23°C (−9.4°F) for at least 7 days. The latter control method is used with success in the Netherlands. Irradiation also kills the larvae.
2) Cleaning (evisceration) of fish and squid as soon as possible after they are caught reduces the number of larvae penetrating into the muscles from the mesenteries.

3) Candling (exposure to a light source) is useful for fishery products where parasites can be visualized.

10. Management of patient—Endoscopic removal of larvae is both diagnostic and therapeutic. Albendazole treatment is effective in managing Anasakiasis conservatively. Intestinal obstruction requires decompression by nasogastric intubation and surgical excision of lesions when necessary.

11. Management of contacts and immediate environment— Examination of others possibly exposed at the same time, or to same fish/squid, may identify other affected persons

12. Special considerations—Reporting: report to local health authority, if required.

[J. Jones, M. Eberhard]

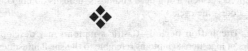

ANTHRAX
(malignant pustule, malignant edema, woolsorter disease, ragpicker disease)

DISEASE	ICD-10 CODE
ANTHRAX	ICD-10 A22

1. Clinical features—An acute bacterial zoonotic disease that historically has been described as occurring in 3 forms: cutaneous, inhalation, or gastrointestinal, depending on the route of exposure. A fourth form, injection anthrax, has been described in recent outbreaks among heroin users in Northern Europe. Systemic illness, including fever, shock, and dissemination to other organs, can occur with any form of anthrax and may include meningitis that is usually fatal.

1) Cutaneous: more than 95% of naturally acquired human cases are cutaneous anthrax, manifested by initial itching of the affected site, followed by a lesion that becomes papular, then vesicular, developing in 2-6 days into a depressed black eschar. Moderate to severe edema usually surrounds the eschar, sometimes with small secondary vesicles. Pain is unusual and, if present, is due to edema or secondary infection. The head, neck, forearms, and hands (exposed areas of the body) are the most common sites of infection. Differential diagnoses include arachnid bites (such as brown recluse in North America), and a variety of other infections

(e.g., staphylococcal or streptococcal cellulitis, dermatomycoses, rickettsialpox, Orf virus, varicella zoster, herpes simplex, vaccinia). Untreated infections may spread to regional lymph nodes and the bloodstream with overwhelming septicemia. Edema associated with cutaneous lesions involving the head and neck can result in respiratory compromise due to compression of the trachea and require intubation. Untreated cutaneous anthrax has a case-fatality rate between 5% and 20%; with effective treatment, however, deaths from cutaneous anthrax are very rare. The lesion evolves through typical local changes even after the initiation of antimicrobial therapy.

2) Inhalation: initial symptoms of inhalation (also referred to as pulmonary) anthrax are mild and nonspecific and may include fever, malaise, and mild cough or chest pain. Symptoms progress to include respiratory distress, stridor, severe dyspnea, hypoxemia, diaphoresis, shock, and cyanosis over 3-4 days. X-ray evidence of mediastinal widening is present in the majority of cases, and pulmonary infiltrates or pleural effusions are usually observed. Maximum case-fatality rate is estimated to be greater than 85%; however early diagnosis and initiation of aggressive combination antimicrobial therapy and supportive care may considerably reduce mortality.

3) Gastrointestinal: gastrointestinal anthrax is rare and difficult to recognize; it tends to occur in outbreaks following consumption of contaminated meat from anthrax-infected animals. Symptoms include abdominal distress characterized by pain, nausea, and vomiting, followed by fever, signs of septicemia, and death in typical cases. The case-fatality rate of gastrointestinal anthrax is estimated to be 40%. A rare oropharyngeal form of primary disease, characterized by edematous lesions, necrotic ulcers, and swelling in the oropharynx and neck, has been described.

4) Injection: patients with anthrax associated with heroin use have not presented with typical symptoms associated with the classic (cutaneous, inhalation, or gastrointestinal) forms of anthrax; however, presentation has been varied. Most patients have serious localized soft tissue infections accompanied by significant soft tissue edema. Fever is not a prominent feature, and pain is less severe than with other serious soft tissue infections. Compartment syndrome may be present. Not all cases have localized injection-related lesions; some cases presented with features more typical of systemic anthrax infection, including hemorrhagic meningitis and multiorgan failure. Differential diagnoses include necrotizing fasciitis, cellulitis, or abscess.

Injection anthrax has a case-fatality rate of 21% in confirmed and probable cases.

2. Causative agent—*Bacillus anthracis*, a Gram-positive, encapsulated, spore-forming, nonmotile rod. Specifically, the spores of *B. anthracis* are the infectious form; vegetative forms of *B. anthracis* rarely transmit disease. *B. anthracis* has 3 main virulence factors: a poly-D-glutamic acid capsule and 2 protein exotoxins—edema toxin and lethal toxin.

3. Diagnosis—Laboratory confirmation is through demonstration of the causative bacilli in blood, lesion exudates or smears, or discharges by direct polychrome methylene blue (McFadyean)-stained smears; or by culture on sheep blood agar or selective media; or through detection of the bacterial deoxyribonucleic acid (DNA), antigens, toxins, or host immune response. Standard diagnosis remains culture of the organism from clinical specimens, but this may be difficult to achieve after antimicrobial treatment is initiated. Rapid detection methods include polymerase chain reaction (PCR), antigen-detection methods including direct fluorescent antibody test (DFA) and immunohistochemistry (IHC), and anthrax lethal toxin detection in serum by mass spectrometry. Sensitivity of these methods may also decline after antimicrobial treatment has been initiated. Serologic assays may be available at national reference laboratories, and a commercial enzyme-linked immunosorbent assay (ELISA) test is available for antibody testing. Rapid assays such as real-time PCR are only available at reference laboratories and laboratories participating in the laboratory response network.

4. Occurrence—In most developed countries, anthrax is an infrequent and sporadic human infection and is primarily an occupational hazard of veterinarians, agriculture and wildlife workers, or workers who butcher animals or process meat, hides, hair, wool, or bone. Human anthrax is endemic in the agricultural regions of the world where anthrax in animals is common, such as sub-Saharan Africa, Asia, South and Central America, and southern and eastern Europe. Outbreaks related to handling and consuming meat from infected livestock have been reported in Africa, Asia, and eastern Europe.

Examples of laboratory-acquired infection exist, and an extensive outbreak occurred in the former USSR in 1979 as the result of an accidental release from a military research institute. Anthrax may also occur through deliberate release of spores. In 2001, spores deliberately released through the postal system in the United States resulted in 11 cutaneous and 11 inhalation cases, including 5 deaths. The remoteness of some of the cases to the original source suggests disease resulted from an exposure to low concentrations of spores through cross-contaminated mail.

5. Reservoir—Animals (normally herbivores, both livestock and wild-life) shed the bacilli in terminal hemorrhages at death. On exposure to the air, vegetative cells sporulate, and the *B. anthracis* spores, which resist adverse environmental conditions and disinfection, contaminate the underlying soil and may remain viable for years. The disease spreads among herbivorous animals through ingestion of spore-contaminated feed or water, and omnivorous and carnivorous animals may become infected through eating meat from infected carcasses. Biting and nonbiting flies may be important in transmission. Infection in livestock may also develop through introduction of animal feed containing contaminated bone meal. Environmental events such as floods or disruption of soil over previous burial sites of infected carcasses may provoke epizootics or may redistribute spores. Scavengers feeding on infected carcasses may also disperse the spores. The skins, hides, hair, and other products from infected animals may pose a risk to those coming in contact with them.

6. Incubation period—The incubation period for cutaneous anthrax is generally 5–7 days, with a range of 1–12 days. The incubation period for inhalation anthrax reported for humans ranges from 1–43 days, although incubation periods of up to at least 60 days may be possible based on studies in animal models. The incubation period for gastrointestinal anthrax is estimated to range from 1–6 days. The incubation period for injection anthrax reportedly ranges from 1–10 days or more.

7. Transmission—The infection can be transmitted through contact with infected livestock or wild animals, with their carcasses, or with their tissues or parts of the animals; or possibly transmitted by biting flies that have fed on such animals. The disease is also transmitted through contact with parts from infected animals such as hair, wool, hides, or bone, or products made from these (e.g., drums, brushes, rugs); or contact with contaminated bone meal used in gardening. Contact with soil contaminated by infected animals is rarely reported as a source of exposure. Reinfection following recovery from a prior infection has rarely been reported. There is limited evidence that seroconversion occurs among people with frequent occupational exposures.

Person-to-person transmission has been rarely reported for cutaneous anthrax, where it requires direct contact with skin lesions. Dried or otherwise processed skins and hides, bones, bone meal, and wool from infected animals may harbor spores for years; they can serve as fomites by which the disease is spread through the trade, resulting in introduction of novel strains, or introduction of anthrax into regions where it was not previously reported.

Cutaneous infection almost always occurs at the site of a preexisting lesion and so is mostly seen on exposed areas of the body (hands, wrists, neck, face). Inhalation anthrax results from inhalation of *B. anthracis* spores, mainly in risky industrial processes (e.g., tanning hides, processing wool or bone) where spore-containing dust or aerosols are generated in an enclosed, poorly ventilated area. The risk of inhalation anthrax is determined not only by bacillary virulence factors, but also by infectious aerosol production and removal rates and by host factors. Anthrax associated with the handling of animal hides outside of an industrial processing plant is rare and is most often of the cutaneous form. Intestinal and oropharyngeal anthrax may arise from ingestion of inadequately cooked meat from such animals; there is no evidence that milk from infected animals transmits anthrax. Injection anthrax has been associated with use of heroin by any route; strains isolated from infections in 2 separate outbreaks in northern Europe have been closely related and genetically related to strains from infected animals in Turkey. The means by which heroin was contaminated with spores remains unknown.

8. Risk groups—Workers involved in industrial processing of hides, wool, or bone; veterinarians; agricultural and wildlife workers in areas with high incidence of epizootic anthrax; and workers who repeatedly enter potentially contaminated areas as part of emergency response activities, such as environmental investigators, remediation workers, and laboratory workers who routinely work with *B. anthracis*. Cases of cutaneous, gastrointestinal, and inhalation anthrax have been reported among persons making or playing contaminated goatskin drums, or participating in events where such drums were played. Heroin injection drug users in northern Europe are the only population of drug users thus far in which cases of injection anthrax have been reported.

9. Prevention—

1) Immunize high-risk persons with a cell-free vaccine prepared from a culture filtrate containing the protective antigen. This vaccine is effective in preventing cutaneous and inhalation anthrax. It is recommended for laboratory workers who routinely work with *B. anthracis* and for workers who handle potentially contaminated industrial raw materials or engage in activities with high potential for production of, or exposure to, *B. anthracis* spore-containing aerosols. It may also be used to protect military personnel against potential exposure to anthrax used as a biological warfare agent. Vaccination may be indicated for veterinarians and other persons handling potentially infected animals in areas with a high incidence of enzootic anthrax. Under certain conditions where threat of deliberate use to cause harm is a concern, first responder organizations may consider vaccination on a voluntary basis. Annual booster injections are recommended if the risk of exposure continues. Vaccines for

administration to humans are produced in the USA and UK (protein-based nonliving vaccines) and China and Russia (live-spore vaccines), and availability is limited outside these countries.

2) Prevention of naturally acquired human anthrax begins with prevention and control in animals. Effective control centers around vaccination of livestock in endemic regions and appropriate procedures in the event of outbreaks of livestock anthrax (correct disposal of carcasses); decontamination of carcass sites and items in contact with the carcasses or sites; vaccination of unvaccinated animals in the affected herd; treatment of symptomatic animals in such herds with penicillin or other suitable antibiotic; and quarantine. (Note that because the animal vaccine is a live vaccine, antibiotics and the vaccine should not be administered simultaneously.)

- Educate employees who handle potentially contaminated animal products about modes of anthrax transmission, signs and symptoms of anthrax, care of skin abrasions, and personal cleanliness. If anthrax is suspected in an animal, do not necropsy the animal; instead, aseptically collect a blood sample for smear and/or culture. Avoid contamination of the area. If a necropsy is inadvertently performed, autoclave, incinerate, or chemically disinfect/fumigate all instruments or materials used.

- Because anthrax spores may survive for years in the soil if carcasses are buried and be a source for new outbreaks—there are many instances on record of outbreaks following disturbance of old burial sites—the preferred disposal techniques for carcasses of animals that die of anthrax and for bedding straw and other contaminated material are incineration at the site of death or removal to an incinerator or rendering plant, taking care to ensure that no contamination occurs en route to the plant. Should these methods prove impossible, after disinfection, such as with formalin, bury carcasses at the site of death as deeply as possible without digging below the local water table level.

- Promptly immunize, and annually reimmunize, all domestic animals at risk. Treat symptomatic animals with penicillin or tetracyclines; immunize them after cessation of treatment. These animals should not be used for food until quarantine and drug clearance times have passed. Treatment in lieu of immunization may be used for animals exposed to a discrete source of infection, such as contaminated commercial feed.

- The affected herd or flock should be quarantined for at least 14 days, preferably 20 days, after the last case is diagnosed.

- Do not sell the hides or other parts of animals infected with anthrax, or use their carcasses as food or feed supplements (bone or blood meal).

3) Control dust and properly ventilate work areas in hazardous industries, especially those handling raw animal materials. Maintain continued medical supervision of employees and provide prompt medical care for all suspicious skin lesions. Workers must wear protective clothing (e.g., gloves, boots, impermeable gowns); adequate facilities must be provided for washing and changing clothes after work. Where possible, workers in at-risk occupations should be vaccinated. Locate eating facilities away from places of work. Vaporized formaldehyde has been used for disinfection of workplaces contaminated with *B. anthracis*. Fumigation with chlorine dioxide or vaporized hydrogen peroxide is also effective.

4) Thoroughly wash, disinfect, or sterilize animal hair, wool, and bone meal—or other feed of animal origin—prior to processing, using disinfecting protocols demonstrated effective against *B. anthracis* spores, such as the Duckering process or irradiation.

5) Control effluents and wastes from rendering plants that handle potentially infected animals and from factories that manufacture products from animal hair, wool, bones, or hides likely to be contaminated. If appropriate, decontaminate.

6) Detailed guidance on prevention, treatment, and control of anthrax in animals and in humans, and on procedures for disinfection and decontamination, is provided in the WHO anthrax guidelines at: http://www.who.int/csr/resources/publications/AnthraxGuidelines2008/en/index.html.

10. **Management of patient—**

1) Isolation: take standard hygienic precautions (wearing disposable gloves, changing dressings, disinfecting clothing and bedding soiled with lesion fluid, washing hands after any of these procedures) for the duration of the lesion or illness in the living patient.

2) Concurrent disinfection of discharges from lesions and articles soiled by the discharges. Hypochlorite is sporicidal and effective when organic matter is not overwhelming and the item is not corrodible; to ensure adequacy of disinfection, free chlorine concentrations should be verified. Hydrogen peroxide, peracetic acid, or glutaraldehyde may be alternative topical decontaminants; formaldehyde, ethylene oxide, and

cobalt irradiation are also effective. Spores require steam sterilization, autoclaving, or burning to ensure complete destruction. Fumigation and chemical disinfection may be used for valuable equipment. Process controls or biological indicators should be used to verify the efficacy of the decontamination methods used. In the event of death, the body fluids of the deceased person should be assumed to have very high concentrations of *B. anthracis* (although antibiotic treatment before death will probably have greatly reduced this) and suitable over-clothing, as well as gloves, should be worn to place the body in a body bag. Bedding is probably best bagged and incinerated rather than simply disinfected. Whether the room should be fumigated depends on the perceived level of contamination beyond bedding.

3) Treatment: initial intravenous therapy with 2 or more antimicrobial agents effective against *B. anthracis* is recommended for treatment of all forms of anthrax, except localized cutaneous anthrax. Ciprofloxacin is the recommended first-line drug of choice, and levofloxacin and moxifloxacin are considered equivalent alternatives to ciprofloxacin. One or two additional antimicrobial agents, such as meropenem, doripenem, imipenem/cilastatin, linezolid, clindamycin, rifampicin, doxycycline, vancomycin, chloramphenicol, penicillin, ampicillin, or amoxicillin should be used to complete the combination regimen. One of the additional agents should have good penetration to the central nervous system; meropenem is recommended as first choice for this purpose in the multidrug regimen, and if meropenem is not available, doripenem and imipenem/cilastatin are considered equivalent alternatives. The other additional agent should be a protein synthesis inhibitor (e.g., linezolid, clindamycin, or doxycycline) to reduce production of exotoxins. Overall duration of antimicrobial therapy should be at least 10-14 days and dependent on patient condition, and therapy may revert to one drug when progression of symptoms ceases and is clinically appropriate. Supportive symptomatic (intensive care) treatment is also important. Obstructive airway disease due to associated edema may complicate cutaneous anthrax of the face or neck, and tracheotomy may be needed. Localized or uncomplicated naturally occurring cutaneous anthrax can be treated with oral ciprofloxacin or doxycycline monotherapy, and treatment for 7-10 days is sufficient. Note that cephalosporins and trimethoprim-sulfamethoxazole should not be used to treat anthrax due to the high

proportion of resistance to these drugs among naturally occurring isolates.

4) Postexposure prophylaxis (PEP): following inhalation exposure to aerosolized *B. anthracis* spores, persons at risk should begin antimicrobial PEP as soon as possible. PEP consists of 3 doses of cell-free vaccine at 0, 2, and 4 weeks in combination with 60 days of antimicrobial treatment. Ciprofloxacin and doxycycline are both recommended first-line choices for PEP; amoxicillin is recommended as an alternative (if isolate is susceptible). The US cell-free vaccine has not been evaluated for safety and efficacy in children younger than 18 years or in adults aged 60 years or older.

11. Management of contacts and the immediate environment—Search for history of exposure to infected animals or animal products and trace to place of origin. In a manufacturing plant, inspect for adequacy of preventive measures. There may be reason to consider deliberate use for human anthrax to cause harm, particularly those with no obvious occupational source of infection, or in other unusual circumstances.

12. Special considerations—

1) Reporting: case reporting is obligatory in many countries. Even a single case of human anthrax, especially of the inhalation variety, is so unusual in industrialized countries and urban centers that it warrants immediate reporting to public health and law enforcement authorities. When naturally occurring, it should also be reported to agricultural or wildlife authorities.

2) Floods in previously infected areas may raise the risk of new cases occurring in livestock.

3) In accordance with The Terrestrial Animal Health Code (World Organisation for Animal Health [OIE], Paris, France, 2007), imported animals or animal products should be accompanied by international veterinary certificates that the animals involved are free from anthrax and were not on-premises quarantined for anthrax at the time of harvesting. Imported bone meal should be sterilized if used as animal feed. Disinfect wool, hair, and hides when indicated and feasible.

4) Measures in case of deliberate use: anthrax has been associated with biological weapons programs and bioterrorism. The general procedures for dealing with deliberate civilian release include the following:

- Anyone who receives a threat about dissemination of anthrax organisms, or a suspicious package or envelope, should immediately notify the relevant local law enforcement authorities and/or those with responsibility for the investigation of deliberately caused biological threats.

- Local and state health departments should also be notified and be ready to provide public health management and follow up as needed.

- If the threat of exposure to deliberately aerosolized anthrax is credible or confirmed, persons at risk should promptly begin PEP as described earlier.

- Primary responders should use an approved, pressure-demand self-contained breathing apparatus, in conjunction with a Level A protective suit, in responding to a suspected biological incident where any of the following information is unknown or the event is uncontrolled: the type(s) of airborne agent(s); the dissemination method; if aerosol dissemination is still occurring or it has stopped, but there is no information on the duration of dissemination; or what the exposure concentration might be. Guidance for protective actions for responders in the event of a wide-area anthrax release has been published by various governments. The US guidance can be found at: http://www.phe. gov/Preparedness/responders/Pages/anthraxguidance.aspx.

- Responders may use a Level B protective suit with an exposed or enclosed, approved pressure-demand self-contained breathing apparatus in a situation in which the suspected biological aerosol is no longer being generated or in which other conditions may present a splash hazard.

- Responders may use a full face piece respirator with a P100 filter or a powered air-purifying respirator with high-efficiency filters, when the following can be determined: an aerosol-generating device was not used to create high airborne concentration, or dissemination was by a letter or package that can be easily bagged.

- Quarantine is not appropriate. Persons who may have been exposed and may be contaminated should be decontaminated with soap and copious amounts of water in a shower.

- All persons who are to be decontaminated should remove clothing and personal effects and place all items in plastic bags clearly labeled with the owner's name, contact telephone number, and inventory of contents. Personal items that are contaminated should be disposed of following local regulations. Personal items may be kept as evidence in

a criminal trial or returned to the owner if the threat is
unsubstantiated.

- If the suspect item associated with an anthrax threat remains
sealed (e.g., unopened envelope), first responders should
not take any action other than notifying the relevant
authority and safely packaging the evidence. Evacuation,
decontamination, and chemoprophylaxis will be dictated by
subsequent epidemiologic and environmental investigation.
For more information on the deliberate use of infectious
agents to cause harm, see "Outbreak Response in Case of
Deliberate Use of Biological Agents to Cause Harm."

[W. Bower, A. Hoffmaster, S. Shadomy]

ARBOVIRAL DISEASES
(arthropod-borne viral diseases)

Introduction—Arboviruses are transmitted to humans primarily
through the bites of infected arthropods (i.e., mosquitoes, ticks, sandflies,
and biting midges). The virus families responsible for most arboviral
infections in humans are *Bunyaviridae*, *Flaviviridae*, *Reoviridae*, and
Togaviridae. More than 100 arboviruses are known to cause human disease.
Although most infections are subclinical, symptomatic illness usually
manifests as 1 of 4 primary clinical syndromes: systemic febrile illness,
polyarthritis and rash, acute central nervous system disease, or hemorrhagic
fever. Some of the arboviruses are covered in separate chapters due to their
international public health importance (e.g., dengue, Japanese encephalitis,
Rift Valley fever, West Nile, and yellow fever viruses). Many arboviral
infections can have more than one primary clinical syndrome. However, the
arboviruses in the following chapter are organized in sections according to
their currently understood most severe clinical presentation.

Most arboviruses are maintained in zoonotic cycles between birds or
small mammals and arthropod vectors. Humans are infected incidentally
and usually do not develop a sustained or high enough level of viremia to
infect arthropod vectors. In a small number of important exceptions (e.g.,
chikungunya, dengue, and yellow fever viruses) humans can be the
primary source of virus amplification and arthropod infection, and the
virus can be spread from person-to-arthropod-to-person (anthroponotic
transmission). Direct person-to-person spread of arboviruses is rare but can
occur through blood transfusion, organ transplantation, intrauterine

transmission, and human milk. Percutaneous and aerosol transmission of arboviruses can occur in the laboratory setting.

The arboviruses are listed in the tables that accompany each section with type of vector and geographical distribution. In some instances, observed cases of disease due to particular viruses have been too few to be certain of the usual clinical course. Viruses recognized to cause human disease only through laboratory exposure or where the only evidence of human infection is based solely on serological surveys are not included.

[M. Fischer, S. L. Hills]

I. ARBOVIRAL FEVERS

VIRUS	ICD-10 CODE	VECTOR	OCCURRENCE
BANZI	ICD-10 A92.8	Mosquito: *Culex* spp.	Africa
BHANJA	ICD-10 A93.8	Tick: *Haemaphysalis intermedia* in Asia, *Hyalomma* spp. in Africa, *Dermacentor* spp. in Europe	Africa, Asia, Europe
BUNYAMWERA	ICD-10 A92.8	Mosquito: *Aedes* spp.	Africa
BWAMBA	ICD-10 A92.8	Mosquito: primarily *Anopheles* spp., but also *Aedes* spp.	Africa
CHANDIPURA	ICD-10 A93.8	Sandfly: *Phlebotomus* and *Sergentomyia* spp. and mosquito: *Aedes* spp., *Anopheles stephensi*, and *Culex tritaeniorhynchus*	Africa, India
CHANGUINOLA	ICD-10 A93.8	Sandfly: *Lutzomyia* spp.	Central and South America
COLORADO TICK FEVER	ICD-10 A93.2	Tick: *Dermacentor andersoni*	Western part of Canada and USA
DUGBE	ICD-10 A93.8	Tick: *Amblyomma* spp.	Africa

VIRUS	ICD-10 CODE	VECTOR	OCCURRENCE
GROUP C VIRUSES (Apeu, Caraparu, Itaqui, Madrid, Marituba, Murutucu, Nepuyo, Oriboca, Ossa, and Restan)	ICD-10 A92.8	Mosquito: *Culex* spp.	South America, Panama, Trinidad, Mexico
HEARTLAND	ICD-10 A93.8	Primary vector unknown, likely ticks	North America
IQUITOS	ICD-10 A93.8	Biting midge (primary vector unknown)	South America
NAIROBI SHEEP DISEASE	ICD-10 A93.8	Tick: primarily *Rhipicephalus appendiculatus*	Africa, India
OROPOUCHE	ICD-10 A93.0	Biting midge: *Culicoides paraensis*	South America, Panama, Trinidad
QUARANFIL	ICD-10 A93.8	Tick: *Argas* spp.	Africa, Middle East
SANDFLY FEVER NAPLES SICILY (Phlebotomus fever, Papatasi fever)	ICD-10 A93.1	Sandfly: *Phlebotomus perniciosus*, *P. perfiliewi*, *P. papatasi* Primarily *P. papatasi*	Europe, Asia, Africa Europe, Asia, Africa
SEMLIKI FOREST	ICD-10 A92.8	Mosquito: *Aedes* spp.	Africa, Asia
SEPIK	ICD-10 A92.8	Mosquito: *Mansonia* spp., *Ficalbia* spp., *Culex sitiens*	Papua New Guinea
SEVERE FEVER WITH THROMBO-CYTOPENIA SYNDROME (Huaiyangshan)	ICD-10 A93.8	Tick (primary vector unknown)	Eastern Asia
SPONDWENI	ICD-10 A92.8	Mosquito: Various species	Africa
TAHYNA	ICD-10 B33.8	Mosquito: *Aedes* and *Culex* spp.	Europe, Asia

VIRUS	ICD-10 CODE	VECTOR	OCCURRENCE
THOGOTO	ICD-10 A93.8	Tick: *Amblyomma, Boophilus, Hyalomma, Rhipicephalus* species	Africa, Europe
USUTU	ICD-10 A92.8	Mosquito: *Culex* spp.	Africa, Europe
VESICULAR STOMATITIS	ICD-10 A93.8	Sandfly: *Lutzomyia* spp.	Americas
WESSELSBRON	ICD-10 A92.8	Mosquito: *Aedes* spp.	Africa
ZIKA	ICD-10 A92.8	Mosquito: *Aedes* spp.	Africa, Asia, Federated States of Micronesia
Rift Valley fever (see "Rift Valley Fever")			

1. **Clinical features**—Febrile illnesses usually lasting a week or less. Initial symptoms include fever, headache, malaise, arthralgia, or myalgia. Occasional symptoms include nausea and vomiting, conjunctivitis, photophobia, or rash. Symptoms usually resolve within a week but may be markedly incapacitating for that time. For most of these viruses, infections are seldom fatal.

Certain clinical features may occur more frequently during infection with specific arboviruses. Sandfly-borne viral fevers often include retro-orbital pain, injected sclerae, and pain in the limbs and back. Severe fever with thrombocytopenia syndrome and Heartland virus infection are characterized by fever, headache, fatigue, leukopenia, and thrombocytopenia. Several viruses (e.g., Colorado tick fever, Bhanja, Thogoto) may occasionally cause central nervous system infection. In vesicular stomatitis, patients typically have pharyngitis, oral mucosal vesicular lesions, and cervical adenopathy.

2. **Causative agents**—Single-stranded ribonucleic acid (RNA) viruses of various families, primarily *Flaviviridae* and *Bunyaviridae*, or double-stranded RNA viruses of the family *Reoviridae*. (See earlier table for specific viruses.)

3. **Diagnosis**—Arboviral infections that cause a febrile syndrome are confirmed most frequently by measurement of virus-specific antibody in serum. Acute-phase specimens should be tested for virus-specific immunoglobulin class M (IgM) antibody. For most arboviral infections, IgM is detectable within the first week after onset of illness and persists for several months, but longer persistence (i.e., years) has been documented. Therefore, a positive IgM test result may reflect a past infection. For Colorado tick fever,

approximately 50% of patients do not develop IgM antibodies until 2–4 weeks after illness onset. Serum immunoglobulin class G (IgG) antibody generally is detectable shortly after IgM and persists for years.

Plaque-reduction neutralization tests can be performed to measure virus-specific neutralizing antibodies. A 4-fold or greater rise in virus-specific neutralizing antibodies between acute- and convalescent-phase serum specimens collected 2–3 weeks apart may be used to confirm recent infection or discriminate between cross-reacting antibodies in primary arboviral infections. In patients who have been infected with another arbovirus from the same virus family in the past (i.e., who have secondary arboviral infections), cross-reactive antibodies in IgM, IgG, and neutralization assays may make it difficult to identify which arbovirus, particularly among flaviviruses, is causing the patient's current illness. Immunization history, date of symptom onset, and information regarding other arboviruses known to circulate in the geographic area that may cross-react in serologic assays should be considered when interpreting results.

Diagnosis can also be made for some viruses (e.g., Colorado tick fever or severe fever with thrombocytopenia syndrome viruses) by testing of serum using molecular methods such as reverse transcription polymerase chain reaction (RT-PCR) or by virus isolation. For most arboviral infections, however, humans usually have low levels of transient viremia and neutralizing antibodies by the time they have clinically apparent infection, so viral culture and testing for nucleic acids are less sensitive for detecting recent infections. Immunohistochemical staining can detect specific viral antigen in fixed tissue.

4. Occurrence—The occurrence of specific arboviruses is dependent on many factors including climate and the relative abundance of susceptible vectors and hosts. Marked seasonality is often observed with arboviral diseases. (See earlier table for geographical distribution of individual viruses.)

Several arboviruses have been recently identified as a source of human infection and febrile disease, including Heartland, Iquitos, Usutu, and severe fever with thrombocytopenia syndrome viruses.

5. Reservoir—Reservoirs for many of the viruses listed have not been identified. Some of these viruses are maintained in a continuous cycle between invertebrate vectors and vertebrate hosts. Identified reservoirs include rodents for group C viruses, small mammals and ticks for Colorado tick fever, rodents and sandflies for the sandfly-borne viral fevers, and primates, sloths, and birds for the sylvatic cycle of Oropouche virus. Humans are usually not involved in the maintenance and spread of these arboviruses; however, humans are an amplifying host for the urban cycle of Oropouche virus, and recent reports suggest that severe fever with thrombocytopenia virus can be transmitted from human to human.

6. Incubation period—Usually 2–14 days for mosquito-borne viruses; 3–4 days for tickborne viruses; and 3–6 days for sandfly-borne viruses.

7. Transmission—By mosquitoes, ticks, biting midges, or sandflies; see earlier table for vectors.

Mosquitoes become infected either when feeding on viremic animals or transovarially. Infected mosquitoes transmit virus to humans during subsequent feeds and typically remain infectious throughout their life. Tick-borne arboviruses are typically acquired by immature ticks feeding on viremic animals; they retain the viruses transstadially and transmit viruses to humans during subsequent feeds. In some cases the cycle is entirely maintained by ticks. Sandfly-borne arboviruses are transmitted transovarially by infected sandflies but may also be acquired by adult sandflies when they feed on infected humans and other animals. They become infective about 7 days after blood feeding, and remain so for their normal lifespan of about 1 month.

Humans may be directly infected with vesicular stomatitis virus through handling of infected animals or their tissues. Rare cases of human-to-human transmission of certain arboviruses have occurred through blood transfusions, transplanted organs, breast-feeding, and the transplacental route. Percutaneous and aerosol transmission of arboviruses can occur in the laboratory setting.

8. Risk groups—Risk of infection is generally determined by exposure to infected vectors and is dependent on many factors including environmental conditions, season, and human activities. In highly endemic areas, adults have often acquired natural immunity following subclinical or mild infection in childhood, and illness occurs mainly in children, visitors, or people new to the area. Patients with immunocompromising conditions may be more susceptible to severe disease. Infection generally results in lifelong immunity.

9. Prevention—

1) Vector prevention measures (see "Arboviral Encephalitides" and "Leishmaniasis").
2) Other prevention measures:

- For vesicular stomatitis viruses, precautions in care and handling of infected animals and their tissues is important.
- For severe fever with thrombocytopenia syndrome virus, precautions should be taken in the care and handling of human acute-phase blood.
- To prevent laboratory infections, precautions should be taken when handling viruses in the laboratory at the appropriate biosafety level. Further information can be found at:

http://www.cdc.gov/biosafety/publications/bmbl5/BMBL5_
sect_VIII_f.pdf.

10. Management of patient—Symptomatic management with analgesics and antipyretics. Standard blood and body substance precautions are sufficient. As a precaution to prevent further transmission, particularly for Oropouche virus, patients should be advised during the first few days after onset of symptoms to avoid further mosquito or sandfly exposure, either by staying in places with screens or by using mosquito nets. In particular for sandflies, very fine screening or mosquito bed nets (10-12 mesh/cm or 25-30 mesh/in, aperture size ≤0.085 cm or ≤0.035 in) should be used, and any sandflies in the residence should be destroyed. To prevent transfusion associated transmission, blood donations (especially from patients infected with Colorado tick fever virus) should be deferred for 6 months.

11. Management of contacts and the immediate environment—A search for unreported or undiagnosed cases wherever the patient lived during the 2 weeks prior to onset should be considered for sporadic or travel-associated cases with exposures in unexpected locations. Identifying and eradicating tick-infested locations and breeding areas of sandflies around dwellings should also be done.

12. Special considerations—

1) Reporting: local health authority may be required to report cases in selected endemic areas or in areas where the virus previously has not been reported. For vesicular stomatitis and Nairobi sheep disease, notify World Organisation for Animal Health (OIE).

2) Epidemic measures: eliminate or treat all potential mosquito breeding places with larvicides. Spraying the inside of all houses in the community with insecticides has shown promise for controlling urban epidemics of some mosquito-borne viruses. Use approved insect repellents for people exposed to bites of vectors. For Nairobi sheep disease, consider immunizing sheep and goats, where available; use acaricides prior to moving potentially exposed animals.

3) International measures: for vesicular stomatitis and Nairobi sheep disease, restrict the movement of infected animals; for others, none except enforcement of international agreements designed to prevent transfer of mosquitoes and infected vertebrates by ships, airplanes, and land transport.

[I. Rabe, S. Yendell]

❖

II. ARBOVIRAL ARTHRITIS AND RASH

VIRUS	ICD-10 CODE	VECTOR	OCCURRENCE
BARMAH FOREST	ICD-10 A92.8	Mosquito: *Culex annulirostris, Aedes vigilax*, and other *Aedes* spp.	Australia
CHIKUNGUNYA	ICD-10 A92.0	Mosquito: *Aedes aegypti, Aedes albopictus* in Asia; other *Aedes* spp. in Africa and Australia	Africa, southeastern Asia, Pacific Islands, Middle East
MAYARO	ICD-10 A92.8	Mosquito: *Haemagogus* spp.	Central America, northern South America, Trinidad
O'NYONG-NYONG	ICD-10 A92.1	Mosquito: *Anopheles* spp.	Africa
ROSS RIVER	ICD-10 B33.1	Mosquito: *Culex annulirostris, Aedes vigilax, Aedes camptorhynchus, Aedes polynesiensis, Aedes pseudoscutellaris* and other *Aedes* spp.	Australia. Sporadic in Papua New Guinea, Pacific Islands
SINDBIS	ICD-10 A92.8	Mosquito: *Aedes* spp. and *Culex* spp.	Africa, northern Europe. Rare in Asia, Australia

   1. Clinical features—Febrile disease characterized by mild-to-severe arthralgia or arthritis, primarily in the wrist, knee, ankle, and small joints of the extremities, lasting days to months. In many patients, onset of arthritis is followed after 1–10 days by a maculopapular rash, usually nonpruritic, affecting mainly the trunk and limbs; the rash may be pruritic with certain viruses (e.g., O'nyong-nyong virus). Buccal and palatal enanthema may occur. In infants, chikungunya viral infections typically cause vesiculobullous lesions. Rashes typically resolve within 7–10 days, and can be followed by a fine desquamation. Myalgia, fatigue, headache, and lymphadenopathy are common. Conjunctivitis, paresthesias, and tenderness of palms and soles occur in a small proportion of cases. With chikungunya, severe congenital infections, mild hemorrhagic manifestations, and rare deaths can occur. Mild hemorrhagic disease symptoms can also occur with Mayaro fever.

Persistence of joint pains, arthritis, myalgia and/or fatigue occurs in 10%–50% of chikungunya cases. Persistence of symptoms may also occur for Ross River and Barmah Forest lasting as long as 12 months, but the arthralgia usually resolves by 7 months.

2. Causative agents—ribonucleic acid (RNA) viruses of the family *Togaviridae*, genus *Alphavirus*. (See earlier table for specific viruses.)

3. Diagnosis—Most commonly diagnosed by serological testing that shows immunoglobulin class M (IgM) antibodies in acute serum samples beginning at approximately 1 week after onset of illness, and a rise in virus-specific titers between acute and convalescent samples. IgM antibodies commonly persist for weeks to months. Diagnosis can also be made for some viruses (e.g., chikungunya, O'nyong-nyong, or Ross River viruses) by molecular methods such as reverse transcription polymerase chain reaction (RT-PCR) on serum or by virus isolation from blood in the first few days of illness.

4. Occurrence—Outbreaks of disease occur during warm and wet conditions that favor proliferation of the mosquito vectors. However, chikungunya outbreaks also have occurred during dry periods as water-holding containers can serve as breeding sites for the vectors of the virus. (See earlier table for the geographic distribution of individual viruses.)

Chikungunya virus caused a major epidemic throughout the Indian Ocean region starting in 2004. During that time, the virus spread to new areas, including temperate areas of Europe, where autochthonous transmission was found to occur. Focal outbreaks of chikungunya continue to occur in the Eastern Hemisphere. In late 2003, an outbreak of Ross River virus disease in Fiji spread to other Pacific islands, including American Samoa, the Cook Islands, and Tonga. Outbreaks of Sindbis virus disease occur in summer and autumn in Europe and South Africa, while Pogosta disease in Finland has a 7-year cycle. Epidemics of O'nyong-nyong virus disease in 1959–1963 and 1996–1997 involved millions of cases throughout eastern Africa. Mayaro outbreaks are relatively small and focal but evidence suggests a high degree of mild clinical illness occurs.

5. Reservoirs—

1) Ross River virus: marsupials, especially kangaroos and wallabies.
2) Barmah Forest virus: natural host is unverified but believed to be opossums and other marsupials.
3) Chikungunya virus: primates.
4) Sindbis virus: birds.
5) Mayaro virus: unverified though nonhuman primates suspected.
6) O'nyong-nyong virus: unknown.

6. Incubation period—From 1–12 days.

7. Transmission—By mosquito; see earlier table for vectors. For chikungunya virus, humans are infectious to mosquitoes for the first few days after onset of illness and, if mobile, can introduce virus into receptive areas.

Health care workers have become infected with chikungunya virus through exposure to infected blood, and neonates have become infected during the intrapartum period. Experimental data also suggest that chikungunya virus may be transmitted by infected organs and tissues. Other modes of transmission, such as through respiratory droplets or particles, have not been documented.

8. Risk groups—Risk of infection is generally determined by exposure to infected vectors and is dependent on many factors including environmental conditions, season, and human activities. In highly endemic areas, adults have often acquired natural immunity following subclinical or mild infection in childhood, and illness occurs mainly in children, visitors, or people new to the area. For chikungunya, both neonates and elderly are at greater risk of severe disease. Underlying medical conditions have also been identified as a risk factor for poor disease outcome. Infection generally results in lifelong immunity.

9. Prevention—General measures applicable to vector and other prevention (see "Arboviral Encephalitides").

10. Management of patient—Symptomatic management with analgesics, antipyretics, and antipruritics. Persistent joint pain might require long-term pain management with anti-inflammatory agents. For patients with disabling peripheral arthritis lasting several months, short-term corticosteroids may be considered.

To prevent further transmission, particularly for chikungunya virus, patients should be advised during the first few days after onset of symptoms to avoid further mosquito exposure, either by staying in places with screens or by using mosquito nets.

11. Management of contacts and the immediate environment—A search for unreported or undiagnosed cases wherever the patient lived during the 2 weeks prior to onset should be considered for sporadic or travel-associated cases with exposures in unexpected locations.

12. Special Considerations—

   1) Reporting: local health authority may be required to report cases in selected endemic areas or in areas where the virus previously has not been reported.
   2) Epidemic measures: eliminate or treat all potential mosquito breeding places with larvicides. Spraying the inside of all houses

in the community with insecticides has shown promise for controlling urban epidemics of some mosquito-borne viruses.

[E. Staples, A. Powers]

III. ARBOVIRAL ENCEPHALITIDES

VIRUS	ICD-10 CODE	VECTOR	OCCURRENCE
BANNA	ICD-10 A83.8	Mosquito (primary vector unknown)	Southeast Asia
CACHE VALLEY	ICD-10 A83.8	Mosquito: *Anopheles*, *Culiseta*, and *Aedes* spp.	North America, Guyana
CALIFORNIA ENCEPHALITIS	ICD-10 A83.5	Mosquito: *Aedes* spp., primarily *A. melanimon*	USA, Canada
EASTERN EQUINE ENCEPHALITIS	ICD-10 A83.2	Mosquito: *Culiseta melanura* (zoonotic cycle); some *Aedes*, *Coquillettidia*, and *Culex* spp. (human transmission)	Americas
EYACH	ICD-10 A84.8	Tick: *Ixodes* spp.	Europe
ILHÉUS	ICD-10 A83.8	Mosquito (primary vector unknown)	Central and South America
JAMESTOWN CANYON	ICD-10 A83.8	Mosquito: *Aedes* and *Culiseta* spp.	North America
KEMEROVO	ICD-10 A84.8	Tick: *Ixodes persulcatus*	Russia

VIRUS	ICD-10 CODE	VECTOR	OCCURRENCE
LA CROSSE	ICD-10 A83.5	Mosquito: *Aedes triseriatus*	USA
LIPOVNIK	ICD-10 A93.8	Tick: *Ixodes ricinus*	Russia
LOUPING ILL	ICD-10 A84.8	Tick: *Ixodes ricinus*	UK, Ireland, Norway
ME TRI	ICD-10 A83.8	Mosquito (primary vector unknown)	Vietnam
MURRAY VALLEY ENCEPHALITIS	ICD-10 A83.4	Mosquito: *Culex annulirostris*	Australia, Papua New Guinea, Indonesia
POWASSAN	ICD-10 A84.8	Tick: *Ixodes* spp., primarily *Ixodes cookei* and *I. scapularis* in North America; *Ixodes persulcatus* and *Haemaphysalis longicornis* in Russia	Canada, USA, Russia
ROCIO	ICD-10 A83.6	Mosquito (primary vector unknown)	Brazil
SNOWSHOE HARE	ICD-10 A83.8	Mosquito: *Aedes* and *Culiseta* spp.	USA, Canada, China, Russia
ST. LOUIS ENCEPHALITIS	ICD-10 A83.3	Mosquito: *Culex* spp.	Americas
TICKBORNE ENCEPHALITIS			
EUROPEAN	ICD-10 A84.1	Tick: *Ixodes ricinus*	From Scandinavia down to the Adriatic region, and east to the Urals, Korea

VIRUS	ICD-10 CODE	VECTOR	OCCURRENCE
FAR EASTERN	ICD-10 A84.0	Tick: *Ixodes persulcatus*	Russia, China, northern Japan
SIBERIAN	ICD-10 A84.8	Tick: *Ixodes persulcatus*	Siberia and the Baltic region
TOSCANA	ICD-10 A93.8	Sandfly: *Phlebotomus* spp.	Southern Europe
TRIVITTATUS	ICD-10 A83.8	Mosquito: *Aedes* spp.	North America
VENEZUELAN EQUINE ENCEPHALITIS	ICD-10 A92.2	Mosquito: Primarily *Culex (Melanoconion)* spp. (enzootic cycle); *Aedes* and *Psorophora* spp. (epizootic cycle)	Americas
WESTERN EQUINE ENCEPHALITIS	ICD-10 A83.1	Mosquito: *Culex Tarsalis*	North and South America
Japanese encephalitis virus (see "Japanese Encephalitis")			
West Nile virus (see "West Nile Virus")			

1. Clinical features—Most arboviral infections are asymptomatic or result in undifferentiated febrile illness. Neurological manifestations include meningitis, encephalitis, or myelitis. Although specific symptoms vary by virus and clinical syndrome, meningitis is characterized by fever, headache, neck stiffness, and other meningeal signs, and arboviral encephalitis produces altered mental status along with variable other neurologic signs including ataxia, tremors, and seizures. Arboviral myelitis results in acute flaccid paralysis.

The severity and long-term outcome of illness varies by virus, syndrome, and patient characteristics such as age and underlying medical conditions. Case-fatality rates vary widely. Among the mosquito-borne viral encephalitides, case-fatality rates for encephalitis caused by Eastern equine encephalitis, Japanese encephalitis (see "Japanese Encephalitis"), and Murray Valley encephalitis viruses are among the highest, with rates often greater than 25%. In contrast, among patients with La Crosse virus encephalitis, fatal cases are rare (<1%). Among the tickborne encephalitis virus subtypes, the Far Eastern subtype causes the most severe disease with a case-fatality rate of 20%-40%. Neurological sequelae following arboviral encephalitis can occur in up to 50% of survivors and may vary from mild peripheral or cranial nerve palsies to spastic quadraparesis. Neuropsychiatric illness or cognitive problems can also occur.

The differential diagnosis of arboviral central nervous system disease is broad and includes many infectious (e.g., viral, bacterial, mycoplasmal, protozoal, or mycotic) and noninfectious (e.g., toxic, metabolic, or postinfectious) causes. Other viral causes of acute neurological illness including herpes simplex, enterovirus, rabies, measles, mumps, Epstein-Barr, varicella zoster, and influenza viruses.

2. Causative agents—Single-stranded ribonucleic acid (RNA) viruses of various families, primarily *Flaviviridae, Togaviridae*, and *Bunyaviridae*, or double-stranded RNA viruses of the family *Reoviridae*. (See earlier table for specific viruses.)

3. Diagnosis—Arboviral infections that cause neuroinvasive disease are confirmed most frequently by measurement of virus-specific antibody in serum or cerebrospinal fluid (CSF). Acute-phase specimens should be tested for virus-specific immunoglobulin class M (IgM) antibody. IgM in CSF is more specific for diagnosing encephalitis than IgM in serum. For most arboviral infections, IgM is detectable within the first weeks after onset of illness and persists for several months, but longer persistence has been documented. Therefore, a positive IgM test result occasionally may reflect a past infection. Serum immunoglobulin class G (IgG) antibody generally is detectable shortly after IgM and persists for years.

Plaque-reduction neutralization tests can be performed to measure virus-specific neutralizing antibodies. A 4-fold or greater rise in virus-specific neutralizing antibodies between acute- and convalescent-phase serum specimens collected 2–3 weeks apart may be used to confirm recent infection or discriminate between cross-reacting antibodies in primary arboviral infections. In patients who have been immunized against or infected with another arbovirus from the same virus family in the past (i.e., who have secondary arboviral infections), cross-reactive antibodies in IgM, IgG, and neutralization assays may make it difficult to identify which arbovirus, particularly among flaviviruses, is causing the patient's illness. Immunization history, date of symptom onset, and information regarding other arboviruses known to circulate in the geographic area that may cross-react in serologic assays should be considered when interpreting results.

Diagnosis can also be made for some viruses by testing of serum or CSF in the first few days of illness by molecular methods such as reverse transcription polymerase chain reaction (RT-PCR) or by virus isolation. For most arboviral infections, however, humans usually have low levels of transient viremia and have neutralizing antibodies by the time they have clinically apparent infection, so viral culture and testing for nucleic acids are less sensitive for detecting infections. Immunohistochemical staining can detect specific viral antigen in fixed tissue.

4. Occurrence—The occurrence of specific arboviruses is dependent on many factors including climate and the relative abundance of susceptible vectors and hosts. Marked seasonality is often observed with arboviral diseases. (See earlier table for geographical distribution of individual viruses.)

5. Reservoirs—A variety of species of birds and mammals (e.g., rodents, squirrels, pigs) act as vertebrate hosts in transmission cycles involving arboviruses; several different reservoir species may be involved in each cycle. Some of these viruses are maintained in a continuous cycle between invertebrate vectors and vertebrate hosts. Humans are usually not involved in the maintenance and spread of most arboviral encephalitides.

6. Incubation period—Usually 3–14 days. Longer incubation periods can occur for tickborne viruses and in immunocompromised people.

7. Transmission—By mosquitoes, ticks, or sandflies; see earlier table for vectors. Mosquitoes become infected either when feeding on viremic animals or transovarially. Infected mosquitoes transmit virus to humans during subsequent feeds and typically remain infectious throughout their life. Tickborne arboviruses are typically acquired by immature ticks feeding on viremic animals; they retain the virus transstadially and transmit virus to humans during subsequent feeds.

Human infection with tickborne encephalitis virus has occurred following consumption of unpasteurized dairy products, such as milk and cheese, from infected goats, sheep, or cows. Rare cases of human-to-human transmission of certain arboviruses have occurred through blood transfusions, transplanted organs, breast-feeding, and the transplacental route. Percutaneous and aerosol transmission of arboviruses can occur in the laboratory setting.

8. Risk groups—Risk of infection is generally determined by exposure to infected vectors and is dependent on many factors including environmental conditions, season, and human activities. In highly endemic areas, adults have often acquired natural immunity following subclinical or mild infection in childhood, and illness occurs mainly in children, visitors, or people new to the area. Risk of neurological illness once infected is typically age related; there is usually a higher risk for more severe disease in older adults. However, this is variable by virus, and clinical illness may be seen more often in children (e.g., La Crosse virus infections). Other factors such as immunosuppression and other underlying medical conditions (e.g., chronic renal failure, hypertension) have been shown to be associated with risk for severe disease for some arboviruses. Infection generally results in lifelong immunity.

9. **Prevention—**

   1) Vector prevention measures:

      - Educate the public about modes of spread and control, including household efforts to reduce vector densities (e.g., eliminating mosquito breeding sites around the home).
      - Avoid exposure to mosquitoes during peak biting hours if possible, or use personal protective measures to decrease exposure to mosquitoes and ticks (e.g., use insect repellent, wear permethrin-impregnated clothing, and cover up with long sleeves and pants while outdoors; see "Malaria" and "Lyme Disease").
      - Screen sleeping and living quarters, use air conditioning if available, or use bed nets. Insecticide-treated bed nets are preferable. In addition, spraying sleeping quarters with an effective insecticide may help lower risk.
      - Implement an integrated vector management program, which should include control of larval mosquitoes through source reduction (removal of larval habitats by removing water-holding containers or draining standing water if feasible) and application of larvicides to known larval habitats and reducing adult mosquitoes through space and residual spraying of appropriate insecticides.

   2) Vaccines:

      - Two safe, effective, inactivated tickborne encephalitis virus vaccines are available in Europe, in adult and pediatric formulations. The adult formulation of one is also licensed in Canada. At least one other tickborne encephalitis vaccine is produced in Russia, but little information is available in the English language literature regarding its safety and effectiveness.
      - See "Japanese Encephalitis" for information on Japanese encephalitis vaccines.

   3) Other prevention measures:

      - Boil or pasteurize milk of susceptible animals in areas where tickborne encephalitis virus occurs.
      - Screening blood and organ donations may be useful in certain settings.

- To prevent laboratory infections, precautions should be taken when handling viruses in the laboratory at the appropriate biosafety level. Further information can be found at: http://www.cdc.gov/biosafety/publications/bmbl5/BMBL5_sect_VIII_f.pdf.
- Although some arboviruses can be transmitted through human milk, transmission is rare; because the benefits of breastfeeding likely outweigh the risk of illness in breastfeeding infants, mothers should be encouraged to breastfeed even in areas of ongoing arboviral transmission.

10. Management of patient—The primary treatment for all arboviral diseases is supportive. Standard blood and body substance precautions are sufficient. Virus is not usually found in blood, secretions, or discharges during clinical disease.

11. Management of contacts and the immediate environment—A search for unreported or undiagnosed cases wherever the patient lived during the 2 weeks prior to onset should be considered for sporadic or travel-associated cases with exposures in unexpected locations. Search for animals excreting tickborne encephalitis virus in milk.

12. Special considerations—

1) Reporting: local health authority may be required to report cases in selected endemic areas or in areas where the virus previously has not been reported.
2) Epidemic measures: use personal protective measures, including mosquito repellents. Eliminate or treat all potential mosquito breeding places. Consider adult mosquito control measures.
3) Specific measures suggested for Venezuelan equine encephalitis virus epidemics include:

   - Determine extent of the infected areas by identifying infected horses and contacts of those animals.
   - Immunize all horses in and surrounding the affected areas and restrict their movement from the affected areas.

[S. L. Hills, M. Fischer]

IV. ARBOVIRAL HEMORRHAGIC FEVERS

DISEASE	ICD-10 CODE	TICK VECTOR	OCCURRENCE
CRIMEAN-CONGO HEMORRHAGIC FEVER	ICD-10 A98.0	*Hyalomma* spp., *Boophilus* and *Rhipicephalus* sp.	Eastern Europe, Middle East, Africa, Central and Southern Asia
KYASANUR FOREST DISEASE	ICD-10 A98.2	*Haemaphysalis spinigera*	India (Karnataka and neighboring states)
ALKHURMA HEMORRHAGIC FEVER	ICD-10 A98.2	*Ornithodoros savignyi, Hyalomma dromedarii*	Saudi Arabia, Egypt, Sudan
OMSK HEMORRHAGIC FEVER	ICD-10 A98.1	*Dermacentor reticulatus (pictus)* and *D. marginatus*	Western Siberia, Russia
Dengue (see "Dengue")			
Yellow fever (see "Yellow Fever")			

1. Clinical features—Crimean-Congo hemorrhagic fever (CCHF) is characterized by sudden onset of fever, myalgia, dizziness, and headache during the prehemorrhagic phase. Vomiting, abdominal pain, and diarrhea occur occasionally, along with hyperemia, congested sclera, and conjunctivitis. Hemorrhagic manifestations develop later and may include petechial rash spreading from the chest and abdomen to the rest of the body, sometimes with large purpuric areas. There may be bleeding from the gums, nose, lungs, uterus, urinary tract, and gastrointestinal tract. Fever is constantly elevated for 5–12 days or may be biphasic. Convalescence is prolonged. Other findings are leukopenia (lymphopenia), thrombocytopenia, elevated liver enzymes aspartate aminotransferase (AST) and alanine transferase (ALT), and elevated clotting factors prothrombin time and activated partial thromboplastin time. The reported case-fatality rate ranges from 2%–30%, with most fatalities occurring 5–14 days after onset of symptoms.

Omsk hemorrhagic fever (OHF) and Kyasanur Forest disease (KFD) have similar clinical presentations. Onset is sudden, with chills, headache, fever, pain in lower back and limbs, arthralgia, and prostration, often associated with conjunctivitis, diarrhea, and vomiting by the third or fourth day. A papulovesicular eruption, sore throat, and conjunctival suffusion may be present. Severe cases are associated with hemorrhages from gums, nose, gastrointestinal tract, uterus, and lungs (rarely from the kidneys). Shock may also occur with, or without, manifest hemorrhage. Leukopenia and thrombocytopenia are marked. The febrile period ranges from 5 days to 2 weeks. In a subset of patients, a biphasic course of illness may occur with an afebrile period of 1-2 weeks, after which a small proportion of patients develop meningoencephalitis (OHF) or neurological manifestations, such as severe headache, mental disturbances, tremors, and vision deficits (KFD). Estimated case-fatality rate is from 1%-3% for OHF and 3-5% for KFD. Convalescence may be prolonged. Disease is nearly identical for Alkhurma hemorrhagic fever (ALKHF), with a large proportion of patients showing both neurological and hemorrhagic clinical manifestations, with central nervous system manifestations being recorded in most of the fatal cases.

2. Causative agents—Crimean-Congo hemorrhagic fever virus is a bunyavirus (genus *Nairovirus*), while Omsk hemorrhagic fever virus, Kyasanur Forest disease virus, and its subtype Alkhurma virus belong to the *Flaviviridae* family.

3. Diagnosis—During the acute phase of disease, virus can be detected by conventional or real-time polymerase chain reaction (PCR), virus isolation, or antigen detection enzyme-linked immunosorbent assay (ELISA; CCHF). Serological diagnosis (immunoglobulin class M [IgM], immunoglobulin class G [IgG]) is made by ELISA. Antibodies may be absent in fatal cases of Crimean-Congo hemorrhagic fever; convalescent sera often have low neutralization antibody titers. Due to the high risk of transmission to health care personnel and laboratory workers, handling of specimens requires trained personnel, good safety procedures, and proper containment laboratories.

4. Occurrence—See the table in this chapter for geographic distribution. Seasonal occurrence correlates with the period of vector activity. CCHF is very often responsible for small nosocomial outbreaks. KFD virus has been recently reported in Karnataka neighboring states (Tamil Nadu and Kerala). The geographic range of Alkhurma virus may be larger than previously known.

5. Reservoirs—Maintained in host tick species. Ixodid ticks (particularly of the genus *Hyalomma*) are the reservoirs for CCHF virus, and domestic animals (sheep, cattle, ostriches, and goats), wild herbivores, hedgehogs, and hares act as amplifying hosts. No animals are known to develop clinical illness when infected with CCHF virus. Hard ticks (*Hemaphysalis spinigera*) are the reservoir of KFD virus, and rodents, shrews, and monkeys likely are capable of amplifying it; KFD virus infection causes epizootics with high fatality in primates. Alkhurma virus has been isolated from soft and hard ticks; the exact epidemiological cycle is unknown. Rodents, such as native water voles (*Arvicola terrestris*) and muskrats (*Ondatra zibethica*) introduced for the fur trade, are known hosts for OHF virus, with Ixodid ticks (particularly *Dermacentor* and *Ixodes* spp.) acting as vectors. Muskrats also develop disease when infected with OHF virus.

6. Incubation period—Usually 3–7 days, with a range of 1–12 days.

7. Transmission—All viruses may be acquired through the bite of infective ticks or by handling or crushing ticks with bare hands. Virus infection may also be acquired by direct contact with the blood or body fluids of viremic animals (livestock, ostriches for CCHF, muskrats for OHF). Drinking raw camel's milk has been suspected in the transmission of ALKHF virus. Human-to-human transmission is also possible during CCHF, and nosocomial infection of medical workers, occurring after exposure to blood and secretions from patients, is an important source of outbreaks. Accidental laboratory infections with CCHF, KFD, and OHF viruses have been described.

Infected ticks remain so for life. Direct transmission of OHF virus from muskrats to humans does occur. OHF, KFD, and ALKHF viruses are not directly transmitted from person to person.

8. Risk groups—Health care workers, abattoir workers, and owners of livestock are at risk of CCHF infection. KFD affects principally young adult males exposed in the forests of Karnataka state, India, during the dry season, from November to June. Farmers and slaughterhouse workers are considered as population-at-risk for CCHF and ALKHF. Shepherds, hunters, and muskrat trappers are at increased risk for OHF. Immunity after infection is probably lifelong.

9. Prevention—

1) Application of insect repellents on clothes in endemic areas; see "Lyme Disease" for preventive measures against ticks.

2) An inactivated mouse brain vaccine has been used in Bulgaria and Russia for Crimean-Congo hemorrhagic fever and for OHF. Tickborne encephalitis vaccine has also been used to protect against OHF, without proof of efficacy. A formalin-inactivated cell-culture KFD vaccine is used in endemic areas of India.

10. Management of patient—

1) For Crimean-Congo hemorrhagic fever:

- Patient isolated in a single room, under negative pressure, if available. Strict droplet, blood, and body fluid precautions needed.

  Persons handling patients who died, or materials contaminated with blood or body fluid from suspect or confirmed CCHF patients, should also take proper safety precautions.

- Bloody discharges are infective; decontaminate with heat or chlorine disinfectants. Carefully dispose of, or disinfect, all blood-contaminated instruments, equipment, linen, clothing, and other objects.
- Treatment: intravenous ribavirin, given early in the course of disease, may be of benefit. Convalescent plasma with a high neutralizing antibody titer is also used, but its effectiveness has not been evaluated.

2) No specific treatment is available for OHF, KFD, and ALKHF; general measures including early hospitalization and symptomatic management of the patients.

11. Management of contacts and the immediate environment—Monitoring of contacts for CCHF; search for missed cases and the presence of infective animals and possible vectors; use of acaricides on livestock and environment.

12. Special considerations—

1) Reporting: individual cases should be reported to local health authority in selected endemic areas, and confirmed cases could be notifiable to national authorities in some countries. These viruses are not listed as agents that must be assessed in terms of potential to cause Public Health Emergencies of International Concern under the International Health Regulations.
2) Epidemic measures: see "Lyme Disease."

[B. Knust, P. E. Rollin]

ARENAVIRAL HEMORRHAGIC FEVERS, NEW WORLD

DISEASE	ICD-10 CODE
JUNIN (ARGENTINIAN) HEMORRHAGIC FEVER	ICD-10 A96.0
MACHUPO (BOLIVIAN) HEMORRHAGIC FEVER	ICD-10 A96.1
GUANARITO (VENEZUELAN) HEMORRHAGIC FEVER	ICD-10 A96.8
SABIA (BRAZILIAN) HEMORRHAGIC FEVER	ICD-10 A96.8
CHAPARE HEMORRHAGIC FEVER	NONE

1. Clinical features—The clinical manifestations of the South American arenaviral hemorrhagic fevers are very similar. They are all acute febrile viral illnesses lasting 6–14 days. Onset is gradual, with malaise, headache, retro-orbital pain, conjunctival injection, and sustained but moderate fever, followed by gastrointestinal signs and symptoms. There may be petechiae and ecchymosis, accompanied by erythema "flushing" of the face, neck, and upper thorax. An enanthem with petechiae on the soft palate is frequent. In the second week of illness, severe infections (20%–30% in Junin infections) result in epistaxis, hematemesis, melena, hematuria, and gingival hemorrhage, or neurologic manifestations (confusion, ataxia, intention tremors and convulsions, and coma). Bradycardia and hypotension with clinical shock are also common findings in severe cases. Progressive leukopenia and thrombocytopenia are characteristic as well as proteinuria. Subclinical infections occur. Case-fatality rates range from 15%–30% in untreated individuals. Around 10% of the patients receiving immune plasma for Junin infection develop a late neurological syndrome with cerebellar signs and cranial nerve palsies. Due to the very limited number of cases described, the full clinical spectrum of Sabia and Chapare infections is unknown.

2. Causative agents—Among the 21 known New World arenaviruses (enveloped ambisense ribonucleic acid [RNA] virus in the genus *Arenavirus*, family *Arenaviridae*) belonging to the Tacaribe complex, 5 have been associated with hemorrhagic fever in humans: Junin virus in Argentina, Machupo virus in Bolivia, Guanarito virus in Venezuela, Sabia virus in Brazil, and recently Chapare virus in Bolivia. These viruses are related to the Old World arenaviruses that include Lymphocytic choriomeningitis, Lassa, and Lujo viruses.

3. Diagnosis—During the acute phase of disease, specific diagnosis is mostly done by virus isolation, RNA detection (conventional or real-time polymerase chain reaction [PCR]), or antigen detection in blood or organs (Machupo infections); in the convalescent phase, immunoglobulin class M (IgM) capture and detection of immunoglobulin class G (IgG) by enzyme-linked immunosorbent assay (ELISA) are very useful. Laboratory studies for virus isolation and neutralizing antibody tests require biosafety level-4 (BSL-4).

4. **Occurrence—**

   1) Argentine hemorrhagic fever was first described among corn harvesters in Argentina in 1955. Since then, the number of cases reported from the endemic areas of the Argentine pampas has ranged from 100–4,000 per year, with an estimated cumulative total of 30,000 symptomatic cases. The region at risk has been expanding northwards and now potentially affects a population of 5 million. Disease occurs seasonally from late February to October, predominantly in males, and 63% of cases are in the age group 20–49 years.

   2) Bolivian hemorrhagic fever occurs sporadically or in epidemics in small villages of the Beni Department of rural northeastern Bolivia. These outbreaks may be associated with high mortality rates; for example in July–September 1994, there were 9 cases with 7 deaths.

   3) Venezuelan hemorrhagic fever was first identified in 1989, with an outbreak of severe hemorrhagic illness in the municipality of Guanarito, Venezuela; 104 cases with 26 deaths occurred between May 1990 and March 1991 among rural residents in Guanarito and neighboring areas. To date, about 200 confirmed cases have been reported. Although the virus continued to circulate in the rodent population, there was an unexplained drop in human cases between 1992 and 2002.

   4) Sabia virus caused a fatal illness with hemorrhage and jaundice in Brazil in 1990, a laboratory infection in Brazil in 1992, and a laboratory infection treated with ribavirin in the USA in 1994.

   5) Chapare virus has been isolated from one fatal hemorrhagic fever case in the Cochabamba region of Bolivia. The geographic distribution and the epidemiology of the disease are unknown.

5. **Reservoir—**

   1) In Argentina, wild rodents of the pampas (*Calomys musculinus* and *Calomys laucha*) are the hosts for Junin virus.

   2) In Bolivia, *Calomys callosus* is the reservoir animal.
      Cane rats (*Zygodontomys brevicauda*) have been shown to be the main reservoir of Guanarito virus.

   3) The reservoir of Sabia and Chapare viruses are not known, although a rodent host is presumed.

Arenaviruses persist in nature by chronically infecting certain rodent species. Rodent infections in the specific rodent species result in long-term virus excretion and lifelong viremia; vertical infection is also common.

6. Incubation period—Usually 6–14 days (in extreme cases 5–21 days).

7. Transmission—Transmission to humans occurs primarily by inhalation of small particle aerosols from rodent excreta containing virus, from saliva, or from rodents disrupted by mechanical harvesters. Viruses deposited in the environment may also be infective when secondary aerosols are generated by farming and grain processing, when ingested, or by contact with cuts or abrasions. Protective immunity of unknown duration follows infection. While uncommon, person-to-person transmission of Machupo virus has been documented in health care and family settings. Fatal scalpel accidents during necropsy, without further person-to-person transmission, have been described. Laboratory infections are described with Junin and Sabia viruses

8. Risk groups—All ages are susceptible. The main human groups at risk are: laboratory workers processing clinical specimens or working in research laboratories; people in contact with, or working with, rodents in endemic areas; and care providers handling infected patients, their secretions, or their excretions, especially in cases of Bolivian hemorrhagic fever, and potentially for the other related viruses.

9. Prevention—Specific rodent control in houses has been successful in Bolivia. In Argentina, human contact most commonly occurs in the fields, and rodent dispersion makes control more difficult. An effective live attenuated Junin vaccine has been administered to more than 150,000 persons in Argentina. In experimental animals, this vaccine is also effective against Machupo, but not Guanarito virus; it is still not known whether it provides effective cross-protection in humans. Education campaigns to avoid rodents and appropriate storage of animal food could have some impact.

10. Management of patient—

1) Isolation: strict isolation during the acute febrile period. Contact and droplet protection is desirable along with other barrier methods.
2) Concurrent disinfection of sputum and respiratory secretions, and blood-contaminated materials.
3) Treatment: convalescent serum given within 8 days of onset has been shown to reduce the case-fatality rate in Argentinian hemorrhagic fever to less than 1%. Ribavirin is likely to be useful. Other compounds (inosine-5 monophosphate dehydrogenate inhibitors, phenothiazines, and myristic acid analogs) were recently shown to inhibit arenavirus replication in cell culture and animals.

11. Management of contacts and immediate environment—Monitoring of contacts and, where feasible, control of rodents.

12. **Special considerations—**

1) Reporting: individual cases should be reported to the local health authority and are notifiable at the national level in several countries. These viruses are not listed as agents that must be assessed in terms of the potential to cause Public Health Emergencies of International Concern under the International Health Regulations. Additionally, isolation of Junin, Machupo, Guanarito, Sabia, and Chapare viruses must be reported to the biosecurity agencies in different countries.

2) Epidemic measures: rodent control, storing of grains and other food in rodent-proof containers, adequate infection control and barrier nursing measures in hospitals and health facilities, availability of ribavirin, and contact tracing and follow-up.

3) During flooding seasons, *Calomys* may become more numerous in homes and food storage areas and increase the risk of human exposures to Machupo virus in Bolivia.

4) Notify the source country and receiving countries of possible exposure by infected travelers.

[P. Rollin, B. Knust, S. Nichol]

ARENAVIRAL HEMORRHAGIC FEVERS, OLD WORLD

DISEASES	ICD-10 CODE
LASSA FEVER	ICD-10 A96.2
LUJO DISEASE	NONE
Lymphocytic choriomeningitis (see "Lymphocytic Choriomeningitis")	

1. **Clinical features—**

1) Lassa fever: patients present, after a gradual onset, with malaise, fever, headache, sore throat, cough, nausea, vomiting, diarrhea, myalgia, and chest and abdominal pain. Fever is persistent or spikes intermittently. Inflammation and exudation of the pharynx and conjunctivae are common. About 80% of human infections are mild or asymptomatic; the remaining cases have severe multisystem disease. Acute illness lasts 1–4 weeks.

Aspartate aminotransferase (AST) levels above 150 and high viremia are poor prognosis indicators for the patient.

In severe cases, hypotension or shock, pleural effusion, hemorrhage, seizures, encephalopathy, and edema of the face and neck are frequent, often with albuminuria and hemoconcentration. Early lymphopenia may be followed by late neutrophilia. Platelet counts are moderately depressed, and platelet function is abnormal. Transient alopecia and ataxia may occur during convalescence, and eighth cranial nerve deafness occurs in 25% of patients, of whom only half recover some function, after 1-3 months.

The overall case-fatality rate is about 1%, but can be as high as 15% among hospitalized cases, and even higher in some epidemics.

Disease is more severe in pregnancy. Fetal loss occurs in more than 80% of cases, and maternal death is frequent, particularly in the third trimester of pregnancy.

Unapparent infections, diagnosed serologically, are common in endemic areas.

2) Lujo disease: the clinical description is similar to that of severe Lassa fever, but is based on only observation of 5 patients, 4 of them with a fatal outcome. The incubation period varied between 7-13 days. The clinical course began with a nonspecific febrile illness, headache, and muscle pain. It then progressed rapidly, becoming more severe with a morbilliform rash on the face and trunk, face and neck swelling, pharyngitis, and diarrhea. Bleeding was not a prominent feature. In the fatal cases, a transient improvement was followed by a rapid deterioration with respiratory distress, neurological signs, and circulatory collapse. Death occurred 10-13 days after onset. Low blood platelet and low white blood cell counts (at the onset, rising later on), and elevated liver function values, were present in all patients.

2. Causative agent—Lassa and Lujo viruses are enveloped ambisense RNA viruses in the genus *Arenavirus*, family *Arenaviridae*. Among viruses in the *Arenavirus* genus, Lassa and Lujo viruses are considered Old World arenaviruses, which includes lymphocytic choriomeningitis virus.

3. Diagnosis—Lassa fever infections are rare and diagnostic reagents are available only at select reference laboratories with biosafety level-4 (BSL-4) capabilities. Lassa fever can be confirmed by direct detection of virus in blood or tissue samples by virus isolation, conventional or real-time polymerase chain reaction (PCR), antigen-detection enzyme-linked immunosorbent assay (ELISA), immunohistochemistry on formalin-fixed tissues, or by detection of virus-specific immunoglobulin class M (IgM) antibodies or rising immunoglobulin class G (IgG) antibody titers. Although a combination of laboratory techniques is recommended, in some instances, such as an individual with a documented clinically compatible illness in an outbreak setting, infection may be confirmed by the presence of IgG reactive antibodies in a single convalescent. Lujo disease can be diagnosed by the same techniques, although the diagnosis experience is based on very few cases.

4. Occurrence—Lassa is endemic in Guinea, Liberia, Sierra Leone, and several regions of Nigeria. Lujo virus has been first isolated from a patient residing in Zambia. Serologically related viruses (of lesser virulence for laboratory hosts) are found in Central African Republic (Mobala virus) and Mozambique and Zimbabwe (Mopeia virus), but these have not yet been associated with human infection or disease.

5. Reservoir—Rodents in the genus *Mastomys* are the reservoir of Lassa virus. The reservoir of Lujo virus is unknown, but likely a rodent, as for other arenaviruses.

6. Incubation period—Commonly 6–21 days.

7. Transmission—Primarily through aerosol or direct contact with excreta of infected rodents deposited on surfaces, such as floors and beds or in food and water. Person-to-person spread may occur during the acute febrile phase when virus is present in secretions and excretions. Nosocomial transmission can occur in hospitals via inoculation with contaminated needles and unprotected contact with the patient's pharyngeal secretions, saliva, blood, or urine. The virus may be excreted in urine for 3–9 weeks from onset of illness. Infection can also spread from person to person by sexual contact through semen for up to 3 months after infection.

8. Risk groups—All ages are susceptible. The main human groups at risk are: health care providers and family members handling infected patients, their secretions, or their excretions; laboratory workers processing clinical specimens or working in research laboratories; and people in contact with, or working with, the rodent reservoir in endemic areas.

9. Prevention—No vaccines are available for human use. For control measures and prevention of infection of hospital and laboratory workers, see Management of Patient in this chapter. In addition, protection of sexual intercourse for 3 months or until semen can be shown to be free of virus. Rodent control measures are important.

10. Management of patient—

1) Institute immediate strict isolation in a private hospital room away from traffic patterns. A negative pressure room and respiratory protection is desirable. Restrict entry of nonessential staff and visitors. Male patients should refrain

from unprotected sexual activity. Dead bodies should be sealed in leak-proof material and cremated or buried promptly in a sealed casket.

2) Strict procedures for isolation and concurrent disinfection of patient's body fluids, excreta, and all objects with which the patient has had contact, including laboratory equipment used to carry out tests on blood. Disinfect everything with 0.5% sodium hypochlorite solution or 0.5% phenol with detergent. As far as possible, effective heating methods (e.g., autoclaving, incineration, boiling, or irradiation) should also be used as appropriate. Thorough terminal disinfection with 0.5% sodium hypochlorite solution or a phenolic compound is adequate; formaldehyde fumigation can be considered.

3) To reduce infectious exposure, laboratory tests should be kept to the minimum necessary for proper diagnosis and patient care. Laboratory testing must be carried out in special high-containment facilities; if there is no such facility, tests should be kept to a minimum and specimens handled by experienced technicians using all available personal protective equipment, such as gloves, gowns, masks, goggles, and biological safety cabinets. When appropriate, serum may be heat-inactivated at 60°C (140°F) for 1 hour. Technicians must be alerted to the nature of the specimens and supervised to ensure appropriate specimen inactivation/isolation procedures.

4) Treatment: ribavirin, most effective within the first 6 days of illness, should be given intravenously for 10 days. The only survivor in the Lujo disease cluster received early treatment with ribavirin.

11. Management of contacts and the immediate environment— Investigate contacts and source of infection. Identify all close contacts in the 3 weeks after the onset of illness: people living with, caring for, testing laboratory specimens from, or having noncasual contact with the patient. Establish close surveillance of contacts as follows: body temperature checks daily for at least 3 weeks after last exposure. In case of temperature above 38.3°C (101°F), contacts should be hospitalized immediately in strict isolation facilities. Postexposure ribavirin prophylaxis could be beneficial in high-risk contacts before onset or immediately after onset of fever.

12. Special considerations—

1) Reporting: Lassa virus is listed as an agent that must be assessed in terms of the potential to cause Public Health Emergencies of International Concern under the International Health Regulations. Individual cases should be reported to the local or national health authority.

2) Epidemic measures: rodent control; storing of grains and other food in rodent-proof containers, infection control and barrier nursing measures in hospitals and health facilities, availability of ribavirin, and contact tracing and follow-up.

3) During disasters, *Mastomys* may become more numerous in homes and food storage areas and increase the risk of human exposures.

4) Notify the source country and receiving countries of possible exposures by infected travelers.

[P. E. Rollin, B. Knust, S. Nichol]

ASCARIASIS
(roundworm infection, ascaridiasis)

DISEASE	ICD-10 CODE
ASCARIASIS	ICD-10 B77

1. Clinical features—Infection with the intestinal helminth *Ascaris lumbricoides* often causes few, or no, overt clinical symptoms. The most frequent complaint of patients infected with *Ascaris* is vague abdominal pain, but some may have pulmonary manifestations (pneumonitis, Löffler syndrome) caused by larval migration (mainly during reinfections) and characterized by wheezing, cough, fever, and signs of eosinophilia and pulmonary infiltration. Live worms, passed in stools or occasionally from the mouth, anus, or nose, are often the first recognized signs of infection. Worm migration may be stimulated by anesthetic agents, fever, or subtherapeutic anthelmintic treatment. Heavy parasite burden may aggravate nutritional deficiency and, if chronic, may affect work and school performance. Serious complications, sometimes fatal, include bowel obstruction by a bolus of worms, particularly in children, or obstruction of bile duct, pancreatic duct, or appendix by one or more adult worms.

2. Causative agent—*A. lumbricoides* is a large intestinal roundworm and is a human parasite. However, *Ascaris suum*, a similar parasite of pigs, is now thought to be the same species, based on molecular studies. The degree of sharing between humans and pigs is still not clear. Ongoing studies are being conducted to elucidate under what conditions and how commonly the infection is shared between the hosts, and what differences and similarities exist between their clinical signs and symptoms.

3. Diagnosis—By identifying typical eggs in standard fecal examination by light microscopy, or adult worms passed from the anus, mouth, or nose. Intestinal worms may be visualized by radiological and sonographic techniques; more rarely, pulmonary involvement may be confirmed by identifying ascarid larvae in sputum or gastric washings.

4. Occurrence—Common and worldwide, with greatest frequency in moist tropical countries where prevalence often exceeds 50%. Prevalence and intensity of infection are usually highest in children aged 3-8 years. Frequently, family members may be infected and reinfected due to shared food, water sources, and hygienic practices.

5. Reservoir—Humans; ascarid eggs in soil.

6. Incubation period—The life cycle from time of infection to adult intestinal stage requires 4-8 weeks for completion. Adult worms can live 1-2 years.

7. Transmission—Eggs are found in warm moist soil where other infected humans have defecated and then undergo development (embryonation) and become infective after 2-3 weeks. May remain infective for several months or years in favorable soil. The disease is transmitted through ingestion of infective eggs from contaminated soil, or from uncooked produce contaminated with soil containing infective eggs, but not directly from person to person or from fresh feces. Transmission occurs mainly in the vicinity of the home, where children defecate in the absence of sanitary facilities; heavy infections in children are frequently the result of ingesting soil. Contaminated soil may be carried long distances on feet or footwear into houses and conveyances; transmission by dust is also possible. Ingested embryonated eggs hatch in the intestinal lumen; the larvae penetrate the gut wall and reach the lungs via the circulatory system. Larvae grow and develop in the lungs, pass into the alveoli 9-10 days after infection, ascend the trachea, and are swallowed, reaching the small intestine 14-20 days after infection, where they grow to maturity, mate, and begin laying eggs 45-60 days after initial ingestion of the embryonated eggs. Eggs passed by gravid females are discharged in feces. The period of communicability lasts as long as mature, fertile worms continue to live in the intestine. The usual life span of adult worms is 12 months; maximum life span may reach 24 months. The female worm can produce more than 200,000 eggs a day.

8. Risk groups—Children in environments with warm, moist climates, and where personal hygiene and sanitation are poor. Use of human feces as fertilizer adds to this risk.

9. **Prevention—**

1) Educate the public in the use of proper toilet facilities and—especially for children—the need to avoid direct contact with contaminated soils.

2) Encourage good hygienic habits in children; in particular, train them to wash hands before eating and handling food.

3) Provide adequate facilities for proper disposal of feces, and prevent soil contamination in areas immediately adjacent to houses, particularly children's play areas.

4) Construct latrines that prevent dissemination of ascarid eggs through overflow, drainage, or otherwise. Treating human feces by composting for later use as fertilizer may not kill all eggs. Night soil and sewage effluents are hazardous, especially where used as fertilizer.

5) In endemic areas, protect food from dirt. Food that has been dropped on the floor should not be eaten unless washed or reheated.

6) The WHO recommends a preventive chemotherapy strategy focused on mebendazole or albendazole treatment of high-risk groups at regular intervals for the control of morbidity due to the soil-transmitted helminths causing ascariasis, trichuriasis, and hookworm disease (http://www.who.int/neglected_diseases/preventive_chemotherapy/pct_manual/en). The action to be taken depends on the prevalence of at least one of these infections among school-age children (usually defined as children aged 5–14 years). The groups to be treated are school-age children (enrolled and nonenrolled); preschool children at least 1 year of age; women of childbearing age, including women in the second and third trimesters of pregnancy and lactating women; and adults in certain high-risk occupations (e.g., tea pickers, miners).

The WHO guidelines call for these groups to be treated 2–3 times a year in high-risk communities (≥50% prevalence of infection among school-age children), and once a year in low-risk communities (≥20% and <50% prevalence of infection among school-age children). When the prevalence of at least one of the above infections among school-age children is less than 20%, large-scale preventive chemotherapy interventions are not recommended; affected individuals should be treated on a case-by-case basis. Extensive monitoring has shown no significant ill effects of treatment in pregnant women, but as a precautionary measure, women in the first trimester of pregnancy should are not treated. Administration of anthelminthics to very young children (1–2 years old) is safe, but some key recommendations should be followed: children should never be forced to swallow tablets;

tablets should be crushed and mixed with water; and treatment should be supervised by trained personnel.

After 5-6 years of periodic deworming according to guidelines discussed earlier, the WHO recommends that soil-transmitted helminth prevalence in school-age children be reassessed, and that more restrictive thresholds be used for making decisions on continued periodic treatment (whqlibdoc. who.int/publications/2011/9789241548267_eng.pdf).

10. **Management of patient—**

1) Sanitary disposal of feces.
2) Treatment: single-dose albendazole or mebendazole, given as either a single dose or over 3 days (albendazole is not US Food and Drug Administration [FDA]-approved for this use). On theoretical grounds, both are contraindicated during the first trimester of pregnancy. Pregnant women in the second or third trimester may want to discuss the decision of whether to delay treatment with their health care provider. Erratic migration of ascarid worms has been reported following mebendazole therapy; this may also occur with other medications, or spontaneously in heavy infections. Single-dose ivermectin is also highly effective against ascaris, but its safety in children weighing less than 15 kg and in pregnant women, remains to be established (it is not US FDA-approved for this use). Single-dose pyrantel pamoate is also effective.

11. **Management of contacts and the immediate environment—** Family members and contacts sharing the same food should be considered contacts and treated. Environmental sources of infection should be sought, particularly on premises of affected families.

12. **Special considerations—**None.

[M. Deming, M. Eberhard]

ASPERGILLOSIS

DISEASE	ICD-10 CODE
ASPERGILLOSIS	ICD-10 B44

1. Clinical features—An opportunistic fungal disease that may present with a variety of clinical syndromes in the human host, ranging from hypersensitivity reactions to direct angioinvasion. It primarily affects the lungs causing 4 main syndromes: allergic bronchopulmonary aspergillosis (ABPA), chronic necrotizing *Aspergillus* pneumonia or chronic necrotizing pulmonary aspergillosis, aspergilloma, and invasive aspergillosis.

ABPA is a hypersensitivity reaction to *Aspergillus* spp. colonization of the tracheobronchial tree that occurs in conjunction with asthma and cystic fibrosis. Up to 5% of adult asthmatics may develop ABPA at some time; increasing evidence suggests that fungal allergy is associated with increasing severity of asthma. It is also estimated that 2%–7% of cystic fibrosis patients reaching adolescence and adulthood develop ABPA. ABPA can lead to permanent lung damage (fibrosis) if untreated. Allergic fungal sinusitis may also occur.

Aspergilloma is a noninvasive form of aspergillosis in which the fungus grows inside a cavity, typically in a previously damaged area of the lung (such as those damaged by tuberculosis, sarcoidosis, or other cavity-causing lung diseases), forming a fungal ball. Aspergillomas may be asymptomatic, or may lead to hemoptysis. In other forms of chronic aspergillosis such as chronic necrotizing pulmonary aspergillosis, symptoms such as weight loss, chronic cough, and fatigue may be slowly progressive over months to years. *Aspergillus* spp. may cause keratitis after minor injury to the cornea, often leading to unilateral corneal opacity and blindness. The organisms may infect the implantation site of a cardiac prosthetic valve or other surgical sites.

Acute invasive aspergillosis usually occurs in persons with significant immunosuppression (e.g., due to hematopoietic stem cell transplant, neutropenia, HIV/AIDS, therapy with corticosteroids and/or other immunosuppressive medications, and solid organ transplantation). A rare inherited condition, chronic granulomatous disease, puts affected people at moderate risk. Invasive aspergillosis primarily involves the lungs and/or sinuses. Symptoms of acute *Aspergillus* sinusitis include fever, facial pain, nasal discharge, and headaches. Symptoms of invasive pulmonary aspergillosis usually include fever, cough, chest pain, and/or breathlessness that do not respond to standard antibiotics. In up to 40% of such cases hematogenous dissemination occurs to the brain or to other organs—including, in particular, the eye, heart, kidneys, and skin—with worsening of the prognosis. In some cases, however, skin infection allows earlier diagnosis and treatment.

Several species of *Aspergillus* produce aflatoxins (mycotoxins); high levels of exposure cause liver necrosis and are associated with hepatic cancer.

2. Causative agents—Of the 180-odd species of *Aspergillus*, about 40 have been reported to cause disease in humans. The species that most commonly cause invasive infection in humans are *Aspergillus flavus*, *Aspergillus fumigatus*, *Aspergillus nidulans*, *Aspergillus niger*, and *Aspergillus terreus*. Common allergenic species include *A. fumigatus*, *Aspergillus clavatus*, and *Aspergillus versicolor*. *A. fumigatus* causes most cases of fungus ball; *A. niger* is the most common fungal cause of external otitis. *A. flavus* and *Aspergillus parasiticus* are the most common aflatoxin producers.

3. Diagnosis—Diagnosis of ABPA in patients with asthma is based on a combination of radiographic, clinical, and laboratory findings, including central bronchiectasis on computerized axial tomography (CAT) scans, infiltrates on chest radiographs, positive *Aspergillus* skin-prick testing, elevated total serum immunoglobulin class E (IgE), elevated serum IgE and/or immunoglobulin class G (IgG) antibodies to *A. fumigatus*, peripheral blood eosinophilia, and positive *Aspergillus* precipitins. In patients with cystic fibrosis, the diagnosis of ABPA is challenging, and consensus criteria have been developed. In acute *Aspergillus* sinusitis, X-rays and computerized tomography (CT) scans are abnormal and culture of specimens obtained during sinus surgery is usually needed to confirm the causative agent. In invasive pulmonary aspergillosis, bronchoscopy may confirm the diagnosis together with microscopy and culture. Sputum cultures have low sensitivity and specificity. The *Aspergillus* galactomannan antigen assay, performed in blood and bronchoalveolar lavage fluid, may help to confirm the diagnosis, especially in patients with hematologic malignancies, but its use is limited in other patient populations, such as solid organ transplant recipients. Antifungal susceptibility testing may be contributory to help detect azole antifungal resistant strains, although no susceptibility breakpoints exist.

4. Occurrence—Worldwide; uncommon and sporadic; occasional outbreaks recognized in health care settings; no distinctive differences in incidence by race or gender. Outbreaks of acute aflatoxicosis (liver necrosis with ascites) have been described in humans in India and Kenya, and in animals, and an association between high aflatoxin levels in foods and hepatocellular cancer has been noted in Africa and southeastern Asia.

5. Reservoir—*Aspergillus* species are ubiquitous in nature, particularly in decaying vegetation, such as in piles of leaves or compost piles. Conidia are commonly present in the air, both outdoors and indoors, and during all seasons of the year. Water and foods may also be contaminated.

6. Incubation period—Probably between 2 days and 3 months.

7. Transmission—By inhalation of airborne conidia. No person-to-person transmission. Rare instances of transmission through contaminated water/spray/aerosols have been documented. People are exposed to aflatoxins by consuming contaminated food.

8. Risk groups—The ubiquity of *Aspergillus* species and the usual occurrence of the disease as an opportunistic infection suggest that most people are naturally immune and do not develop disease caused by *Aspergillus*. Immunosuppressive or cytotoxic therapy increase susceptibility, and invasive disease is seen primarily in those with prolonged neutropenia or corticosteroid treatment. Transplant recipients, patients with HIV/AIDS infection and persons with chronic granulomatous disease are also susceptible.

9. Prevention—High efficiency particulate air filtration and other air quality improvement measures may decrease the incidence of invasive aspergillosis in hospitalized patients with profound and prolonged neutropenia. Antifungal prophylaxis might be considered for high-risk conditions, such as construction sites in health care settings. Special caution (Filtering Face Piece 2 [FFP2] type protective mask) should be taken during transport of high-risk patients inside hospitals.

10. Management of patient—

1) Ordinary cleanliness. Terminal cleaning of patient environment.
2) Treatment: ABPA is treated with steroids by aerosol or by mouth, especially during attacks, and treatment is usually prolonged. Itraconazole is useful in reducing the amount of steroids needed. The role of voriconazole in the treatment of ABPA remains to be determined. Surgical resection, if possible, is the treatment of choice for patients with aspergilloma who cough blood, but it is best reserved for single cavities. Asymptomatic patients may require no treatment; oral itraconazole or voriconazole may help symptoms but do not kill the fungi within the cavity. Voriconazole (intravenous [IV] or orally) is the treatment of choice in tissue-invasive forms. Alternatives include liposomal amphotericin B (IV only), posaconazole (only oral), and echinocandins such as caspofungin (IV only). Immunosuppressive therapy should be discontinued or reduced as much as possible. Endobronchial colonization should be treated by measures to improve bronchopulmonary drainage and aerosolized amphotericin. In sinusitis, surgery may be of help. Treatment with voriconazole, amphotericin B, posaconazole or caspofungin is usually effective, although relapse is common.

11. Management of contacts and the immediate environment—Not ordinarily indicated.

12. Special considerations—Aflatoxins, which are produced by several *Aspergillus* species and are highly carcinogenic, could be used deliberately to cause harm through contamination of water and/or food.

[A. Litvintseva, M. Brandt]

BABESIOSIS

DISEASE	ICD-10 CODE
BABESIOSIS	ICD-10 B60.0

1. Clinical features—The clinical spectrum ranges from asymptomatic to life threatening. Common manifestations include fever, other nonspecific flu-like symptoms (e.g., chills, sweats, myalgia, fatigue), and hemolytic anemia; thrombocytopenia also is common. Severe cases can be associated with hemodynamic instability, acute respiratory distress, renal failure, hepatic compromise, disseminated intravascular coagulation, altered mental status, and death. Even persons with asymptomatic infection may have low-level parasitemia for months, sometimes for longer than a year, making transmission via blood transfusion a year-round concern.

2. Causative agents—Intraerythrocytic protozoan parasites of the *Babesia* genus. In the USA, the identified zoonotic agents include, predominantly, *Babesia microti*; also, *Babesia duncani* (formerly, the WA1-type parasite) and related organisms, as well as *Babesia divergens*-like parasites. In Europe, the identified agents include *B. divergens* and the EU1 agent (*B. venatorum*); also, *B. microti*. In other regions of the world, various *Babesia* species and strains have been identified.

3. Diagnosis—Acute cases with patent parasitemia are diagnosed through light-microscopic identification of intraerythrocytic *Babesia* parasites on Wright- or Giemsa-stained blood smears. In some circumstances, distinguishing *Babesia* species from *Plasmodium falciparum* can be difficult. Some *Babesia* species (e.g., *B. microti* and *B. duncani*) are morphologically indistinguishable from one another. Confirmation of the diagnosis/species by a reference laboratory should be considered; adjunctive molecular and serologic testing should be tailored to the setting and *Babesia* species. If indicated by the epidemiologic and clinical context, the possibility of coinfection with *Borrelia burgdorferi* (Lyme disease) or *Anaplasma phagocytophilum* (human granulocytic anaplasmosis) should be considered.

4. Occurrence—Overall, most of the documented zoonotic cases in the world have occurred in the USA, some have occurred in Europe, and relatively few in various other regions. However, the geographic distribution of zoonotic transmission of *Babesia* parasites (in general and for particular species) is inadequately understood; underrecognition, misdiagnosis (e.g., as malaria), and underreporting of cases are common. Increased awareness among clinicians and laboratorians is needed. In the USA, most documented cases have been acquired in the Northeast (particularly, but not exclusively, in parts of New England and in New Jersey and New York) and the upper Midwest (Minnesota and Wisconsin).

5. Reservoir—White-footed mice (*Peromyscus leucopus*) and other small mammals for *B. microti* in the USA; cattle for *B. divergens* in Europe; not definitively established for some zoonotic *Babesia* species.

6. Incubation period—Variable; in part dependent on host, parasite, and epidemiologic factors. Around 1-3 weeks or longer for tickborne transmission, and from weeks to months for transfusion-associated transmission. Symptoms may appear or recrudesce many months (even >1 year) after initial exposure, particularly in the context of immunosuppression or surgical splenectomy.

7. Transmission—Tickborne in nature, although the tick bite typically is not noticed, and the tick vector has not been identified for some *Babesia* species. The vectors include *Ixodes scapularis* for *B. microti* in the USA (typically, the nymphal stage, during warm spring/summer months) and *Ixodes ricinus* for *B. divergens* and the EU1 agent (*B. venatorum*) in Europe. Nymphal *I. scapularis* ticks become infected by feeding on infected white-footed mice (*P. leucopus*) or other small mammals (e.g. voles, *Microtus pennsylvanicus*). Adult *I. scapularis* ticks typically feed on white-tailed deer (*Odocoileus virginianus*), which are not infected with *B. microti*.

Person-to-person transmission may occur via blood transfusion (documented for *B. microti* and *B. duncani*), even months to more than 1 year after the donor became infected; asymptomatic, undiagnosed parasitemia may be protracted. Transfusion-associated transmission is not inherently restricted by season or geographic region. Rare instances of congenital/perinatal transmission have been reported.

8. Risk groups—Persons who are asplenic, immunocompromised, elderly, born prematurely, or otherwise debilitated are at increased risk for symptomatic infection, which can be severe.

9. Prevention—

    1) Educate the public about personal protective measures to reduce the risk for tick exposures/bites. Control rodents around human

habitation and use tick repellents. (See "Lyme Disease" and Tickborne Spotted Fevers section in "Rickettsioses".)

2) No *Babesia* tests have been licensed yet for screening blood donors in the USA.

10. Management of patient—

1) Blood and body fluid precautions.

2) Treatment: most asymptomatic persons do not require treatment. Symptomatic persons typically are treated with a combination of 2 antimicrobial agents. In a controlled clinical trial restricted to adults with non–life-threatening *B. microti* infection, combination therapy with atovaquone plus azithromycin had comparable efficacy to clindamycin plus quinine and was better tolerated. However, clindamycin plus quinine remains the standard of care for severe babesiosis, such as in patients with hemodynamic instability, organ-system dysfunction, or a high proportion of parasitized red blood cells (e.g., ≥10%). Such patients also may require or benefit from vasopressor therapy, mechanical ventilation, dialysis, or exchange transfusion.

11. Management of contacts and the immediate environment—

1) Cases occurring in a new geographic area deserve careful study (e.g., to identify/characterize the *Babesia* species, tick vector, and reservoir hosts).

2) Investigations of potential transfusion-associated cases require medical and public health attention. The implicated blood donor should be investigated promptly and refrain from future donations. In addition, recipients of cellular blood components from all potentially relevant donations from the implicated donor should be promptly evaluated for evidence of *Babesia* infection.

12. Special considerations—Reporting: reporting requirements/criteria vary by country and local jurisdiction.

[B. L. Herwaldt]

BALANTIDIASIS
(balantidiosis, balantidial dysentery)

DISEASE	ICD-10 CODE
BALANTIDIASIS	ICD-10 A07.0

1. **Clinical features**—An infection of the colon characteristically producing diarrhea or dysentery, accompanied by abdominal colic, tenesmus, nausea, and vomiting. Occasionally the dysentery resembles that due to amebiasis, with stools containing much blood and mucus but relatively little pus. Peritoneal or urogenital invasion is rare.

2. **Causative agent**—*Balantidium coli*, a large ciliated protozoan.

3. **Diagnosis**—Identification of trophozoites or cysts of *B. coli* in fresh feces, or trophozoites in material obtained by sigmoidoscopy.

4. **Occurrence**—Worldwide. The incidence of human disease is low, and epidemics have rarely been identified except for occasional water-borne epidemics occurring in areas of poor sanitation. Environmental contamination with swine feces may result in higher incidence.

5. **Reservoir**—Swine, and possibly other animals such as rats and nonhuman primates. Laboratory pigs may carry this parasite.

6. **Incubation period**—Unknown; may be only a few days.

7. **Transmission**—Through ingestion of contaminated food or water containing cysts from feces of infected hosts; in epidemics, mainly through fecally contaminated water. Sporadic transmission by transfer of feces to mouth via hands or contaminated water or food. Transmissible for as long as infection persists.

8. **Risk groups**—Individuals debilitated by other diseases may have serious, and even fatal, infections.

9. **Prevention**—

   1) Educate the general public in personal hygiene, especially on the need for handwashing before handling food, before eating, and after toilet use.
   2) Educate and supervise food handlers through health agencies.
   3) Dispose of feces in a sanitary manner.
   4) Minimize contact with swine feces.
   5) Protect public water supplies against contamination with swine feces. Diatomaceous earth and sand filters remove all cysts, but

ordinary water chlorination does not destroy cysts. Small quantities of water are best treated by boiling.

10. Management of patient—Treatment: tetracycline for 10 days eliminates infection; metronidazole and iodoquinol are also effective.

11. Management of contacts and the immediate environment—Microscopic examination of feces of household members and other suspected contacts. Also investigate contact with swine; consider treating infected pigs with tetracycline.

12. Special considerations—None.

[A. Gabrielli, L. Savioli]

BARTONELLOSIS
(Oroya fever, Verruga peruana, Carrión's disease)

DISEASE	ICD-10 CODE
OROYA FEVER	ICD-10 A44.0
VERRUGA PERUANA	ICD-10 A44.1

1. Clinical features—A bacterial infection with 2 clinical forms: a life-threatening febrile anemia (Oroya fever) and a benign dermal eruption (Verruga peruana). Asymptomatic infection and a carrier state may both occur. Oroya fever is characterized by irregular fever, headache, myalgia, arthralgia, pallor, severe hemolytic anemia (macrocytic or normocytic, usually hypochromic), and generalized nontender lymphadenopathy. Verruga peruana has a preeruptive stage characterized by shifting pains in muscles, bones, and joints; the pain, often severe, lasts minutes to several days at any one site. The dermal eruption may be miliary with widely disseminated small hemangioma-like nodules, or nodular with fewer—but larger—deep-seated lesions, most prominent on the extensor surfaces of the limbs. Individual nodules, particularly near joints, may develop into tumor-like masses with an ulcerated surface. Atypical cases with milder manifestations (prolonged splenomegaly and mild anemia) may occur.

Verruga peruana may be preceded by Oroya fever or by an asymptomatic infection, with an interval of weeks to months between the stages. The case-fatality rate of untreated Oroya fever ranges from 10%–90%; death is often associated with protozoal and bacterial superinfections, including salmonella septicemia. Verruga peruana has a prolonged course but seldom results in death.

2. Causative agent—*Bartonella bacilliformis*.

3. Diagnosis—Isolation of the organisms from blood is usually achieved through bacteriological culture of blood using specific agar medium enriched with rabbit or sheep blood. An application of cell-culture-based techniques and specifically designed liquid media can improve the cultivation of the bacteria from clinical specimens. A chemically modified, insect-based liquid medium has been reported to enhance detection of bacteria in clinical samples. Molecular techniques, particularly conventional and real-time polymerase chain reaction (PCR) assays, have been successfully used for detection and identification of *Bartonella* deoxyribonucleic acid (DNA) in most types of clinical materials, including tissues and body fluids. Nonspecific histological stains may provide presumptive evidence of infection. More specific immunohistological methods have been used for the detection of *Bartonella* species in valvular and other tissues. Several techniques are available, including a capture enzyme-linked immunosorbent assay (ELISA), direct immunofluorescence using fluorescein-conjugated polyclonal antibodies, and immunoperoxidase staining. Use of indirect immunofluorescence assays for detection of *Bartonella* antibodies provide the most common and convenient serologic method.

4. Occurrence—Historically limited to mountain valleys of southwestern Colombia, Ecuador, and Peru, at altitudes between 600–2,800 meters (2,000–9,200 ft), where the sandfly vector is present. During the past 2 decades, Peruvian outbreaks have been documented at lower altitudes between highlands and jungle, while coastal lowlands in Ecuador have become endemic.

5. Reservoir—Humans. In endemic areas, the asymptomatic carrier rate may reach 5%. There is no known animal reservoir.

6. Incubation period—Usually 16–22 days, occasionally 3–4 months.

7. Transmission—Through the bite of sand flies of the genus *Lutzomyia* (Family *Phlebotomidae*). Species are not identified for all areas; *Lutzomyia verrucarum* is important in Peru. These insects feed only from dusk to dawn. Blood transfusion, particularly during the Oroya fever stage, may transmit infection. No other direct person-to-person transmission. Recovery from untreated Oroya fever almost invariably gives permanent immunity to this form; the verruga stage may recur. Humans are infected by the sand fly and for a long period; the agent may be present in blood for weeks before, and, up to several years after, clinical illness. Duration of infectivity of the sand fly is unknown.

8. Risk groups—The disease is milder in children than in adults. Oroya fever is most common in immunologically naive persons, such as tourists.

9. Prevention—

1) Control sand flies (see Prevention under Cutaneous and Mucosal Leishmaniasis section in "Leishmaniasis").
2) Avoid known endemic areas after sundown; apply insect repellent (e.g., N,N-diethyl-meta-toluamide [DEET]) to exposed parts of the body; and use fine-mesh bednets, preferably insecticide-treated. For more information on insecticide-treated mosquito nets, see "Malaria." Further information on WHO-recommended nets can be found at: http://www.who.int/whopes/en.
3) Blood from residents of endemic areas should not be used for transfusions until it has tested negative.

10. Management of patient—

1) Blood and body fluid precautions. The infected individual should be protected from sandfly bites (see Prevention in this chapter).
2) Treatment: Oroya fever: chloramphenicol plus another anti-biotic (beta-lactam preferred) for 14 days; oral fluoroquinolones are an alternative but must be used with caution in children. Successful treatment does not eliminate risk for development of dermal eruption. Verruga peruana: rifampin for 14 days; aminoglycosides are an alternative.

11. Management of contacts and the immediate environment— Intensify protection in areas where sand flies are present, after identification of localities where post-sundown exposure of infected persons to sand flies could have occurred during the preceding 3–8 weeks.

12. Special considerations—Report to local health authority is required in selected some areas.

[P. Mead]

BEJEL
(Njovera, nonvenereal endemic syphilis)

DISEASE	ICD-10 CODE
BEJEL	ICD-10 A65

1. Clinical features—A chronic skin and tissue disease characterized by an eruption on skin and mucous membranes, usually without an evident primary sore, as seen in yaws.

During the primary stage, lesions are painless, tiny papules or ulcers that appear on the mouth and lips and often go undetected. Secondary lesions are characterized by shallow, painless mucous patches of the mouth, soon followed by moist papules in skinfolds and by drier lesions on the trunk and extremities. Other secondary skin lesions are macular or papular, often hypertrophic, and frequently circinate; lesions resemble those of venereal syphilis. Plantar and palmar hyperkeratoses occur frequently, often with painful fissuring; alopecia and patchy depigmentation/hyperpigmentation of the skin are common. Inflammatory or destructive lesions of skin, long bones, and nasopharynx are late manifestations. Unlike venereal syphilis, bejel rarely shows neurological or cardiovascular involvement. The case-fatality rate is low.

2. Causative agent—*Treponema pallidum* subsp. *endemicum*, a spirochete.

3. Diagnosis—See "Yaws." Based on clinico-epidemiological findings in the field. Confirmed by dark-field and direct fluorescent antibody (DFA) microscopic examination of lesion exudate during early disease. Molecular methods using poymerase chain reaction (PCR) and deoxyribonucleic acid (DNA) sequencing have been developed to detect *Treponema pallidum* subsp. endemic-specific sequences in lesion exudate. Nontreponemal serological tests for syphilis are reactive in the early stages and remain so for many years, then gradually tend toward reversal, while treponemal tests remain positive for life despite adequate treatment.

4. Occurrence—A common disease of childhood in localized areas with poor socioeconomic conditions and primitive sanitary and dwelling arrangements. Low-level transmission in a few areas in the eastern Mediterranean, including the Middle East; major foci exist in the Sahel region (southern border of the Sahara desert). Bejel should be considered in the evaluation of a reactive syphilis serology in any person who has emigrated from an endemic area.

5. Reservoir—Humans.

6. Incubation period—From 2 weeks to 3 months.

7. Transmission—Through direct or indirect contact with infectious early lesions of skin and mucous membranes; the shared use of eating and drinking utensils and generally unsatisfactory hygienic conditions. Congenital transmission does not occur.

Patients are contagious until moist eruptions of skin and mucous patches disappear, which sometimes takes several weeks or months.

8. Risk groups—Children aged between 2 and 15 years appear to be most susceptible.

9. Prevention—See "Yaws." Measures apply to all nonvenereal treponematoses.

10. Management of patient—Treatment: for patients with active disease and their contacts, treat with a single intramuscular injection of benzathine penicillin G or single-dose oral treatment with azithromycin. There are no reports of azithromycin treatment failures for the nonvenereal treponematoses. Avoid intimate contact and contamination of the environment until lesions are healed.

11. Management of contacts and the immediate environment—Treat all family contacts; those with no active disease should be regarded as latent cases. In low-prevalence areas, treat all active cases and all close contacts, including children.

12. Special considerations—Reporting: report to local health authority required in some endemic areas.

[A. Pillay]

BLASTOMYCOSIS
(North American blastomycosis, Gilchrist's disease)

DISEASE	ICD-10 CODE
BLASTOMYCOSIS	ICD-10 B40

1. Clinical features—A granulomatous systemic mycosis that primarily affects the lungs and is often subclinical. Hematogenous dissemination may occur, and in the majority of cases involves skin, bones, and genitourinary tract. Pulmonary blastomycosis may be acute or chronic. Acute infection, which often goes unrecognized, presents with the sudden onset of fever, cough, and a pulmonary infiltrate on chest X-ray. The acute disease usually resolves spontaneously after 1–3 weeks of illness. More commonly, there is an indolent onset of pulmonary infection that evolves into chronic disease. Some patients exhibit extrapulmonary infection during or after the resolution of pneumonia. Disseminated disease is more common in the immunocompromised. Cough and chest ache may be mild or absent, so patients may present with infection already spread to other sites, particularly the skin, and less often to bone, prostate, or epididymis. Cutaneous lesions begin as erythematous papules that become verrucous, crusted, or ulcerated, and spread slowly. Most commonly, cutaneous lesions are located on the face and distal extremities. Constitutional symptoms such as weight loss, weakness, and low-grade fever are often present. Untreated disseminated or chronic pulmonary blastomycosis can eventually progress to death.

2. Causative agent—*Blastomyces dermatitidis* (teleomorph *Ajellomyces dermatitidis*), a dimorphic fungus.

3. Diagnosis—Confirmed by culture, deoxyribonucleic acid (DNA) probe, or by visualizing the fungus through direct microscopic examination of unstained smears of sputum and lesional material, which shows characteristic "broad-based" budding forms of the fungus, often dumbbell-shaped. An enzyme immunoassay (EIA) test is commercially available for detection of antigen in urine, serum, or bronchoalveolar lavage. Serological tests have some limitations, as sensitivity and specificity vary with the test employed. The immunodiffusion test is more sensitive and specific than the complement fixation (CF) test, and antibodies against A antigen have been reported in 52%–80% of patients with blastomycosis. There is no commercially available skin test for blastomycosis.

4. Occurrence—Uncommon. Endemic in some areas in North America, including the southeastern and southern United States, especially those bordering the Mississippi and Ohio river basins, the Midwestern states and Canadian provinces that border the Great Lakes, and a small area in New York and Canada along the St. Lawrence River. Outside North America, well-documented autochthonous cases have been reported in Africa, and occasional cases have been reported in Central America, South America, India, and the Middle East.

5. Reservoir—Moist soil, particularly in wooded areas along waterways, and in undisturbed places, such as under porches or sheds. Disease is common in dogs and has also been reported in cats, a horse, a captive African lion, and a sea lion, but animals do not appear to directly transmit the disease to humans.

6. Incubation period—Probably weeks to months. For symptomatic infections, median is 45 days.

7. Transmission—Inhalation of conidia in spore-laden dust, typically of the mold or saprophytic growth forms. No person-to-person transmission.

8. Risk groups—Rare in children; males are more frequently affected than females.

9. Prevention—Preventive measures not yet fully understood.

10. Management of patient—Treatment: itraconazole is the drug of choice; amphotericin B is indicated in severely ill patients or those with brain lesions, followed by itraconazole after the patient's condition has stabilized.

11. Management of contacts and the immediate environment—Investigation of contacts and source of infection not beneficial unless clusters of disease occur.

12. Special considerations—Immunocompromised persons are more likely to have disseminated disease.

[M. Roy]

BOTULISM

DISEASE	ICD-10 CODE
BOTULISM	ICD-10 A05.1

1. Clinical features—Botulism is a severe neuroparalytic illness resulting from irreversible blockade of acetylcholine release from presynaptic nerve endings by botulinum toxin. Beyond infancy (i.e., >1 year) it manifests as bilateral cranial nerve palsies followed by bilateral descending flaccid paralysis. Signs and symptoms typically include some or all of the following: ptosis, diplopia, blurred vision, dysphagia, dysarthria, and ophthalmoplegia. Autonomic symptoms such as constipation commonly occur. Patients maintain their baseline mental status. Gastrointestinal symptoms, including nausea, vomiting, and diarrhea, can occur in foodborne botulism. Illness may include respiratory failure and death if mechanical ventilation and supportive care are not provided. Most patients recover if diagnosed and treated promptly, but recovery may take months, and some have residual weakness.

Symptoms in infants younger than 1 year typically start with constipation and may include poor suck, altered cry, weakness, and loss of head control. Infant botulism ranges from a mild illness with gradual onset to severe paralysis and respiratory failure. Mortality from infant botulism is rare, about 0.1% during 2000–2009 in the USA, where 85% of all reported infant botulism cases occur.

2. Causative agent—Botulinum toxin is a potent neurotoxin that is one of the most lethal substances known. Botulinum toxin is produced by *Clostridium botulinum* but is also produced by some strains of *Clostridium butyricum*, *Clostridium baratii*, and *Clostridium argentinense*. These gram-positive, spore formers are present in the environment but only grow and produce toxin under specific conditions in food products (see Transmission in this chapter), in contaminated wounds, and in the intestinal tract of infants and adults with structurally or functionally compromised intestinal tracts (e.g., intestinal surgery, antibiotic use). Of the 7 recognized serotypes of botulinum toxin, (types A–G), the most common serotypes associated with naturally occurring human illness are A, B, E, and F.

3. Diagnosis—Botulism is clinically diagnosed and laboratory confirmed. Other neurological disorders resembling botulism in noninfants include myasthenia gravis and Guillain-Barré syndrome, and in infants, sepsis and electrolyte imbalances. Illnesses confused with botulism can be hard to differentiate in the early workup. Botulism should be considered, and antitoxin administered, early in the workup as more common diseases are evaluated. Routine hospital laboratory studies are not helpful in diagnosing botulism but may help rule out other illnesses. Electromyography can support the clinical diagnosis of botulism.

1) Foodborne: confirmed by detecting botulinum toxin in serum, stool, or gastric aspirate, or through culture of botulinum toxin producing clostridia from gastric aspirate or stool in a clinically compatible case. Laboratory confirmation of a foodborne case can also be achieved by detecting botulinum toxin in a food source known to have been consumed by the patient. Botulism is considered confirmed in persons with a consistent clinical syndrome who consumed a food item implicated in a laboratory-confirmed case.

2) Infant intestinal: confirmed by detecting botulinum toxin in clinical specimens (serum or stool) or by isolating botulinum toxin producing clostridia from stool specimens from an infant younger than 1 year.

3) Wound: confirmed by culture of botulinum toxin producing clostridia from a wound or detection of botulinum toxin in serum in a patient with history of a contaminated wound or injection drug use within 2 weeks before onset of symptoms.

4) Other: a designation as "other" botulism occurs when a clinically compatible case is laboratory confirmed in a patient aged 1 year or older who has no history of ingestion of suspect food and has no wounds. Some of these cases are suspected to be adult intestinal colonization cases due to complicating medical factors and/or prolonged excretion of botulinum toxin producing clostridia in stool.

4. Occurrence—Botulism is likely underrecognized and underreported. Although the worldwide incidence is unknown, cases have been reported from the Americas, Africa, Asia, Australia, Europe, and the Middle East. Outbreaks of foodborne botulism occur when food is prepared by methods that do not destroy spores and is preserved under conditions that permit toxin formation. The foods implicated reflect local eating habits and food-preservation procedures. Although primarily reported in the USA, infant and wound botulism have been reported in other countries.

5. Reservoir—Botulinum toxin producing clostridia are ubiquitous in soil. Spores are frequently recovered from agricultural products, including honey and vegetables, and are also found in dust, soil, lake and marine sediments, and the intestinal tracts of animals, including fish. Toxin is produced only under conditions that promote spore germination, growth, and toxin production.

6. Incubation period—Generally, the shorter the incubation period, the more severe the disease. Neurological symptoms of foodborne botulism usually appear within 12–72 hours of toxin ingestion, but onset can range from 2 hours to 8 days. The incubation periods of botulism due to intestinal colonization in infants is estimated to be up to 30 days, but for adults is unknown (see Transmission in this chapter); the incubation period for iatrogenic botulism is unclear. For wound botulism, the incubation period is generally 4–14 days. The 3 known cases of inhalational botulism occurred among laboratory workers with a work-related exposure to botulinum neruotoxin; patients had neurological symptoms similar to those in foodborne botulism and recovered within 2 weeks of the exposure.

7. Transmission—Person-to-person transmission does not occur. Mode of transmission varies by transmission category.

1) Foodborne: occurs by ingestion of preformed toxin in contaminated food. Spores of botulinum toxin producing clostridia present in food germinate and produce the toxin before the food is eaten; sufficient heating inactivates the toxin. Growth and toxin formation require an anaerobic environment, moisture, neutral-to-alkaline pH, and an energy source such as sugar or protein. These conditions are most often present in lightly preserved foods (such as fermented, lightly salted, or smoked fish and meat products) and in inadequately processed, home-preserved foods (such as home-canned vegetables and garlic in oil) that are low in sugar, salt, and acid. Outbreaks have been linked to foods that have been inadequately stored, such as frozen chili product, chilled commercial soup, and flash pasteurized carrot juice. Occasionally, commercially prepared foods or restaurant-prepared foods are involved. However, foodborne botulism is more often due to home-canned vegetables such as green beans;

home-canned tomatoes, formerly considered too acidic to support growth of *C. botulinum*, have been linked to botulism cases. Outbreaks have occurred following consumption of uneviscerated fish, baked potatoes, improperly handled commercially produced pot pies, pruno (an alcoholic beverage produced illicitly in prisons), sautéed onions, fermented bean curd, and minced garlic in oil.

In Canada and the USA (specifically Alaska), outbreaks have been associated with seal meat, fermented whale blubber, salmon, salmon eggs, and other traditional foods that are processed and consumed without cooking. In Europe, most cases are associated with sausages and smoked or preserved meats; in Japan, with fermented fish. Foodborne transmission could hypothetically be used by bioterrorists for intentional exposure.

2) Intestinal (infant and adult): occurs after ingestion of botulinum spores rather than by ingestion of preformed toxin. Ingested spores germinate and produce botulinum toxin in the colon. Colonization is believed to occur in infants because normal bowel flora that compete with *C. botulinum* have not been fully established. Sources of spores for infant botulism include honey and dust, although the source is unknown in most cases. Adult intestinal botulism is poorly understood but typically occurs in adults who have altered intestinal flora because of antimicrobial use or because of anatomical or functional bowel abnormalities.

3) Wound: occurs when a wound is contaminated by *C. botulinum* spores that germinate and produce toxin inside the wound. Since the 1990s, wound botulism has emerged among chronic drug abusers in some parts of Europe and North America, primarily in dermal abscesses from subcutaneous or intramuscular injection (skin or muscle "popping") of black-tar heroin. Wound botulism also results from contamination of wounds or open fractures with soil or gravel.

4) Inhalational: inhalation of aerosolized botulinum neurotoxin has been documented only once, among laboratory workers. This transmission mode could hypothetically be used by bioterrorists for intentional exposure.

5) Iatrogenic: commercial preparations of botulinum toxin are injected for cosmetic and other indications, including ophthalmological disorders, movement disorders, neuromuscular disorders, and pain. Laboratory confirmed iatrogenic botulism has occurred after injection of high doses of an unapproved botulinum toxin product.

8. Risk groups—Susceptibility to foodborne botulism is general. Persons who eat improperly home-preserved foods are at increased risk of foodborne botulism.

Almost all infants hospitalized with intestinal botulism are younger than 6 months. Infants younger than 1 year who are fed honey are at increased risk for infant botulism. Adult intestinal colonization is rare and poorly understood. Suspected risk factors include use of antimicrobial agents or presence of an anatomical or functional bowel abnormality. Persons who use injection drugs, particularly black-tar heroin, are at increased risk of wound botulism. Persons who receive very high doses of botulinum toxin for therapeutic purposes may be at increased risk of iatrogenic botulism.

9. **Prevention—**

1) Foodborne botulism can be prevented by sound food preparation practices, including proper retort canning of commercially canned foods.

- Home-preserved foods should be prepared following directions such as those provided by the US Department of Agriculture (http://nchfp.uga.edu/publications/publications_ usda.html) so that bacterial spores are inactivated and toxin is not produced.
- Commercial heat pasteurization alone may not kill all spores, so a second barrier to organism growth and toxin production, such as acidification, should be considered for these products (e.g., vacuum-packed pasteurized and hot-smoked products).
- Proper storage can prevent the growth of *C. botulinum* and toxin formation. Consumers should read and follow all manufacturer's recommendations for storage of food products, including temperature and shelf-life.
- Boiling of foods for 10 minutes may destroy the toxin; however, if food is suspected of containing botulinum toxin it should be discarded since there is a risk that uniform heating will not occur throughout the product.

2) Infants should not be fed honey. This may prevent some cases of infant botulism.

3) Adult intestinal colonization is poorly understood, and prevention strategies are not known.

4) Wound botulism can be prevented by not using injection drugs (specifically black-tar heroin) and by thorough cleaning of wounds contaminated by soil.

5) Iatrogenic botulism may be prevented by using commercially manufactured therapeutic botulinum toxin and by avoiding injections above doses recommended by the manufacturer and for conditions not approved by regulators.

10. Management of patient—

1) Immediate access to an intensive care unit is essential so that impending respiratory failure—the usual cause of death—can be detected and managed promptly. Most botulism patients require hospitalization, and some require mechanical ventilation that can last for weeks to months.

2) Treatment for botulism includes meticulous supportive care and botulinum antitoxin. Infant botulism can be treated with human-derived botulinum antitoxin or equine-derived botulinum antitoxin. Noninfant botulism is treated with equine-derived botulinum antitoxin. Antitoxin is most effective when given early in the clinical course because it can limit progression of the disease, although it does not reverse existing paralysis. Mechanical ventilation may be required. The role of antibiotics for wound botulism and adult intestinal colonization botulism is unclear. Antibiotics are not used to treat foodborne botulism or infant botulism, and in these cases, should be used only to treat secondary infections. Stool should be collected for testing of both suspect infant and noninfant botulism as soon as possible, but treatment should not be withheld pending test results. Clinical specimens collected for noninfant botulism include serum, which should always be obtained before antitoxin administration. Other clinical specimens collected for noninfant botulism, including stool, and when indicated, vomitus, gastric aspirates, and wound specimens, should be collected as soon as possible.

3) In addition to the measures described in the previous paragraph, in wound botulism, wounds should be debrided or drained. Antibiotics can be considered, as appropriate for the clinical situation, after wound debridement or drainage.

4) Aminoglycosides and other medications such as anticholinergic medications may worsen botulism symptoms by causing a synergistic neuromuscular blockade. They should not be used in patients with botulism.

5) Botulism is not contagious; Standard Precautions for infection control should, however, be followed during inpatient hospital care.

11. Management of contacts and the immediate environment—

1) A thorough history should be taken to determine the type of botulism suspected.

2) If foodborne botulism is suspected, an immediate public health investigation should be launched to identify the implicated food. Persons known to have eaten an implicated food should be

monitored for signs and symptoms of botulism and, if these develop, should be treated promptly. Food samples should be collected promptly, stored in sealed containers, and sent to a reference laboratory for testing. If food that may be contaminated is spilled, the spill should be wiped up using a dilute bleach solution (1/4 cup bleach for each 2 cups of water).

3) Additional cases should be actively sought when more than one case of botulism occurs; one case may be the harbinger of a larger outbreak.

12. Special considerations—

1) Reporting: reporting of suspected and confirmed cases is obligatory in most countries; an immediate telephone report to public health authorities is indicated.

2) Outbreaks: a single case of suspected foodborne botulism should immediately raise suspicion of an outbreak. Home-preserved foods are the most common sources of foodborne botulism. However, in the rare situations when restaurant food or widely distributed commercially preserved food is contaminated, many people may be exposed, posing a major public health threat. Food implicated by epidemiological or laboratory findings may require immediate recall. An immediate search for persons sharing the suspect food and for any remaining food from the same source should be performed. Suspected foods along with clinical specimens should be submitted for laboratory examination. International common source outbreaks have occurred from widely distributed commercial products; international efforts may be required to recover and test implicated foods.

3) Deliberate use: attempts to develop and use botulinum toxin as a bioweapon have been made. Although these attempts have been unsuccessful so far, foodborne, waterborne, and aerosolized toxin exposures could all hypothetically be caused intentionally. Outbreaks associated with commercial food products should be investigated with the possibility of intentional contamination in mind. The occurrence of several seemingly unrelated cases in the same time frame should raise the question of deliberate use of botulinum toxin. Suspicion of inhalational botulism, outside of a laboratory setting, would indicate intentional use.

[A. K. Rao, K. A. Jackson]

BRUCELLOSIS
(undulant fever, Malta fever, Mediterranean fever)

DISEASE	ICD-10 CODE
BRUCELLOSIS	ICD-10 A23

1. **Clinical features**—A systemic bacterial disease that has an acute or insidious onset, with continued, intermittent, or irregular fever of variable duration, headache, weakness, profuse sweating, arthralgia, myalgia, fatigue, anorexia, and weight loss. Localized suppurative infections of organs, including liver and spleen, may occur, as well as chronic localized infections; subclinical infection has been reported. The disease may last days, months, or occasionally a year or more, if not adequately treated.

Osteoarticular complications occur in 20%–60% of cases; sacroiliitis is the most frequent joint manifestation. Genitourinary involvement is seen in 2%–20% of cases, with orchitis and epididymitis as common manifestations. Recovery is usual, but disability is often pronounced. Neurobrucellosis is a less common but more severe manifestation that occurs in 3%–7% of cases. The case-fatality rate of untreated brucellosis is 2% or less, and usually results from endocarditis caused by *Brucella melitensis* (most virulent) infection. Part of, or the entire original syndrome, may reappear as relapses.

2. **Causative agents**—*Brucella abortus*, *B. melitensis*, *Brucella suis*, *Brucella canis*, *Brucella ceti*, and *Brucella pinnipedialis* (nov. sp.).

3. **Diagnosis**—Microbiological isolation of *Brucella* species from blood, bone marrow, or other tissues or discharges is considered the gold standard for patient diagnosis. Several polymerase chain reaction (PCR) assays are currently available for isolates to identify *Brucella* at the species level. A 4-fold rise in titer on an agglutination assay is the serologic method of choice in diagnosing acute, noncomplicated cases of brucellosis caused by *B. abortus, B. melitensis,* or *B. suis.* For chronic, complicated, or neurobrucellosis cases, serologic assays other than agglutination, such as enzyme-linked immunosorbent assay (ELISA), are recommended. Serologic tests to detect *B. canis* antibodies are not performed routinely by diagnostic laboratories.

4. **Occurrence**—Worldwide, especially in Mediterranean countries, the Middle East, Africa, central Asia, India, central and South America, and Mexico. Sources of infection and responsible organism vary according to geographic area. Cases are increasingly documented in nonendemic regions subsequent to international travel to endemic areas and import of infected livestock.

5. Reservoirs—Cattle, swine, goats, and sheep are most common. Infection can occur in camels, bison, elk, equids, caribou, and some species of deer. *B. canis* is an occasional problem in laboratory dog colonies and kennels; a small percentage of pet dogs and a higher proportion of stray dogs have positive *B. canis* antibody titers. Coyotes have been found to be infected. Marine mammals can be infected with *B. ceti* (whales, porpoises, dolphins) and *B. pinnipedialis* (seals, sea lions, walruses).

6. Incubation period—Variable and difficult to ascertain; 1–2 months is commonplace, with a range of 5 days to 5 months.

7. Transmission—Contact through mucous membranes and breaks in the skin with animal tissues, blood, urine, vaginal discharges, aborted fetuses, and especially placentas; and ingestion of undercooked meat, raw milk, and dairy products (unpasteurized cheese) from infected animals. Airborne infection has been reported in laboratory and slaughterhouse workers. Isolated cases of infection with *B. canis* occur in animal handlers from contact with dogs, and with *B. suis* in hunters from contact with feral swine and other game animals. Rare cases of infection with newly described marine-associated *Brucella* spp. have been reported. A small number of cases have resulted from accidental self-inoculation of *B. abortus* strain 19 animal vaccine, or with the attenuated *B. abortus* RB51 cattle vaccine; the same risk is present when *B. melitensis* Rev-1 vaccine is handled. Person-to-person transmission is rare—possibly sexually transmitted. Breastfeeding women may transmit infections to their infants.

8. Risk groups—Brucellosis is predominantly an occupational disease of those working with infected animals or their tissues, especially farm workers, veterinarians, and slaughterhouse workers. Medical personnel in endemic regions may be at risk when participating in activities characterized by gross exposure to contaminated fomites or tissues or massive bleeding, such as certain obstetric procedures. Brucellosis is among the most common laboratory-acquired bacterial infections. The high communicability in the laboratory warrants biosafety level 3 precautions. Persons consuming undercooked meat and unpasteurized dairy products are at increased risk.

9. Prevention—Prevention of human brucellosis rests on the elimination of the infection among domestic animals.

1) Educate the public (especially tourists) regarding the risks associated with consuming undercooked meat or unpasteurized dairy products.
2) Educate farmers and workers in slaughterhouses, meat processing plants, and butcher shops about the nature of the disease and the risk in handling carcasses and products from potentially

infected animals—particularly products of parturition—together with proper operation of slaughterhouses to reduce exposure. Give emphasis to the importance of appropriate use of personal protective equipment and ventilation.

3) Educate hunters to use protective outfits (gloves, clothing) when handling feral swine or other potentially infected wildlife (elk, bison, moose, and caribou/reindeer); to practice good hygiene, such as handwashing, when possible; to avoid eating meat from animals that appear sick; and to bury animal remains.

4) Search for infection among livestock by serological testing or testing of cow's milk (ring test); eliminate infected animals (segregation and/or slaughtering). Infection among swine usually requires slaughter of the herd. In high prevalence areas, immunize young goats and sheep with *B. melitensis* Rev-1 vaccine, and immunize calves and, sometimes, adult animals with *B. abortus* strain 19. Since 1996, RB51 has largely replaced strain 19 for immunization of cattle against *B. abortus* in the USA.

5) Pasteurize milk and dairy products from cows, sheep, and goats. Boiling milk is effective when pasteurization is impossible. Do not eat meat from animals that appear ill.

6) Exercise care in handling and disposal of placenta, uterine discharges, and fetuses. Disinfect contaminated areas.

10. **Management of patient—**

1) Isolation: draining and secretion precautions if there are draining lesions; otherwise none.

2) Concurrent disinfection of purulent discharges.

3) Treatment: the treatment of choice is a combination of doxycycline and rifampicin, or streptomycin, for at least 6 weeks. The streptomycin-containing regimen is generally associated with a lower rate of relapse, although may be less effective in treating neurobrucellosis, due to low penetration into cerebrospinal fluid and potential for neurotoxicity. Doxycycline for 6 weeks in combination with gentamicin for 7 days may be an acceptable alternative. Trimethoprim-sufamethoxazole-containing regimens can be effective, but relapses occur in up to 30% of cases. Relapses also occur in about 5%–15% of patients with uncomplicated infections treated with doxycycline and rifampicin and are due to sequestered rather than resistant organisms; patients should be treated again with the original regimen. Monotherapy should be avoided, as relapse rates can be as high as 50%. Arthritis may occur in recurrent cases.

4) Rev-1 is resistant to streptomycin and RB51 to rifampicin in vitro. This must be taken into account when treating human infections caused by animal Rev-1 vaccines.

11. Management of contacts and immediate environment—Trace infection to the common or individual source, usually infected domestic goats, swine, or cattle, or raw milk or dairy products from cows and goats. Test suspected animals, and remove animals with evidence of infection. Disinfect affected areas.

12. Special considerations—

1) Reporting: case report to local health authorities; obligatory in most countries.
2) Epidemic measures: search for common vehicle of infection, usually raw milk or milk products—especially cheese—from an infected herd. Recall incriminated products; stop production and distribution unless pasteurization is instituted.
3) The potential to infect humans and animals through aerosol exposure, combined with a low infectious dose of 10–100 organisms, has led to *Brucella* species being considered as potential biological weapons.

[M. Guerra]

BURULI ULCER

DISEASE	ICD-10 CODE
BURULI ULCER	ICD-10 A31.1

1. Clinical features—Classically presents as a chronic painless skin ulcer, with undermined edges and a necrotic white or yellow base ("cotton wool" appearance). Secondary bacterial infection may occur, causing the ulcer to become painful. Most lesions are located on the extremities and tend to be seen more frequently on lower rather than upper extremities. It often starts as a painless nodule or a papule, which eventually ulcerates. Other presentations may be seen, such as indurated plaques or edematous lesions; the latter represents a rapidly disseminated form that does not pass through a nodular stage. Bones and joints may be affected by direct spread from an overlying cutaneous lesion, or through the bloodstream. Long-neglected or poorly managed patients usually present with scars that are sometimes hypertrophic or keloid, with partially healed areas or disabling contractures, especially for lesions that cross joints. Marjolin ulcers (squamous cell carcinoma) may develop in unstable or chronic non-pigmented scars.

The differential diagnosis includes the following, by dermatologic manifestation:

1) Minor infections: insect bites and a variety of dermatological conditions.
2) Nodules: cysts, lipomas, boils, onchocercomas, lymphadenitis, mycoses.
3) Plaques: leprosy, cellulites, mycoses, psoriasis.
5) Edematous forms: cellulites, elephantiasis, actinomycosis.
6) Ulcers: tropical phagedenic ulcer, diabetic ulcer, leishmaniasis, neurogenic ulcer, yaws, squamous cell carcinoma, pyoderma gangrenosum, noma.

2. **Causative agent**—*Mycobacterium ulcerans*, an acid-fast bacillus, is a slow-growing environmental mycobacterium. *M. ulcerans* secretes mycolactone, a virulence factor that destroys tissues and locally suppresses immune activity. Three variants of cytopathic mycolactones may be produced by *M. ulcerans*, the type and amount varying by strain. African strains, which produce the greatest number and amount (and most potent variant) of mycolactone, are associated with the more severe forms of disease.

3. **Diagnosis**—An experienced clinician in endemic areas can usually diagnose on clinical grounds. Swabs, fine-needle aspirates, and biopsy specimens can be sent to the laboratory for confirmation by the Ziehl-Neelsen stain for acid-fast bacilli, culture, polymerase chain reaction (PCR), and histopathology. PCR is the most common method of diagnosis. Histopathologically, active lesions have contiguous coagulation necrosis of subcutaneous fat and acid-fast bacilli present.

4. **Occurrence**—*M. ulcerans* infection has been reported in more than 30 countries, mostly tropical, and tends to be seen most frequently in children younger than 15 years in rural areas. The global burden of the disease is yet to be determined. Based on the available data, Africa is the continent most affected, although disease also occurs in Australia, Japan, and South America. Numbers of reported cases have been increasing over the last 25 years, most strikingly in western Africa, where *M. ulcerans* disease is second only to tuberculosis in terms of mycobacterial disease prevalence following the elimination of leprosy as a public health problem in these countries. In some endemic districts and communities, it is the most prevalent mycobacterial disease.

5. Reservoir—Evidence points to the fauna, flora, and other ecological aspects of tropical or subtropical wetlands. The bacterium has been identified as a commensal organism in insects, snails, and fish; further studies are needed to clarify their roles as natural hosts for *M. ulcerans*. In Australia, it has been described not only in humans but also in native animals including the koala (*Phascolarctos cinereus*), the brushtail and ringtail possums (family *Phalangeridae*), and the long-footed potoroo (*Potorous longipes*). Infection has been reported in a domesticated alpaca (*Lama pacos*); all of these, except for those in the potoroo, occurred in focal areas where human cases were known to have occurred.

6. Incubation period—About 2-3 months; however, anecdotal observations have suggested that *M. ulcerans* infections could exhibit longer periods of latency. Similarly to tuberculosis, it is believed that only a small proportion of infected people develop clinically apparent disease.

7. Transmission—The mode of transmission is mostly speculative, but regular contact with a contaminated aquatic environment, and local trauma to the skin, have been shown to be risk factors. In most studies, a significant number of patients had antecedent trauma at the site of the ulcer. Environmental changes that promote flooding, such as deforestation, dam construction, and irrigation systems, are often associated with outbreaks of Buruli ulcer. Lack of protected water supplies contributes to dependence on pond water for domestic use and potential exposure; aerosols arising from stagnant waters may disseminate *M. ulcerans*. Studies have shown a significant association between *M. ulcerans* in the environment and Buruli ulcer cases in neighboring villages, and recent evidence suggests insects may play a role in transmitting infection to humans through bites. Human-to-human transmission of Buruli ulcer is exceptional; cases have rarely developed in caregivers of patients. Factors that probably determine the type of disease are dose of agent, depth of inoculation, and host immunological response. Bacillus Calmette-Guérin (BCG) neonatal vaccination appears to protect against *M. ulcerans* osteomyelitis in patients with skin lesions.

8. Risk groups—Those who reside in, or travel to, wetlands in endemic areas. Population increases in rural wetlands can place populations at risk during manual farming activities in those areas. HIV infection is not a risk factor for *M. ulcerans* infection but may exacerbate the clinical course of the disease.

9. Prevention—

1) Health education on the disease for populations at risk.
2) Provision of a protected water supply.
3) Avoidance of insect bites and wearing protective clothing covering the extremities.

4) BCG neonatal vaccination may provide short-term prophylaxis.

5) Prompt cleansing of abrasions or wounds antiseptically.

10. Management of patient—

1) Early detection and reporting of suspicious skin lesions to the nearest health facility for screening will facilitate early treatment and help avoid complications and deformities.

2) Treatment: 8 weeks of combination antimicrobial therapy with rifampicin and an aminoglycoside (streptomycin) or rifampicin and clarithromycin for all patients. Combined antibiotic therapy has been shown to be effective in treating early, limited disease. For more advanced disease, surgical excision and skin graft may be required. For surgical cases, at least 4 weeks of antimicrobial therapy should be completed before the initial surgery to minimize *M. ulcerans* bacteremia and reduce the extent of surgical excision. Antibiotic treatment abates recurrence. In some patients, physiotherapy is needed to prevent disability.

3) Rehabilitation: provision of rehabilitation for those deformed by the disease is important in helping to minimize the long-term disability that can occur in association with advanced disease.

11. Management of contacts and the immediate environment— Although not considered transmissible from person to person, screening activities for other cases within the community may be indicated due to possible common exposure risks.

12. Special considerations—

1) Although neither notifiable nor contagious from person to person, it is recommended that cases be reported to local health authorities so that the geographic distribution can be clearly defined.

2) International measures: endemic countries should coordinate efforts across borders. Further information can be found at: http://www.who.int/buruli/en. It can also be found from WHO Collaborating Centres, which provide support as required, at: http://apps.who.int/whocc/Detail.aspx?cc_ref=BEL-40&cc_code= bel&cc_city=antwerp& and http://apps.who.int/whocc/Detail. aspx?cc_ref=AUS-95&cc_ref=aus-95&.

[D. Blaney]

❖

CAMPYLOBACTER ENTERITIS

DISEASE	ICD-10 CODE
CAMPYLOBACTER ENTERITIS	ICD-10 A04.5

1. **Clinical features**—The disease is characterized by diarrhea (which may be bloody) abdominal pain, fever, malaise, and nausea, sometimes with vomiting. A prodromal period of fever and malaise may precede diarrhea by a day or more. Severe abdominal pain may be mistaken for acute appendicitis or inflammatory bowel disease. Symptoms usually persist for several days to 2 weeks. Gross or occult blood with mucus and white blood cells is often present in liquid stools. Extraintestinal infection is rare, usually occurring in immunocompromised patients. Rare postinfectious complications include reactive arthritis (~1% of cases) and Guillain-Barré syndrome (~0.1% of cases). Postinfectious irritable bowel syndrome has also been linked to *Campylobacter* infection. The number of campylo-bacteriosis cases is comparable to or higher than the number of cases of nontyphoidal salmonellosis in most developed countries. Many infections are asymptomatic, and most are self-limited. Case-fatality rates have been estimated from 0.01% to 1%.

2. **Causative agents**—*Campylobacter jejuni* and, less commonly, *Campylobacter coli* are the usual causes of *Campylobacter* diarrhea. Several subtyping methods are available that may be helpful for epidemiological purposes, especially in outbreak settings. Other *Campylobacter* species, including *Campylobacter lari*, *Campylobacter fetus*, and *Campylobacter upsaliensis*, have been associated with illness in both normal and immunocompromised hosts.

3. **Diagnosis**—Definitive diagnosis is based on isolation of the organisms from clinical specimens using selective media, microaerobic growth conditions, and incubation at 42°C (107.6°F). Standard culture methods may not detect all strains of *C. fetus* and *C. upsaliensis*. Bacteremia is detected in fewer than 1% of patients. Visualization of motile and curved, spiral, or S-shaped rods similar to those of *Vibrio cholerae* by stool phase contrast or dark-field microscopy can provide rapid presumptive evidence for *Campylobacter* enteritis. Culture-indepen-dent nucleic acid and antigen-based methods for detection of *C. jejuni* and, in some cases, *C. coli* in stool specimens have also been developed for early diagnosis. The relatively low specificity described to date for antigen-based diagnostic methods suggest that high false positive rates may limit the usefulness of these tests. Diagnosis through whole genome sequencing is likely to be available also at central hospital level in many countries in the near future.

4. Occurrence—*Campylobacter* is an important cause of diarrheal illness worldwide. In industrialized countries, males and children younger than 5 years have the highest incidence of illness, though all age groups can be affected. In developing countries, illness is confined largely to children younger than 2 years. *Campylobacter* is a major cause of traveler's diarrhea. Common-source outbreaks are rarely detected. Those that are detected are most often associated with unpasteurized dairy products, undercooked poultry, and nonchlorinated water. In temperate areas, most cases occur in the warmer months, when there is a significant rise in the *Campylobacter* prevalence in chicken.

5. Reservoir—Animals, most frequently poultry and cattle. Puppies, kittens, other pets, swine, sheep, rodents and birds may also be sources of human infection. In many countries, raw poultry meat is commonly contaminated with *C. jejuni*.

6. Incubation period—Usually 2–5 days, with a range of 1–10 days, depending on dose ingested.

7. Transmission—Through ingestion of the organisms in under-cooked meat (particularly poultry), unpasteurized dairy products, or other contaminated food or water, or from direct contact with infected animals, especially puppies, kittens, and farm animals. Water is an important vehicle, and "viable but not culturable" forms of *Campylobacter* can be found in water sources contaminated with animal feces. The infectious dose can be as little as 500 organisms or even fewer. Infected persons not treated with antibiotics may excrete organisms for 2–7 weeks, but this shedding is of little epidemiologic importance, as person-to-person transmission is uncommon.

8. Risk groups—Persons with immunocompromising conditions have increased risk of infection, severe or invasive disease, and relapse or recurrence. Decreased stomach acidity is a risk for infection. Mechanisms of immunity are not well understood, but lasting immunity to serologically related strains follows infection. In developing countries, most people appear to develop immunity within the first 2 years of life.

9. Prevention—

1) Control and prevention measures at all stages of the food chain, from agricultural production to processing, manufacturing, and preparation of foods in both commercial establishments and private homes.
2) Pasteurize all milk, and chlorinate or boil water supplies. Thoroughly cook all food of animal origin, especially poultry, which should reach a minimum internal temperature of 165°F. Avoid cross-contamination; for example, do not use the same cutting board for raw and cooked products, and do not allow

drippings from raw poultry to contaminate foods that are cooked or that will be eaten raw.

3) Reduce prevalence of *Campylobacter* in meat through specific interventions. Comprehensive control programs and hygienic measures (e.g., attention to biosecurity, changes of boots and clothes, full rather than partial depopulation of poultry houses followed by thorough cleaning and disinfection) can help prevent spread of organisms in poultry and animal farms. Vaccines and competitive exclusion are being investigated as control measures. The use of fly screens in chicken houses seems to reduce prevalence of *Campylobacter*-positive flocks significantly. Good slaughtering, handling, and processing practices, which can include testing of carcasses, can reduce contamination of carcasses and meat products. Further reduction of contamination can be achieved through freezing, chemical carcass decontamination, or irradiation.

4) Recognize, prevent and control *Campylobacter* infections among domestic animals and pets. Puppies and kittens with or without diarrhea are possible sources of infection. Keep pets away from food preparation surfaces like cutting boards and counter tops. Stress hand washing after animal contact.

5) Minimize contact with poultry and their feces. Stress hand washing after contact with poultry and their environment when contact cannot be avoided. Keep backyard poultry out of the kitchen. Promote and use the WHO Five Keys to Safer Food to achieve good preparation practices in commercial and domestic kitchens (http://www.who.int/foodsafety/consumer/5keys/en).

10. **Management of patient—**

1) Isolation: Enteric precautions for hospitalized patients. Exclude symptomatic individuals from food handling or care of people in hospitals, custodial institutions, and day care centers; exclude asymptomatic culture-positive individuals only if hand washing and personal hygiene practices are unreliable. Stress proper hand washing.

2) Concurrent disinfection: Cleaning of areas and articles soiled with stool. In communities with an adequate sewage disposal system, feces can be discharged directly into sewers without preliminary disinfection, though terminal disinfection is required.

3) Treatment: None generally indicated except rehydration and electrolyte replacement in cases with dehydration (see "Cholera and Other Vibrioses"). *C. jejuni* and *C. coli* organisms are susceptible in vitro to many antimicrobial agents, including erythromycin, tetracyclines and quinolones (though resistance

has increased), but treatment is usually not indicated. Antimicrobial agents can reduce the duration of symptoms if given early in the illness and are indicated in invasive cases.

4) Worldwide incidence of fluoroquinolone resistance has increased markedly in the last 20 years, which is thought to be related at least in part to veterinary use of fluoroquinolones. Methods for susceptibility testing vary, but resistance rates greater than 50% have been reported from Europe and the Middle East and greater than 80% from Southeast Asia. Resistance should be suspected in patients who acquired infection in areas of high resistance or whose infections have failed to resolve after treatment with fluoroquinolones. Some but not all studies have reported longer durations of illness and increased likelihood of hospitalization in those with resistant organisms.

11. Management of contacts and the immediate environment—

1) Investigation of contacts and source of infection is useful only to detect outbreaks; investigate outbreaks to identify contaminated food (unpasteurized dairy products are an especially commonly identified source) or water sources to which others may have been exposed. Note that only a small proportion of campylobacteriosis can be linked to a common source by methods currently available.

12. Special considerations—

1) Reporting: obligatory case report in several countries.
2) Risk of common-source outbreaks when mass feeding and poor sanitation coexist.

[B. Mahon, M. Patrick]

CANDIDIASIS
(moniliasis, thrush, candidosis)

DISEASE	ICD-10 CODE
CANDIDIASIS	ICD-10 B37

1. Clinical features—A mycosis usually confined to the superficial layers of skin or mucous membranes, presenting clinically as oral thrush, intertrigo, vulvovaginitis, paronychia, or onychomycosis. Ulcers or pseudo-membranes may form in the esophagus, stomach, or intestine. Invasive candidiasis, including candidemia, usually occurs in patients with specific risk factors for infection, such as central venous catheters, immunosuppression, antibiotic therapy, abdominal surgery, or critical illness. Repeated clinical skin or mucosal eruptions are common. Candidemia may be uncomplicated or may disseminate and cause deep-seated infection in many organs, including the eyes, kidneys, liver, spleen, heart, and central nervous system.

2. Causative agents—*Candida albicans*, *Candida* (formerly *Torulopsis) glabrata*, *Candida parapsilosis, Candida tropicalis*, and *Candida krusei* are most common. Numerous less common species, such as *Candida dubliniensis*, have also been reported to cause disease.

3. Diagnosis—Requires both laboratory and clinical evidence of candidiasis. The single most valuable laboratory test is microscopic demonstration of pseudohyphae or yeast cells in infected tissue or normally sterile body fluids. Culture confirmation is important, but isolation from sputum, bronchial washings, stools, urine, mucosal surfaces, skin, or wounds is not proof of a causal relation to the disease as the organism may be part of the transient flora. Severe or recurrent oropharyngeal infection in an adult with no obvious underlying cause should suggest the possibility of HIV infection. Polymerase chain reaction (PCR) may play a role in early detection of candidemia. Specific biomarkers (i.e., beta-D-glucan) could be useful for starting empirical therapy in some classes of high-risk critically ill patients.

4. Occurrence—Worldwide. *Candida* species are often part of the normal flora.

5. Reservoir—Humans.

6. Incubation period—Variable, 2-5 days for thrush in infants.

7. Transmission—Contact with secretions or excretions of mouth, skin, vagina, and feces, from patients or carriers; by passage from mother to neonate during childbirth; and by endogenous spread. The role of spread by the sexual route is limited, although some studies have demonstrated significant asymptomatic male genital colonization with species of *Candida*, more commonly in male sexual partners of infected women.

8. Risk groups—Oral thrush is a common, usually benign condition during the first few weeks of life. Clinical disease occurs when host defenses are low. Diabetics, those with HIV infection, and those treated with broad-spectrum antibiotics or corticosteroids are predisposed to superficial candidiasis. Women in the third trimester of pregnancy are prone to vulvovaginal candidiasis. Factors predisposing to invasive candidiasis include: immunosuppression, indwelling intravenous catheters, neutropenia, hematological malignancies, burns, postoperative complications, and very low birth weight in neonates. Urinary tract candidiasis usually arises as a complication of prolonged catheterization of the bladder or renal pelvis.

The frequent isolation of *Candida* species from sputum, throat, feces, and urine in the absence of clinical evidence of infection suggests a low level of pathogenicity or some level of immunity. Local factors contributing to superficial candidiasis include interdigital intertrigo and paronychia on hands with excessive water exposure (e.g., cannery and laundry workers or dishwashers) and intertrigo in moist skinfolds of obese individuals.

9. Prevention—To prevent systemic spread, early detection and local treatment of any infection in the mouth, esophagus, or urinary bladder of those with predisposing systemic factors as described (see Risk Groups in this chapter). Fluconazole chemoprophylaxis decreases the incidence of invasive candidiasis following hematopoietic stem cell transplantation in some studies of high-risk critically ill patients and liver transplant recipients and in very low birth weight neonates. Posaconazole is effective in preventing invasive candidiasis in hematopoietic stem cell transplant recipients with graft-versus-host disease and in patients with prolonged, chemotherapy-induced neutropenia.

10. Management of patient—

1) Concurrent disinfection: of secretions and contaminated articles.
2) Treatment: improving conditions or reducing risk factors for candidiasis; for example, removal of indwelling central venous catheters may facilitate cure. Preemptive fluconazole treatment could be initiated in some critically ill patients with a high degree of *Candida* species colonization and multiple risk factors for candidemia. Topical nystatin or an azole (miconazole, clotrimazole, ketoconazole, fluconazole) is useful in many forms of superficial candidiasis. Oral clotrimazole troches or nystatin suspension are effective for treatment of oral thrush. Itraconazole suspension or fluconazole are effective in oral and esophageal candidiasis. A number of newer antifungals, such as voriconazole, posaconazole, and the echinocandins (caspofungin, micafungin, and anidulafungin) are also effective in oropharyngeal and esophageal candidiasis,

but their use should generally be reserved for patients with disease refractory to standard therapy. Vaginal infection may be treated with oral fluconazole or topical clotrimazole, miconazole, butoconazole, terconazole, tioconazole, or nystatin. For most patients with invasive candidiasis, fluconazole or an echinocandin is recommended as initial therapy for most adult patients. Treatment may be adjusted once the infecting species is known; transition from an echinocandin to fluconazole is recommended for stable patients with isolates likely to be susceptible to fluconazole.

11. Management of contacts and the immediate environment— Investigation of contacts and source of infection is not beneficial in sporadic cases.

12. Special considerations—Outbreaks are most frequently due to contaminated intravenous solutions and thrush in nurseries for newborns. Outbreaks of *C. parapsilosis* fungemia in neonatal intensive care units have been linked to transmission from health care workers. Concurrent disinfection and terminal cleaning, comparable to that used for epidemic diarrhea in hospital nurseries, is recommended (see "*E. Coli* Diarrheal Diseases").

[M. Brandt, F. Ndowa, A. A. Cleveland]

CAPILLARIASIS

DISEASE	ICD-10 CODE
INTESTINAL CAPILLARIASIS	ICD-10 B81.1
HEPATIC CAPILLARIASIS	ICD-10 B83.8
PULMONARY CAPILLARIASIS	ICD-10 B 83.8

1. Clinical features—Capillariasis is a zoonotic parasitic disease caused by infection with 3 different Capillaria species. Clinical features depend on the location in the human body where the worm resides—intestines, liver, and respiratory tract.

1) Intestinal capillariasis is an enteropathy with fever, eosinophilia, massive protein loss due to diarrhea, and a malabsorption syndrome, leading to progressive weight loss and emaciation. Fatal cases are characterized by the presence of great numbers of parasites in the small intestine together with ascites, pleural transudate, and abnormalities in electrolytes. Case-fatality rates of

10% have been reported. Subclinical cases also occur but usually become symptomatic over time.

2) Hepatic capillariasis is an uncommon and occasionally fatal infection of the liver. The picture is that of an acute, or subacute, hepatitis, with hepatomegaly and marked eosinophilia resembling that of visceral larva migrans; the organism can disseminate to the lungs and other viscera.

3) Pulmonary capillariasis is associated with fever, cough, shortness of breath, and other symptoms of lower respiratory tract infection. Eggs may appear in the sputum in 4 weeks; symptoms may appear earlier or later. Pneumonitis may be severe; heavy infections may be fatal.

2. Causative agents—Intestinal capillariasis is a caused by infection with *Capillaria philippinensis*; hepatic capillariasis by *Capillaria hepatica* (*Hepaticola hepatica*); and pulmonary capillariasis by *Capillaria aerophila* (*Thominx aerophila*).

3. Diagnosis—Diagnosis of intestinal capillariasis is based on clinical findings plus the identification of eggs, larvae, or adult parasites in the stool. The eggs resemble those of *Trichuris trichiura*. Jejunal biopsy may show worms in the mucosa. Hepatic capillariasis is diagnosed by demonstrating eggs or the parasite in a liver biopsy or at necropsy (eggs are not passed in stool), while pulmonary capillariasis is diagnosed by demonstrating eggs in the sputum or through eggs seen on bronchial biopsy.

4. Occurrence—Intestinal capillariasis is endemic in the Philippines and in Thailand; cases have been reported from Egypt, Japan, the Republic of Korea, and Taiwan (China). Isolated cases have also been reported from Colombia, India, Indonesia, and the Islamic Republic of Iran. The disease was first described in the early 1960s in Luzon, Philippines, where more than 1,800 cases have been seen since 1967.

Since hepatic capillariasis was identified as a human disease in 1924, about 30 cases have been reported from Africa, North and South America, Asia, Europe, and the Pacific area. This form appears to be more common in children younger than 3 years.

About 11 human cases of pulmonary capillariasis have been documented from the Islamic Republic of Iran, Morocco, and Russia; animal infection has been reported in North and South America, Europe, Asia, and Australia.

5. Reservoir—

1) Intestinal: unknown; possibly aquatic birds. Fish are considered intermediate hosts.

2) Hepatic: primarily rats and other rodents, but also a large variety of domestic and wild mammals. The adult worms live and produce eggs in the liver.

3) Pulmonary: cats, dogs and other carnivorous mammals.

6. Incubation period—For intestinal capillariasis, the incubation period in humans is unknown. For hepatic capillariasis, the incubation period is 3–4 weeks. For pulmonary disease, the incubation period is also unknown, however it is currently thought to be 25–40 days.

7. Transmission—

1) Intestinal: *C. philippinensis* is transmitted to humans through ingestion of raw or inadequately cooked small fish, eaten whole. The life cycle of the parasite begins with fish-eating birds or humans passing unembryonated eggs in their stool into the environment. The eggs then become embryonated, develop infective larvae, and are eaten by freshwater fish. In the fish, these eggs hatch in the intestine, and the larvae then penetrate the intestine to migrate to the tissues, which when eaten uncooked by humans (or by birds, monkeys, Mongolian gerbils), completes the infection cycle. Once ingested by humans, the adult nematodes reside in the small intestine and deposit unembryonated eggs. In rare instances, these become embryonated and can result in auto- and hyperinfection. *C. philippinensis* is not transmitted directly from person to person.

2) Hepatic: *C. hepatica* is transmitted to humans primarily through the ingestion of embryonated eggs in fecally contaminated (from rodents, or possibly pigs, carnivores, nonhuman and human primates) food, water, or soil. The adult worms produce fertilized eggs that remain in the liver of the host animal (e.g., rodents) until its death and decomposition, or eaten by a predator. When an infected liver is eaten, the eggs are freed by digestion, reach the soil in the feces, and develop to the infective stage in 2–4 weeks. When ingested by a suitable host, including humans, embryonated eggs hatch in the intestine; larvae migrate through the wall of the gut and are transported via the portal system to the liver, where they mature and produce eggs. Spurious findings of unembryonated eggs in human stools after consumption of infected liver—raw or cooked—occurs; however, since these eggs are not embryonated, infection cannot be established. The infection is not transmitted from person to person.

3) Pulmonary: humans become infected with *C. aerophila* through the ingestion of infective eggs in soil, or in soil-contaminated food or water. The larvae migrate from the intestine (humans, cats,

dogs, and other carnivorous mammals) to the lungs and live in tunnels in the epithelial lining of the trachea, bronchi, and bronchioles where they develop into the adult stage. Adults lay fertilized eggs, which are sloughed into the air passages, coughed up, swallowed, and discharged in the feces. In the soil, larvae develop in the eggs and remain infective for a year or longer.

8. Risk groups—Men aged 20–45 years appear to be particularly at risk of intestinal capillariasis, while hepatic capillariasis appears to affect malnourished children more often than any other group (especially <3 years), and children appear to be the main risk group for pulmonary capillariasis. Unsanitary environments, poor hygiene, and rodent infestation increase the risk of infections.

9. Prevention—

1) Avoid eating uncooked fish or other aquatic animal life in known endemic areas.
2) Avoid ingestion of dirt, whether directly (pica), in contaminated food or water, or on hands.
3) Protect water supplies and food from soil contamination.
4) Provide adequate facilities for the disposal of feces.

10. Management of patient—Treatment: mebendazole or albendazole are the drugs of choice for intestinal capillariasis. Thiabendazole and albendazole kill the worms in the liver. Mebendazole, albendazole, and thiabendazole are the choice for pulmonary capillariasis.

11. Management of contacts and the immediate environment—Stool examination for all family members of those with intestinal capillariasis and others with common exposure to raw or undercooked fish, with treatment of infected individuals.

12. Special considerations—None.

[V. J. Lee, M. Ho]

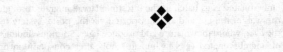

CAT SCRATCH DISEASE
(cat scratch fever, benign lymphoreticulosis)

DISEASE	ICD-10 CODE
CAT SCRATCH DISEASE	ICD-10 A28.1

1. **Clinical features**—A subacute, usually self-limited bacterial disease characterized by malaise, granulomatous lymphadenitis, and variable patterns of fever. Often preceded by a cat scratch, lick, or bite that produces a red papular lesion with involvement of a regional lymph node, usually within 2 weeks; may progress to suppuration. The papule at the inoculation site can be found in 50%–90% of cases. Parinaud oculoglandular syndrome (granulomatous conjunctivitis with pretragal adenopathy) can occur after direct or indirect conjunctival inoculation; approximately 10% of cases may be complicated by systemic disease including prolonged high fever, malaise, fatigue, myalgia, arthralgia, weight loss, or hepatosplenomegaly. Rarely neurological complications such as encephalopathy and optic neuritis can also occur. Bacteremia, hepatic vascular proliferation resulting in blood-filled spaces in the liver (peliosis hepatis), and bacillary angiomatosis due to this infection may occur among young children and among immunocompromised persons, particularly those with HIV infection. Cat scratch disease (CSD) can be clinically confused with other diseases that cause regional lymphadenopathies (e.g., tularemia, brucellosis, tuberculosis, plague, pasteurellosis, and lymphoma).

2. **Causative agent**—*Bartonella* (formerly *Rochalimaea*) *henselae* has been implicated epidemiologically, bacteriologically, and serologically as the causal agent of most cases of CSD.

3. **Diagnosis**—Clinically compatible illness combined with serological evidence of antibody to *Bartonella henselae* by immunofluorescence assay (IFA) or enzyme immunoassay (EIA). Antibodies usually become detectable within 1–2 weeks of symptom onset. Cross-reactivity occurs with other species, in particular *B. quintana*. Histopathological examination of affected lymph nodes may show consistent characteristics but is not diagnostic. Immunodetection and polymerase chain reaction (PCR) are highly efficient in detecting *Bartonella* in biopsies or aspirates of lymph nodes. Although *Bartonella* can be isolated from blood or lymph node aspirates using blood agar in 5% CO_2, yield is low in patients with CSD and a prolonged incubation of up to 45 days may be required. Cell-based culture systems may be more sensitive but require special laboratory capabilities and are not widely available.

4. **Occurrence**—Worldwide, but uncommon; more common in children and young adults. Familial clustering rarely occurs. Most cases are seen during the late summer, autumn, and winter months.

5. Reservoir—Domestic cats are the main vectors and reservoirs for *B. henselae*; no evidence of clinical illness in cats even when chronic bacteremia has been demonstrated. Cat fleas and ticks may be infected, but their role in transmission to humans is not well defined.

6. Incubation period—Variable, usually 3–14 days from inoculation to primary lesion and 5–50 days from inoculation to lymphadenopathy.

7. Transmission—More than 90% of patients give a history of scratch, bite, lick, or other exposure to a healthy, usually young, cat or kitten. Dog scratch or bite, monkey bite, and contact with rabbits, chickens, or horses have also been reported prior to the syndrome, but cat involvement was not excluded in all cases. Cat fleas (*Ctenocephalides felis*) transmit *Bartonella henselae* among cats but play no clear role in direct transmission to humans. Not transmitted from person to person.

8. Risk groups—Children and young adults appear to be at greatest risk of infection.

9. Prevention—Thorough cleaning of cat scratches and bites may help. Flea control is very important to prevent continuing infection of cats.

10. Management of patient—Treatment: treatment of uncomplicated disease in immunocompetent patients is generally not indicated, although azithromycin may lead to faster resolution of swelling in patients with extensive lymphadenitis. Doxycycline and rifampin are recommended for treatment of CSD-associated retinitis. Based on ease of administration, low cost, and efficacy, oral erythromycin or doxycycline for 3–4 months are considered the initial agents of choice for treatment of patients with bacillary angiomatosis or peliosis hepatis, with longer courses indicated for immunocompromised patients with HIV infection. Needle aspiration of suppurative lymphadenitis may be required for relief of pain, but incisional biopsy of lymph nodes may be avoided.

11. Management of contacts and the immediate environment—None.

12. Special considerations—None.

[P. Mead]

CHANCROID
(ulcus molle, soft chancre)

DISEASE	ICD-10 CODE
CHANCROID	ICD-10 A57

1. **Clinical features**—An acute, sexually transmitted bacterial infection usually localized in the genital area and characterized clinically by a single, or multiple, painful, necrotic ulcers that bleed on contact. Chancroid ulcers are more frequently found in uncircumcised men, on the foreskin or in the coronal sulcus, and may cause a phimosis. These lesions are frequently accompanied by painful, swollen, and suppurating regional lymph nodes. In women, asymptomatic carriage is rare, but minimally symptomatic or painless lesions may occur on the vaginal wall or cervix. Extragenital lesions have been reported. Chancroid ulcers, like other genital ulcers, are associated with an increased risk of HIV infection.

2. **Causative agent**—*Haemophilus ducreyi*, a Gram-negative coccobacillus

3. **Diagnosis**—Culture and polymerase chain reaction (PCR) tests are the preferred tests for definitive diagnosis, although PCR is not commonly available. Culture diagnosis is by isolation of the organism from lesion exudates on a selective medium incorporating vancomycin into chocolated horse blood agar enriched with fetal calf serum IsoVitaleX and activated charcoal. *H. ducreyi* grows best at 33°C.

4. **Occurrence**—Most prevalent in tropical and subtropical regions, including Africa and South East Asia, where incidence may be higher than that of syphilis. Incidence has declined significantly in many regions where syndromic case management of genital ulcer disease is utilized. The disease is much less common in temperate zones, where it may occur in small outbreaks. In industrialized countries, outbreaks and some endemic transmission have occurred, but principally among high-risk groups.

5. **Reservoir**—Humans.

6. **Incubation period**—From 3–5 days, up to 14 days.

7. **Transmission**—Through direct sexual contact with open lesions and pus from buboes. Auto-inoculation to nongenital sites may occur in infected persons. Beyond the neonatal period, sexual abuse must be considered when chancroid is found in children. The disease is communicable until the lesions are healed and the organism is cleared from discharging regional lymph nodes. Nonsexual transmission may occur from contact with open lesions.

8. Risk groups—It is more often diagnosed in uncircumcised men, sex workers, and clients of sex workers. In industrialized countries, cases are frequently linked to sex work, travel, or exposure to persons from endemic regions.

9. Prevention—

1) See "Syphilis."
2) Perform serological follow-up for syphilis and HIV in all patients.

10. Management of patient—

1) Avoid sexual contact until all lesions are healed.
2) Treatment: single-dose therapy with azithromycin or ceftriaxone is effective and should be considered for cases where compliance is a concern. Multiday courses of erythromycin and ciprofloxacin are curative; however, ciprofloxacin should be reserved for non-pregnant adults. Fluctuant inguinal nodes may require incision and drainage. Lesions typically heal in 1–2 weeks. HIV-infected and uncircumcised cases may require prolonged or repeat therapy.

11. Management of contacts and the immediate environment—Examine and empirically treat all sexual contacts exposed within 10 days preceding onset of symptoms.

12. Special considerations—

1) Reporting: case report obligatory in many countries.
2) Epidemic measures: empiric treatment of high-risk groups including sex workers, contacts to sex workers, and patients with genital ulcers may be required to control outbreaks. Periodic presumptive treatment of sex workers and their clients has resulted in reduced incidence in some settings.
3) International measures: see "Syphilis."

More information can be found at:

- http://www.cdc.gov/std/treatment
- http://www.who.int/topics/sexually_transmitted_infections/en

[M. M. Taylor]

CHLAMYDIAL INFECTIONS

DISEASE	ICD-10 CODE
CHLAMYDIAL DISEASE, SEXUALLY TRANSMITTED	ICD-10 A56
NONSPECIFIC URETHRITIS	ICD-10 N34.1
Conjunctivitis (see "Conjunctivitis/Keratitis")	
Lymphogranuloma venereum (see "Lymphogranuloma Venereum")	
Pneumonia due to *Chlamydia pneumoniae* (see "Pneumonia")	
Pneumonia due to *Chlamydia trachomatis* (see "Pneumonia")	
Psittacosis (see "Psittacosis")	

1. Clinical features—Most chlamydial infections are asymptomatic. Symptomatic infections are difficult to distinguish clinically from gonorrhea and manifest in males primarily as urethritis (moderate or scanty mucopurulent discharge, dysuria, urethral itching), and in females as cervicitis (mucopurulent endocervical discharge, cervical friability). Rectal infection (asymptomatic or with symptoms of proctitis) can be acquired through receptive anal intercourse, or possibly via contiguous spread from the vagina. Less common manifestations of chlamydial infection include epididymitis in males; urethral syndrome (dysuria and pyuria), perihepatitis (Fitz-Hugh-Curtis syndrome), and bartholinitis in females; and conjunctivitis (acquired through contact with infected genital secretions) in either sex.

In women, untreated infection can ascend from the cervix to the uterus, fallopian tubes, and ovaries, causing pelvic inflammatory disease (PID), which may be asymptomatic (i.e., subclinical) or acute, with abdominal and pelvic pain, and adenexal, uterine, and cervical motion tenderness. Both subclinical and acute PID can lead to long-term sequelae of chronic pelvic pain, ectopic pregnancy, and infertility. Infection during pregnancy has been associated with preterm delivery and can result in conjunctival and pneumonic infection of the newborn.

Chlamydial infection has been associated with an increased risk of HIV acquisition. Reactive arthritis occurs as a sequela in a minority of chlamydial infections.

2. Causative agent—*Chlamydia trachomatis* serovars B and D through K are responsible for sexually acquired genital infections in the adult and perinatally transmitted infections of the neonate and infant.

While *C. trachomatis* is the most frequently isolated causal agent of non-gonococcal urethritis (NGU) in men (isolated in 15%–40% of cases), other agents have been implicated. These include: *Mycoplasma genitalium*

(15%–25% of NGU cases in the USA), *Trichomonas vaginalis*, herpes simplex virus, adenovirus, *Ureaplasma urealyticum*, and enteric bacteria.

3. Diagnosis—Culture is technically difficult and not as sensitive as molecular assays. Antigen detection using enzyme immunoassay (EIA) has been shown not to be as sensitive as the molecular assays. Nucleic acid amplification tests offer excellent sensitivity (usually well above 90%) and high specificity. Nucleic acid amplification tests can be used with noninvasive and minimally invasive specimens, including vaginal swabs (patient- or provider-collected) and urine specimens.

4. Occurrence—Common worldwide. Since infection is often asymptomatic, identification of infections is linked to availability of screening programs; extension of screening has likely contributed to recently observed increases in case reports in many countries.

5. Reservoir—Humans.

6. Incubation period—Poorly defined, probably 7–14 days or longer.

7. Transmission—Sexual contact with the penis, vagina, mouth, or anus of an infected partner. Neonatal infection results from exposure to the mother's infected cervix. Infected individuals are presumed to be infectious. Without treatment, infection can persist for months.

8. Risk groups—Sexually active persons, especially adolescents and young adults, and those with concurrent or multiple recent sex partners. Geographic and racial/ethnic disparities in chlamydia prevalence have been observed in some countries. Reinfection (with the same or different strains of chlamydia) is common and associated with increased risk of PID and long-term sequelae in women.

9. Prevention—

1) Health and sex education, same as for syphilis (see "Syphilis"), with emphasis on use of a condom.
2) Screening of women for *C. trachomatis* has been shown to reduce the risk of pelvic inflammatory disease. Routine, periodic screening for chlamydia is recommended for defined groups in some countries. In the USA, chlamydia screening is recommended yearly for all sexually active women aged 25 years and younger, older women with risk factors (e.g., new or multiple sex partners), and men who have receptive anal sex, and is recommended at the first prenatal care visit for all pregnant women. More frequent screening may be performed based on patient risk factors. Newer tests for *C. trachomatis* infection enable use of noninvasive or minimally invasive specimens, including vaginal swabs (patient- or clinician-collected) and urine.

10. **Management of patient—**

1) Appropriate antibiotics render discharges noninfectious. Patients should abstain from sexual activity until they and their sex partners have completed antibiotic treatment; the index patient and all partners should adhere to abstinence for 7 days after receiving a single-dose regimen, or until completion of a 7-day course of antibiotics.

2) Treatment: doxycycline for 7 days; or a single dose of azithromycin. Azithromycin enables provision of single-dose directly observed therapy. Erythromycin, levofloxacin, and ofloxacin are alternative treatment options. Dosing frequency and gastrointestinal side effects may limit patient compliance for erythromycin. Erythromycin is the recommended drug of choice for infants, and azithromycin or amoxicillin are recommended for pregnant women.

3) Because repeat infections are common, all patients diagnosed with chlamydia should be rescreened approximately 3 months after treatment.

4) If laboratory testing for chlamydia is not available, patients with nonspecific (nongonococcal) urethritis and their sex partners should be managed as though their infections were due to chlamydia, especially since many chlamydia-negative cases respond to the recommended treatment.

11. Management of contacts and the immediate environment— Evaluation and treatment of all sex partners within 60 days before symptom onset or diagnosis (or the most recent sex partner if the last sexual contact was >60 days before symptom onset or diagnosis) is recommended. While all partners should be encouraged to seek medical evaluation, patient delivery of antibiotic therapy to their partners is an option for partner management in some jurisdictions. The mothers of infants who have chlamydial infection and the sex partners of these women should be evaluated and treated.

12. Special considerations—Reporting: case report is required in some countries.

Further information can be found at:

- http://www.cdc.gov/std/treatment
- http://www.who.int/topics/sexually_transmitted_infections/en

[R. Gorwitz, E. Torrone]

CHOLERA AND OTHER VIBRIOSES

DISEASE	CAUSATIVE AGENT	ICD-10 CODE
CHOLERA	Toxigenic *Vibrio cholerae* serogroups O1 and O139	ICD-10 A00
VIBRIO PARAHAEMOLYTICUS INFECTION	*Vibrio parahaemolyticus*	ICD-10 A05.3
VIBRIO VULNIFICUS INFECTION	*Vibrio vulnificus*	ICD-10 A05.3
OTHER *VIBRIO* INFECTIONS	Other non O1 and O139 serogroups of *V. cholerae, Vibrio mimicus, Vibrio alginolyticus*, and others	ICD-10 A05.81

Of the more than 200 recognized *Vibrio cholerae* serogroups, only cholera toxin-producing O1 and O139 serogroups have caused large epidemics and are defined as causing cholera.

Infection with other *Vibrio* species has been associated with sporadic diarrhea and rare outbreaks, as well as with wound and septicemic infections. These include *Vibrio parahaemolyticus, Vibrio vulnificus,* and other vibrios, such as *Vibrio cholerae* of serogroups other than O1 and O139 (*Vibrio mimicus, Vibrio alginolyticus, Vibrio fluvialis, Vibrio furnissii,* and *Grimontia hollisae*). The main *Vibrio* diseases are profiled later.

I. CHOLERA

1. **Clinical features**—An acute bacterial enteric disease characterized in its severe form by sudden-onset, profuse, painless watery stools. Massive loss of fluids is caused by release of an enterotoxin that affects the small intestine. Nausea and profuse vomiting occur early in the course of illness. In most cases, infection is asymptomatic or causes mild diarrhea, especially with organisms of the El Tor biotype; asymptomatically infected persons can transmit the infection.

In untreated severe disease, rapid dehydration, acidosis, circulatory collapse, hypoglycemia in children, and renal failure can lead rapidly to death. In severely dehydrated cases (cholera gravis), death may occur within a few hours, and the case-fatality rate may reach 50%. With proper and timely rehydration, case-fatality rates should be less than 1%.

2. **Causative agent**—Toxigenic *Vibrio cholerae* serogroups O1 and O139. Serogroup O1 occurs as 2 biotypes—classical and El Tor—each of

which occurs as 3 serotypes (Inaba, Ogawa and, rarely, Hikojima). The clinical illnesses caused by *V. cholerae* O1 and O139 are alike because these 2 serogroups produce similar enterotoxins; however, infections caused by serogroup O1 of the classical biotype are associated with more severe disease, although these strains are not currently circulating. In recent years, an El Tor variant that has characteristics of both the classical and El Tor biotypes and may be more virulent than older El Tor strains has emerged in Asia and spread to Africa and the Caribbean.

In any single epidemic, one particular serogroup and biotype tends to be dominant, but serotype switching (e.g., from Inaba to Ogawa or Ogawa to Inaba) is commonly seen in cholera epidemics worldwide and is thought to be driven primarily by the development of population immunity to the circulating serotype.

3. Diagnosis—The etiology is confirmed by isolation of *V. cholerae* serogroups O1 or O139 from a stool specimen. Ideally, serogroup O139 isolates and all *V. cholerae* isolates from sporadic illness should be tested for cholera toxin production or cholera toxin gene sequences (*ctxA*). Strains of *V. cholerae* O1 or O139 that do not possess the cholera toxin gene can cause acute watery diarrhea but do not cause cholera or epidemic disease. In nonendemic areas, organisms isolated from initial suspected cases should be confirmed in a reference laboratory.

For clinical purposes, a quick presumptive diagnosis can be made by dark-field or phase microscopic visualization of vibrios in stool moving like "shooting stars," inhibited by preservative-free, serotype-specific antiserum. When acute and convalescent serum specimens are collected, a presumptive diagnosis can be based on the demonstration of a significant rise in titer of anticholera toxin or vibriocidal antibodies. One-step dipstick tests for rapid antigen detection of *V. cholerae* O1 and O139 are available and have shown promise in initial field evaluations; however, these tests do not yield isolates for subtyping or antimicrobial resistance testing that may be useful for some epidemiologic and treatment decisions and are not recommended for individual patient diagnosis.

In epidemics, once laboratory confirmation and antibiotic susceptibility have been established, it is unnecessary to confirm all subsequent cases. A shift should then be made to primary use of proposed WHO clinical case definitions for cholera surveillance, as follows:

1) Disease unknown in area: severe dehydration or death from acute watery diarrhea in a patient aged 5 years or older.
2) Endemic cholera: acute watery diarrhea with or without vomiting in a patient aged 5 years or older.
3) Epidemic cholera: acute watery diarrhea with or without vomiting in any patient.

Prolonged outbreaks should include periodic laboratory confirmation and antimicrobial susceptibility testing of a small proportion of cases to monitor for antimicrobial resistance.

4. **Occurrence**—Cholera is one of the oldest and best-understood epidemic diseases. Epidemics and pandemics are strongly linked to the consumption of unsafe water and food, poor hygiene, poor sanitation, and crowded living conditions. Typical settings for cholera are periurban slums where basic urban infrastructure is missing and rural areas where the population depends on surface water sources for drinking and where *V. cholerae* are endemic in the environment. Man-made or natural disasters (e.g., floods) resulting in population movements and overcrowded refugee camps are potentially fertile ground for explosive outbreaks with high case-fatality rates.

During the 19th century, cholera spread repeatedly, through 6 pandemic waves, from the Gulf of Bengal to most of the world. During the first half of the 20th century, the disease was confined largely to Asia. During the latter half of the 20th century, the epidemiology of cholera was marked by: (a) the global spread of the seventh pandemic of cholera caused by *V. cholerae* O1 El Tor; (b) the recognition of environmental reservoirs of cholera, such as on the shore of the Gulf of Bengal and along the US coast of the Gulf of Mexico; and (c) the appearance for the first time in 1992 of large explosive epidemics of cholera in southeast Asia caused by *V. cholerae* organisms of a non-O1 serogroup (*V. cholerae* serogroup O139).

Outbreaks can also occur on a seasonal basis in endemic areas of Asia and Africa. Cases of cholera are regularly imported into industrialized countries. However, safe water and adequate sanitation limit the potential for outbreaks, and secondary transmission in developed countries is exceedingly rare.

In 2012, 48 countries reported 254,393 cases of cholera, including 3,034 deaths, to WHO—an overall case-fatality rate of 1.2%. These numbers represent a 58% decrease in reported cases compared to 2011. From 2001–2009, more than 90% of cholera cases were reported from Africa, including 98% of cases and 99% of deaths during 2009. In October 2010, a cholera epidemic began in Haiti, with over 600,000 cases and 7,500 deaths reported during the first 2 years of the epidemic. In 2012, 49% of all reported cases originated from this outbreak. Globally, actual numbers of cholera cases and deaths are likely to be much higher because of limited surveillance and underreporting.

5. **Reservoir**—Reservoirs include both humans and the environment. Observations in Australia, Bangladesh, and the USA have found environmental reservoirs for toxigenic *V. cholerae* O1, primarily in association with copepods or other zooplankton in brackish water or estuaries.

6. **Incubation period**—From a few hours to 5 days, usually 2–3 days.

7. Transmission—Through ingestion of an infective dose in contaminated water or food. Water is usually contaminated by feces of infected individuals. Contamination of drinking water can occur at the source, during transportation, or during storage at home. Food may also be contaminated by soiled hands, either during preparation or while eating. In funeral ceremonies of persons who have died of cholera, transmission may occur through consumption of food and beverages prepared by family members after they handled the corpse. *V. cholerae* O1 and O139 can persist in water for long periods and multiply in moist leftover food.

Beverages prepared with contaminated water and sold by street vendors, ice, and even commercial bottled water have been implicated as vehicles in cholera transmission, as have cooked vegetables and fruit "freshened" with untreated wastewater. Cases are often attributed to raw or undercooked seafood.

Cholera is communicable for as long as stools are positive for *V. cholerae*: from symptomatic individuals usually only a few days after recovery; and from asymptomatic individuals between 7–14 days. While intermittent shedding occasionally persists for several months, chronic carriage is rare.

8. Risk groups—

   1) Increased risk: lowest socioeconomic groups, particularly people without access to safe drinking water and adequate sanitation; gastric achlorhydria. Persons with blood group O are more vulnerable to severe cholera if infected.
   2) Reduced risk: breastfed infants.

Cholera infection provides short-term protection against reinfection, particularly by a homologous strain. In endemic areas, most people acquire antibodies by early adulthood. It appears that clinical infection with *V. cholerae* O1 of the classical biotype confers protection against either classical or El Tor biotypes but that an initial infection with biotype El Tor results in only a modest level of protection that is limited to El Tor infections. Additionally, some studies indicate that the Inaba serotype confers stronger protection than does the Ogawa serotype. Infection with O1 serogroup strains affords no protection against O139 infection, and vice versa.

9. Prevention—

   1) Prevention of cholera and its spread relies on the interruption of fecal-oral transmission through ensuring access to safe, potable drinking water; proper sanitation and waste disposal; and appropriate hygiene including handwashing. Raw fruits and vegetables, food from street vendors, and raw or undercooked seafood should be avoided. (See additional prevention measures discussed for typhoid fever in "Typhoid Fever and Paratyphoid Fever.")

2) Two oral vaccines are prequalified by WHO and are available in many countries but not in the USA: Dukoral (Crucell, the Netherlands, http://www.crucell.com) and Shanchol (Shantha Biotechnics, India, http://www.shanthabiotech.com). In vaccine trials, efficacy for persons receiving 2 doses was 65% after 5 years of follow-up. No country or territory requires vaccination against cholera as a condition for entry, though some countries recommend cholera vaccine for international travelers.

3) Measures that inhibit or otherwise compromise the movement of people and foods or other goods are not epidemiologically justified and have never proven effective in controlling cholera.

4) WHO does not advise routine screening or quarantine of travelers coming from cholera-affected areas. For further information, the WHO statement relating to international travel and trade to and from countries experiencing outbreaks of cholera can be found at: http://www.who.int/cholera/choleratravelandtradeadvice161107.pdf.

10. **Management of patient—**

1) Hospitalization with enteric precautions is desirable for severely ill patients; strict isolation is not necessary. Less severe cases can be managed on an outpatient basis with oral rehydration. Antimicrobials are clinically indicated for patients who are severely dehydrated or who are moderately dehydrated but with continued profuse volume loss in whom rehydration needs would be difficult to meet; their injudicious use increases the risk of development of antimicrobial resistant strains. Cholera wards can function well even when crowded, without hazard to staff and visitors, provided standard procedures are observed for handwashing and cleanliness and for the circulation of staff and visitors.

2) Treatment: the cornerstone of cholera treatment is timely and adequate rehydration. Patients presenting with mild or moderate dehydration can be treated successfully by oral rehydration solution (ORS) therapy alone. Only severely dehydrated patients or patients with severe vomiting and those who are unable to drink ORS will need intravenous rehydration. Patients who survive hypovolemic shock and severe dehydration may develop complications, such as hypoglycemia, that must be recognized and treated promptly.

Mild and moderate volume depletion should be corrected with oral solutions, replacing over 4-6 hours a volume matching the estimated fluid loss (~5% of body weight for mild dehydration and 7% for moderate dehydration). Continuing losses are replaced by giving, over 4 hours, a volume of oral solution equal to 1.5 times the stool volume lost in the previous 4 hours. In children 14 years and younger, daily supplementation with 30 mg elemental zinc during illness has been shown to reduce both duration and severity of cholera.

Severely dehydrated patients or patients in shock should be given rapid intravenous (IV) rehydration of 100 mL/kg with a balanced multi-electrolyte solution containing approximately 130 mEq/L of sodium, 4 mEq/L of potassium, 3 mEq/L of calcium, 110 mEq/L of chloride, and 28 mEq/L of lactate. Ringer's lactate is preferred for initial intravenous rehydration, but normal saline can be used in an emergency if ringer's lactate is not available. The initial fluid replacement should be 30 mL/kg in the first hour for infants and in the first 30 minutes for persons older than 1 year, after which the patient should be reassessed. The next 70 mL/kg should be given over 5 hours for infants and over 2.5 hours for older children and adults. After circulatory collapse has been effectively reversed, most patients can continue on oral rehydration to complete the 10% initial fluid deficit replacement and to match continuing fluid loss.

In moderate or severe cases, appropriate antimicrobial agents can shorten the duration of diarrhea, reduce the volume of rehydration solutions required, and shorten the duration of vibrio excretion. Adults are given a single 300 mg dose of doxycycline as first-line therapy. Where tetracycline-resistant strains of *V. cholerae* are prevalent, alternative antimicrobial regimens include azithromycin, erythromycin, or ciprofloxacin. Azithromycin and erythromycin are acceptable alternatives to doxycycline for children and pregnant women. Since individual strains of *V. cholerae* O1 or O139 may be resistant to any of these antimicrobials, knowledge of the susceptibility of local strains to these agents, if available, should always guide the choice of antimicrobial therapy.

3) Concurrent disinfection: feces and vomit from patients should be disposed in a sanitary manner to prevent contamination of water sources and food. In communities with a modern and adequate sewage disposal system, feces can be discharged directly into the sewers without preliminary disinfection. Linens and articles used by patients can be disinfected with a chlorine solution (0.05%) or by boiling for at least 5 minutes.

11. **Management of contacts and the immediate environment—**

1) Surveillance of persons who shared food and drink with a cholera patient for 5 days from last exposure. Chemoprophylaxis is rarely advisable—often by the time it can be delivered to contacts of a case, the targeted individuals have either already acquired the

infection or have little chance of acquiring it from the case in question. However, chemoprophylaxis of institutionalized populations, such as those in jail, who may be rapidly accessible following the identification of an index case, has been successfully accomplished. The same antimicrobials used for treatment can be used for chemoprophylaxis, with attention to the resistance patterns of circulating strains. Mass chemoprophylaxis of whole communities is never indicated, as it wastes resources and can quickly lead to antibiotic resistance.

2) Investigate possibilities of infection from polluted drinking water and contaminated food. Meal companions for the 5 days before illness onset should be interviewed. A search by stool culture for unreported cases is recommended only among household members or those exposed to a possible common source in a previously uninfected area.

12. **Special considerations—**

1) Reporting: under the International Health Regulations (IHR), governments are required to report cholera cases and outbreaks or epidemics of acute watery diarrhea to WHO when they are unusual or unexpected or when they present significant risk of international spread or of international travel or trade restrictions. The reporting as cholera caused by non-O1 or non-O139 serogroups of *V. cholerae* is not correct (even if these strains possess the cholera toxin gene) and therefore leads to confusion. In addition, nontoxigenic *V. cholerae* O1 should not be reported as cholera.

2) Epidemic measures:

- Educate the population at risk concerning the need to seek appropriate treatment for dehydration without delay.
- Provide effective treatment facilities.
- Adopt emergency measures to ensure a safe water supply.
- Chlorinate public water supplies, even if the source water appears uncontaminated. Chlorinate or boil water used for drinking, cooking, and washing dishes and food containers, unless the water supply is already adequately chlorinated. Households that store drinking water should ensure that protective storage containers are used to prevent recontamination of treated water by hands or objects during storage.
- Ensure careful preparation and supervision of food and drinks. After cooking food or boiling water, protect against contamination by flies and unsanitary handling; leftover foods should be thoroughly reheated (70°C/158°F for at least

15 minutes) before ingestion. Persons with diarrhea should not prepare food or haul water for others.

- Food served at funerals of cholera victims may be particularly hazardous if the body has been prepared for burial by persons in contact with the diseased person without stringent precautions; this practice should be discouraged during epidemics, and handwashing promoted.
- Initiate a thorough investigation designed to find the predominant vehicle(s) of infection and circumstances (time, place, and person) of transmission, and plan control measures accordingly.
- Provide appropriate safe facilities for sewage disposal.

Oral cholera vaccines may be used as an additional public health tool in outbreak control but should not replace other recommended control measures or detract from clinical management of cases. Priority measures during cholera outbreaks should focus on access to lifesaving treatment (ORS in particular) and provision of safe drinking water.

3) Disaster implications: outbreak risks are high in endemic areas if large groups of people are crowded together without sufficient quantities of safe water, adequate food handling, or sanitary facilities.

4) Measures applicable to ships, aircraft, and land transport arriving from cholera areas are to be applied within the framework of the IHR.

5) International travelers: No country is authorized under the IHR to require proof of cholera vaccination as a condition of entry, and the International Certificate of Vaccination no longer provides a specific space for recording cholera vaccination. Immunization with either of the oral vaccines can be recommended for individuals traveling to areas of endemic or epidemic cholera but should not replace the need to be sure that drinking water is safe.

Further information can be found at: http://www.who.int/csr/disease/cholera.

II. *VIBRIO PARAHAEMOLYTICUS* INFECTION (*Vibrio parahaemolyticus* infection)

1. Clinical features—An intestinal disorder characterized by watery diarrhea and abdominal cramps in most cases, often with nausea, vomiting, and headache. About one quarter of patients experience a dysentery-like illness with bloody or mucoid stools. Wound infections can also occur. Typically, it is a disease of moderate severity lasting 1-7 days; systemic infection and death rarely occur.

2. Causative agent—*Vibrio parahaemolyticus* is a natural inhabitant of estuarine and marine environments. Isolates may be subtyped into O and K serotypes. Over 30 different O:K serotypes are found in the USA, but O3:K6, O4:K12, and O6:K18 have been identified from recent outbreaks. Clinical isolates from humans are generally (but not always) capable of producing a characteristic hemolytic reaction (the "Kanagawa phenomenon") and carriage of 2 hemolysin genes correlate with diarrheal disease. Over 90% of isolates from ill persons carry one or both of these genes in contrast to less than 1% of isolates from food or environmental sources.

3. Diagnosis—By isolation of *V. parahaemolyticus* from stool, blood, or other clinical specimen. No serodiagnostic or rapid tests have been developed.

4. Occurrence—Sporadic cases and common-source outbreaks are reported in many parts of the world, particularly Japan, southeastern Asia, and the USA. Cases occur primarily in warm months. In 1998, two large outbreaks caused by serotype O3:K6, a common strain in Asia, occurred in the USA linked to consumption of raw oysters. This strain eventually emerged in South America and Africa causing additional large outbreaks. Other genotypically similar serotypes, such as O4:K68 and O1:K untypeable have also spread worldwide and together are referred to as the *V. parahaemolyticus* "pandemic clone."

5. Reservoir—Marine coastal environs are the natural habitat. During the cold season, organisms are found in marine silt; during the warm season, they are found free in coastal waters and in fish and shellfish.

6. Incubation period—Usually about 24 hours but can range from 4-96 hours.

7. Transmission—By ingestion of raw or inadequately cooked seafood, especially oysters or other shellfish. Not normally communicable from person to person.

8. Risk groups—Those with decreased gastric acidity, liver disease, or immunosuppression.

9. Prevention—

    1) Educate consumers about the risks associated with eating raw or undercooked seafood, especially oysters and other shellfish. Consumers in high-risk groups should not eat raw or undercooked seafood.

    2) Educate seafood handlers and processors on the following preventive measures:

- Ensure that seafood reaches temperatures adequate to kill the organism by cooking it to an internal temperature of 145°.
- Handle cooked seafood in a manner that precludes contamination from raw seafood or contaminated seawater.
- Keep all seafood, raw and cooked, adequately refrigerated.
- Avoid use of seawater in food handling areas (e.g., on cruise ships).

3) Several methods of postharvest processing of oysters (high hydrostatic pressure, heat-cool pasteurization, individual quick-freezing) can reduce but may not eliminate vibrio contamination.

4) Wash wounds that have been exposed to sea or brackish waters with soap and clean water.

5) Monitor shellfish and coastal waters for pathogenic *V. para-haemolyticus*.

10. Management of patient—

1) Enteric precautions.
2) Treatment: rehydration as appropriate. For septicemia or wound infection, effective antimicrobials (aminoglycosides, third-generation cephalosporins, fluoroquinolones, tetracycline) and supportive care.

11. Management of contacts and the immediate environment— Trace source of contamination and take measures to prevent transmission to humans.

12. Special considerations—Reporting: case report to local health authority is recommended and in some countries obligatory. Recognition and reporting of cases associated with recent shellfish consumption is especially important for follow-up investigation.

III. INFECTION WITH *VIBRIO VULNIFICUS*

1. Clinical features—Typically produces septicemia in persons with chronic liver disease, chronic alcoholism, hemochromatosis, or immunocompromising conditions. Intestinal infection rarely occurs. Fever, chills, and hypotension are common, as are distinctive bullous skin lesions that progress to necrotic ulcers. About 50% of patients with septicemia die. *Vibrio vulnificus* can also cause wound infection when preexisting or new skin lesions are exposed to sea or brackish water or to sea life; these infections range from mild, self-limited lesions to rapidly progressive cellulitis, myositis, and septicemia. Others can be infected and can develop gastroenteritis but do not usually present with septicemia.

2. Causative agent—*V. vulnificus* is halophilic and is commonly found in marine environments. Three biogroups have been identified. Biogroup 1 is an opportunistic human pathogen usually associated with the consumption of raw oysters, although wound infections can occur after trauma and exposure to a contaminated marine environment. Biogroup 2 strains are rarely found outside of Europe and are isolated predominantly from diseased eels but are occasionally isolated from human septicemia and wound infections acquired from handling eels. Biogroup 3 has been isolated only from Israeli patients with wound infections and bacteremia. These cases are associated with exposure to live fish (tilapia and carp) grown in aquaculture environments.

3. Diagnosis—*V. vulnificus* infection is usually diagnosed by isolation of the organism from blood or a wound usually on blood agar. No serodiagnostic or rapid tests have been developed.

4. Occurrence—It is the most common agent of serious infections caused by *Vibrio* species in North America, and has been reported in many areas of the world (e.g., Israel, Japan, the Republic of Korea, Spain, Taiwan [China], and Turkey).

5. Reservoir—*V. vulnificus* is a free-living autochthonous element of flora of estuarine environments. It is recovered from estuarine waters and from shellfish, particularly oysters. During summer, it can often be isolated routinely from oysters.

6. Incubation period—Usually 12-72 hours after eating raw or undercooked seafood.

7. Transmission—Through ingestion of raw or undercooked seafood, after exposure of wounds to marine or estuarine water (e.g., in boating accidents), or from occupational wounds (in oyster shuckers, fishermen). Not transmitted directly from person to person.

8. Risk groups—Persons with cirrhosis, hemochromatosis, and other chronic liver disease, or immunocompromising conditions are at increased risk for the infection and for the septicemic form of disease.

9. Prevention—Same as for *Vibrio Parahaemolyticus* Infection section in this chapter. Avoid seawater exposure of open wounds. Wash wounds that have been exposed to sea or brackish waters with soap and clean water.

10. Management of patient—Same as for *Vibrio Parahaemolyticus* Infection section in this chapter.

11. Management of contacts and the immediate environment—Trace source of contamination and take measures to prevent transmission to humans.

12. **Special considerations—**

1) Reporting: case report to local health authority recommended and in some countries obligatory. Recognition and reporting of cases associated with recent shellfish consumption is especially important for investigation.

2) A potential hazard in environmental disaster situations, such as hurricanes, in which wounds and exposure to sea water are widespread among those at risk. Healthy persons with a wound can develop infection, but their risk is much lower than for people in the risk groups.

IV. INFECTION DUE TO OTHER *VIBRIOS*

1. **Clinical features**—Infection with vibrios other than those discussed earlier causes a range of clinical syndromes. *Vibrio cholerae* of serogroups other than O1 and O139, as well as *Vibrio mimicus*, nontoxigenic *V. cholerae* O1, and others, cause gastroenteritis that ranges from mild to severe, but they have not caused large epidemics. *Vibrio alginolyticus* causes otitis externa, otitis media, and cellulitis. Other less commonly identified vibrios cause wound and septicemic illnesses.

2. **Causative agents**—Isolates of *V. cholerae* O1 and O139 that do not produce cholera toxin are known to occur but, as is the case with nontoxigenic non-O1/O139 strains, these strains do not cause large cholera epidemics but are usually associated with sporadic diarrheal disease. Isolates of non-O1/non-O139 *V. cholerae* can cause illness because they can possess a variety of virulence factors, sometimes including production of cholera toxin. However, cholera toxin–producing strains of non-O1 *V. cholerae* are rarely encountered. In the United States, toxigenic strains of *V. cholerae* serogroups O75 and O141 are associated with sporadic cholera-like illness that is usually attributed to consumption of undercooked seafood; on average fewer than 10 cases a year are detected. Some *V. cholerae* strains that do not agglutinate in O1 or O139 antiserum and produce a heat-stable enterotoxin (ST) are referred to as nonagglutinable-ST strains. Certain other species in the family *Vibrionaceae* can cause human illness, including diarrhea, septicemia, and other extraintestinal infections. These include *V. mimicus, Grimontia hollisae* (formerly *V. hollisae*), *Vibrio furnissii, Vibrio fluvialis, V. alginolyticus,* and *Photobacterium damselae* (formerly *Vibrio damsela*). Some strains of *V. mimicus* produce cholera toxin and have been associated with outbreaks of severe watery diarrhea. Most septicemic infections occur in immuno-compromised individuals or persons with underlying liver disease.

3. Diagnosis—Diagnosis is by isolation of the organism from clinical specimens. No serodiagnostic or rapid tests have been developed.

4. Occurrence—Other vibrios are uncommon causes of diarrheal, wound, and septicemic illness, mainly in tropical and coastal areas. Most are of little public health importance, though small outbreaks have been reported.

5. Reservoir—Vibrios are found in aquatic environments worldwide, particularly in brackish and salt waters. Vibrio counts vary seasonally, peaking in warm seasons. In brackish waters, they are often found adherent to chitinous zooplankton and shellfish. Isolates can survive and multiply in a variety of foods.

6. Incubation period—12-24 hours.

7. Transmission—Cases of gastroenteritis are usually linked to consumption of raw or undercooked seafood, particularly shellfish. In tropical endemic areas, some infections may be due to ingestion of surface waters. Wound infections arise from environmental exposure, usually to brackish or salt water or to sea life. In high-risk hosts, septicemia may result from a wound infection or from ingestion of contaminated seafood.

8. Risk groups—The immunosuppressed; alcoholics. Septicemia develops most commonly in persons with immunocompromising conditions, chronic liver disease, or severe malnutrition.

9. Prevention—Same as for *Vibrio Parahaemolyticus* Infection section in this chapter.

10. Management of patient—Same as for *Vibrio Parahaemolyticus* Infection section in this chapter.

11. Management of contacts and the immediate environment—Trace source of contamination and take measures necessary to prevent transmission to humans.

12. Special considerations—

1) Reporting: report to national health authority is recommended and mandatory in some areas.
2) The reporting of non-O1/non-O139 *V. cholerae* infections or of nontoxigenic *V. cholerae* O1 infection as cholera is inaccurate and leads to confusion.

[J. M. Brunkard, B. Mahon, J. Routh, E. Mintz]

CHROMOMYCOSIS
(dermatitis verrucosa)

DISEASE	ICD-10 CODE
CHROMOMYCOSIS	ICD-10 B43

1. **Clinical features**—A chronic spreading mycosis of the skin and subcutaneous tissues, usually of the lower extremities, although other areas can be involved. The initial lesion appears as a papule or a nodule. Progression to contiguous tissues is slow, over a period of years, with eventual large, nodular, verrucous, or even cauliflower-like masses. Invasion to muscle or bone can occur, although disseminated disease is rare. Rarely is a cause of death.

2. **Causative agents**—Dematiaceous fungi, including *Fonsecaea* (*Phialophora*) *pedrosoi*, *Phialophora verrucosa*, *Cladosporium carrionii*, *Rhinocladiella aquaspersa*, *Botryomyces caespitatus*, *Exophiala spinifera*, and *Exophiala jeanselmei*.

3. **Diagnosis**—Microscopic examination of scrapings or biopsies from lesions shows characteristic muriform cells—large, brown, thick-walled rounded cells that divide by fission in 2 planes. Confirmation of diagnosis should be made by biopsy and attempted cultures of the fungus.

4. **Occurrence**—Worldwide; most common in tropical and subtropical regions, particularly Latin America, the Caribbean, Asia, and Africa.

5. **Reservoir**—Wood, soil, and decaying vegetation.

6. **Incubation period**—Unknown; likely months to years.

7. **Transmission**—Inoculation via superficial, minor penetrating trauma/injuries (e.g., usually a sliver of contaminated wood or other material). Not transmitted from person to person.

8. **Risk groups**—Primarily a disease of barefoot rural agricultural workers in tropical regions, probably due to frequent traumatic inoculation. The disease is most common among men aged 30-50 years.

9. **Prevention**—Protect against small puncture wounds by wearing shoes or protective clothing.

10. **Management of patient—**

1) Disinfection of discharges from lesions and soiled articles.
2) Treatment: chromomycosis is not easy to cure medically, and multiple long-term treatment approaches are often used. Itraconazole is the treatment of choice, but its effectiveness appears to depend on the etiologic agent. Terbinafine, oral 5-fluorocytosine, or voriconazole have also been used. Oral flucytosine has been shown to benefit some patients, but relapse and development of resistance have been common. Large lesions may respond better when flucytosine is combined with amphotericin B. Small lesions are sometimes cured by surgical excision or cryotherapy alone.

11. **Management of contacts and the immediate environment—** None.

12. **Special considerations—**None.

[M. Brandt]

COCCIDIOIDOMYCOSIS
(valley fever, San Joaquin fever, desert fever, desert rheumatism, coccidioidal granuloma)

DISEASE	ICD-10 CODE
COCCIDIOIDOMYCOSIS	ICD-10 B38

1. **Clinical features**—The primary infection may be entirely asymptomatic or may resemble an acute influenza-like illness with fever, chills, cough, rash, and (rarely) pleuritic pain. About 1 in 5 clinically recognized cases (an estimated 5% of all primary infections) develop erythema nodosum. Primary infection may heal completely without detectable sequelae; may leave fibrosis, a pulmonary nodule that may or may not have calcified areas; may leave a persistent thin-walled cavity; or, most rarely, may progress to the disseminated form of the disease.

Less than 1% of symptomatic coccidioidomycosis becomes disseminated. Disseminated coccidioidomycosis is a progressive, severe granulomatous disease characterized by lesions in nearly any part of the body, especially in subcutaneous tissues, skin, bone, and meninges. Coccidioidal meningitis can resemble tuberculous meningitis but runs a more chronic course. Disseminated infection is uniformly fatal without treatment.

2. Causative agent—*Coccidioides immitis* and *posadasii*, dimorphic fungi. *Coccidioides* grow in soil and culture media as a saprophytic mold that reproduces by arthroconidia; in tissues and under special conditions, the parasitic form grows as spherical cells (spherules) that reproduce by formation of endospores. The 2 species cannot be distinguished morphologically.

3. Diagnosis—Through demonstration of characteristic coccidioidal spherules on microscopic examination, or through culture of sputum, pus, urine, cerebrospinal fluid, or biopsies of skin lesions or organs. Handling cultures of the agent is extremely hazardous and must be carried out in a class II biological safety cabinet under biosafety level 3 (BSL-3) containment. Clinical specimens should be handled under BSL-2 containment.

Serology: the precipitin test detects immunoglobulin class M (IgM) antibody, which appears 1–2 weeks after symptoms appear and persists for 3–4 months. CF tests detect mostly immunoglobulin class G (IgG) antibody, which appears 1–2 months after clinical symptoms start and persists for 6–8 months. Enzyme immunoassay tests are also available and detect IgM or IgG. Serial serological tests may be helpful in monitoring response to therapy; serological tests may be negative in the immunocompromised. Detection of antigen in serum or urine is useful in making the diagnosis and following the results of treatment; however, there is cross-reactivity with histoplasmosis and blastomycosis antigen.

4. Occurrence—Primary infections are common in the arid and semiarid endemic areas of the Western Hemisphere: in the USA from central/southern California to southern Texas, northern Argentina, north-eastern Brazil, Colombia, Mexico, Paraguay, Venezuela, and Central America. Dusty fomites from endemic areas can transmit infection. Disease has occurred in people who have merely traveled through endemic areas. High frequency of subclinical infection has been indicated by the high prevalence of positive skin tests in endemic areas.

Infection is seasonal and most frequent following rainy seasons during hot and dry periods, especially after wind and dust storms. Infects humans, cattle, cats, dogs, horses, burros, sheep, swine, wild desert rodents, coyotes, chinchillas, llamas, and other animal species.

5. Reservoir—Soil; especially in and around rodent burrows in endemic areas.

6. Incubation period—In primary infection, 1–4 weeks. Dissemination may develop insidiously years after the primary infection, sometimes without recognized symptoms of primary pulmonary infection.

7. Transmission—Inhalation of infective arthroconidia from soil and in laboratory accidents from cultures. *Coccidioides* is highly infectious; disease may occur after inhalation of only a few arthroconidia. While the parasitic form is normally not infective, accidental inoculation of infected pus, or culture suspension into the skin or bone, can result in granuloma formation. No direct person-to-person or animal-to-human transmission. *Coccidioides* spp. from skin abscesses or fistulas may change, rarely, from the parasitic to the infective saprophytic form.

8. Risk groups—Coccidioidomycosis is an important disease among persons with potential occupational exposure and those who are visiting or have moved into endemic areas. The disease affects all races and age groups, although the elderly are most frequently affected. Persons at highest risk for disseminated infection include pregnant women in the third trimester, persons of African or Filipino race/ethnicity, and immunocompromised persons, especially those with HIV or an organ transplant. Reactivation can occur in those who become immunosuppressed therapeutically or through HIV infection.

9. Prevention—In endemic areas: no practical prevention measures have been identified.

10. Management of patient—

1) Discharges and soiled articles must be disinfected. Terminal cleaning.
2) Treatment: primary coccidioidomycosis usually resolves spontaneously after days or weeks without therapy, and the benefit of treating primary pulmonary disease is controversial. Amphotericin B intravenous (IV) is used in severe pulmonary infections. Fluconazole is currently the agent of choice for meningeal infection. Fluconazole, itraconazole, and ketoconazole have been useful in chronic, nonmeningeal coccidioidomycosis. Posaconazole, a newer antifungal agent, has been shown to be of benefit in salvage studies of severe and disseminated infection.

11. Management of contacts and the immediate environment— In cases appearing in nonendemic areas, residence, work exposure, and travel history should be obtained.

12. Special considerations—

1) Reporting: case report to local health authority may be required.
2) Outbreaks occur when groups of susceptible persons are infected by airborne arthroconidia.
3) Possible hazard if large groups of susceptible persons are forced to move through or live in dusty conditions in areas where the fungus is prevalent.

4) *Coccidioides* arthroconidia have low potential use as a weapon. See "Anthrax" for general measures to be taken when confronted with a deliberate threat, such as that posed by *Coccidioides* arthroconidia.

[M. Brandt]

COMMON COLD AND OTHER ACUTE VIRAL RESPIRATORY DISEASES

DISEASE	ICD-10 CODE
COMMON COLD	ICD-10 J00
OTHER ACUTE FEBRILE RESPIRATORY ILLNESSES	ICD-10 J01-J06; J12
Influenza (see "Influenza")	
SARS (see "SARS, MERS, and Other Coronavirus Infections")	
Streptococcal pharyngitis (see "Streptococcal Diseases")	

Numerous acute respiratory illnesses of known and presumed viral etiology are grouped here. Clinically, infections of the upper respiratory tract (above the epiglottis) can be designated as acute viral rhinitis or acute viral pharyngitis (common cold), and infections involving the lower respiratory tract (below the epiglottis) can be designated as croup (laryngotracheitis), acute viral tracheobronchitis, bronchitis, bronchiolitis, or acute viral pneumonia. These respiratory syndromes are associated with a large number of viruses, which can produce a wide spectrum of acute respiratory illness and differ in etiology between children and adults.

The illnesses, caused by known agents, have important common epidemiological attributes, such as reservoir and mode of transmission. Many of the viruses invade any part of the respiratory tract; others show a predilection for certain anatomical sites. Some predispose to bacterial complications. Morbidity and mortality from acute respiratory diseases are especially significant in children. In adults, relatively high incidence and resulting disability, with consequent economic loss, make acute respiratory diseases a major health problem worldwide. As a group, acute respiratory diseases are one of the leading causes of death from any infectious disease.

Several other infections of the respiratory tract are presented as separate chapters, because they are sufficiently distinctive in their manifestations and occur in regular association with a single infectious agent: examples include influenza, psittacosis, hantavirus pulmonary syndrome, chlamydial pneumonia, vesicular pharyngitis (herpangina), epidemic myalgia (pleurodynia), and severe acute respiratory syndrome (SARS) and other coronavirus infections. Symptoms of upper respiratory tract infection, mainly pharyngotonsillitis, can be produced by bacterial agents, among which group A streptococcus is the most common. Viral infections should be differentiated from bacterial or other infections for which specific antimicrobial measures are available.

I. COMMON COLD (acute viral rhinitis, rhinitis, coryza [acute])

1. Clinical features—An acute catarrhal infection of the upper respiratory tract characterized by coryza, sneezing, lacrimation, irritation of the nasopharynx, chills, and malaise lasting 2–7 days. Fever is uncommon in children older than 3 years and rare in adults. White blood cell counts are usually normal. Illness may be accompanied by laryngitis, tracheitis, or bronchitis and may predispose to more serious complications, such as sinusitis and otitis media. Fatalities are not associated with common colds, although severe illness may progress through a catarrhal phase, such as in debilitated persons, or with secondary infections. Disability due to common colds is important, because it affects work performance and industrial and school absenteeism.

2. Causative agents—Rhinoviruses, of which there are more than 100 recognized serotypes, are the major known causal agents of the common cold in adults; they account for about 30%–50% of infections, especially in the autumn. Coronaviruses are responsible for about 10%–15% of common colds in adults. Other known respiratory viruses account for a small proportion of common colds in adults. In infants and children, parainfluenza viruses, respiratory syncytial virus (RSV), adenoviruses, certain enteroviruses, and coronaviruses may cause illnesses similar to the common cold (see Other Acute Febrile Respiratory Illnesses section in this chapter). The cause of about half of common colds has not been identified.

3. Diagnosis—Cell or organ culture studies of nasal secretions may show a known virus. Specific clinical, epidemiological, and other manifestations aid differentiation from similar diseases due to toxic, allergic, physical, or psychological stimuli. Polymerase chain reaction (PCR) methods can also be used to detect respiratory viruses.

4. Occurrence—Worldwide, both endemic and epidemic. In temperate zones, incidence rises in autumn, winter, and spring; in tropical settings, incidence is highest in the rainy season. Many people have 1–6 colds yearly. Incidence is highest in children younger than 5 years and gradually declines with increasing age.

5. Reservoir—Humans.

6. Incubation period—Between 12 hours and 5 days, usually 48 hours, varying with the agent.

7. Transmission—Presumably through direct contact or exposure of mucous membranes to respiratory droplets, and indirect transmission through hands and articles freshly soiled by nose and throat discharges of an infected person. Contaminated hands carry rhinovirus, RSV, and probably other similar viruses to the mucous membranes of the eye or nose. Nasal washes taken 24 hours before onset and for 5 days after onset have produced symptoms in experimentally infected volunteers. Inapparent infections occur; some viruses, notably rhinoviruses and adenoviruses, have been detected in asymptomatic persons.

8. Risk groups—Susceptibility is universal.

9. Prevention—

1) Practice good personal hygiene, such as covering the mouth when coughing and sneezing, sanitary disposal of oral and nasal discharges, and frequent handwashing.
2) When possible, avoid crowding in living and sleeping quarters, especially in institutions, in barracks, and onboard ships. Provide adequate ventilation.
3) Oral live adenovirus vaccines are administered to US military recruits to prevent adenovirus type 4 and 7 infections, but are not indicated in civilian populations because of the low incidence of specific disease.
4) Avoid smoking and passive smoke exposure. The risk of pneumonia increases among infected children exposed to passive smoke.

10. Management of patient—

1) Implement contact precautions in children's hospital wards, adding droplet precautions for specific pathogens (i.e., adenovirus and rhinovirus). Outside hospitals, ill people should avoid direct and indirect exposure to others, particularly young children, older adults, or patients with underlying conditions. See "Influenza" and chapters on other respiratory pathogens.
2) Disinfect eating and drinking utensils; sanitary disposal of oral and nasal discharges.

3) Treatment: none. Indiscriminate use of antibiotics is to be discouraged; they should be reserved for patients with group A streptococcal pharyngitis and patients with identified bacterial complications such as otitis media, sinusitis, or pneumonia. There is a lack of consensus regarding the use of aerosolized ribavirin to treat infants with RSV infection. No clear improvement in clinical outcomes attributed to the use of aerosolized ribavirin is consistent across all studies. Cough medicines, decongestants, and antihistamines are of questionable effectiveness, and may be detrimental, especially in children.

11. Management of contacts and the immediate environment— Personal hygiene and infection control practices (see Prevention and Management of Patient under Common Cold section in this chapter) among cases and contacts will reduce potential transmission.

12. Special considerations—None.

II. OTHER ACUTE FEBRILE RESPIRATORY ILLNESSES

1. Clinical features—Viral diseases of the respiratory tract may be characterized by fever, cough, increased respiratory rate, chills, headache, general aches, malaise, anorexia, and, occasionally, gastrointestinal symptoms. Localizing signs also occur at various sites in the respiratory tract, either alone or in combination, such as rhinitis, pharyngitis or tonsillitis, laryngitis, laryngotracheitis, bronchitis, bronchiolitis, pneumonitis, or pneumonia. There may be associated conjunctivitis. Upper respiratory tract infection symptoms and signs usually subside in 2–5 days without complications. Lower respiratory tract infections may be severe or complicated by bacterial infections.

2. Causative agents—Viruses considered etiologic agents of acute febrile respiratory illnesses are: RSV; parainfluenza virus, types 1, 2, 3, 4; human metapneumovirus; adenoviruses; rhinoviruses; certain coronaviruses; certain enteroviruses, including some types of coxsackievirus groups A and B, and echoviruses. Influenza virus (see "Influenza") can produce a similar clinical picture. Some of these agents tend to cause more severe illnesses; others are more commonly detected in certain age groups and populations. RSV, the major viral respiratory tract pathogen of early infancy, produces illness with greatest frequency during the first 2 years of life; it is the major known causal agent of bronchiolitis and is a cause of pneumonia, croup, bronchitis, otitis media, and febrile upper respiratory tract illness. The parainfluenza viruses are the major known causal agents of croup and also cause pneumonia, bronchitis, bronchiolitis, and febrile upper respiratory tract illness, particularly in children. Human metapneumovirus also causes upper and lower respiratory tract illness in children. RSV, parainfluenza viruses, and human metapneumovirus may cause symptomatic disease in adults, particularly older adults, persons with chronic cardiopulmonary conditions or immunosuppression.

Adenoviruses are associated with several forms of respiratory disease; types 4 and 7 are common causes of acute respiratory disease in non-immunized military recruits.

3. Diagnosis—Depends on isolation of the causal agent from respiratory secretions in appropriate cell or organ cultures and identification of viral antigen in nasopharyngeal cells by fluorescent antibody (FA), enzyme-linked immunosorbent assay (ELISA), and radioimmunoassay tests, and/or antibody studies of paired sera. PCR methods can also be used to detect respiratory viruses in respiratory specimens, such as nasopharyngeal or oropharyngeal swab specimens.

4. Occurrence—Worldwide. Seasonal in temperate zones, with greatest incidence during autumn and winter, and occasionally spring. In tropical zones, respiratory infections tend to be more frequent in wet and in colder weather. In large communities, some viral illnesses are constantly present, usually with little seasonal pattern; others tend to occur in seasonal outbreaks (e.g., RSV).

Annual incidence is high, particularly in infants and children, with 2–6 episodes per child per year, and depends on the number of susceptibles and the virulence of the virus.

5. Reservoir—Humans. Some viruses produce inapparent infections; Some cause similar infections in many animal species, but are thought to be of minor importance as sources of human infections.

6. Incubation period—From 1–10 days, depending on the viral pathogen.

7. Transmission—Directly through oral contact or droplet spread; indirectly from hands, handkerchiefs/tissues, eating utensils, or other articles freshly soiled with respiratory discharges of an infected person. Enteroviruses and adenoviruses may be transmitted by the fecal-oral route. Outbreaks of illness due to adenovirus have been related to swimming pools.

Infections are communicable shortly prior to, and for the duration of, active disease; limited information is available about subclinical or asymptomatic infections.

8. Risk groups—Susceptibility is universal. Illness is more frequent and more severe in infants, children, and older adults. Infection induces specific antibodies that are usually short-lived. Reinfection with RSV and parainfluenza viruses is common, but illness is generally milder. Individuals with compromized cardiac, pulmonary, or immune systems are at increased risk of severe illness. Those at high risk of RSV-related complications include infants and children younger than 2 years who have congenital heart disease, or required medical treatment for chronic lung disease within 6 months of the RSV season, and premature infants of under 35 weeks gestation at birth. HIV-infected children have a greater risk of hospitalization for RSV-associated lower respiratory illness and a higher case-fatality rate, which may be related to heightened susceptibility to coinfection with other pathogens, including bacteria and *Pneumocystis jiroveci*.

9. **Prevention—**

1) As for common cold. See Prevention under Common Cold section.

2) Infants at high risk of RSV-related complications (see Risk Groups under Other Acute Febrile Respiratory Illnesses section in this chapter), may benefit from palivizumab prophylaxis. Palivizumab is a monoclonal antibody preparation against RSV that is given monthly (intramuscular [IM]) in some countries during the course of the RSV season. Palivizumab has reduced RSV-related hospitalization by about half in such infants.

10. **Management of patient—**Same as for common cold. See Management of Patient under Common Cold section in this chapter.

11. **Management of contacts and the immediate environment—** Same as for common cold. See Management of Contacts and the Immediate Environment under Common Cold section in this chapter.

12. **Special considerations—**None.

[M. Iwane]

CONJUNCTIVITIS/KERATITIS

DISEASE	ICD-10 CODE
CONJUNCTIVITIS, BACTERIAL	ICD-10 A48.4
KERATOCONJUNCTIVITIS, ADENOVIRAL	ICD-10 B30.0
KERATOCONJUNCTIVITIS, MICROSPORIDIAL	ICD-10 B60.8†H19.2*
HEMORRHAGIC CONJUNCTIVITIS, ADENOVIRAL and ENTEROVIRAL	ICD-10 B30.1 (Adenoviral) ICD-10 B30.3 (Enteroviral)
CHLAMYDIAL CONJUNCTIVITIS	ICD-10 A74.0
Gonococcal conjunctivitis (see "Gonococcal Infections")	
Trachoma (see "Trachoma")	

I. CONJUNCTIVITIS, BACTERIAL (pinkeye, "sticky eye," Brazilian purpuric fever)

1. Clinical features—A clinical syndrome beginning with lacrimation, irritation, and hyperemia of the palpebral and bulbar conjunctivae of one or both eyes, followed by edema of eyelids and mucopurulent discharge. In severe cases, ecchymoses of the bulbar conjunctiva and marginal infiltration of the cornea with mild photophobia may occur. Nonfatal (except as noted later), the disease may last from 2 days to 2–3 weeks; many patients have no more than hyperemia of the conjunctivae and slight exudate for a few days.

2. Infectious agents—*Haemophilus influenzae* biogroup *aegyptius* (Koch-Weeks bacillus) and *Streptococcus pneumoniae* appear to be the most important; *H. influenzae* type b, *Moraxella* and *Branhamella* spp., *Neisseria meningitidis*, and *Corynebacterium diphtheriae* may also produce the disease. *H. influenzae* biogroup *aegyptius*, gonococci (see "Gonococcal Infections"), *S. pneumoniae*, *Streptococcus viridans*, various Gram-negative enteric bacilli and, rarely, *Pseudomonas aeruginosa* may produce the disease in newborn infants.

3. Diagnosis—Diagnosis through microscopic examination of a stained smear. Culture to exclude other causative agent.

4. Occurrence—Widespread and common worldwide, particularly in warmer climates; frequently epidemic. Infection due to other organisms occurs throughout the world, often associated with acute viral respiratory disease during cold seasons. Occasional cases of systemic disease have occurred among children in several communities in Brazil 1–3 weeks after conjunctivitis due to a unique invasive clone of *H. influenzae* biogroup *aegyptius*. This severe Brazilian purpuric fever (BPF) had a 70% case-fatality rate among more than 100 cases recognized over a wide area of Brazil covering 4 states. The causal agent has been isolated from conjunctival, pharyngeal, and blood cultures.

5. Reservoir—Humans. Carriers of *H. influenzae* biogroup *aegyptius* and *S. pneumoniae* are common in many areas during interepidemic periods.

6. Incubation period—Usually 24–72 hours.

7. Transmission—Contact with discharges from conjunctivae or upper respiratory tracts of infected people; contaminated fingers, clothing, and other articles, including shared eye-makeup applicators, multiple dose eye medications, and inadequately sterilized instruments such as tonometers. Eye gnats or flies may transmit the organisms mechanically in some areas, but their importance as vectors is undetermined and probably differs from area to area.

8. Risk groups—Children younger than 5 years are most often affected; incidence decreases with age. The very young, the debilitated and the aged are particularly susceptible to staphylococcal infections. Immunity after attack is low grade and varies with the infectious agent.

9. Prevention—Personal hygiene, hygienic care, and treatment of affected eyes.

10. Management of patient—

1) Drainage and secretion precautions. Children should not attend school during the acute stage.
2) Concurrent disinfection of discharges and soiled articles. Terminal cleaning.
3) Treatment: local application of an ointment or drops containing fusidic acid, chloramphenicol, ciprofloxacin, gentamycin, or combination antibiotics such as polymyxin B with neomycin or trimethoprim is generally effective. For BPF, systemic treatment is required; isolates are sensitive to both ampicillin and chloramphenicol and resistant to trimethoprim-sufamethoxazole. Oral rifampicin may be more effective than local chloramphenicol in eradication of the causal clone and may be useful in prevention among children with Brazilian purpuric fever clone conjunctivitis (see "Gonococcal Infections").

11. Management of contacts and the immediate environment— Usually not beneficial for conjunctivitis but must be undertaken for BPF.

12. Special considerations—

1) Reporting: report to local health authority obligatory for epidemics in some countries; no case report for classic disease.

2) Epidemic measures:

- Prompt and adequate treatment of patients and their close contacts.
- In areas where insects are suspected of mechanically transmitting infection, measures to prevent access of eye gnats or flies to the eyes of sick and well people.
- Insect control, according to the suspected vector.

II. KERATOCONJUNCTIVITIS, ADENOVIRAL (epidemic keratoconjunctivitis, shipyard conjunctivitis, shipyard eye)

1. Clinical features—An acute viral disease of the eye, with unilateral or bilateral inflammation of conjunctivae and edema of the lids and periorbital tissue. Onset is sudden with pain, photophobia, and blurred vision, and occasionally low-grade fever, headache, malaise, and tender preauricular lymphadenopathy. Approximately 7 days after onset in about half the cases, the cornea exhibits several small, round subepithelial infiltrates; these may eventually form punctate erosions that stain with fluorescein. Duration of acute conjunctivitis is about 2 weeks; it may continue to evolve, leaving discrete subepithelial opacities that may interfere with vision for a few weeks. In severe cases, permanent scarring may result.

2. Causative agents—Typically, adenovirus types 8, 19, and 37 are responsible, though other adenovirus types have been involved. Most severe disease has been found in infections caused by types 8, 5, and 19.

3. Diagnosis—Confirmed by recovery of virus from appropriate cell cultures inoculated with eye swabs or conjunctival scrapings; virus may be visualized through fluorescent antibody (FA) staining of scrapings or through immune electron microscopy; viral antigen may be detected by enzyme-linked immunosorbent assay (ELISA) testing. Serum neutralization or hemagglutination inhibition tests may identify type-specific titer rises.

4. Occurrence—Presumably worldwide. Both sporadic cases and large outbreaks have been reported from Asia, Europe, the Pacific Islands, and North America.

5. Reservoir—Humans.

6. Incubation period—Between 5 and 12 days, but in many instances longer.

7. Transmission—Direct contact with eye secretions of an infected person and, indirectly, through contaminated surfaces, instruments, or solutions. The infection is communicable from late in the incubation period to 14 days after onset. Prolonged viral shedding has been reported.

8. Risk groups—Trauma, even minor, and eye manipulation increase the risk of infection. There is usually complete type-specific immunity after adenoviral infections.

9. **Prevention**—

1) Ensure personal hygiene and avoid sharing towels, eye droppers, eye makeup, and toilet articles. Educate patients to minimize hand-to-eye contact.
2) Wash hands properly before doing any ophthalmologic procedures, such as examining patient, and properly sterilize instruments after use. Use clean gloves to examine eyes. Any ophthalmic medicines or droppers that have come in contact with eyelids or conjunctivae must be discarded. Medical personnel with overt conjunctivitis should not have physical contact with patients.
3) With persistent outbreaks, patients with epidemic keratoconjunctivitis should be seen in physically separate facilities.
4) Use safety measures such as goggles in high-risk areas.

10. **Management of patient**—

1) Drainage and secretion precautions; patients must use separate towels and linens during the acute stage.
2) Infected medical personnel or patients should not come in contact with uninfected patients.
3) Concurrent disinfection of conjunctival and nasal discharges and articles soiled therewith. Terminal cleaning.
4) Treatment: none during the acute phase. If residual opacities interfere with the patient's ability to work, topical corticosteroids may be administered by a qualified ophthalmologist.

11. Management of contacts and the immediate environment—In outbreaks, the source of infection should be identified and precautions taken to prevent further transmission.

12. **Special considerations**—

1) Reporting: obligatory report to local health authority of epidemics in some countries; no individual case report.
2) Epidemic measures: strictly apply prevention recommendations discussed earlier and organize convenient facilities for prompt diagnosis, with no or minimal contact between infected and uninfected individuals.

III. HEMORRHAGIC CONJUNCTIVITIS ADENOVIRAL (pharyngoconjunctival fever), ENTEROVIRAL (Apollo 11 disease, acute hemorrhagic conjunctivitis)

1. Clinical features—In adenoviral hemorrhagic conjunctivitis, lymphoid follicles usually develop, the conjunctivitis lasts 7–15 days, and there are frequently small subconjunctival hemorrhages. In one adenoviral syndrome, pharyngoconjunctival fever (PCF), there is upper respiratory disease and fever with minor corneal epithelial inflammation (epithelial keratitis). In enteroviral acute hemorrhagic conjunctivitis (AHC), onset is sudden, with redness, swelling, and pain often in both eyes; the course of the inflammatory disease is 4–6 days, during which subconjunctival hemorrhages appear on the bulbar conjunctiva as petechiae that enlarge to form confluent subconjunctival hemorrhages. Large hemorrhages gradually resolve over 7–12 days. In major outbreaks of enteroviral origin, there has been a low incidence of a polio-like paralysis, including cranial nerve palsies, lumbosacral radiculomyelitis, and lower motor neuron paralysis.

Neurological complications start a few days to a month after conjunctivitis, and often leave residual weakness.

2. Causative agents—Adenoviruses and picornaviruses. Most adenoviruses can cause PCF, but types 3, 4, and 7 are the most common causes. The most prevalent picornavirus type is enterovirus 70; this and a variant of coxsackievirus A24 have caused large outbreaks of AHC.

3. Diagnosis—Laboratory confirmation of adenovirus infections is through isolation of the virus from conjunctival swabs in cell culture, rising antibody titers, detection of viral antigens through immunofluorescence (IF), or identification of viral nucleic acid with a deoxyribonucleic acid (DNA) probe. Enterovirus infection is diagnosed by isolation of the agent, immunofluorescence, demonstration of a rising antibody titer, or polymerase chain reaction (PCR).

4. Occurrence—Widespread and common worldwide, especially in warmer climates. PCF occurs during outbreaks of adenovirus-associated respiratory disease or as summer epidemics in temperate climates associated with swimming pools. Smaller outbreaks have occurred in Europe, usually associated with eye clinics.

5. Reservoir—Humans.

6. Incubation period—For adenovirus infection, 4–12 days, with an average of 8 days. For enteroviral infection, 12 hours to 3 days.

7. Transmission—Direct or indirect contact with discharge from infected eyes. Person-to-person transmission is most noticeable in families, where high attack rates often occur. Adenovirus can be transmitted in poorly chlorinated swimming pools and also transmitted through respiratory droplets. Large AHC epidemics are often associated with overcrowding and low hygienic standards, especially among school children, which can result in rapid dissemination of AHC throughout communities. Adenovirus infections may be communicable up to 14 days after onset, picornavirus at least 4 days after onset.

8. **Risk groups**—Institutional populations associated with overcrowding.

9. **Prevention**—No effective treatment; prevention is critical.

   1) Personal hygiene should be emphasized, including use of nonshared towels and avoidance of overcrowding.
   2) Maintain strict asepsis in eye clinics; proper handwashing before examining patients and doing procedures. Eye clinics must ensure high-level disinfection of potentially contaminated equipment.
   3) Adequate chlorination of swimming pools. Closing schools may be necessary in an outbreak.

10. **Management of patient**—

    1) Drainage and secretion precautions; restrict contact with cases while disease is active (e.g., children should not attend school).
    2) Concurrent disinfection of conjunctival discharges and articles and equipment soiled therewith. Terminal cleaning.

11. **Management of contacts and the immediate environment**— Locate other cases to determine whether a common source of infection is involved.

12. **Special considerations**—

    1) Reporting: obligatory report of epidemics to local health authority in some countries.
    2) Epidemic measures: organize adequate facilities for the diagnosis and symptomatic treatment of cases; improve standards of hygiene and limit overcrowding wherever possible.

IV. CHLAMYDIAL CONJUNCTIVITIS (inclusion conjunctivitis, paratrachoma, neonatal inclusion blennorrhea, "sticky eye")

1. **Clinical features**—In the newborn, an acute conjunctivitis with purulent discharge, usually recognized within 5-12 days after birth. The acute stage usually subsides spontaneously in a few weeks; inflammation of the eye may persist for more than a year if untreated, with mild scarring of

the conjunctivae and infiltration of the cornea (micropannus). Chlamydial pneumonia (see "Pneumonia" and "Chlamydial Infections") occurs in some infants with concurrent nasopharyngeal infection. Gonococcal infection must be ruled out.

In children and adults, an acute follicular conjunctivitis is seen typically with preauricular lymphadenopathy on the involved side, hyperemia, infiltration, and a slight mucopurulent discharge, often with superficial corneal involvement. In adults, there may be a chronic phase with scant discharge and symptoms that sometimes persist for more than a year if untreated. The agent may cause symptomatic infection of the urethral epithelium and the cervix, with or without associated conjunctivitis.

2. Causative agents—*Chlamydia trachomatis* of serovars D through K. Feline strains of *Chlamydia psittaci* have also caused acute follicular keratoconjunctivitis in humans.

3. Diagnosis—Laboratory methods to assist diagnosis include isolation in cell culture, antigen detection using IF staining of direct smears, enzyme immunoassay (EIA) methods, and DNA probe.

4. Occurrence—Sporadic cases of conjunctivitis are reported worldwide among sexually active adults. Neonatal conjunctivitis due to *C. trachomatis* is common and occurs in 15%–35% of newborns exposed to maternal infection. Among adults with genital chlamydial infection, 1 in 300 develops chlamydial eye disease.

5. Reservoir—Humans for *C. trachomatis*; cats for *C. psittaci*.

6. Incubation period—In newborns, 5–12 days, ranging from 3 days to 6 weeks; in adults, 6–19 days.

7. Transmission—Generally transmitted in adults during sexual intercourse; the genital discharges of infected people are infectious. In the newborn, conjunctivitis is usually acquired by direct contact with infectious secretions during transit through the birth canal. In utero infection may also occur. The eyes of adults become infected by the transmission of genital secretions to the eye, usually by the fingers. Children may acquire conjunctivitis from infected newborns or other household members; cases in children should be assessed for sexual abuse as appropriate. Outbreaks reported among swimmers in nonchlorinated pools have not been confirmed by culture and may be due to adenoviruses or other known causes of "swimming pool conjunctivitis."

The disease is communicable while genital or ocular infection persists; carriage on mucous membranes has been observed for as long as 2 years after birth.

8. Risk groups—Diabetics and infants of infected mothers.

9. **Prevention—**

1) Correct and consistent use of condoms to prevent sexual transmission; prompt treatment of persons with chlamydial urethritis and cervicitis, including pregnant women.
2) General preventive measures as for other sexually transmitted infections (STIs); see "Syphilis."
3) Sanitary control of swimming pools; ordinary chlorination suffices.
4) Identification of infection in high-risk pregnant women by culture or antigen detection. Treatment of cervical infection in pregnant women will prevent subsequent transmission to the infant. Erythromycin base is usually effective, but frequent gastrointestinal (GI) side effects interfere with compliance and treatment must be observed to ensure completion. If compliance is a problem, consideration may be given to the use of other macrolides.
5) Routine prophylaxis for gonococcal ophthalmia neonatorum is effective against chlamydial infection and should be practiced. The method of choice is a single application into the eyes of the newborn within 1 hour after delivery of one of the following: povidone-iodine (2.5% solution); tetracycline 1% eye ointment; erythromycin 0.5% eye ointment; or silver nitrate eye drops (1%). Ocular prophylaxis does not prevent nasopharyngeal colonization and risk of subsequent chlamydial pneumonia. Penicillin is ineffective against chlamydiae.

10. **Management of patient—**

1) Drainage and secretion precautions for the first 96 hours after starting treatment.
2) Aseptic techniques and proper handwashing by personnel appear to be adequate to prevent nursery transmission.
3) Treatment: for ocular and genital infections, tetracycline, erythromycin, or ofloxacin is effective. Azithromycin is an effective single-dose therapy. Oral treatment of neonatal ocular infections with erythromycin for 2 weeks is recommended to eliminate the risk of chlamydial pneumonia as well.

11. **Management of contacts and the immediate environment—** All sexual contacts of adult cases, and parents of neonatally infected infants, should be examined and treated. Infected adults should be investigated for evidence of ongoing infection with gonorrhea or syphilis.

12. **Special considerations—**Reporting: case report of neonatal cases obligatory in many countries.

V. MICROSPORIDIA KERATOCONJUNCTIVITIS

1. Clinical features—Clinical symptoms include foreign body sensations, moderate to intense pain, redness, light sensitivity, excessive tearing, swelling of eyelid, itchiness, and impaired eyesight. Ocular manifestations include superficial punctate keratoconjunctivitis and corneal stromal keratitis. Duration of symptoms lasts between 4 days and 18 months. Disease commonly causes symptoms in immunocompromised patients but also has been documented in immunocompetent persons.

2. Causative agents—Microsporidia, obligate, intracellular, spore-forming protozoae belonging to the phylum Microspora. Keratoconjunctivitis is caused by genus *Encephalitozoon* and stromal keratitis is caused by genus *Nosema* and *Microsporidium. Vittaforma corneae* (syn. *Nosema corneum)* cause keratoconjunctivitis and urinary tract infections in human.

3. Diagnosis—By corneal scraping/conjunctival smear for microsporidia. Culture to exclude other causative agents. Laboratory methods to assist diagnosis include light microscopy using various stains including gram stains (microsporidia spores are Gram-positive and stain dark violent and become readily visible under the microscope), modified trichrome stains (e.g., trichrome blue), Warthin-Starry silver stains, Giemsa, and chemofluorescent agents like Calcoflur.

V. corneae and *Nosema* spp. measure 1.5–4 μm under the microscope. Immunofluorescence assays (IFAs) and molecular techniques are emerging methods for diagnosis. Transmission electron microscopy is the gold standard for identifying specific species.

4. Occurrence—Cases of microsporidial keratoconjunctivitis are reported worldwide among immunocompromised humans but cases in immunocompetent persons are seen in India and Singapore.

5. Reservoir—Unclean contaminated river water; contaminated rain, soil, and mud.

6. Incubation period—Usually from 2–30 days.

7. Transmission—Generally through contact with mud, soil, river water, and rain water contaminated with spores of *V. corneae* and *Nosema* spp. Predisposing factors include exposure to contaminated river water, rain, soil, and mud during swimming and outdoors activities such as cricket, rugby, soccer, and golf. It can occur both in immunocompromised and immunocompetent individuals. Person-to-person transmission has not been reported.

8. Risk groups—Those in contact with unclean contaminated river water, contaminated rain, soil, and mud.

9. **Prevention**—Avoid playing on very muddy, waterlogged pitches, in unclean rivers, and contaminated rain, and avoid contact with soil and mud. If that cannot be avoided, regular thorough washing of faces and eyes immediately after contact with mud, soil, and unclean water sources is advised.

10. **Management of patient**—

   1) Corneal debridement to reduce the load of spores.
   2) Treatment: in immunocompetent persons, ciprofloxacin eye drops with or without chlorhexidine 0.02% and oral T. albendazole and T. itraconazole. In immunocompromised persons, topical fumidil B. and oral T. albendazole and T. itraconazole

11. **Management of contacts**—None.

12. **Special considerations**—None.

[M. Maznieda]

CRYPTOCOCCOSIS
(torula)

DISEASE	ICD-10 CODE
CRYPTOCOCCOSIS	ICD-10 B45

1. **Clinical features**—Primary pulmonary infection, in immunocompetent persons, commonly presents with fever and dry cough. In immunocompromised persons, signs and symptoms often develop after hematogenous spread to the meninges, with subacute or chronic meningitis and include headache, visual disturbance, and confusion. Other sites of disseminated infection include the kidneys, prostate, bone, and skin (pustules, papules, plaques, ulcers, or subcutaneous masses). Untreated meningitis leads to death within weeks to months.

2. **Causative agents**—*Cryptococcus neoformans* var. *neoformans* and var. *grubii*, and *Cryptococcus gattii*.

3. **Diagnosis**—Cryptococcal meningitis diagnosis is aided by the evidence of the characteristic capsular halo or budding forms on microscopic examination of cerebrospinal fluid (CSF) mixed with India ink. Tests for antigen in serum and CSF are highly sensitive and specific. Diagnosis is confirmed through histopathology or culture (media containing cycloheximide

inhibit the agent and should not be used). *Cryptococcus* can be stained using Gomori-methenamine silver or periodic acid-Schiff staining; mucicarmine helps differentiate it from other yeasts, especially *Blastomyces* and *Histoplasma*.

4. Occurrence—Cases of *C. neoformans* occur worldwide and tend to follow the AIDS epidemic in a given country or region. Infection is more frequent in adults than in children, and in males slightly more frequently than in females. *C. gattii* is more frequent in tropical or subtropical regions, such as Australia, Africa, tropical South America, and the southern Pacific coast of the USA. Recent reports have described *C. gattii* emergence in British Columbia, Canada, and the Pacific Northwest USA.

5. Reservoir—Saprophytic growth in the environment. *C. neoformans* can be isolated consistently from old pigeon nests and pigeon droppings and from soil in many parts of the world. Foliage and bark of many species of trees have yielded *C. gattii*. Infection also occurs in cats, dogs, horses, camelids, and other animals.

6. Incubation period—Unknown for *C. neoformans* and 2–13 months for *C. gattii*. Pulmonary disease may precede brain infection by months or years.

7. Transmission—Presumably by inhalation of the fungal spores. No person-to-person or animal-to-person transmission.

8. Risk groups—Susceptibility is increased during corticosteroid or other immunosuppressive therapy and by immune deficiency disorders (especially HIV infection).

9. Prevention—

1) There are no data that demonstrate that specific measures to avoid exposure are of any benefit in preventing infection.
2) Fluconazole antifungal prophylaxis for patients with HIV has been shown to reduce the incidence of infection, but not overall survival.

10. Management of patient—

1) Concurrent disinfection of discharges and contaminated dressings. Terminal cleaning.
2) Treatment: the combination of amphotericin B and 5-flucytosine is the therapy of choice for disseminated infection, including meningitis, but has some toxicity; lipid formulation of amphotericin B can help avoid nephrotoxicity. For meningitis, consolidation therapy follows induction and is often long-term; fluconazole is used after an initial course of amphotericin B and 5-flucytosine. Management of elevated intracranial pressure in

patients with meningeal involvement, through manometry and periodic therapeutic lumbar punctures, is essential.

11. Management of contacts and the immediate environment—None.

12. Special considerations—Reporting: report to local health authority is required in some areas as a possible manifestation of AIDS. Within the USA, *C. gattii* is a notifiable disease in Oregon and Washington states.

[S. Lockhart]

CRYPTOSPORIDIOSIS

DISEASE	ICD-10 CODE
CRYPTOSPORIDIOSIS	ICD-10 A07.2

1. Clinical features—This parasitic infection affects epithelial cells of the gastrointestinal (GI), biliary, and respiratory tracts. The major symptom is diarrhea, which may be profuse and watery and is associated with cramping abdominal pain. The diarrhea is preceded by anorexia and vomiting in children, but general malaise, fever, anorexia, nausea, and vomiting occur less often in adults. Symptoms often wax and wane but remit in less than 30 days in most immunologically healthy people. Immunocompetent people may have asymptomatic or self-limited symptomatic infections; it is not clear whether reinfection and latent infection with reactivation can occur. Immunodeficient individuals generally clear their infections when factors contributing to immunosuppression (including malnutrition or intercurrent viral infections such as measles) are ameliorated or controlled. In those with HIV infection, the clinical course may vary, and asymptomatic periods may occur, but the infection usually persists throughout the illness unless highly active antiretroviral therapy is successful. Symptoms of cholecystitis may occur in biliary tract infections; the relationship between respiratory tract infections and clinical symptoms is unclear.

2. Causative agent—*Cryptosporidium hominis* and *Cryptosporidium parvum*, coccidian protozoa, are the 2 species most often associated with human infection.

3. Diagnosis—Generally through identification of oocysts in fecal smears or of life cycle stages of the parasites in intestinal biopsy sections. Oocysts are small (4–6 μm) and may be confused with yeast unless appropriately stained. Most commonly used stains include auramine-rhodamine, a modified acid-fast stain, and safranin-methylene blue. More sensitive immunobased enzyme-linked immunosorbent assays (ELISAs) are also available. A fluorescein-tagged monoclonal antibody is useful for detecting oocysts in stool and in environmental samples. Infection with this organism is not easily detected unless looked for specifically. Serological assays may help in epidemiological studies. Molecular tests, such as polymerase chain reaction (PCR), are increasingly being used.

4. Occurrence—Worldwide. *Cryptosporidium* oocysts have been identified in human fecal specimens from more than 50 countries. In industrialized countries, prevalence of infection is less than 1%–4.5% of individuals surveyed by stool examination. In developing regions, prevalence ranges from 3%–20%.

5. Reservoir—Humans and various animals. The parasite infects more than 45 vertebrate species including birds, fish, reptiles, and mammals.

6. Incubation period—Variable; 1–12 days is the likely range, with an average of about 7 days.

7. Transmission—Fecal-oral, which includes person-to-person, animal-to-person, waterborne, and foodborne transmission. Outbreaks have been reported in day care centers around the world and have also been associated with: drinking water (at least 3 major outbreaks involved public water supplies); recreational use of water including waterslides, swimming pools, and lakes; and consumption of contaminated beverages.

The parasite infects intestinal epithelial cells and multiplies initially by meiogony (schizogony), followed by a sexual cycle resulting in fecal oocysts. Oocysts, the infectious stage, appear in the stool at the onset of symptoms and are infectious immediately upon excretion. Excretion continues in stools for several weeks after symptoms resolve; outside the body, oocysts may remain infective for 2–6 months or longer in a moist environment. Oocysts are highly resistant to chemical disinfectants used to purify drinking water. One or more autoinfectious cycles may occur in humans.

8. Risk groups—Children younger than 2 years, animal handlers, travelers, men who have sex with men, and close personal contacts of infected individuals (families, health care and day care workers) are particularly prone to infection. Hospital experience indicates that 10%–20% of AIDS patients develop the infection at some time during their illness. In immunodeficient persons, especially those infected with HIV, who may be unable to clear the parasite, the disease has a prolonged and fulminant clinical course contributing to death.

9. Prevention—

1) Educate the public in personal hygiene, especially on the need for handwashing before handling food, before eating, and after toilet use.

2) Dispose of feces in a sanitary manner; use care in handling animal or human excreta.

3) Have those in contact with calves and other animals with diarrhea (scours) wash their hands carefully.

4) Boil drinking water supplies for 1 minute; chemical disinfectants are not effective against oocysts in drinking water. Filters capable of removing particles 0.1–1.0 μm in diameter should be considered.

10. Management of patient—

1) For hospitalized patients, enteric precautions in the handling of feces, vomitus, and contaminated clothing and bed linen; exclusion of symptomatic individuals from food handling and from direct care of hospitalized and institutionalized patients; and release to return to work in sensitive occupations when asymptomatic. Stress proper handwashing.

2) Exclude infected children from day care facilities until diarrhea stops.

3) Concurrent disinfection of feces and articles soiled therewith. In communities with modern and adequate sewage disposal systems, feces can be discharged directly into sewers without preliminary disinfection. Terminal cleaning. Heating to 45°C (113°F) for 20 minutes (or, more conservatively, 50°C–60°C for 30 min) or to 64.2°C (147.5°F) for 2 minutes is effective, as is chemical disinfection with 10% formalin or 5% ammonia solution.

4) Rehydration, when indicated, has been proven effective. Fluid and electrolyte replacement with oral rehydration solutions or intravenous fluids is essential. It may be difficult to clear infection while the patient is taking immunosuppressive drugs, and in the case of severe persistent symptoms, it may be necessary to consider if it is possible to safely reduce or stop their use until the infection has cleared.

5) Treatment: nitazoxanide can be used to treat cryptosporidiosis in patients aged 1 year and older.

11. Management of contacts and the immediate environment—

1) Microscopic examination of feces in household members and other suspected contacts, especially if symptomatic. Contact with cattle or domestic animals warrants investigation.

2) If waterborne transmission is suspected, large volume water sampling filters can be used to look for oocysts in the water.

12. Special considerations—

1) Reporting: report to local health authority; case report to local health authorities required in some countries.

2) Epidemic measures: epidemiological investigation of clustered cases in an area or institution to determine source of infection and mode of transmission; search for common vehicle, such as recreational water, drinking water, raw milk, or other potentially contaminated food or drink; and institution of applicable prevention or control measures. Control of person-to-person or animal-to-person transmission requires emphasis on personal cleanliness and safe disposal of feces.

[M. Arrowood, M. Eberhard, A. Gabrielli, L. Savioli]

CYCLOSPORIASIS

DISEASE	ICD-10 CODE
CYCLOSPORIASIS	ICD-10 A07.8

1. **Clinical features**—An infection of the upper small bowel with a clinical syndrome that consists of watery diarrhea, nausea, anorexia, abdominal cramps, fatigue, myalgia, and weight loss; fever is rare. Persistence of symptoms, with remittance and relapse episodes, is typical: if untreated, diarrhea in the immunocompetent usually lasts for 10–24 days, but is self-limited; in the immunocompromised, who appear more susceptible to infection, diarrhea can last for months in some patients. *Cyclospora* infection occurring in individuals who are not treated or not treated promptly is also associated with chronic complications including Guillain-Barré syndrome and Reiter's syndrome. Health care providers should consider the diagnosis of *Cyclospora* infection in persons with prolonged diarrheal illness and should request stool specimens so that specific tests for this parasite can be made.

2. **Causative agent**—*Cyclospora cayetanensis*, a sporulating coccidian protozoan.

3. **Diagnosis**—Identification in the stools of the 8–10 micrometer size oocysts, about twice the size of *Cryptosporidium parvum*, in wet mount under phase contrast microscopy. A modified acid-fast stain or modified safranin technique can be used. Organisms autofluoresce under ultraviolet illumination.

4. **Occurrence**—*Cyclospora* is endemic in many developing countries. The disease is most common in tropical and subtropical countries, where

asymptomatic infections are not infrequent. It has also been associated with diarrhea in travelers to Asia, the Caribbean, and Latin America.

5. Reservoir—Humans. Several *Cyclospora* spp. are known to infect primates; whether this is the case for *C. cayetanensis* is still unclear.

6. Incubation period—Approximately 1 week.

7. Transmission—Occurs either through drinking (or swimming in) contaminated water or through consumption of contaminated fresh fruits and vegetables. *Cyclospora cayetanensis* has been responsible for multiple foodborne outbreaks in North America linked to various types of fresh produce imported from developing countries. Raspberries, basil, and lettuce are among the incriminated vehicles. *Cyclospora* oocysts in freshly excreted stool are not infectious; they require days to weeks outside the host to sporulate and become infectious, making person-to-person transmission unlikely. The mechanism of contamination of water and food has not been fully elucidated. Mean duration of organism shedding was 23 days in Peruvian children.

8. Risk groups—Those with HIV and HIV/tuberculosis (TB) coinfection are particularly susceptible to infection.

9. Prevention—Produce should be washed thoroughly before it is eaten, although this practice does not eliminate the risk of cyclosporiasis. *Cyclospora* is resistant to chlorination.

10. Management of patient—Treatment: can be treated with a 7–10 day course of oral trimethoprim-sulfamethoxazole, shown to cure about 90% of cases. Patients with HIV infection may require higher dosage and longer treatment. Ciprofloxacin is less effective than trimethoprim-sulfamethoxazole but is the treatment of choice for patients who cannot tolerate sulfa drugs. In all patients, fluid and electrolyte balance should be monitored and maintained. In patients who are not treated, illness can be protracted, with remitting and relapsing symptoms.

11. Management of contacts and the immediate environment—Search for site of infection of index case; identify others exposed. Intensify preventive measures.

12. Special considerations—Reporting: in jurisdictions where formal reporting mechanisms are not yet established, clinicians and laboratory workers who identify cases of cyclosporiasis are encouraged to inform the appropriate health departments.

[M. Arrowood, M. Eberhard, A. Gabrielli, L. Savioli]

CYTOMEGALOVIRUS DISEASE

DISEASE	ICD-10 CODE
CYTOMEGALOVIRUS DISEASE	ICD-10 B25
CONGENITAL CYTOMEGALOVIRUS INFECTION	ICD-10 P35.1

1. **Clinical features**—While infection with cytomegalovirus (CMV) is common, it often passes undiagnosed as a febrile illness without specific characteristics. Serious manifestations of infection vary depending on the age and immunocompetence of the individual.

The most severe form of the disease develops in approximately 10% of infants infected in utero, who show signs and symptoms of severe generalized infection, especially involving the central nervous system and liver. Lethargy, convulsions, jaundice, petechiae, purpura, hepatosplenomegaly, chorioretinitis, intracerebral calcifications, intrauterine growth restriction, and pulmonary infiltrates may occur. Survivors may show mental retardation, microcephaly, motor disabilities, hearing loss, and/or evidence of chronic liver disease. Death may occur in utero; the neonatal case-fatality rate is high for severely affected infants.

Primary infection in an immunocompetent person acquired later in life is usually asymptomatic but may cause a syndrome clinically and hematologically similar to Epstein-Barr virus mononucleosis and hepatitis, distinguishable by virological or serological tests and the absence of heterophile antibodies. Disseminated infection, with pneumonitis, retinitis, gastrointestinal (GI) tract disorders (gastritis, enteritis, colitis), and hepatitis occurs in immunodeficient and immunosuppressed patients, including those with AIDS.

CMV is a common cause of post-transplant infection, both for solid organ and bone marrow transplants; symptomatic infection occurs in about 10%–40% of transplant recipients.

2. **Causative agent**—Human (beta) herpesvirus 5 (human CMV), a member of the subfamily Betaherpesvirus of the family *Herpesviridae*; includes 4 major genotypes and many strains, although there often is cross-antigenicity among genotypes and strains.

3. **Diagnosis**—Optimal diagnosis in the newborn is through virus isolation or polymerase chain reaction (PCR), usually from urine or saliva, in the first 2–3 weeks of life. A strongly positive CMV-specific immunoglobulin class M (IgM) antibody test at birth can also be helpful, but commercial assays vary in sensitivity and specificity. Diagnosis of CMV disease in the adult is made difficult by the high frequency of asymptomatic and recurrent infections. Multiple diagnostic modalities should be used if possible. Virus

isolation, CMV antigen detection (which can be done within 24 hours), and CMV deoxyribonucleic acid (DNA) detection by PCR or in situ hybridization, can be used to demonstrate virus in organs, blood, respiratory secretions, or urine. Serological studies can be done to demonstrate the presence of CMV specific IgM antibody, seroconversion (4-fold rise in immunoglobulin class G [IgG] antibody titer), or IgG antibody avidity. Interpretation of the results requires knowledge of the patient's clinical and epidemiological background.

4. **Occurrence**—Worldwide, the birth prevalence of congenital CMV infection is approximately 0.6% and tends to be higher in countries with high CMV seroprevalence. The reported birth prevalence of congenital CMV infection in developing countries ranges from 0.6%–6.1%, higher than in developed countries (0.2%–2.0%). Seroprevalence among young adults varies from 30% in highly industrialized countries to almost 100% in some developing countries; it is higher among women than among men and is related to socioeconomic status or ethnic group in some countries.

5. **Reservoir**—Humans are the only known reservoir of human CMV; strains found in many animal species are not infectious for humans.

6. **Incubation period**—The incubation period for horizontally transmitted infections is not known. Illness following a transplant of an infected allograft, or transfusion with infected blood, begins within 3–8 weeks. Perinatal or early postnatal infection from breast milk is usually demonstrable 3–12 weeks after birth.

7. **Transmission**—Intimate exposure through mucosal contact with infectious tissues, secretions, and excretions, including saliva, breast milk, cervical secretions, and semen. Transmission through sexual intercourse is common and is reflected by the almost universal infection of men who have many male sexual partners. Viremia may be present in asymptomatic people, so the virus may be transmitted by blood transfusion, probably associated with leukocytes. The fetus may be infected in utero from either a primary maternal infection, maternal reinfection with a new CMV strain, or reactivation of latent maternal infection. Most intrauterine infections are due to maternal reactivation or reinfection. Fetal infection with manifest disease at birth occurs most commonly following maternal primary infection but has also been reported in populations with high seroprevalence, in whom recurrent infections are more likely. Perinatal transmission through exposure to infected cervical secretions at delivery, or early postnatal transmission via breast milk, may occur among infants born to CMV-seropositive mothers.

Virus is excreted in urine and saliva for many months and may persist or be episodic for several years following primary infection. Many children in day care centers excrete CMV; this may represent a community reservoir. Children with congenital CMV infection may excrete virus as long as 5–6 years. Adults appear to excrete virus for shorter periods. CMV persists as a latent infection. Excretion recurs with immunodeficiency and immunosuppression.

8. Risk groups—Fetuses, infants born prematurely or with a very low birth weight, patients with immunosuppressive conditions, including persons with HIV infection, those on immunosuppressive drugs, and especially organ allograft recipients (kidney, heart, bone marrow) are more susceptible to overt and severe disease.

9. Prevention—

1) Take care in handling diapers/nappies; wash hands after diaper changes and toilet care of newborns and infants.

2) Health care personnel should follow standard precautions. Workers in day care centers and preschools should observe strict standards of hygiene, including handwashing after contact with urine or saliva.

3) CMV transmission through transfusion of blood products to newborns or immunocompromised persons can be prevented by freezing red blood cells in glycerol before administration, by removal of the buffy coat, by filtration to remove white blood cells, or by use of CMV antibody-negative donors. However, screening of blood products for CMV may not be routinely performed in all countries or may not be a feasible strategy in countries with high CMV seroprevalence.

4) Avoid transplanting organs from CMV-seropositive donors to seronegative recipients. If unavoidable, hyperimmune immune globulin (IG), or prophylactic or preemptive administration of antivirals, may be helpful. Antivirals are also helpful in seropositive bone-marrow transplant recipients who carry latent CMV.

10. Management of patient—

1) Standard precautions should be followed in health care settings.

2) Treatment: the drugs of choice for prophylaxis and treatment of CMV disease include ganciclovir intravenous (IV) or valganciclovir, administered orally. Alternatively, cidofovir IV (together with probenecid), foscarnet IV and fomivirsen have been approved for the treatment of CMV retinitis in immunocompromised persons. Ganciclovir, valganciclovir, cidofovir, and foscarnet may also be helpful—especially when combined with anti-CMV immune globulin—for pneumonitis and possibly GI disease in immunocompromised persons; these drugs are licensed for use in CMV infections occurring after organ transplantation. For newborns with congenital CMV and severe symptomatic or central nervous

system disease, antiviral treatment with ganciclovir or oral valganciclovir may be effective, but safety data are limited.

11. Management of contacts and the immediate environment— None, because of the high prevalence of asymptomatic shedders in the population.

12. Special considerations—None.

[T. M. Lanzieri, S. R. Bialek]

DENGUE

DISEASE	ICD-10 CODE
DENGUE FEVER	ICD-10 A90
DENGUE HEMORRHAGIC FEVER	ICD-10 A91

DENGUE FEVER, DENGUE HEMORRHAGIC FEVER/ DENGUE SHOCK SYNDROME, SEVERE DENGUE

1. Clinical features—Dengue is a mild to moderately severe acute febrile illness that usually follows three phases: febrile, critical, and convalescent. Patients with dengue often have sudden onset of fever, which lasts for 2-7 days and may be biphasic. Other signs and symptoms include intense headache, myalgia, arthralgia, bone pain, retro-orbital pain, anorexia, vomiting, macular or maculopapular rash, and minor hemorrhagic manifestations, including petechiae, ecchymosis, purpura, epistaxis, bleeding gums, hematuria, or a positive tourniquet test. Some patients have injected oropharynx and facial erythema in the first 24-48 hours after onset. Warning signs of progression to severe dengue occur in the late febrile phase, around the time of defervescence, and include persistent vomiting, severe abdominal pain, mucosal bleeding, difficulty breathing, signs of hypovolemic shock, and rapid decline in platelet count with an increase in hematocrit (hemoconcentration).

The critical phase of dengue begins at defervescence and typically lasts 24-48 hours. Most patients clinically improve during this phase, but those with significant plasma leakage develop severe dengue as a result of a marked increase in vascular permeability. Initially, physiologic compensatory mechanisms maintain adequate circulation, which narrows pulse pressure as diastolic blood pressure increases. Patients may appear to be well despite early signs of shock. However, once hypotension develops, systolic blood pressure rapidly declines, and irreversible shock and death may ensue despite resuscitation. Patients with severe plasma leakage have pleural effusions or ascites, hypoproteinemia, and hemoconcentration. Patients can also develop hemorrhagic manifestations, including severe frank hemorrhage, hematemesis, hematochezia, melena, or menorrhagia, especially if they have prolonged shock. Patients with severe dengue may also present clinically as hepatitis, myocarditis, pancreatitis, and encephalitis.

The convalescent phase begins when plasma leakage subsides, and extravasated fluids (intravenous, pleural, abdominal) reabsorb, hemodynamic status stabilizes, and diuresis ensues. The hematocrit stabilizes or may fall because of the dilutional effect of the reabsorbed fluid, and the white cell count usually starts to rise, followed by a slow recovery of platelet count. Patients may develop a generalized erythematous rash with circular areas of nonerythematous skin. This convalescent-phase rash may desquamate and be pruritic.

Laboratory findings commonly include leucopenia, thrombocytopenia, hyponatremia, elevated aspartate aminotransferase and alanine aminotransferase, and a normal erythrocyte sedimentation rate. Some patients may have an elevated partial thromboplastin time and a decreased fibrinogen level (with a normal prothrombin time).

Differential diagnosis includes chikungunya and other epidemiologically relevant diseases listed under "Arboviral Fevers"; influenza; measles; rubella; malaria; leptospirosis; melioidosis, typhoid; scrub typhus; and other systemic febrile illnesses, especially those accompanied by rash.

Dengue hemorrhagic fever (DHF) and dengue shock syndrome (DSS) are now classified as subsets of severe dengue according to the 2009 WHO Guidelines. Timely identification of dengue patients with warning signs is critical to ensure proper anticipatory guidance and initiation of supportive treatment. Severe dengue can occur in both children and adults.

2. Causative agents—Dengue viruses (DENV) are flaviviruses and include 4 types (serotypes; DENV -1, -2, -3, -4). All 4 DENV serotypes can cause dengue and have been associated with severe dengue, including DHF/DSS with a fatal outcome. It is important to note, however, that the majority (~75%) of DENV infections are asymptomatic in both children and adults. Long-term, serotype-specific protective immunity is produced by infection with each serotype, but there is no long-term, cross-protective immunity following infection. An increased risk of severe dengue is associated with the presence of heterotypic antibody and with viral strains that have greater virulence and/or epidemic potential. DENV serotypes can be further defined into genotypes based on differences in the envelope gene sequence; molecular epidemiologic studies may assist in tracking disease transmission patterns.

3. Diagnosis—Laboratory confirmation of the clinical diagnosis of dengue can be made using a single serum specimen obtained during the febrile phase of the illness (days 0-7 after onset of fever) with diagnostic testing to detect DENV and immunoglobulin class M (IgM) anti-DENV. DENV viremia occurs for 5-6 days before and after fever onset. Molecular diagnostics by nucleic acid amplification, such as by reverse transcriptase polymerase chain reaction (RT-PCR), can detect DENV ribonucleic acid (RNA) with a higher sensitivity than virus isolation by cell culture, and multiplex RT-PCR provides serotype-specific results. Molecular diagnostics are now available in many dengue endemic areas. DENV can also be detected by an immunoassay for the nonstructural protein 1 (NS1) antigen; a soluble antigen present during the viremic period. While somewhat less sensitive than DENV detection by RT-PCR, NS1 antigen detection tests have become commercially available in many dengue endemic areas. Detection of IgM anti-DENV in the febrile phase may indicate a current or recent DENV infection, or in some settings, infection with another flavivirus because of antibody cross-reactivity. IgM anti-DENV becomes detectable in about 30% of dengue patients on the third day after fever onset and in almost all patients 6-7 days after fever onset. IgM capture anti-DENV enzyme-linked immunosorbent assay (ELISA) testing is widely available, and evaluation studies have identified commercially available microplate tests with high sensitivity and specificity, and low cross-reactivity with other flaviviruses.

Testing for immunoglobulin class G [IgG] anti-DENV is not useful for dengue diagnosis since a high proportion of persons in endemic areas have preexisting, cross-reactive IgG antibody from previous DENV infections (secondary DENV infection).

4. Occurrence—Dengue virus transmission has now become endemic in most countries located in the tropics and subtropics. In dengue endemic areas, transmission occurs year-round with peak disease incidence usually occurring during the rainy season and in areas of high *Aedes aegypti* prevalence. Most dengue endemic areas experience epidemic cycles at 2-5 year intervals, with disease incidence exceeding the expected annual increase in incidence. In most endemic areas, more than one DENV serotype will circulate over time, and usually 2 or more serotypes circulate simultaneously. In some island nations, DENV is reintroduced periodically and produces large epidemics, but with little or no transmission between introductions. In addition, places such as Taiwan and Queensland have annual DENV introductions with transmission and disease occurring only during a single dengue season. All tropical and subtropical regions of Asia, the Americas, the Caribbean, Oceania, and Africa should be considered at risk for dengue. Areas that border dengue endemic regions (e.g., northern Argentina and Brazil, USA-Mexico border) may experience DENV introductions and epidemics. Epidemics may occur wherever vectors are present and DENV is introduced, whether in urban or rural areas. Good risk maps for dengue are available, as well as mapping programs with real-time reporting of reported dengue activity.

5. Reservoir—Where endemic, DENV is maintained in a human/ *Ae. aegypti* mosquito cycle, in which human infections are either with or without symptoms. There is a sylvatic monkey/mosquito cycle, which may spill over into human populations of southeastern Asia and western Africa.

6. Incubation period—From 3-14 days, commonly 4-7 days.

7. Transmission—Bite of infective mosquitoes, principally *Ae. aegypti*. This is a day-biting species, with increased biting activity for 2 hours after sunrise and several hours before dusk. Dengue outbreaks have been attributed to *Ae. aegypti* and to a lesser extent, *Aedes albopictus*. The latter is a periurban species abundant in Asia that has now spread to the USA, the Caribbean, Central and South America, the Pacific, parts of southern Europe, and Africa. *Ae. albopictus* is less anthropophilic than *Ae. aegypti* and hence a less efficient epidemic vector. Other *Aedes* spp. mosquitoes associated with DENV transmission include *Aedes polynesiensis* and several species of the *Aedes scutellaris* complex. Each of these species has a particular ecology, behavior, and geographical distribution. Patients are infective for mosquitoes during their period of viremia, from shortly before, until the end of the febrile period. The mosquito becomes infective 8-12 days after the viremic blood-meal and remains so for life. Because of the approximately 7-day viremia in infected persons, bloodborne transmission is possible through exposure to infected blood, organs, or other tissues. In addition, perinatal DENV transmission occurs with the highest risk among infants born to mothers acutely ill around the time of delivery.

8. Risk groups—People of all ages living in dengue endemic areas should be considered at risk of infection. In most areas, disease incidence is highest in children, although increasing numbers of adult cases are being reported from both rural and urban areas. Perinatal DENV transmission can occur with most reported cases being febrile, but temperature instability can also occur similar to other perinatal infections. Other findings have included hemorrhagic manifestations, hepatomegaly, and hypotension. In addition, infants infected with DENV at 6-12 months of age, and born to mothers previously infected with DENV, are at increased risk for severe dengue. This is thought to occur because of waning levels of transplacentally transferred maternal IgG anti-DENV and immune enhanced DENV infection.

Persons from dengue nonendemic areas traveling to dengue endemic areas for recreation, work, or to live are at risk for DENV infection and dengue. Dengue is the leading cause of febrile illness among travelers to the Caribbean, South America, and south central/southeast Asia.

9. Prevention—

    1) Presently no vaccine, chemoprophylaxis, or antiviral agent is available to prevent or treat dengue; prevention of bites from

the vector mosquito is the only means of prevention. Vector control includes public education and community programs to eliminate mosquito vector larval habitats, which for *Ae. aegypti* include water-holding containers close to or inside human habitation (e.g., old tires, flowerpots, trash, food, or water storage containers). Community surveys to determine the density of vector mosquitoes and identify productive larval habitats should complement plans for the elimination, management, or treatment of mosquito production sites with appropriate larvicides. Communities should be educated about personal protection against day-biting mosquitoes by using repellents, screening, and protective clothing (see "Malaria"). Prevention measures are required year-round; once increased dengue activity is identified it is usually too late for reactive vector control activities to be effective.

2) Because vector control and personal protection have generally been ineffective in preventing seasonal and epidemic increases in dengue or mitigating an epidemic once it has begun, timely identification of cases and good clinical management of dengue patients to prevent mortality and morbidity is essential. This should include ongoing education of the public about dengue and warning signs, ongoing education of health care professionals in best clinical practices, evaluation of health care practices related to clinical outcomes, and planning by health care facilities to meet demands placed upon them by the annual seasonal increase in cases or by periodic epidemics.

10. **Management of patient—**

1) Standard/bloodborne infection precautions. Until the fever subsides, prevent access of day-biting mosquitoes to patients by screening the sickroom or using a mosquito bed net, preferably insecticide-impregnated, or by spraying quarters with a knockdown adulticide or residual insecticide.

2) Treatment: there is no specific antiviral therapy for dengue. During the febrile phase, patients should be kept well hydrated and avoid use of aspirin (acetylsalicylic acid), aspirin-containing drugs, and other nonsteroidal anti-inflammatory drugs (e.g., ibuprofen) to control fever. Additional supportive care is required if the patient becomes dehydrated or develops warning signs for severe disease at the time of fever defervescence. Early recognition of shock (compensated or decompensated) and intensive supportive therapy for severe dengue can reduce risk of death from approximately 10% to less than 1%. During the critical phase, maintenance of fluid volume and hemodynamic

status is central to management of severe cases. Patients should be monitored for early signs of shock, occult bleeding, and resolution of plasma leak to avoid prolonged shock, end organ damage, and fluid overload. Patients with refractory shock may require intravenous colloids and/or blood or blood products after an initial trial of intravenous isotonic crystalloids. Reabsorption of extravascular fluid occurs during the convalescent phase with stabilization of hemodynamic status and diuresis. It is important to watch for signs of fluid overload; the patient's hematocrit stabilizes or may drop due to dilutional effect of reabsorbed fluid.

11. Management of contacts and the immediate environment—Determine patient's place of residence during the 2 weeks before onset of illness and search for unreported or undiagnosed cases residing there and in neighboring households.

12. Special considerations—

1) Reporting: obligatory reporting of dengue cases according to national health authority regulations. Dengue is a reportable condition in the USA and in most dengue-endemic countries. Dengue is a reportable condition under the International Health Regulations.

2) The 2009 WHO clinical case definition for dengue states that "dengue is one disease entity with different clinical presentations and often with unpredictable clinical evolution and outcome." Criteria for dengue warning signs are:

- live in/travel to dengue endemic area plus fever and 2 of the following criteria:

  o Nausea, vomiting
  o Rash
  o Aches and pains
  o Tourniquet test positive
  o Leukopenia

- Warning signs, which include: abdominal pain or tenderness, persistent vomiting, clinical fluid accumulation, mucosal bleeding, lethargy/restlessness, liver enlargement greater than 2 cm, increase in hematocrit test concurrent with rapid decrease in platelet count

3) Epidemic measures: epidemics can be extensive and affect a high percentage of the population. Response should include establishing enhanced surveillance for acute febrile illness or conducting seroincidence surveys to determine the extent of

the epidemic; ensuring availability of dengue diagnostic testing; ensuring appropriate medical care for cases and surge capacity in medical facilities to handle the increase in cases; coordinating community messages to ensure persons with symptoms seek medical attention; conducting vector surveys and source reduction activities; providing education in use of mosquito repellents for people exposed to vector mosquitoes; and where appropriate, applying indoor residual spraying to reduce adult mosquito populations guided by information from the vector surveys.

4) Improve international surveillance and exchange of data between countries.

Further information can be found at:

- http://www.cdc.gov/dengue
- http://www.who.int/tdr/publications/training-guideline-publications/dengue-diagnosis-treatment/en
- http://www.healthmap.org/dengue/index.php

[H. Margolis, K. Tomashek, E. Hunsperger, J. Muñoz]

DIPHTHERIA

DISEASE	ICD-10 CODE
DIPHTHERIA	ICD-10 A36

1. Clinical features—An acute bacterial disease primarily involving the mucous membrane of the upper respiratory tract (nose, tonsils, pharynx, larynx), skin, or rarely other mucous membranes (e.g., conjunctivae, vagina, or ear). Inapparent infections (colonization) outnumber clinical cases. The characteristic lesion, caused by reaction to a potent exotoxin, is an asymmetrical adherent greyish white membrane with surrounding inflammation. In moderate to severe cases of respiratory diphtheria, the throat may be moderately to severely sore with enlarged and tender cervical lymph nodes and, together with marked swelling of the neck, can give rise to a "bull neck" appearance. Pharyngeal membranes may extend into the trachea or progress to cause airway obstruction. Nasal diphtheria can be mild and chronic with one-sided serosanguinous nasal discharge and excoriations. The lesions of cutaneous diphtheria are variable and may be indistinguishable from impetigo. Absorption of diphtheria toxin can lead to myocarditis, with heart block and progressive congestive failure beginning about 1 week after onset. Neurologic complications may occur about 2 weeks after onset of illness and include polyneuropathies that can mimic Guillain-Barré syndrome. The case-fatality rate is 5%-10% for respiratory diphtheria even with treatment and has changed little in the past 50 years.

Respiratory diphtheria should be suspected in the differential diagnosis of membranous pharyngitis that includes streptococcal pharyngitis, Vincent angina, infectious mononucleosis, oral syphilis, oral candidiasis, and adenoviruses.

2. **Causative agent**—Toxin-producing strains of *Corynebacterium diphtheriae*. There are 4 biotypes: gravis, mitis, intermedius, and belfanti. Toxin production results when bacteria are infected by corynebacteriophage containing the diphtheria toxin gene *tox*. Nontoxigenic strains may cause sore throat but rarely produce membranous lesions; however, they are increasingly associated with infective endocarditis.

3. **Diagnosis**—Presumptive diagnosis is based on observation of an asymmetrical, adherent grayish membrane associated with tonsillitis, pharyngitis, or a serosanguinous nasal discharge. The diagnosis is confirmed by bacteriological examination of lesions. If respiratory diphtheria is strongly suspected, specific treatment with antitoxin and antibiotics should be initiated without awaiting laboratory confirmation by culture and continued even if the laboratory report is negative. Delay in starting treatment is associated with increased risk for complications and death.

4. **Occurrence**—A disease of colder months in temperate zones. In the tropics, seasonal trends are less distinct; inapparent, cutaneous, and wound diphtheria are much more common. Diphtheria epidemics can occur in susceptible populations. In 1990, for example, a massive outbreak began in Russia after diphtheria immunization was stopped, and it spread to all countries of the former Soviet Union and Mongolia where immunizations had also been stopped. The outbreak was responsible for more than 150,000 reported cases and 5,000 deaths between 1990 and 1997.

In Ecuador, an outbreak of about 200 cases occurred in 1993-1994; about 50% of cases occurred in persons aged 15 years or older. In both epidemics, control was achieved through mass immunization campaigns. More recently, outbreaks have occurred in Haiti, Sudan, Indonesia, Thailand, and Lao People's Democratic Republic.

5. **Reservoir**—Humans.

6. **Incubation period**—Usually 2-5 days, occasionally longer.

7. **Transmission**—Contact with a patient or carrier; more rarely, contact with articles soiled with discharges from lesions of infected people including raw milk that has served as a vehicle. Period of communicability

is variable, until virulent bacilli have disappeared from discharges and lesions; usually 2 weeks or less, seldom more than 4 weeks for respiratory diphtheria. The rare chronic carrier may shed organisms for 6 months or more. Effective antibiotic therapy promptly terminates shedding.

8. Risk groups—Occurs primarily in nonimmunized or underimmunized children younger than 15 years but may be found among adult population groups with low vaccination coverage. Infants born to immune mothers have passive protection, which is usually lost before the sixth month. Disease or inapparent infection may induce long-lasting or lifelong immunity but do not always do so.

Immunization with diphtheria toxoid produces prolonged but not lifelong immunity. Immunity wanes with increasing age. Serosurveys in developed countries indicate that more than 40% of adults lack protective levels of circulating antibodies. Older adults may have immunological memory and may be protected against disease after exposure. Immunity induced by diphtheria toxoid protects against toxin-mediated systemic disease but not against colonization in the nasopharynx.

9. Prevention—

1) Educational measures are important: inform the public, particularly parents of young children, of the hazards of diphtheria and the need for active immunization.

2) The only effective control is widespread active immunization with diphtheria toxoid. Immunization should be initiated in infancy with a formulation containing diphtheria toxoid, tetanus toxoid, and either diphtheria/tetanus and acellular pertussis vaccine (DTaP) or diphtheria/tetanus and whole-cell pertussis vaccine (DTwP). Some currently available formulations combine DTwP or DTaP with one or more of the following: *Haemophilus influenzae* type B vaccine, inactivated poliomyelitis vaccine, or hepatitis B vaccine.

3) The schedule recommended in developing countries is at least 3 primary doses intramuscular (IM) at 6, 10, and 14 weeks of age; and a diphtheria/tetanus and whole-cell pertussis vaccine (DTP) booster at 1–6 years of age. The following schedules are recommended for use in industrialized countries (some countries may recommend different ages or dosages):

   ● Recommended immunization schedule for persons aged 0–18 years: vaccination is recommended with a primary series of diphtheria toxoid combined with other antigens, such as DTaP, or DTaP–*Haemophilus influenzae* type b (Hib), DTaP-HB-inactivated polio vaccine. The first 3 doses are given at 4-week to 8-week intervals beginning when the infant is 6–8 weeks of age;

a fourth dose is given 6–12 months after the third dose. This schedule should not entail restarting immunizations because of delays in administering scheduled doses. A fifth dose is given at 4–6 years of age, prior to school entry; this dose is not necessary if the fourth dose was given after the fourth birthday. If the pertussis component of DTP is contraindicated, diphtheria/tetanus vaccine (DT) for children should be substituted. A booster dose with an adult formulation, tetanus, diphtheria, and acellular pertussis (Tdap; or tetanus and diphtheria [Td] if Tdap is unavailable), is recommended at 11–18 years of age.

- Previously unvaccinated persons older than 7 years: because adverse reactions may increase with age, a preparation with a reduced concentration of diphtheria toxoid (adult Td) is usually given after the seventh birthday for booster doses. For a previously unimmunized person, a primary 3-dose series of adsorbed tetanus and diphtheria toxoids (Td) is advised. Two doses are given at a 4- to 8-week interval, and the third dose is given 6 months to 1 year after the second dose. If the person is aged 10 years or older, a dose of Tdap may be substituted for a single Td dose in the series. Limited data from Sweden suggest that the 3-dose Td regimen may not induce protective diphtheria antibody levels in most adults, and additional doses may be needed.

- Active protection should be maintained by administering a dose of Td every 10 years thereafter. A 1-time dose of Tdap may be substituted for the next Td dose in persons aged 19–64 years, for added protection against pertussis.

4) Special efforts should be made to ensure that those who are at higher risk of patient exposure, such as health workers, are fully immunized and receive a booster dose of Td every 10 years.

5) For those who are severely immunocompromised or infected with HIV, diphtheria immunization is indicated, with the same schedule and dose as for immunocompetent persons, even though immune response may be suboptimal.

10. Management of patient—

1) Droplet precautions (face mask) for pharyngeal diphtheria and contact isolation for cutaneous diphtheria, until 2 cultures from both throat and nose (and skin lesions in cutaneous diphtheria), taken at least 24 hours apart and at least 24 hours after cessation of antibiotic therapy, fail to grow *C. diphtheriae*. Where culture is impractical, droplet precautions may end after 14 days of appropriate antibiotic therapy (see Treatment in Management of Patient in this chapter).

2) Concurrent disinfection of all articles in contact with patient and all articles soiled by discharges of patient. Terminal cleaning.

3) Treatment: diphtheria antitoxin is the specific treatment for respiratory diphtheria. Sensitivity testing (skin or eye testing) should be undertaken before giving antitoxin. After completion of tests to rule out hypersensitivity, a single dose of antitoxin should be given intramuscularly immediately after bacteriological specimens are taken, without waiting for results. Antibiotics are not a substitute for antitoxin but will eliminate *C. diphtheriae* and halt toxin production, and reduce communicability. Procaine penicillin G (IM) or parenteral erythromycin is recommended until the patient can swallow comfortably. Oral erythromycin or oral penicillin V may be substituted for a recommended total treatment period of 14 days.

4) Prophylactic treatment of carriers: A single dose of benzathine penicillin G (IM) or a 7–10 day course of erythromycin has been recommended.

11. **Management of contacts and the immediate environment—**

1) All close contacts, (e.g., householders) should have swabs taken from nose and throat for culture of *C. diphtheriae,* and should be kept under surveillance for 7 days. A single dose of benzathine penicillin (IM) or a 7–10 day course of erythromycin is recommended for all close contacts, regardless of immunization status. Contacts who do not receive prophylaxis should be monitored for 7 days and treated as diphtheria if symptoms develop.

2) Adult contacts whose occupations involve handling food (especially milk) or close association with nonimmunized children should be excluded from that work until treated as described later and until bacteriological examination proves them not to be carriers.

3) Previously immunized contacts should receive a booster dose of diphtheria toxoid if more than 5 years have elapsed since their last dose, and in nonimmunized contacts, a primary series should be initiated; use Td, DT, DTP, DTaP or DTP-Hib, DTP-HepB-IPV, or Tdap combination vaccine, depending on the contact's age and indication for other components.

4) Searching for carriers by culture of nasal and throat specimens, other than among close contacts, is neither useful nor indicated if provisions mentioned earlier are carried out.

12. **Special considerations—**

1) Reporting: case report to local health authority obligatory in most countries.

2) Outbreaks can occur when social or natural conditions lead to crowding of susceptible groups, especially infants and children. This frequently occurs when there are large-scale movements of susceptible populations.

3) Epidemic measures:

- Immunize the largest possible proportion of the population group involved, especially infants and preschool children. In an epidemic involving adults, immunize groups that are most affected or at high risk. Repeat immunization procedures 1 month later to provide at least 2 doses to recipients.

- Identify close contacts and define population groups at special risk. In areas with appropriate facilities, carry out a prompt field investigation of reported cases to verify the diagnosis and to determine the biotype and toxigenicity of *C. diphtheriae*.

4) People traveling to or through countries where either respiratory or cutaneous diphtheria is common should receive primary immunization if necessary, or a booster dose of Td for those previously immunized.

[T. S. P. Tiwari]

DRACUNCULIASIS
(guinea worm disease, dracunculiasis)

DISEASE	ICD-10 CODE
DRACUNCULIASIS	ICD-10 B72

1. Clinical features—An infection of the subcutaneous and deeper tissues by a large nematode. A blister appears, often on a lower extremity (especially the foot) when the gravid, adult (60–100 cm long) female worm is ready to discharge its larvae. Burning and itching of the skin in the area of the lesion, and frequently fever, nausea, vomiting, diarrhea, dizziness, generalized urticaria, and eosinophilia, may accompany or precede vesicle formation. After the vesicle ruptures, the worm discharges larvae whenever the affected part is immersed in fresh water. The prognosis is good unless bacterial infection of the lesion occurs; such secondary infections may produce arthritis, synovitis, ankylosis, and contractures of the involved limb.

Tetanus infections may occur via the site of the lesion. Infection may be life-threatening as a result of complications from secondary infections.

2. **Causative agent**—*Dracunculus medinensis*, a nematode.

3. **Diagnosis**—By visual recognition of the adult worm protruding from a skin lesion. For programmatic purposes (not clinical use), *Dracunculus* can also be identified by microscopic identification of larvae within a worm specimen and the species determined by polymerase chain reaction (PCR).

4. **Occurrence**—Under eradication. In Africa, remains in 4 countries south of the Sahara: Ethiopia, Chad, Mali, and South Sudan. As of 2013, infection had been eliminated from 16 formerly endemic countries by the Guinea Worm Eradication Program.

5. **Reservoir**—Humans.

6. **Incubation period**—Approximately 10-14 months.

7. **Transmission**—Larvae discharged by the female worm into stagnant fresh water are ingested by minute crustacean copepods (*Cyclops* spp.). In about 2 weeks, the larvae develop into the infective stage. People swallow the infected copepods in drinking water from infested wells, ponds, and other stagnant surface water. The larvae are liberated in the stomach, cross the duodenal wall, migrate through the connective tissue, and become adults. The female, after mating, grows and develops to full maturity, then migrates to the subcutaneous tissues (most frequently of the legs). The period of communicability lasts from rupture of vesicle until larvae have been completely evacuated from the uterus of the gravid worm, likely a few days to a few weeks. In water, the larvae are infective for the copepods for about 3-5 days. After ingestion by copepods, the larvae become infective for people after 12-14 days at temperatures above 25°C (77°F). No direct person-to-person transmission.

8. **Risk groups**—Susceptibility is universal. Multiple and repeated infections may occur in the same person.

9. **Prevention**—In addition to disease surveillance and prevention of patients with emerging worms from contaminating water supplies, the provision of uncontaminated water from protected wells and flowing surface water sources, filtered drinking water, treatment of stagnant sources of drinking water with the insecticide temephos, and health education of the populations at risk, are leading to eradication of the disease.

1) Provide health education programs in endemic communities to convey 3 messages:

- Guinea worm infection comes from drinking unsafe water.
- In endemic areas, people with blisters or ulcers should not enter any source of drinking water.
- Drinking water should be filtered through fine mesh cloth (e.g., nylon gauze with a mesh size of 100 μm) or through pipe filters (with the same mesh size) to remove copepods.

2) Provide safe water. Construct and maintain protected water sources, such as boreholes, protected wells, and rainwater catchments, to provide uncontaminated water. Provide filter cloths and pipe filters to at-risk populations along with training on their proper use.

3) Eliminate copepod populations in ponds, tanks, reservoirs, and wells within 14 days of suspected contamination by applying temephos, where feasible.

10. Management of patient—

1) Prevent patients with emerging worms from entering and contaminating drinking water sources.

2) Treatment: wrap the emerging worm around a piece of gauze or a small stick and slowly pull the worm out, a few centimeters per day. Clean the wound and provide local treatment with antibiotic ointment and occlusive bandaging. Give tetanus toxoid if available. Aseptic surgical extraction just prior to worm emergence is only possible on an individual basis but not applicable as a public health measure of eradication. Drugs, such as thiabendazole, albendazole, ivermectin, and metronidazole, have no therapeutic value.

11. Management of contacts and the immediate environment—
Obtain information as to source of drinking water at probable time of infection (~1 year previously). Obtain information about contamination of possible drinking water supplies at time of worm emergence and treat these sources with temephos within about 14 days of contamination, if feasible. Search for other cases.

12. Special considerations—

1) Reporting: case report to local health authority required wherever the disease occurs, as part of the WHO eradication program.

2) Epidemic measures: wherever cases are identified, field survey to determine prevalence, discover sources of infection, and guide control/eradication measures as described under "Infection Prevention and Control."

3) Further information can be found at: http://www.cdc.gov/ parasites/guineaworm and http://www.who.int/dracunculiasis/ en.

[S. Roy, M. Eberhard]

E. COLI DIARRHEAL DISEASES

DISEASE	ICD-10 CODE
SHIGA TOXIN-PRODUCING E. COLI	ICD-10 A04.3
ENTEROTOXIGENIC E. COLI	ICD-10 A04.1
ENTEROPATHOGENIC E. COLI	ICD-10 A04.0
ENTEROINVASIVE E. COLI	ICD-10 A04.2
INTESTINAL E. COLI INFECTION, OTHER	ICD-10 A04.4

I. SHIGA TOXIN-PRODUCING E. COLI (STEC)
(verotoxin-producing E. coli E. coli O157:H7, enterohemorrhagic E. coli)

1. Clinical features—The diarrhea may range from mild and non-bloody to stools that are virtually all blood; abdominal cramps are often severe. The most severe manifestation of STEC infection is hemolytic uremic syndrome (HUS), a thrombotic microangiopathy occurring in both children and adults that is characterized by hemolytic anemia, thrombocytopenia, and acute renal dysfunction. The term D+HUS is used to describe HUS that follows a diarrheal illness, and it may be associated with neurologic abnormalities. STEC is the primary cause of D+HUS. Adults with D+HUS are often misdiagnosed as having thrombotic thrombocytopenic purpura (TTP), a different thrombotic microangiopathy unrelated to STEC infection. Most D+HUS patients with an identified etiology show evidence of infection with STEC that produce Shiga toxin 2 (Stx2). Stx2 is produced by virtually all STEC O157 strains causing human illness. STEC O157 causes the most D+HUS cases worldwide. About 15% of young children and a much smaller proportion of adults with STEC O157 diarrhea develop D+HUS. However, in an outbreak in Germany of a rare enteroaggregative STEC O104:H4 infections, principally among adults, the reported percentage who developed D+HUS was 22%. About 55% of patients with STEC O157 D+HUS require dialysis and 5% die; rates vary for other serotypes.

2. Causative agent—STEC is a heterogeneous group of bacteria that express potent cytotoxins called Shiga toxins 1 and 2 (Stx1 and Stx2 are also called verocytotoxins or verotoxins). Stx1 is essentially identical to the toxin produced by *Shigella dysenteriae* 1; D$^+$HUS is also a complication of *S. dysenteriae* 1 infection. STEC that produce certain Stx2 subtypes (e.g., Stx2a and Stx2d) tend to be more virulent. In North America, approximately 70% of D$^+$HUS cases have laboratory evidence of antecedent STEC infection; approximately 95% of these are STEC O157. The percentage of D$^+$HUS attributable to STEC O157 in industrialized countries is generally 50% or greater, but ranges from nearly 100% in the UK to approximately 20%–80% in other European countries to less than 20% in Australia. Over 70 STEC serogroups have been isolated from ill persons. After O157, the most common serogroups isolated from persons with diarrheal illness in North America are O26, O111, O103, O45, O145, and O121. STEC strains vary considerably in their virulence, from strains of no apparent human virulence detected primarily in animals to others causing severe human disease and outbreaks. The pathogenesis of STEC is complex and involves several virulence factors. In addition to the Shiga toxins, STEC must also express intestinal adherence factors to cause disease. A common adherence factor among STEC is intimin (encoded by *eae*; see EPEC section in this chapter).

3. Diagnosis—*Escherichia coli* O157:H7 infections are diagnosed by culturing the organism on a specialized selective isolation medium such as cefixime-tellurite sorbitol MacConkey Agar or CHROMAgar O157 (CHROM) and confirming that the strain is biochemically identified as *E. coli* and either has the O157 antigen and produces Stx or has the H7 antigen. Non-O157 STEC infections may be diagnosed by testing fecal specimens for Shiga toxin using an immunoassay or cell culture that detects all STEC serotypes including O157:H7. Alternately, polymerase chain reaction (PCR) for Stx1 and Stx2 genes may be used to test growth from an agar plate. A positive result from a Shiga toxin assay, in the absence of simultaneous isolation or molecular detection of *E. coli* O157:H7, should be followed up with determination of serogroup at a reference laboratory. Specimens should be collected as close to the onset of symptoms as possible to avoid loss of the phages that carry the Stx genes. Positive findings should be reported promptly for patient management, and to public health authorities for the detection and control of outbreaks.

4. Occurrence—An important problem in North America, Europe, Japan, Australia, and the southern cone of South America. Their importance in the rest of the world is less well-established.

5. Reservoir—Cattle are the most important reservoir of STEC O157; cattle also harbor many non-O157 STEC. Other ruminants, including sheep, goats, and deer, may carry STEC. Humans may serve as a reservoir for person-to-person transmission.

6. Incubation period—2-10 days, with a median of 3-4 days for most serotypes. In the *E. coli* O104:H4 outbreak in Germany in 2011, the median incubation was 8 days.

7. Transmission—Mainly through ingestion of food contaminated with ruminant feces and direct contact with animals or their environment. Outbreaks, including cases of hemorrhagic colitis, HUS, and death, have occurred from beef (usually as inadequately cooked hamburgers); produce (including lettuce, apple cider, raw spinach, coleslaw, sprouts, and melons); and unpasteurized cows' milk. Outbreaks in children have been associated with petting zoos. Direct person-to-person transmission can occur in families, child care centers, and custodial institutions. Waterborne transmission occurs both from contaminated drinking water and from recreational waters. The infectious dose is very low. The duration of excretion of the pathogen is typically 1 week or less in adults, but 3 weeks in one-third of children. Prolonged carriage is uncommon.

8. Risk groups—Infections and D⁺HUS occur in persons of all ages. Children 1-4 years are most frequently diagnosed with infection and, in general, are at greatest risk of developing HUS. Older adults are at highest risk of death from D⁺HUS.

9. Prevention—

1) Investigate measures to limit the prevalence of carriers in cattle herds. Decrease the carriage and excretion of STEC O157 in cattle on farms, through improved farm management practices, especially in the days just before slaughter and with particular emphasis on reducing super-shedders (i.e., animals that excrete $>10^4$ colony forming units of STEC O157/g of feces).

2) Manage slaughterhouse operations to minimize contamination of meat by animal hides and intestinal contents.

3) Decrease contamination with animal feces of foods consumed with no or minimal cooking, including considerations about location of animal farming, agricultural produce fields, and their water sources.

4) Pasteurize milk, other dairy products, juices, and ciders.

5) Wash fruits and vegetables, particularly if eaten raw. Peel raw fruits when possible.

6) Avoid consumption of raw sprouts, especially by those most susceptible to severe complications of foodborne infections (young children, the elderly, pregnant women, and persons with compromised immune systems).

7) Cook beef adequately, especially ground beef, to an internal temperature of 70°C (160°F). Do not rely on cooking until all pink color is gone. Use a meat thermometer.

8) Protect, purify, and chlorinate public water supplies; chlorinate swimming pools. When the safety of drinking water is doubtful, boil it.

9) Wash hands thoroughly and frequently using soap, in particular after contact with farm animals or the farm environment.

10) Strengthen control measures for exhibits that allow contact with animals or their environment in public settings, such as fairs, farm tours, petting zoos, camps, and schools, and educate populations at risk about the risks associated with attending such events.

11) Ensure adequate hygiene and frequent handwashing with soap in child care centers and in petting zoos and other animal displays.

10. Management of patient—

1) The following recommendations apply to all diarrheagenic *E. coli* (i.e., STEC, ETEC, EPEC, EIEC, enteroaggregative *E. coli* [EAEC], and diffuse-adherence *E. coli* [DAEC]): general enteric precautions should be taken, including instructing family members to thoroughly wash hands after defecation, after caring for infected persons, and before handling food or caring for other persons, and to properly dispose of soiled diapers/ nappies and human waste. Disinfect contaminated articles by washing in hot water. In communities with an adequate sewage disposal system, feces can be discharged directly into sewers without preliminary disinfection. Fluid replacement is the cornerstone of treatment for diarrhea.

2) Data from observational studies suggest that some antimicrobial agents increase the risk of HUS. Most experts do not use an antimicrobial agent to treat persons with STEC O157 or other virulent STEC infections because no benefit has been proven, and harm is possible.

3) For O157 and other virulent STEC infections, prompt rehydration is beneficial to attenuate the severity of colitis and the possible resulting D+HUS, and to monitor for development of D+HUS (a rising platelet count suggests a lower risk, a leukocyte count $\geq 13,000/\mu L$ in the first 3 days of illness suggests a higher risk). Hospitalization may have an added benefit of reducing secondary spread.

4) There is no clear evidence to support the use of complement inhibitors or plasma exchange therapy in D+HUS.

11. Management of contacts and the immediate environment—

1) Because of the small infective dose, infected persons should not be employed to handle food or to provide child or patient care until 2 successive negative fecal samples or rectal swabs are

obtained (collected 24 hours apart and not sooner than 48 hours after the last dose of antimicrobials).

2) When feasible, persons with diarrhea should not handle food that will be eaten by others and should not care for children within their own homes until diarrhea ceases and 2 successive stool cultures are negative.

3) Cultures of asymptomatic contacts should generally be confined to food handlers, attendants, and children in child care centers and other settings where the spread of infection is particularly likely.

4) Culture of suspected foods, livestock feces, and agricultural environmental samples can be useful in some settings, particularly outbreaks, especially when laboratories use selective broth enrichment, immunomagnetic separation methods, and plating on selective media.

12. **Special considerations—**

1) Reporting: case report of STEC infection to local health authority is obligatory in many countries. The potential severity of this infection calls for early involvement of local health authorities to identify the source and apply appropriate preventive measures.

2) Epidemic measures:

- Report at once to the local health authority any group of persons with acute bloody diarrhea, D+HUS, or TTP (TTP clusters may be misdiagnosed HUS cases), even in the absence of identification of the causal agent.

- Initiate epidemiologic investigations to: (a) identify specific transmission vehicle(s) (e.g., food, water, animal contact); (b) evaluate for ongoing person-to-person transmission; and (c) implement control measures.

- Collaborate with regulatory agencies to trace the source of suspected food and recall any implicated product to prevent additional cases.

- If a waterborne outbreak is suspected, issue an order to boil water and chlorinate suspected water supplies adequately under competent supervision, or do not use them.

- If a swimming-associated outbreak is suspected, close pools or beaches until chlorinated or shown to be free of fecal contamination, and until adequate toilet facilities are provided to prevent contamination of water by bathers.

- If a milkborne outbreak is suspected, evaluate the possibility of postpasteurization contamination, and assure that people only consume milk that is pasteurized or boiled.

- Prophylactic administration of antimicrobial agents is not recommended.
- Publicize the importance of hand washing after defecation; provide equipment for proper hand washing with soap and individual paper towels in public venues.

3) Disaster implications: a potential problem where personal hygiene and environmental sanitation are deficient (see "Typhoid Fever").

Further information can be found at:

- http://whqlibdoc.who.int/hq/1994/WHO_FNU_FOS_94.5.pdf
- http://www.who.int/foodsafety/publications/consumer/manual_ keys
- http://www.cdc.gov/mmwr/pdf/rr/rr6004.pdf

II. ENTEROTOXIGENIC *E. COLI* (ETEC)

1. Clinical features—Enterotoxigenic *E. coli* (ETEC) strains are an important cause of diarrhea in developing countries, particularly among young children. ETEC are a frequent cause of travelers' diarrhea. The severity of illness can range from mild watery diarrhea to severe cholera-like purging, as the enterotoxigenic strains may behave like *Vibrio cholerae* in producing a profuse watery diarrhea without blood or mucus. Abdominal cramping, vomiting, acidosis, prostration, and dehydration can occur; low-grade fever may or may not be present; symptoms usually last less than 5 days, but may last longer in previously unexposed travelers. ETEC are responsible for significant rates of morbidity and mortality among children in developing countries, where mortality rates may be as high as 16%-32% in children 4 years old or younger.

2. Causative agent—ETEC are a heterogeneous group of noninvasive *E. coli* that colonize the small intestine and produce a heat-labile enterotoxin (LT), a heat-stable enterotoxin (ST), or both toxins (LT/ST). Serotypes O6:H16 and O169:H41 have been implicated in most North American ETEC outbreaks, but more than 20 O antigens and more than 30 H antigens have been identified. *E. coli* enterotoxins have been purified and sequenced and are on plasmids. Strains that produce ST only or ST in combination with LT have caused most North American ETEC outbreaks.

3. Diagnosis—Infections are usually diagnosed only during outbreak investigations because few clinical laboratories have the resources to routinely perform the specialized tests required to isolate and identify ETEC. ETEC strains are most often identified by PCR detection of the ST and LT genes, but immunoassays for the identification of ST or LT from culture supernatants are available from at least 2 commercial sources. Testing for ETEC typically is available only through reference or public health laboratories. Reporting of ETEC isolations provides a retrospective diagnosis.

4. Occurrence—An infection detected primarily in developing countries and in travelers returning from these countries. The role of ETEC as a cause of sporadic diarrhea in developed countries is largely unknown because most clinical laboratories do not test for these organisms. During the first 3 years of life, children in developing countries experience multiple ETEC infections that lead to the acquisition of immunity; consequently, illness in older children and adults occurs less frequently. ETEC is also a major cause of travelers' diarrhea in people from industrialized countries who visit developing countries. ETEC transmission has also occurred on cruise ships. WHO estimates that ETEC causes as many as 380,000 deaths annually in children younger than 5 years.

5. Reservoir—Humans. Although ETEC infections occur in animals, people constitute the reservoir for strains causing diarrhea in humans.

6. Incubation period—Incubations as short as 10–12 hours have been observed in outbreaks and in volunteer studies with certain LT-only and ST-only strains. The incubation period of LT/ST diarrhea in volunteer studies has usually been 24–72 hours.

7. Transmission—Through contaminated food and water. Transmission via contaminated weaning foods may be particularly important in infants. Direct contact transmission through feces-contaminated hands is believed to be rare. The period of communicability lasts for the duration of excretion of ETEC, which may be prolonged.

8. Risk groups—Children younger than 5 years in developing countries; travelers visiting developing countries. Multiple infections with different serotypes are required to develop broad-spectrum immunity against ETEC. Preexisting malnutrition, including micronutrient deficiency, can lead to more severe infections.

9. Prevention—

1) For general measures for prevention of fecal-oral spread of infection, see "Typhoid Fever."
2) Travelers to areas where the safety of the water and food supply is uncertain should be advised to drink only bottled or canned beverages and boiled or bottled water; travelers should avoid ice, raw produce including salads, and fruit they have not peeled themselves. Cooked foods should be eaten hot.
3) For adult travelers going for short periods to high-risk areas where it is not easy to obtain safe food or water, the use of prophylactic bismuth subsalicylate may be considered.

Although some physicians provide prophylactic antimicrobial agents, these can actually increase the risk of enteric infection. A much preferable approach is to initiate very early treatment, near the onset of diarrhea (e.g., after the second or third loose stool). Packets of oral rehydration salts can be added to boiled or bottled water and ingested to maintain fluid balance.

10. **Management of patient—**

   1) See general recommendations for all diarrheagenic *E. coli* in the STEC section in this chapter.
   2) Treatment: electrolyte-fluid therapy to prevent or treat dehydration is the most important measure (see "Cholera and Other Vibrioses"). Most people do not require any other treatment. For severe travelers' diarrhea in adults, early treatment with an antimicrobial agent such as a fluoroquinolone (e.g., ciprofloxacin or norfloxacin) for 5 days. Fluoroquinolones are used as initial treatment because many ETEC strains worldwide are resistant to other agents. However, if local strains are known to be sensitive, trimethoprim-sulfoxazole or doxycycline for 5 days can be used. Feeding should be continued according to the patient's appetite.

11. **Management of contacts and the immediate environment—**

   1) When feasible, persons with diarrhea should not handle food that will be eaten by others and should not care for young children until diarrhea ceases.
   2) Ill food handlers with ETEC isolated from stool should have 2 negative stool cultures taken 24 hours apart and at least 48 hours after receipt of antimicrobial agents before handling food.

12. **Special considerations—**

   1) Reporting: since infection is rarely confirmed by culture, ETEC is generally not a notifiable infection.
   2) Epidemic measures: epidemiological investigation is indicated to determine how transmission is occurring. In an outbreak setting, ETEC testing should be considered if the clinical presentation is compatible and the results of bacterial cultures for routine enteric pathogens are negative.

III. ENTEROPATHOGENIC *E. COLI* (EPEC)

   1. Clinical features—Infection is mainly among children younger than 2 years, in whom it causes watery diarrhea with mucus, fever, and dehydration. It can be severe and prolonged or persistent, and in developing countries may be associated with high case-fatality rates.

2. Causative agent—EPEC strains have traditionally been defined as certain *E. coli* serotypes epidemiologically associated with severe diarrhea in infants but that do not produce Shiga toxin or enterotoxin and are not invasive. Traditional EPEC strains that have caused outbreaks fall into these serogroups: O55, O111, O114, O119, O125, O127, O128, O142, and O157 (non-Shiga toxin-producing O157:H45). These strains demonstrate a distinct pattern of localized adherence to HeLa and Hep-2 cells and have the chromosomal locus of enterocyte effacement, which mediates the attaching-and-effacing phenotype and for which the intimin gene (*eae*) serves as a marker. Located on the EPEC adherence factor plasmid, the pilin subunit of the bundle-forming pilus (bfpA) gene encodes a fimbrial adhesion that mediates the localized Hep-2 adherence pattern. The term "typical EPEC" has been suggested for those organisms harboring both the EPEC adherence factor plasmid and the locus of enterocyte effacement pathogenicity island and therefore have both *eae* and bfpA markers (usually detected by PCR). More recently, atypical EPEC have been implicated as enteric pathogens; these strains possess *eae* but not bfpA. Many STEC and *Escherichia albertii* also have the *eae* gene and express intimin.

3. Diagnosis—EPEC infection is diagnosed by culturing diarrheal fecal specimens for *E. coli* that possess *eae*, that exhibit localized adherence in Hep-2 or HeLa cells, or that demonstrate the attaching-and-effacing phenotype. No commercial tests are available. Testing for EPEC typically is available only through reference or public health laboratories. Antimicrobial susceptibility testing can inform treatment because most EPEC strains are multiply resistant. Reporting of EPEC isolations provides a retrospective diagnosis. The laboratory should provide the clinician an explanation of the clinical significance of EPEC in infantile diarrhea and refer the clinician to the reference or public health laboratory or the health department for further information.

4. Occurrence—Since the late 1960s, EPEC has largely disappeared as an important cause of outbreaks of infant diarrhea in North America and Europe. However, it remains a major agent of infant diarrhea in less developed areas of South America, sub-Saharan Africa, and Asia. Atypical EPEC may be common in both developed and developing countries, but not all cause diarrhea.

5. Reservoir—Humans.

6. Incubation period—As short as 9-12 hours in adult volunteer studies. It is not known whether the same incubation period applies to infants who acquire infection through natural transmission.

7. Transmission—Through contaminated infant formula, weaning foods, and water. In infant nurseries, transmission by fomites and by contaminated hands can occur if handwashing techniques are compromised. Outbreaks due to contaminated water and rice have been reported. The infection is communicable for the duration of excretion, which may be prolonged.

8. Risk groups—EPEC infection is uncommon in breastfed infants. Although susceptibility to clinical infection appears to be confined to infants in nature, it is not known whether this is because of immunity or age-related or other host factors. The induction of diarrhea in some adult volunteers suggests that specific immunity may be important in susceptibility.

9. Prevention—

1) The safest way to feed an infant younger than 6 months is to breastfeed exclusively. If the infant is fed formula prepared from commercial powder, the powder should be reconstituted with hot water at a temperature of at least 158°F (70°C). This precaution will kill most pathogens in the water and those with which the infant formula may have become contaminated during manufacturing or through handling after opening. To ensure that the water is hot enough (≥158°F [70°C]), prepare formula within 30 minutes after boiling the water for at least 1 minute.

2) Prevention of hospital outbreaks depends on washing hands between handling babies and maintaining high sanitary standards in the facilities in which babies are held. Provide individual equipment for each infant, including thermometers and stethoscopes, whenever possible. Clean and disinfect equipment that must be shared, like scales, between each use.

3) Practice rooming-in for mothers and infants in maternity facilities, unless there is a firm medical indication for separation. If mother or infant has a gastrointestinal or respiratory infection, keep the pair together but isolate them from healthy individuals. In special care facilities, separate infected infants from those who are premature or ill in other ways.

4) Train health professionals to support mothers to breastfeed and to safely prepare powdered formulas used to feed infants.

5) Ensure adequate hygiene and frequent handwashing with soap in child care centers.

10. Management of patient—

1) See general recommendations for all diarrheagenic *E. coli* in the STEC section in this chapter.

2) Treatment: electrolyte-fluid replacement (oral or intravenous [IV]) is the most important measure (see "Cholera"). In children younger than 5 years, give 20 mg (for children <6 months 10 mg) elemental zinc per day for 10–14 days. Most cases do not require any other treatment. For severe enteropathogenic infant diarrhea,

oral trimethoprim-sufamethoxazole ameliorates the severity and duration; it should be administered in 3–4 divided doses for 5 days. Because many EPEC strains are resistant to a variety of antimicrobial agents, selection should be based on the sensitivity of locally isolated strains. Feeding, including breastfeeding, must continue.

11. Management of contacts and the immediate environment— Discharged babies should be followed up, hand washing promoted, and safe feeding practices reinforced among mothers. The immediate environment should be thoroughly cleaned and disinfected. Also, see Epidemic Measures under EPEC section in this chapter.

12. Special considerations—

1) Reporting to local health authority: obligatory report of epidemics to local health authority in some countries. Two or more concurrent cases of diarrhea requiring treatment for these symptoms in a nursery or among those recently discharged should be interpreted as a possible outbreak requiring investigation.

2) Epidemic measures: for nursery epidemics, the following:

- All babies with diarrhea should be placed in one nursery under enteric precautions. Admit no more babies to the contaminated nursery. Promptly move each new infected infant to the single nursery used for these infants. Separate clean nurseries should be created for exposed or ill and healthy babies. For babies exposed in the contaminated nursery, provide separate medical and nursing personnel skilled in the care of infants with communicable diseases. Infected infants should be promptly discharged as soon as medically possible. Thorough cleaning and terminal disinfection is necessary after the discharge of infected babies, their mothers, and contacts. Observe contacts for at least 2 weeks after the last case leaves the nursery. Put into practice the prevention recommendations, insofar as feasible, during the emergency.

- Conduct a thorough epidemiological investigation into the distribution of cases by time, place, person, and exposure to risk factors, to determine how transmission is occurring.

Further information can be found at: http://www.who.int/foodsafety/publications/micro/pif2007/en/index.html.

IV. ENTEROINVASIVE E. COLI (EIEC)

1. Clinical features—This inflammatory disease of the gut mucosa and submucosa closely resembles that produced by *Shigella*. The organisms possess the same plasmid-dependent ability to invade and multiply within epithelial cells. EIEC is much more likely to cause watery diarrhea than dysentery (90% vs. 10% of patients). The O antigens of EIEC may cross-react with *Shigella* O antigens. Illness begins with severe abdominal cramps, malaise, watery stools, tenesmus, and fever.

2. Causative agent—EIEC strains invade cells of the colon by a pathogenic mechanism similar to that of *Shigella* but do not produce enterotoxins or demonstrate adherence in cell culture. They are associated with a few characteristic serogroups including O124, O143, and O164.

3. Diagnosis—EIEC cannot be distinguished from commensal *E. coli* strains by routine phenotypic screening techniques. Many are nonmotile and fail to decarboxylate lysine; however, some are motile or lysine positive. Most are lactose-nonfermenting. EIEC can be identified by various in vivo assays (invasiveness of guinea pig or rabbit conjunctiva [Sereny test], cell culture invasion assays), immunoassay, and nucleic acid-based assays (PCR assays) for the *ipaC* or *ipaH* invasion-related factors, but no commercial kits or reagents are available. Plasmid deoxyribonucleic acid (DNA) electrophoresis may be used to detect the large 120- to 140-MDa plasmid associated with invasiveness, but this plasmid is easily lost when the isolate is subcultured. Because of shared invasiveness-related characteristics, all of the above assays also detect *Shigella* strains. Testing for EIEC typically is available only through reference or public health laboratories. Reporting of EIEC isolations provides a retrospective diagnosis.

4. Occurrence—EIEC infections are endemic in developing countries and cause about 1%-5% of diarrheal episodes among people visiting treatment centers. Rarely, infections and outbreaks of EIEC diarrhea have been reported in industrialized countries.

5. Reservoir—Humans. There are no known animal hosts.

6. Incubation period—Incubation periods as short as 10 and 18 hours have been observed in volunteer studies and outbreaks, respectively.

7. Transmission—The scant available evidence suggests that EIEC is transmitted by contaminated food. It is communicable for as long as EIEC strains are excreted.

8. Risk groups—Children living in endemic areas. Travelers to developing countries where the disease is endemic.

9. Prevention—Same as for ETEC section in this chapter.

10. Management of patient—Same as for ETEC section in this chapter. For the rare cases of severe diarrhea, treat using antimicrobials effective against local *Shigella* isolates.

11. Management of contacts and the immediate environment— Same as for ETEC section in this chapter.

12. Special considerations—Few clinical or public health laboratories can diagnose EIEC, thus few patients are tested for this agent.

V. INTESTINAL E. COLI INFECTION, OTHER (enteroaggregative E. coli [EAEC], diarrhea caused by diffuse-adherent E. coli [DAEC])

1. Clinical features—EAEC is a cause of epidemic and sporadic diarrhea, yet its role as an enteric pathogen is not fully understood. EAEC is associated with persistent infant diarrhea (continuing unabated for ≥14 days). EAEC has also been associated with acute diarrhea. Diarrhea is watery with mucous. Bloody diarrhea has been reported in 3%-31%.

The pathogenicity of DAEC is uncertain. They have been implicated as a cause of diarrhea in some studies but not in others. The ability to cause epithelial cells to secrete a high amount of chemokine IL-8 seems to be linked to disease for certain strains. In a retrospective case-control study, the majority of infected children had watery diarrhea without blood or fecal leukocytes.

2. Causative agent—EAEC strains are a heterogeneous group of bacteria defined by their ability to adhere to Hep-2 cells in a pattern resembling stacked bricks. EAEC strains vary considerably in their virulence with subsets of pathogenic strains identified through studies and outbreak investigations. The pathogenesis of EAEC is complex and involves the production of various adhesins and accessory proteins that mediate adherence throughout the entire intestinal tract; the elaboration of one or more enterotoxins, cytotoxins, and proteases that mediate cytopathic effects on the epithelium; and the induction of cellular factors that may lead to mucosal inflammation. The adherence of EAEC to the intestinal epithelium results in increased mucus secretion, which forms a biofilm that entraps the bacteria onto the small intestinal epithelium. The adhesins for many EAEC have not been identified.

DAEC strains comprise a heterogeneous group of organisms that exhibit a diffuse pattern of adherence to Hep-2 cells in culture. A recent study showed that DAEC was significantly associated with diarrheal disease in children older than 12 months of age but not in children younger than 12 months of age. This finding is consistent with the fact that the cellular receptor (decay-accelerating factor or CD55) for the adhesion produced by most DAEC (F1845 adhesin) is not expressed until about 1 year of age. Binding of the bacteria to this receptor induces a cytopathic effect and is accompanied by activation of signal transduction cascades. Independently of this binding, DAEC may cause diarrhea by impairing the activities and reducing the abundance of brush-border-associated enzymes (sucrase-isomaltase and dipeptidylpeptidase intravenous [IV]). A role has been proposed for DAEC in inflammatory bowel disease by promoting proinflammatory responses through the interaction of their adhesions with host membrane-bound receptors.

3. Diagnosis—EAEC can be identified by cell culture adherence assays and nucleic acid-based assays for the various adherence-related genes, but no commercial kits or reagents are available. Most EAEC encode one or more cytotoxin/enterotoxins that are believed to be responsible for watery diarrhea with mucus. Other diagnostic tools include a DNA probe and PCR assays. A few studies suggest that there is an inflammatory component to EAEC infection that may help to distinguish it from ETEC or EPEC.

DAEC can be identified by cell culture adherence assays and nucleic acid-based assays for the genes that encode diffuse adherence, but no commercial kits or reagents are available. The diffuse adherence pattern of many DAEC strains on Hep-2 cells is mediated by the F1845 fimbrial adhesin. The *daaC* gene, which encodes a component essential for the expression of the F1845 adhesin, has been identified and a specific DNA probe to it has been shown to react with 75% of the DAEC isolates tested. PCR assays are also available to detect the *daaC* gene as well as genes for other Afa and Dr adhesins.

Testing for EAEC and DAEC typically is available only through reference or public health laboratories. Reporting of EAEC and DAEC isolations provides a retrospective diagnosis.

4. Occurrence—EAEC is associated with both acute and persistent diarrhea among children and adults in developing and developed countries. Reports associating EAEC with infant diarrhea, including persistent diarrhea, have come from countries in Latin America, Asia, and sub-Saharan Africa. Studies in Europe and the USA suggest that EAEC may be responsible for a proportion of diarrheal disease in developed countries; it has been more frequently identified in children with than without diarrhea in a few studies. EAEC have also been associated with diarrhea in HIV-infected adults and international travelers to developing countries. A small number of outbreaks have been reported. EAEC is a cause of traveler's diarrhea, responsible for 10%–20% of such cases in some analyses.

Preliminary evidence suggests that DAEC may be more pathogenic in children of preschool age than in infants and toddlers. Two DAEC strains failed to cause diarrhea when fed to volunteers, and no outbreaks have been recognized.

5. Reservoir—Likely humans, possibly animals.

6. Incubation period—The incubation period for EAEC is estimated to be 20–48 hours. Incubation periods as short as 8–18 hours have been observed. The incubation period for DAEC is not known.

7. Transmission—EAEC is transmitted by the fecal-oral route. The high inoculum required for disease suggests a food or water vehicle as the likely mode of transmission. The mode of transmission for DAEC is not known.

8. Risk groups—For EAEC, infants and young children, particularly malnourished children living in developing countries, HIV-infected persons, and international travelers to developing countries. Little is known about host risk factors for DAEC.

9. Prevention—General enteric precautions are advised. Travelers should be advised to drink only bottled or canned beverages and boiled or bottled water; travelers should avoid ice, raw produce including salads, and fruit they have not peeled themselves. Cooked foods should be eaten hot. Antimicrobial agents are not recommended for prevention of travelers' diarrhea. Packets of oral rehydration salts can be added to boiled or bottled water and ingested to maintain fluid balance.

10. Management of patient—

1) See general recommendations for all diarrheagenic *E. coli* in the STEC section in this chapter.
2) Treatment can follow recommendations for travelers' diarrhea of unknown cause: (a) orally administered electrolyte-containing solutions usually can prevent or treat dehydration and electrolyte abnormalities; (b) antimotility agents should not be administered to children with bloody diarrhea; (c) continued feeding of young children should be encouraged, particularly in developing country settings; (d) for an episode of severe watery diarrhea in a traveler to a resource-limited country, antibiotic therapy can be helpful. Azithromycin or a fluoroquinolone have been the most reliable agents, although fluoroquinolones are not approved for individuals less than 18 years of age for this indication. Reports suggest that EAEC strains are often resistant to antimicrobial agents commonly used to treat gastroenteritis; therefore, whenever possible, the choice of an antimicrobial agent should be based on the sensitivity of locally isolated strains.

11. Management of contacts and the immediate environment— See ETEC section in this chapter.

12. Special considerations—Optimal detection methodologies are lacking, and identification of truly pathogenic strains remains difficult.

[R. K. Mody, C. O'Reilly, P. M. Griffin]

EBOLA-MARBURG VIRAL DISEASES

(African hemorrhagic fever, Ebola virus hemorrhagic fever, Marburg virus hemorrhagic fever)

DISEASE	ICD-10 CODE
EBOLA HEMORRHAGIC FEVER	ICD-10 A98.4
MARBURG HEMORRHAGIC FEVER	ICD-10 A98.3

1. Clinical features—Severe acute viral illnesses, usually with sudden onset of fever, malaise, myalgia, and headache, followed in most cases by pharyngitis, vomiting, diarrhea, and maculopapular rash. In severe and fatal forms, a hemorrhagic diathesis is often accompanied by hepatic damage, renal failure, central nervous system (CNS) involvement, and terminal shock with multiorgan dysfunction. Laboratory findings usually show lymphopenia, severe thrombocytopenia, and transaminase elevation (aspartate aminotransferase [AST]>alanine transferase [ALT]), sometimes with hyperamylasemia, elevated creatinine, and blood urea nitrogen levels during the final renal failure phase. Case-fatality rates for Ebola infections in well-studied outbreaks in Africa have ranged from 32% to nearly 88%. In Marburg outbreaks, case-fatality rates have ranged from 22%–90%.

2. Causative agents—Ebola and Marburg viruses are negative stranded ribonucleic acid (RNA) viruses in the family *Filoviridae*. Pleomorphic virions with branched, circular, or coiled shapes are frequent on electron microscopy preparation and may reach micrometers in length. Five Ebola virus species have been identified, and viruses in 4 of these (*Zaire ebolavirus, Sudan ebolavirus, Tai Forest ebolavirus,* and *Bundibugyo ebolavirus*) have been shown to cause disease in humans. The fifth Ebola species, *Reston ebolavirus,* which originated in the Philippines, causes fatal hemorrhagic disease in nonhuman primates. A single Marburg virus species, *Marburg marburgvirus,* has been identified.

3. Diagnosis—Ebola or Marburg infection can be confirmed by direct detection of virus in blood or tissue samples by virus isolation, conventional or real-time polymerase chain reaction (PCR), antigen-detection enzyme-linked immunosorbent assay (ELISA), immunohistochemistry on formalin-fixed tissues, or detection of virus-specific immunoglobulin class M (IgM) antibodies or rising immunoglobulin class G (IgG) antibody titers. For a proper diagnosis, a combination of laboratory techniques, clinical evaluation, and epidemiological investigation is always recommended.

4. Occurrence—Ebola disease was first recognized in 1976. The largest outbreak to date—in Guinea, Liberia, Sierra Leone, Nigeria, and

Senegal—was ongoing at the time of writing and, unlike other outbreaks, was not contained by the initial response in rural areas where it appears to have emerged, and spread across international borders and to major urban areas in West Africa. Significant outbreaks and sporadic or small clusters of cases since 1976 include:

Year	Location	Cases
1976	Democratic Republic of Congo	318 cases, 280 deaths
1976	Sudan	284 cases, 151 deaths
1977	Democratic Republic of Congo	1 fatal case
1979	Sudan	34 cases, 22 deaths
1994	Ivory Coast	1 mild case
1994–1996	Gabon, Republic of South Africa	3 outbreaks (149 cases, 97 deaths); a fatal secondary infection occurred in a nurse in South Africa
1995	Democratic Republic of Congo	315 cases, 250 deaths
2000–2001	Uganda	425 cases, 224 deaths
2001–2003	Gabon, Republic of Congo	Several outbreaks (300 cases, 254 deaths); high numbers of deaths were simultaneously reported among wild animals in the region, particularly nonhuman primates
2004	Sudan	17 cases, 7 deaths
2007	Democratic Republic of Congo	264 cases, 187 deaths
2007–2008	Uganda	131 cases, 42 deaths
2008–2009	Democratic Republic of Congo	32 cases, 15 deaths
2011	Uganda	1 fatal case
2012	Uganda	2 outbreaks, 31 cases, 21 deaths
2012	Democratic Republic of Congo	53 cases, 36 deaths
2014	Guinea, Liberia, Sierra Leone, Nigeria, Senegal	3,707 confirmed, probable, and suspected cases; 1,848 deaths (as of 8/31/2014)

Antibodies have been found in residents of other areas of sub-Saharan Africa; their relation to the Ebola virus species is unknown. Laboratory infections have been reported in the UK and Russia.

Reston virus has been isolated from cynomolgus monkeys (*Macaca fascicularis*) imported to the USA in 1989, 1990, and 1996, and to Italy in 1992, all from the same export facility in the Philippines; many of these monkeys died. In the USA in 1989, 4 animal handlers with daily exposure to these monkeys developed specific antibodies but were asymptomatic. In 2008, Reston virus was isolated from domestic swine experiencing severe disease in the Philippines. Porcine reproductive and respiratory disease syndrome was also present in this pig population. Several animal handlers were asymptomatically infected and developed Ebola antibodies.

Marburg disease was first recognized in laboratory outbreaks in which workers had been exposed to African green monkeys *Chlorocebus tantalus* (formerly *Cercopithecus aethiops*) imported from Uganda, and in outbreaks since then in sub-Saharan Africa:

Year	Location	Cases
1967	Germany, Yugoslavia	31 cases, 7 deaths
1975	South Africa	3 cases, 1 death
1980	Kenya	2 cases, 1 death
1987	Kenya	1 fatal case
1998–2000	Democratic Republic of Congo	≥154 cases, 128 deaths
2005	Angola	252 cases, 227 deaths
2007	Uganda	4 cases, 2 deaths
2008	Netherlands, USA	2 cases among tourists from Netherlands (fatal) and USA after a trip in Uganda
2012	Uganda	23 cases, 15 deaths

5. Reservoir—Forest-dwelling fruit bats are believed to be the reservoir of Ebola viruses, and viral ribonucleic acid (RNA) has been detected in 3 bat species in central Africa (*Hypsignathus monstrosus*, *Epomops franqueti*, and *Myonycteris torquata*). Cave-dwelling fruit bats are believed to be the reservoir of Marburg virus, and numerous virus isolates have been acquired from a particular species, *Rousettus aegyptiacus*. Ebola and Marburg viruses have been identified in multiple species of nonhuman primates in which highly lethal outbreaks have occurred, although these are likely incidental hosts and not reservoirs of these viruses. Swine, responsible for the Reston virus epidemic in 2008 in the Philippines, are considered intermediary hosts.

6. Incubation period—Probably 5-15 days for both Ebola and Marburg disease.

7. Transmission—Ebola infection of index cases seems to occur as follows:

1) In central Africa, while manipulating infected wild mammals found dead in the rainforest.
2) For Reston virus, while handling infected cynomolgus monkeys (through direct contact with their infected blood or fresh organs) or while handling infected pigs (through direct contact with secretions and fresh organs).

Marburg infection of index cases seems to occur when people are in close contact with bats or spending time in bat-inhabited confined areas, such as caves or mines.

Person-to-person transmission of Ebola and Marburg diseases occurs through direct contact with infected blood, urine, vomiting, diarrhea, secretions, organs, or semen. Risk is highest during the late stages of illness, when the patient is vomiting, having diarrhea, or hemorrhaging, and during funerals with unprotected body preparation. Under natural conditions, airborne transmission among humans has not been documented. Nosocomial infections have been frequent; virtually all patients who have acquired infection from contaminated syringes and needles died. Transmission through semen appears to be rare but has occurred up to 7 weeks after clinical recovery. Risk during the asymptomatic incubation period is negligible. The diseases are not communicable before the febrile phase, and communicability increases with stage of illness, as long as blood and secretions contain virus. For both viruses, the semen may remain infectious for several weeks or months (e.g., Ebola virus was isolated from the seminal fluid on the 61st but not on the 76th day after onset of illness in a laboratory-acquired case).

8. Risk groups—All ages are susceptible. The main human groups at risk are patients who are injected with contaminated needles and syringes that are not properly sterilized; caregivers in affected communities (often women) and health care workers handling infected patients, their secretions, or their excretions; laboratory workers processing clinical specimens or working in research laboratories; people working with wildlife, in particular nonhuman primates in central Africa or bats; and people working in bat-inhabited locations, such as mines.

9. Prevention—No vaccines are currently approved for human use. For control measures as well as prevention of infection of patients and hospital and laboratory workers, see Management of Patient in this chapter. In addition: protection of sexual intercourse for 3 months or until semen can be shown to be free of virus.

10. **Management of patient—**

1) Strict procedures for isolation of patients and their body fluids and excreta must be maintained. Institute immediate strict isolation in a private hospital room away from traffic patterns. Entry of nonessential staff and visitors should be restricted. All persons entering the patient's room should wear gloves and gowns to prevent contact with contaminated items or environmental surfaces. Face shields or masks (N95 or N99) and eye protection should be worn to prevent contact with blood, other body fluids, secretions (including respiratory droplets), or excretions. The need for additional barriers depends on the potential for fluid contact, as determined by the procedure performed and the presence of clinical symptoms that increase the likelihood of contact with body fluids from the patient. Recourse to a negative pressure room and respiratory protection is desirable. To reduce infectious exposure, laboratory tests should be kept to the minimum necessary for proper diagnosis and patient care and only performed where full infection control measures are correctly implemented. Technicians must be alerted to the nature of the specimens and supervised to ensure application of appropriate specimen inactivation/isolation procedures. Dead bodies should be sealed in leak-proof material and cremated or buried promptly in a sealed casket, while respecting as much as possible religious or cultural burial practices to avoid unnecessary conflicts with affected families and local communities, which may otherwise compromise the outbreak response.

2) Patient's excreta, sputum, blood, and all objects with which the patient has had contact, including needles and syringes as well as laboratory equipment used to carry out tests on blood, must be disinfected with 0.5% sodium hypochlorite solution or 0.5% phenol with detergent, and, as far as possible, effective heating methods—such as autoclaving, incineration, boiling, or irradiation—should be used as appropriate. Laboratory testing must be carried out in special high-containment facilities; if there is no such facility, tests should be kept to a minimum and specimens handled by experienced technicians using all available personal protective equipment, such as gloves, gowns, masks, goggles, and biological safety cabinets. When appropriate, serum may be heat-inactivated at 60°C (140°F) for 1 hour. Thorough terminal disinfection with 0.5% sodium hypochlorite solution or a phenolic compound is adequate; formaldehyde fumigation can be considered.

3) No specific antiviral treatment is available as yet for either Ebola or Marburg disease.

11. Management of contacts and the immediate environment—Identify all close contacts (people living with, caring for, testing laboratory specimens from, or having noncasual contact with the patient) in the 3 weeks after the onset of illness. Establish, at home when practical, close surveillance of contacts as follows: body temperature checks at least 2 times daily for at least 3 weeks after last exposure. In case of temperature above 38.3°C (101°F), hospitalize immediately in strict isolation facilities while initiating diagnostic testing. Determine patient's place of residence during the 3 weeks prior to onset; search for unreported or undiagnosed cases.

12. Special considerations—Reporting: in many countries, Ebola and Marburg virus infections are reportable as "viral hemorrhagic fever." Suspected cases should be reported to the national health authorities and to a WHO Collaborating Center (Hamburg, Salisbury, Atlanta, Winnipeg, Johannesburg) for diagnostic support. Occurrence of Ebola or Marburg infections likely constitutes an International Health Regulations notifiable event to WHO. Additionally, isolation of Ebola or Marburg viruses must be reported to the national biosecurity agencies in several countries.

[P. E. Rollin, B. Knust, S. Nichol]

ECHINOCOCCOSIS

DISEASE	ICD-10 CODE
CYSTIC ECHINOCOCCOSIS	ICD-10 B67.0-B67.4
ALVEOLAR ECHINOCOCCOSIS	ICD-10 B67.5-B67.7
POLYCYSTIC ECHINOCOCCOSIS	ICD-10 B67.9

1. Clinical features—The larval stages (hydatid cyst or solid/multi-vesiculated lesions) of *Echinococcus* spp. tapeworm produce disease in humans and animals; disease characteristics depend upon the infecting species. Cysts/lesions usually develop in the liver or the lungs but also develop in other viscera, nervous tissue, or bone. They can be cystic, alveolar, and/or polycystic.

1) Cystic: larval stages of the tapeworm Echinococcus granulosus, the most common Echinococcus species, cause cystic echino-coccosis or hydatid disease. Hydatid cysts enlarge slowly and require several years for development. Developed cysts range from 1-15 cm in diameter but may be larger. Infections may be

asymptomatic until cysts cause noticeable mass effect; signs and symptoms vary according to location, cyst size, cyst type, and numbers. Ruptured or leaking cysts can cause severe anaphylactoid reactions and may release protoscolices that can produce secondary echinococcosis. One or several cysts, typically spherical, thick-walled and consisting of a single cavity (unilocular), are most frequently found in the liver and lungs, although they may occur in other organs. Differential diagnoses include benign tumor, malignancies, amebic abscesses, and congenital cysts.

2) Alveolar: a highly invasive, destructive disease. Lesions are usually found in the liver; because a thick laminated cyst wall does not restrict their growth, they expand at the periphery to produce solid, tumor-like masses. Metastases can result in secondary cysts and larval growth in other organs. Clinical manifestations depend on the size and location of cysts but are often confused with hepatic carcinoma and cirrhosis.

3) Polycystic: this disease occurs in the liver, lungs, and other viscera. Symptoms vary depending on cyst size and location. The polycystic lesion is unique in that the germinal membrane proliferates externally to form new cysts and internally to form septae that divide the cavity into numerous microcysts. Brood capsules containing many protoscolices develop in the microcysts.

2. Causative agents—

1) Cystic: *E. granulosus*.
2) Alveolar: *Echinococcus multilocularis*.
3) Polycystic: *Echinococcus vogeli* and *Echinococcus oligarthrus*.

3. Diagnosis—

1) Cystic: based on signs and symptoms compatible with a slowly growing tumor, a history of residence in an endemic area, and an association with canines. Ultrasonography, computerized tomography, and serological testing are useful for supporting diagnosis, with ultrasonography the method of first choice. WHO has developed a classification of ultrasound images of liver cystic echinococcosis for diagnostic and prognostic purposes and determination of the type of intervention required (see specific treatment). Definitive diagnosis in seronegative patients, however, requires microscopic identification from specimens obtained at surgery or by percutaneous aspiration; the potential risks of this (anaphylaxis, spillage) can be avoided by ultrasound guidance and anthelminthic coverage. Species identification is based on finding thick laminated cyst walls and protoscolices as well as on the structure and measurements of protoscolex hooks.

Molecular techniques are now available to identify the species from biopsies.

2) Alveolar: diagnosis is often based on histopathology, that is, evidence of the thin host layer and multiple microvesicles formed by external proliferation. Humans are an abnormal host, and the lesions rarely produce brood capsules, protoscolices, or calcareous bodies. Serodiagnosis using purified or recombinant *E. multilocularis* antigen is highly sensitive and specific. A staging and classification system proposed by WHO, named PNM, is based on:

- hepatic localization of the parasite (P)
- extrahepatic involvement of neighboring organs (N)
- metastases (M)

3) Polycystic: immunodiagnosis using a purified antigen of *E. vogeli* does not always allow differentiation from alveolar echinococcosis (which does not co-occur in South America). The causative agents are distinguished by the form and size of their rostellar hooks from protoscolices.

4. Occurrence—

1) Cystic: all continents except Antarctica; depends on close association of humans and infected dogs. Especially common in grazing countries where dogs eat viscera containing cysts. Transmission has been eliminated in Iceland and greatly reduced in Tasmania (Australia), Cyprus, and New Zealand. Control programs exist in Argentina, Brazil, China, Kenya (Turkana district), Spain, Uruguay, and other countries, including those of the Mediterranean basin.

2) Alveolar: distribution is limited to areas of the Northern Hemisphere (China, Russia, northern Japan, Turkey, central Europe, Alaska, Canada, and rarely the north central USA). The disease is usually diagnosed in adults.

2) Polycystic: Central and South America.

5. Reservoir—

1) Cystic: the domestic dog and other canids, definitive hosts for *E. granulosus*, may harbor thousands of adult tapeworms in their intestines without signs of infection. Intermediate hosts include herbivores, primarily sheep, cattle, goats, pigs, horses, camels, and other animals.

2) Alveolar: adult tapeworms are largely restricted to wild animals such as foxes, racoon dogs, and coyotes, and the associated disease is commonly maintained in nature in fox-rodent cycles. Dogs and cats can be sources of human infection if hunting wild

(and rarely domestic) intermediate hosts such as rodents, including voles, lemmings, and mice.

2) Polycystic: natural definitive hosts are bush dogs (for *E. vogeli*) and wild felids (for *E. oligarthrus*), while intermediate hosts are rodents. Domestic dogs can act as occasional definitive hosts for *E. vogeli*.

6. Incubation period—12 months to years, depending on number and location of cysts and how rapidly they grow.

7. Transmission—

1) Cystic: human infection often takes place directly with hand-to-mouth transfer of eggs after association with infected dogs or indirectly through contaminated food, water, soil, or fomites. In some instances, flies have dispersed eggs after feeding on infected feces. Adult worms in the small intestines of canines produce eggs containing infective embryos (oncospheres); these are passed in feces and may survive for several months in pastures or gardens. When ingested by susceptible intermediate hosts, including humans, eggs hatch, releasing oncospheres that migrate through the mucosa and are bloodborne to organs, primarily the liver (first filter), then the lungs (second filter), where they form cysts. Strains of *E. granulosus* vary in their ability to adapt to infect various hosts as well as their infectivity to humans. Not directly transmitted from person to person or from one intermediate host to another. Dogs become infected by eating animal viscera containing hydatid cysts and begin to pass eggs 5-7 weeks later. Most canine infections resolve spontaneously by 6 months; however some adult worms may survive up to 2-3 years. Dogs may become infected repeatedly. Sheep and other intermediate hosts are infected while grazing in areas contaminated with dog feces containing parasite eggs.

2) Alveolar: ingestion of eggs passed in the feces of dogs and cats that have fed on infected rodents. Fecally soiled dog hair, harnesses, and environmental fomites also serve as vehicles of infection.

3) Polycystic: ingestion of eggs passed in the feces of definitive hosts that have hunted or fed on infected rodents.

8. Risk groups—Children, who are more likely to have close contact with infected dogs and less likely to have adequate hygienic habits, are at greater risk of cystic echinococcosis, especially in rural areas. Alveolar echinococcosis usually affects adults.

9. **Prevention—**

1) Avoid ingestion of raw vegetables and water that may have been contaminated with the feces of infected dogs. Emphasize basic hygiene practices such as handwashing and washing of fruits and vegetables. Educate those at risk on avoidance of exposure to dog feces.

2) Interrupt transmission from intermediate to definitive hosts by preventing access of dogs to potentially contaminated (uncooked) viscera and through inspection of livestock carcasses and organs after slaughter, and condemnation and safe disposal of infected viscera. Disposal should be by incineration or deep burial.

3) Periodically treat high-risk dogs, and all dogs in high-risk areas, with praziquantel; encourage responsible dog ownership and implement programs for the reduction of dog populations in compliance with principles of animal welfare.

4) Field and laboratory personnel must observe strict safety precautions to avoid ingestion of tapeworm eggs.

10. **Management of patient—**Treatment: based on WHO classification of liver cysts. In some instances, surgical resection of isolated cysts is the most common treatment. Other cyst types may first be treated by percutaneous techniques such as Puncture, Aspiration, Injection, Reaspiration (PAIR). PAIR consists of the percutaneous drainage of echinococcal cysts located in the abdomen with a fine needle or a catheter, followed by the killing of remaining protoscolices with a protoscolicide and by the reaspiration of protoscolicide solution. It is a minimally invasive technique of lesser risk than surgery, recommended for the treatment of certain cysts (http://whqlibdoc.who.int/hq/2001/WHO_CDS_CSR_APH_2001.6.pdf). Treatment with mebendazole and albendazole has also proved successful and may be the preferred treatment in many cases. If a primary cyst ruptures, praziquantel, a protoscolicidal agent, reduces the probability of secondary cysts. Other cyst types may not need a surgical, percutaneous, or medical intervention but should be followed for a long period of time.

In alveolar echinococcosis, radical surgical excision is less often successful and must be followed by chemotherapy. Mebendazole or albendazole for a limited period after surgery, or long-term (several years) for inoperable patients, may prevent progression of the disease; presurgical chemotherapy is indicated in rare cases.

Albendazole has been used for chemotherapy in polycystic echinococcosis.

11. **Management of contacts and the immediate environment—** Examine families and associates for suspicious cysts or tumors using

ultrasound, chest X-ray, and other imaging techniques. Check dogs kept in and around houses for infection, by autopsy, coproantigen, or copro-polymerase chain reaction (PCR) techniques. Determine beliefs, practices, and behaviors affecting risk of infection, and educate populations at risk.

12. Special considerations—Control the movement of dogs from known enzootic areas.

[M. Eberhard, F. Meslin, P. Kern, P. Schantz, S. Magnino, B. Abela-Ridder]

EHRLICHIOSIS

DISEASE	ICD-10 CODE
EHRLICHIOSIS	ICD-10 A79.8

DISEASE IN HUMANS	CAUSATIVE AGENTS	RESERVOIRS	GEOGRAPHIC DISTRIBUTION OF HUMAN ILLNESS
EHRLICHIOSIS	*Ehrlichia chaffeensis*, *Ehrlichia ewingii*, and *Ehrlichia muris* (or a closely related organism)	White-tailed deer and dogs, small rodents	North and South America
ANAPLASMOSIS	*Anaplasma phagocytophilum*	Ruminants, deer, field rodents, dogs	North America, Asia, Europe
SENNETSU FEVER	*Neorickettsia sennetsu*	Trematodes that live in aquatic hosts such as snails, insects, and fish	Western Japan, Malaysia
NEOEHRLICHIOSIS	*Neoehrlichia mikurensis*	Wild rodents, dogs	Northern Europe and Asia

1. Clinical features—Acute, febrile illnesses caused by a group of small, pleomorphic, obligate intracellular, bacteria that survive and reproduce in the phagosomes of mononuclear or polymorphonuclear leukocytes of the infected host. The organisms are sometimes observed within these cells in the peripheral blood. The clinical spectrum of ehrlichioses infections ranges from mild illness to severe, life-threatening, or fatal disease. Ehrlichiosis caused by *Ehrlichia chaffeensis* affects primarily mononuclear phagocytes, while Ehrlichiosis caused by *Ehrlichia ewingii,* and anaplasmosis caused by *Anaplasma phagocytophilum,* affect the neutrophils.

Ehrlichiosis caused by *E. chaffeensis* presents with nonspecific symptoms, including fever, headache, malaise, and myalgia. It may be confused clinically with Rocky Mountain spotted fever, although rash is less commonly reported. Laboratory findings include leukopenia, thrombocytopenia, and elevation of 1 or more hepatocellular enzymes. Encephalitis or meningitis may occur. Infection with *E. chaffeensis* can be severe, and a 1.9% case-fatality rate is reported. There is no current evidence for persistent infection in humans.

Symptoms of *E. ewingii* and *Ehrlichia muris* (or a closely related organism) infections are usually nonspecific, and commonly include fever, headache, anorexia, nausea, myalgia, and vomiting. To date, these infections have not been reported to be associated with fatalities.

Anaplasmosis, caused by *A. phagocytophilum,* is characterized clinically by acute and usually self-limited fever, headache, malaise, and myalgia. Common laboratory findings may include thrombocytopenia, leukopenia, and increased hepatic transaminases. Meningoencephalitis is rare. Illness ranges from mild to severe, with a 0.6% case-fatality rate. Coinfections with *Borrelia burgdorferi, Babesia* spp., and tickborne encephalitis viruses may occur, because *Ixodes* species of ticks transmit all these organisms. There is no current evidence for persistent infection in humans.

Sennetsu fever, caused by *Neorickettsia sennetsu* is characterized by the sudden onset of fever, chills, malaise, headache, muscle and joint pain, sore throat, and sleeplessness. Generalized lymphadenopathy with tenderness of the enlarged nodes is common. Atypical lymphocytosis with postauricular and posterior cervical lymphadenopathy is similar to that seen in infectious mononucleosis. The course is usually benign; fatal cases have not been reported. Infection with *Neoehrlichia mikurensis* has recently been described in Europe and Asia. General clinical features have included recurrent fever, erysipelas-like rashes, arthralgias, sepsis, and thromboembolisms. Most severe illnesses have occurred in immunocompromised people.

The veterinary pathogens *Ehrlichia canis* and an *Anaplasma platys*–like agent have been reported to infect a few humans in Venezuela. Clinically, the patients were asymptomatic or showed signs compatible with ehrlichiosis. These etiologies have not been reported from other areas.

Differential diagnosis for all these infections includes various viral syndromes, Rocky Mountain spotted fever, sepsis, toxic shock syndrome, gastroenteritis, meningoencephalitis, tularemia, Colorado tick fever, tickborne encephalitis, babesiosis, Lyme borreliosis, leptospirosis, hepatitis, typhoid fever, murine typhus, and blood malignancies.

2. Causative agents—See table in this chapter. These organisms are members of the family *Anaplasmataceae*, order *Rickettsiales*.

3. Diagnosis—Based on clinical and laboratory findings and 4-fold change in antibody titer detected by using organism-specific antigens or *E. chaffeensis* as surrogate antigen for *E. ewingii* and *E. muris*. Blood smear examination is not recommended as the most sensitive method of detection, but in some cases blood smears or buffy coat smears could be examined for characteristic inclusions (morulae) during the acute stage of illness, when the percentage of infected cells is generally low (<1%). Other, highly sensitive diagnostic techniques, especially during the acute febrile phase of illness, include deoxyribonucleic acid (DNA) amplification by polymerase chain reaction (PCR) assay. Culture and immunohistochemistry of blood marrow or necropsy tissues can be used for diagnosis in fatal cases.

4. Occurrence—See table in this chapter for geographical distribution of human illness. The distribution of the organisms in their reservoirs can extend beyond the areas where human cases occur. Travel-associated infections have been reported.

5. Reservoirs—See table in this chapter. A number of vertebrate reservoirs have been identified for each pathogen, and the ecology can be complex.

6. Incubation period—7-14 days for human ehrlichioses and anaplasmosis; 14 days for Sennetsu fever.

7. Transmission—*E. chaffeensis* is transmitted through the bite of a tick; *Amblyomma americanum* in North America, and possibly *Amblyomma cajenennse* in southern and central America. *A. americanum* transmits *E. ewingii*. *E. canis* is transmitted by *Rhipicephalus sanguineus*. *E. muris* and similar organisms have been identified in *Ixodes persulcatus* and *Haemaphysalis flava* ticks in some parts of the world, and in *Ixodes scapularis* in the upper midwestern USA. The vectors of *A. phagocytophilum* are *Ixodes* spp., including *Ixodes scapularis*, *Ixodes ricinus*, *Ixodes pacificus*, *Ixodes trianguliceps*, *Ixodes spinipalpis*, and *Ixodes persulcatus* ticks. The means of transmission are not fully elucidated for Sennetsu fever, although ingestion of an uncooked trematode-parasitized aquatic host is suspected.

Blood transfusions donated during the eclipse phase of infections with both *A. phagocytophilum* and *E. ewingii* have caused infections in blood recipients. No evidence of other person-to-person transmission.

8. Risk groups—Older or immunocompromised individuals are likely to suffer more serious illness. Reinfection is rare. Approximately 12%–14% of patients with these diseases report concurrent conditions that appear to be immunosuppressive, and patients with immunosuppressive conditions have been shown to experience a more severe clinical course.

9. Prevention—Measures to avoid tick bites (see "Lyme Disease" and Tickborne Spotted Fevers section of "Rickettsioses") should be employed to prevent ehrlichioses and anaplasmosis. Preventive measures have not yet been established for Sennetsu fever; however, consumption of raw fish and fish products should be avoided in endemic areas.

10. Management of patient—

1) Remove any attached ticks. Rapid removal of ticks may reduce the likelihood of transmission of infectious organism. Effective transmission of agents probably requires 24 or more hours of attachment.

2) Treatment: doxycycline is the drug of choice for adults and children of all ages, particularly because Rocky Mountain spotted fever is a primary differential diagnosis for these diseases and effective alternative treatments are not available for that infection. Delay in treatment can result in death. The pediatric dose is 2.2 mg/kg twice a day, continued for 3 days after resolution of fever (usually a 5- to 10-day course). The adult dose is 100 mg twice a day. Rifampin has been used to treat ehrlichiosis and anaplasmosis in pregnant patients but is not effective against Rocky Mountain spotted fever. If symptoms worsen, expert opinion should be consulted regarding the need for possible doxycycline use during pregnancy.

11. Management of contacts and the immediate environment—None.

12. Special considerations—Reporting: case reporting to local health authority required in most countries.

[J. McQuiston, W. Nicholson]

ENTEROBIASIS
(pinworm infection, oxyuriasis)

DISEASE	ICD-10 CODE
ENTEROBIASIS	ICD-10 B80

1. Clinical features—A common intestinal helminthic infection that may range from asymptomatic to recurrently symptomatic. The most common clinical feature is perianal itching which may lead to disturbed sleep, irritability, and secondary infection of scratched skin. Other clinical manifestations include vulvovaginitis, salpingitis, and pelvic and liver granulomata. Appendicitis and enuresis have also been reported as possible associated conditions.

2. Causative agent—*Enterobius vermicularis*, a small intestinal nematode helminth, also called pinworm, that can be seen with naked eye as a tiny white thread. The male worm measures 2-4 mm in length, while the female measures 8-12 mm. The worm is oviparous, and the adults are found in the lumen of the caecum and appendix and occasionally in ascending colon and ileum.

3. Diagnosis—The diagnosis can be made by demonstrating the presence of worms or their eggs. Adult worms can be seen in the perianal region 2-3 hours after the infected person goes to sleep. Eggs can be demonstrated by applying transparent adhesive tape (tape swab or pinworm paddle) to the perianal region and examining the tape or paddle microscopically for eggs; material for examination is best obtained in the morning before bathing or passage of stools. Examination should be repeated 3 or more times before accepting a negative result. Eggs are sometimes found on microscopic stool and urine examination, nail washings, and bed linen. Female worms may be found in feces and in the perianal region during rectal or vaginal examinations. There is no serological test available for diagnosis.

4. Occurrence—Worldwide, affecting all socioeconomic classes, with high rates in some areas. It is the most common worm infection in countries with a temperate climate; prevalence is highest in school-age children (in some groups near 50%), followed by preschoolers, and is lowest in adults except for mothers of infected children.

5. Reservoir—Humans. Pinworms of other animals are not transmissible to humans.

6. Incubation period—The incubation period ranges between 1 and 2 months. Symptomatic disease with high worm burdens results from successive reinfections occurring within months of initial exposure.

7. Transmission—By direct transfer of infective eggs by hand from anus to mouth of the same or another person or indirectly through clothing, bedding, food, or other articles contaminated with parasite eggs. Dustborne infection is possible in heavily contaminated households and institutions. Eggs become infective within a few hours after being deposited on perianal skin by migrating gravid females; eggs survive less than 2 weeks outside the host. Larvae from ingested eggs hatch in the small intestine; young worms mature in the cecum and upper portions of the colon. Gravid worms usually migrate actively from the rectum and may enter adjacent orifices. People who are infected with pinworm can transfer the parasite to others as long as there is a female pinworm depositing eggs on the perianal skin. A person can also self-reinfect or be reinfected by eggs from another person.

8. Risk groups—Differences in frequency and intensity of infection are due primarily to differences in exposure. Infection often occurs in more than 1 family member. Prevalence can be high in domiciliary institutions. Those most likely to be infected with pinworm are children younger than 18 months, people who take care of infected children, and people who are institutionalized. In these groups, the prevalence can reach up to 50%.

9. Prevention—

1) Educate the public in personal hygiene—particularly the need to wash hands with soap and water after defecation, after changing of diapers, and before eating or preparing food. Keep nails short; discourage nail biting and scratching the anal area.
2) Daily morning bathing with showers (or stand-up baths) preferred to tub baths.
3) Change to clean underclothing, nightclothes, and bed sheets frequently, preferably after bathing.
4) Reduce overcrowding in living accommodations.
5) Provide adequate toilets; maintain cleanliness in these facilities.

10. **Management of patient—**

1) Change bed linen and underwear of infected person daily for several days after treatment, avoiding aerial dispersal of eggs. Use closed sleeping garments. Eggs on discarded linen are killed by exposure to temperatures of 55°C (131°F) for a few seconds; either boil bed clothing or use a washing machine on hot cycle, and dry on hot setting. Plush and other children's toys must be cleansed similarly. Clean and vacuum sleeping and living areas daily for several days after treatment.

2) Treatment: albendazole, mebendazole, or pyrantel pamoate. All these drugs are given as 1 dose. Treatment to be repeated after 2-4 weeks to ensure treatment of possible reinfection. Concurrent treatment of the whole family may be advisable if several members are infected. Some experts routinely treat all family members whether symptomatic or not, without prior testing (considering the low cost, safety, and efficacy of therapy).

11. **Management of contacts and the immediate environment—**

1) Remove sources of infection through treatment of cases.
2) Examine all members of an affected family or institution.
3) Clean and vacuum house daily for several days after treatment of cases.

12. **Special considerations—**Multiple cases in schools and institutions can best be controlled through systematic treatment of all infected individuals and household contacts.

[M. Eberhard, A. Gabrielli, A. Montresor, L. Savioli]

ENTEROVIRUS DISEASES

DISEASE	CAUSATIVE AGENTS	ICD-10 CODE
ENTEROVIRAL VESICULAR PHARYNGITIS	*Enterovirus A* serotypes CV-A1 to 10, 16, 22, and EV-A71	ICD-10 B08.5
ENTEROVIRAL VESICULAR STOMATITIS WITH EXANTHEM	Predominantly CV-A16 and EV-A71, but includes other *Enterovirus A* serotypes. Less frequently associated with *Enterovirus B* serotypes CV-B2 and CV-B5	ICD-10 B08.4
ENTEROVIRAL LYMPHONODULAR PHARYNGITIS	*Enterovirus A* serotype CV-A10	ICD-10 B08.8
MYALGIA, EPIDEMIC	Predominantly associated with *Enterovirus B* serotypes CV-B1 to 3, 5, 6, and E-1, 6. Sporadically associated with other *Enterovirus A* and *B* serotypes	ICD-10 B33.0
VIRAL CARDITIS	Primarily *Enterovirus B* serotypes CV-B1 to 5, CV-A9 and CV-A23, but occasionally *Enterovirus A* serotypes CV-A4 and CV-A16, *Enterovirus C* serotype CV-A1, and other enteroviruses	ICD-10 B33.2
Enteroviral hemorrhagic conjunctivitis (see "Conjunctivitis/Keratitis")		
Meningitis (see "Meningitis")		

I. ENTEROVIRAL VESICULAR STOMATITIS WITH EXANTHEM (hand, foot, and mouth disease), ENTEROVIRAL VESICULAR PHARYNGITIS (herpangina)

1. **Clinical features**—Hand, foot, and mouth disease is a brief, usually mild, febrile illness with papulovesicular rashes over the palms and soles, with or without multiple painful mouth ulcers. Sometimes, the rash may be of maculopapular type without vesicles. It may also involve the buttocks, knees, or elbows, particularly in younger children and infants. In the 2012 CV-A6 outbreaks in North America and Europe, patients most typically had perioral and perirectal papules in addition to vesicles on the dorsum of their hands. The skin lesions, which heal spontaneously without scarring, may last for 3–5 days after the onset of illness. Secondary bacterial skin infection is very unusual.

Herpangina is characterized by a brief, generally mild, febrile illness with multiple painful mouth ulcers that predominantly affect the posterior oral cavity, including the anterior pharyngeal folds, uvula, tonsils, and soft palate. In some children, the ulcers may affect other parts of the mouth, including the buccal mucosa and tongue. The oral lesions may persist for 3–5 days after the onset of illness.

The most common clinical problems associated with these 2 closely related conditions are odynophagia and dehydration. The odynophagia may be severe in young children and result in inadequate fluid intake and dehydration. Recent epidemics of hand, foot, and mouth disease and herpangina in Asia have shown that infection caused by EV-A71, in contrast to that caused by other enteroviruses, may be associated with central nervous system (CNS) complications, including aseptic meningitis, encephalitis, and acute flaccid paralysis. Children with CNS involvement (encephalitis and acute flaccid paralysis), particularly those aged 5 years or younger, are at risk of acute severe, and sometimes fatal, cardiac dysfunction and pulmonary edema. The warning signs of CNS involvement and systemic complications include persistent fever for more than 48 hours, body temperature higher than 39°C, recurrent vomiting, unexplained irritability, lethargy, myoclonus, focal limb weakness, truncal ataxia, nystagmus, signs of respiratory distress, and skin mottling.

Important differential diagnoses for hand, foot, and mouth disease and herpangina include herpetic gingivostomatitis, aphthous stomatitis, and scabies infestation. Patients with herpetic gingivostomatitis are usually febrile and toxic. The gingiva is typically inflamed and may be bleeding. There may be circumoral ulcers or vesicles without extremity involvement, and associated cervical lymphadenopathy. Aphthous stomatitis is characterized by larger, ulcerative lesions of the lips, tongue, and buccal mucosa that are painful but lack constitutional symptoms. It is benign and noncontagious, and commonly affects older children and adults. Recurrence is common. Scabies infestation may sometimes be confused with hand, foot, and mouth disease because it also causes pustules, vesicles, or nodular lesions over the hands and feet. Intense itch and interdigital space involvement are useful clinical clues to the parasitic infestation.

2. Causative agents—See the table in this chapter. The enteroviruses often cocirculate, usually with one predominant serotype, during outbreaks of hand, foot, and mouth disease, and herpangina, and result in clinically indistinguishable skin and mucosal lesions.

3. Diagnosis—To date, more than a 100 different enterovirus serotypes have been described. With such a large number of serotypes and overlapping clinical syndromes, cross-reactivity will confound the interpretation of any results, limiting the usefulness of serology for confirmatory diagnosis. Current diagnostic tools for identification of enteroviruses involve detection of viral ribonucleic acid (RNA) via molecular amplification by the reverse transcription polymerase chain reaction (RT-PCR). These methods (e.g., RT-PCR, multiplex RT-PCR, real-time RT-PCR) typically target the 5' untranslated region of the enterovirus genome to identify the genus, and one or more of the structural genes (VP1 predominantly, VP2, and VP4) for molecular typing ("serotyping"). These methods are useful as they can be performed directly on primary clinical specimens and identify the probable causative agent. However, for a confirmatory diagnosis, virus isolation (preferably from the infected site) by cell culture, followed by molecular typing can be performed. Since this may not be possible for most cases, virus isolation and molecular identification from secondary sites (e.g., throat swabs, feces, blood) will provide information on the likely causative agent.

4. **Occurrence**—Worldwide, sporadic, and epidemic occurrence. In temperate regions, the peak incidence is during summer and early autumn, whereas in the tropics, the conditions occur throughout the year. Since 1997, epidemics of hand, foot, and mouth disease have been reported in many parts of Asia; the occurrence is perennial or cyclical with an interval of 2-3 years.

5. **Reservoir**—Human.

6. **Incubation period**—Usually 3-5 days.

7. **Transmission**—Direct contact with nasal and oral secretions, vesicular fluid, and stools of infected individuals, as well as contaminated articles such as toys and surfaces, is the most important route of transmission. Spread through aerosol droplets may occur. Asymptomatic individuals, including adults, are an important source of infection. There is no reliable evidence of spread through insects, water, food, or sewage. The disease is most contagious during the first week of illness. Viral shedding may occur for as long as 2 and 11 weeks in throat secretions and stools, respectively.

8. **Risk groups**—These diseases frequently occur in outbreaks among groups of children (e.g., in nursery schools, child care centers, and large households with many young children).

9. **Prevention**—Limit person-to-person contact, where practicable, by measures such as crowd reduction and isolating infected children. Promote handwashing with soap and water, and other hygienic measures.

10. **Management of patient**—

   1) Enteric precautions: wash hands with soap and water before and after leaving room; wear gloves and gown when tending to patient.
   2) Concurrent disinfection of nose and throat discharges. Wash or discard soiled articles. Give careful attention to prompt handwashing when handling discharges, feces, and soiled articles.

3) Treatment: analgesia, antipyretics, intravenous rehydration. No specific antiviral is available; early recognition and intervention of CNS and systemic complications; supportive management. Intravenous immunoglobulin (IVIG) has been used to treat cases with CNS and systemic complications, but the clinical benefit is uncertain in the absence of randomized clinical trials.

4) Risk communication: educate parents, guardians, and child caregivers to bring the child to the nearest clinic or hospital if the following warning signs of CNS and systemic complications occur: refusal to eat or drink; persistent vomiting or drowsiness; startling or myoclonic jerks.

11. Management of contacts and the immediate environment— Follow up contacts for clinical signs of hand, foot, and mouth disease. Clean contaminated surfaces and soiled articles, first with soap and water, and then disinfect them with a dilute solution of chlorine-containing bleach (1 part of product to 20 parts of water; ~3,000 ppm) at a contact time of at least 5 minutes. This is a very effective way to inactivate the virus, especially in institutional settings such as child care centers.

12. Special considerations—

1) Reporting: obligatory report of epidemics in some countries.

2) Epidemic measures: give general notice to physicians/health care providers of increased incidence of the disease, together with a description of onset, clinical characteristics, and precautions. Isolate diagnosed cases and all children with fever, pending diagnosis, with special attention to proper handling of respiratory secretions and feces.

II. MYALGIA, EPIDEMIC (epidemic pleurodynia, Bornholm disease, devil's grippe)

1. Clinical features—Pleurodynia is an uncommon complication of *Enterovirus B* infection. It is characterized by paroxysmal spasmodic pain in the chest or abdomen, which may be intensified by movement, and is usually accompanied by fever and headache. The pain tends to be more abdominal than thoracic in infants and young children, while the reverse applies to older children and adults. Most patients recover within 1 week of onset, but relapses occur; no fatalities have been reported. It is important to differentiate from more serious medical or surgical conditions. Complications occur infrequently and include orchitis, pericarditis, pneumonia, and aseptic meningitis.

Localized epidemics are characteristic. During outbreaks of epidemic myalgia, cases of *Enterovirus B* (serotypes CV-B1 to 5) myocarditis of the newborn have been reported. While myocarditis in adults is a rare complication, the possibility should always be considered.

2. **Causative agents**—See the table in this chapter.

3. **Diagnosis**—See Diagnosis under Enteroviral Vesicular Stomatitis With Exanthem section in this chapter.

4. **Occurrence**—An uncommon disease, occurring in summer and early autumn; usually in youths aged 5–15 years, but all ages may be affected. Multiple cases in a household can occur frequently. Outbreaks have been reported in Europe, Australia, New Zealand, and North America.

5. **Reservoir**—Humans.

6. **Incubation period**—Usually 3–5 days.

7. **Transmission**—Directly by fecal-oral or respiratory droplet contact with an infected person, or indirectly by contact with articles freshly soiled with feces or throat discharges of an infected person. *Enterovirus B* (serotypes CV-B1 to 5) has been found in sewage and flies, though the relationship to transmission of human infection is not clear. Stools may contain virus for several weeks.

8. **Risk groups**—No specific risk group.

9. **Prevention**—Avoid fecal-oral contact and/or respiratory droplet contact with infected persons and/or associated materials.

10. **Management of patient**—

1) Ordinarily limited to enteric precautions. Because of possible serious illness in the newborn, if a patient in a maternity unit or nursery develops an illness suggestive of enterovirus infection, precautions should be instituted at once. Individuals with suspected enterovirus infections (including health personnel) should be excluded from visiting maternity and nursery units and from contact with infants and women near term.

2) Prompt and safe disposal of respiratory discharges and feces; wash or dispose of soiled articles. Careful attention must be given to prompt, thorough handwashing when handling discharges, feces, and soiled articles.

3) Treatment: no specific treatment exists. Nonsteroidal anti-inflammatory drugs and analgesics (other than aspirin) are used for the symptomatic relief of pleurodynia.

11. **Management of contacts and the immediate environment**— Common hygiene measures aid in the prevention of the oral-fecal transmission of *Enterovirus B*; contaminated surfaces and articles can be disinfected as stated in Enteroviral Vesicular Stomatitis With Exanthem section in this chapter.

12. **Special considerations—**

1) Reporting: obligatory report of epidemics to the local health authority.
2) Epidemic measures: general notice to physicians and health care providers of the presence of an epidemic and the necessity for differentiation of cases from more serious medical or surgical emergencies.

III. VIRAL CARDITIS (enteroviral carditis)

1. **Clinical features—**An acute or subacute viral myocarditis or pericarditis, occurring as a manifestation of infection with enteroviruses, especially *Enterovirus B*. The enteroviruses are commonly identified etiologies of myocarditis. The myocardium is affected, particularly in neonates, in whom fever and lethargy may be followed rapidly by heart failure with pallor, cyanosis, dyspnea, tachycardia, and enlargement of heart and liver. Heart failure may be progressive and fatal, or recovery may take place over a few weeks; some cases run a relapsing course over months and may show residual heart damage (dilated cardiomyopathy). In young adults, pericarditis is the more common manifestation, with acute chest pain, disturbance of heart rate, and often dyspnea. It may mimic myocardial infarction but is frequently associated with pulmonary or pleural manifestations (pleurodynia). The disease may be associated with aseptic meningitis; hepatitis; orchitis; pancreatitis; pneumonia; hand, foot, and mouth disease; rash; or epidemic myalgia (see Myalgia, Epidemic section in this chapter).

2. **Causative agents—**See the table in this chapter.

3. **Diagnosis—**See Diagnosis under Enteroviral Vesicular Stomatitis With Exanthem section in this chapter.

4. **Occurrence—**The enteroviruses have long been known to be important causes of acute myocarditis. The true incidence of acute myocarditis is unknown, as is the true incidence of an enterovirus etiology. The etiology of most cases of myocarditis is probably not determined. However it is estimated that enteroviruses may cause 25%–35% of cases of myocarditis for which a cause is found. This estimate is based on serological study, nucleic-acid hybridization, and PCR-based studies of endomyocardial biopsy and autopsy specimens

5. **Reservoir; 6. Incubation period; 7. Transmission—**Same as for Myalgia, Epidemic section in this chapter.

8. Risk groups—Neonates, young infants, and young adults are susceptible to *Enterovirus B*-associated myocarditis.

10. Management of patient—Treatment: no specific antiviral available; supportive care with use of inotropes; IVIG have been used with uncertain clinical benefit in the absence of randomized clinical trials.

11. Management of contacts and the immediate environment; 12. Special considerations—Same as for Myalgia, Epidemic section in this chapter.

[A. Kiyu, M. H. Ooi, D. Perera, M. J. Cardosa, F. G. L. Ong]

EPSTEIN-BARR VIRUS INFECTIONS

DISEASE	ICD-10 CODE
MONONUCLEOSIS, INFECTIOUS	ICD-10 B27
BURKITT'S LYMPHOMA	ICD-10 C83.7
NASOPHARYNGEAL CARCINOMA	ICD-10 C11
OTHER MALIGNANCIES POSSIBLY RELATED TO EPSTEIN-BARR VIRUS	
HODGKIN'S DISEASE	ICD-10 C81
NON-HODGKIN'S LYMPHOMAS	ICD-10 B21.2, C83.0, C83.8, C83.9, C85

I. MONONUCLEOSIS, INFECTIOUS (gammaherpesviral mononucleosis, mononucleosis due to Epstein-Barr virus [EBV], glandular fever, monocytic angina, kissing disease)

1. Clinical features—An acute viral syndrome characterized clinically by fever, sore throat (often with exudative pharyngotonsillitis), lymphadenopathy (especially posterior cervical), and splenomegaly; characterized hematologically by mononucleosis and lymphocytosis of 50% or greater, including 10% or more atypical cells; and characterized serologically by the presence of EBV antibodies. Recovery usually occurs in a few weeks, but a very small proportion of individuals can take months to regain their former level of energy. There is no evidence that this is due to abnormal persistence of the infection in a chronic form.

In young children the disease is generally mild and more difficult to recognize. Jaundice occurs in about 4% of infected young adults, although

95% have abnormal liver function tests; splenomegaly occurs in 50%. Duration is from one to several weeks; the disease is rarely fatal and is more severe in older adults.

The causal agent, EBV, is also closely associated with the pathogenesis of several lymphomas and nasopharyngeal cancer (see Nasopharyngeal Carcinoma section in this chapter). Fatal immunoproliferative disorders involving a polyclonal expansion of EBV infected B-lymphocytes may occur in persons with an X-linked recessive immunoproliferative disorder; they can also occur in persons with acquired immune defects, including those with HIV, transplant recipients, and persons with other conditions requiring long-term immunosuppressive therapy.

A syndrome resembling infectious mononucleosis is caused by cytomegalovirus, and accounts for 5%–7% of the "mono syndrome" (see "Cytomegalovirus Disease"); other rare causes are toxoplasmosis and herpesvirus type 6 (see "Exanthema Subitum") following rubella. A mononucleosis-like illness may occur early in HIV-infected patients; differentiation depends on laboratory results that include the EBV immunoglobulin class M (IgM) test.

2. Causative agent—EBV, also called human (gamma) herpesvirus 4. It is closely related to other herpesviruses morphologically, but distinct serologically; it infects and transforms B-lymphocytes.

3. Diagnosis—Laboratory diagnosis may include the finding of a lymphocytosis exceeding 50% (including ≥10% abnormal forms) and abnormalities in liver function tests (aspartate aminotransferase [AST]). EBV antibody tests are not usually needed to diagnose infectious mononucleosis; however, antibody tests may be beneficial in identifying the cause of illness, particularly in those individuals who do not have a typical case of infectious mononucleosis. Because of their poor sensitivity and specificity, the use of heterophile antibody tests is no longer recommended in the diagnosis of EBV infections. The most beneficial EBV antibody tests include measuring antibodies to the viral capsid antigen (VCA) and the EBV nuclear antigen (EBNA). A positive anti-VCA IgM response or a high anti-VCA immunoglobulin class G (IgG) response coupled with a negative anti-EBNA response is indicative of a current or recent EBV infection. The presence of both anti-VCA and anti-EBNA antibodies during a period of 4 weeks after onset of clinical symptoms suggests evidence of a past EBV infection. In rare cases, individuals with active EBV infections may not have detectable EBV-specific antibodies. Since most adults have been infected with EBV, they will have elevated anti-VCA and anti-EBNA antibody titers for years.

4. Occurrence—Worldwide. Typical infectious mononucleosis occurs primarily in industrialized countries, where age of infection is delayed until older childhood and young adulthood, so that it is most commonly recognized in high school and college students. About 50% of those infected develop clinical infectious mononucleosis; the others are mostly asymptomatic. Infection is common and widespread in early childhood in developing countries, and in socioeconomically depressed population groups in some industrialized countries, where it is usually mild or asymptomatic.

5. Reservoir—Humans.

6. Incubation period—From 4-6 weeks.

7. Transmission—Person-to-person spread by the oropharyngeal route, via saliva. Young children may be infected by saliva on the hands of nurses and other attendants and on toys, or by prechewing of baby food by the mother, a practice in some countries. Kissing facilitates spread among young adults. Spread may also occur via blood transfusion to susceptible recipients, but ensuing clinical disease is uncommon. Reactivated EBV may play a role in the interstitial pneumonia of HIV-infected infants and in hairy leukoplakia and B-cell tumors in HIV-infected adults.

The period of communicability is prolonged; pharyngeal excretion may persist in cell-free form for a year or more after infection; 15%-20% or more of EBV antibody-positive healthy adults are long-term oropharyngeal carriers.

8. Risk groups—Reactivation of EBV may occur in immunodeficient individuals and may result in elevated antibody titers to EBV, and possibly in the development of lymphomas. Infection confers a high degree of resistance; immunity from unrecognized childhood infection may account for low rates of clinical disease in older populations of lower socioeconomic groups.

9. Prevention—Use hygienic measures, including handwashing, to avoid salivary contamination from infected individuals through intimate or other contact; avoid drinking beverages from a common container in order to minimize contact with saliva.

10. Management of patient—

1) Concurrent disinfection of articles soiled with nose and throat discharges.
2) No specific treatment. Nonsteroidal anti-inflammatory drugs, or steroids given in small doses in decreasing amounts over about a week, are of value in severe toxic cases and in patients with severe oropharyngeal involvement and airway encroachment.

11. Management of contacts and the immediate environment—None.

12. Special considerations—None.

II. BURKITT'S LYMPHOMA (BL, African Burkitt's lymphoma, endemic Burkitt's lymphoma, Burkitt tumor)

Burkitt's lymphoma (BL) is a tumor of B cell origin characterized by the activation of the c-MYC oncogene. Three distinct clinical types of BL have been described by the WHO: endemic (African), sporadic (nonendemic), and immunodeficiency-associated. They all have similar histopathological features with germinal centroblasts and similar clinical behavior but differ in epidemiology, clinical presentation, EBV association, and genetics. The translocation of most endemic cases involves the heavy chain joining region while in sporadic cases the heavy chain switch region is most often involved. Translocations in BL are likely followed by several other additional genetic abnormalities, which are commonly found in all BL cases, in order for tumorigenesis to occur.

The endemic type occurs in regions where altitudes are typically below 1,000 m (~3,000 ft) and rainfall above 1,000 mL (~40 in) a year, such as in equatorial Africa and lowland Papua New Guinea. The incidence rates in these areas are around 50 per year per million children younger than 18 years, with peak incidence occurring in children around 6 years old. BL accounts for more than 90% of childhood lymphomas and commonly present with jaw and facial bone involvement.

Sporadic BL is much less common and is seen mostly in North America, Europe, and East Asia. Incidence rates vary but have been reported to be around 3 per million (children and adults combined) per year in North America and Western Europe; they account for around 30% of all childhood lymphomas and less than 1% of adult lymphomas. Incidence rates peak for children around 11 years old and for adults around 30 years old. Patients commonly present with abdominal disease.

The immunodeficiency-associated type is mostly seen in patients with HIV and less commonly in patients with organ transplant and hereditary immunodeficiency, such as familial X-linked immunodeficiency. Patients usually present with nodal and central nervous system (CNS) disease. In patients with BL and HIV, cluster of differentiation 4 glycoprotein (CD4) counts are typically high and they present during the early stages of HIV infection.

EBV plays an important pathogenic role in almost all of the cases for endemic BL, where EBV infection occurs in infancy and where malaria, an apparent cofactor, is holoendemic. For sporadic BL, EBV association rates vary geographically and are not well characterized; rates range from under 25% in North America to 85% in northern Brazil, and disease is not malaria-related. In HIV-associated BL, EBV positivity has been reported to be around 30%–40%. In general, the estimated time range of tumor development is 2–12 years from primary EBV infection, but is much shorter in patients with HIV.

BL is a highly aggressive tumor, but can nevertheless be cured in 90% of cases with intensive multiple-agent chemotherapy. Prevention of EBV infection early in life and control of malaria (see "Malaria") might reduce tumor incidence in Africa and Papua New Guinea. Subunit vaccines against EBV are in the trial stage. Cases should be reported to a tumor registry.

III. NASOPHARYNGEAL CARCINOMA

Nasopharyngeal carcinoma is a malignant tumor of the epithelial cells of the nasopharynx that usually occurs in adults aged 20–40 years. Incidence is particularly high (~10-fold when compared with the general population) among groups from China (Taiwan and southern China), even in those who have moved elsewhere. This risk decreases in subsequent generations after emigration from Asia.

Immunoglobulin class A (IgA) antibody to the EBV viral capsid antigen in both serum and nasopharyngeal secretions is characteristic of the disease and has been used in China as a screening test for the tumor. Its appearance may precede the clinical appearance of nasopharyngeal carcinoma by several years and its reappearance after treatment heralds recurrence.

The serological and virological evidence relating EBV to nasopharyngeal carcinoma is similar to that for BL (high EBV antibody titers, genome in tumor cells); this genetic relationship has been found without respect to the geographical origin of the patient. The tumor occurs worldwide, but is highest in southern China, southeastern Asia, northern and eastern Africa, and the Arctic. Male cases outnumber female cases by about a 2:1 ratio. Chinese with HLA-2 and SIN-2 antigen profiles have a particularly high risk.

EBV infection occurs early in life in settings where nasopharyngeal carcinoma is most common, yet the tumor does not appear until 20–40 years old, which suggests the occurrence of some secondary reactivating factor, with epithelial invasion later in life. Repeated respiratory infections or chemical irritants, such as nitrosamines in dried foods, may play a role. The higher frequency of the tumor in persons of southern Chinese origin without respect to later residence, and the association with certain human leukocyte antigen (HLA) haplotypes, suggest a genetic susceptibility. A lower incidence among those who have migrated to the USA and elsewhere suggests that one or more environmental factor(s)—suspected are the nitrosamines present in smoked fish and other foods—may be associated cofactors. Early detection in highly endemic areas (screening for EBV IgA antibodies to viral capsid antigen) permits early treatment. A subunit vaccine against EBV infection is under study. Chemotherapy after early recognition is the only specific therapy for nasopharyngeal carcinoma. Cases should be reported to a tumor registry.

IV. OTHER MALIGNANCIES POSSIBLY RELATED TO EBV

Hodgkin's disease is a tumor of the lymphatic system occurring in 4 histological subtypes: nodular sclerosis, lymphocyte predominance, mixed cellularity, and lymphocyte depletion. The histology shows the presence of a highly specific but nonpathognomonic cell, the Reed-Sternberg cell, also seen in cases of infectious mononucleosis. The cause of Hodgkin's disease is not certain, but laboratory and epidemiological evidence associates EBV in at least half the cases. The disease is more common in industrialized countries, but age-adjusted incidence is relatively low. It is more common in higher socioeconomic settings, in smaller families, and in Caucasians compared to Americans of African origin.

Hodgkin's disease may develop after infectious mononucleosis and occur some 10 years later; Hodgkin's disease in older adults, if EBV-associated, is thought to be the result of virus reactivation in the presence of a naturally deteriorating immune system. The high frequency of EBV found in cases of Hodgkin's disease diagnosed among HIV-infected patients and the relatively short incubation period appear related to the severe immunodeficiency of HIV infection; whether the presence of EBV in the tumor cell is cause or effect is not known. Among HIV-infected patients, particularly those infected through intravenous (IV) drug use, a higher proportion of Hodgkin's disease is EBV-associated. Cases should be reported to a tumor registry.

For non-Hodgkin's lymphomas (NHL), the incidence of lymphomas in AIDS patients is about 50–100 times that in the general population. While these lymphomas may be related to EBV, HIV is the virus most associated with NHL tumors such as high grade and CNS lymphomas. Since 1980, NHL has shown a dramatic increase among young, single white men with AIDS in the USA. About 4% of AIDS patients present with lymphoma, and perhaps 30% will eventually develop lymphoma if untreated for their HIV infection and survival is sufficiently long. Whether EBV is a causal factor in EBV-associated lymphomas in HIV-infected patients, or simply enters the tumor cell after it has been formed, is not clear, but accumulating evidence points to the former possibility. A marked increase in NHL not explained by the increase in AIDS patients has been noted in recent years. The disease commonly occurs in the presence of other forms of immunodeficiency, such as those in post-transplant patients, people given immunosuppressive drugs, and people with inherited forms of immunodeficiency. There are few epidemiological indications as to the risk factors responsible. Altered antibody patterns to EBV, characteristic of those seen in immunodeficiency states, occur in many cases of NHL; these changes have been shown to precede the development of NHL. Molecular techniques have demonstrated the EBV genome in 10%–15% of tumor cells of the spontaneous form of NHL. Cases should be reported to a tumor registry.

[D. L. Heymann, B. Wilcke, E. K. Yeoh, K. W. Yeoh]

ERYTHEMA INFECTIOSUM
(fifth disease)

DISEASE	ICD-10 CODE
ERYTHEMA INFECTIOSUM	ICD-10 B08.3

1. **Clinical features**—A usually mild childhood viral exanthematous disease, with low-grade or no fever, occurring sporadically or in epidemics. Characteristic is a striking erythema of the cheeks (slapped cheek appearance), frequently associated with a lace-like rash on the trunk and extremities, which fades but may recur for 1–3 weeks or longer on exposure to sunlight or heat (e.g., bathing). Itch may occur on the rash-affected skin and on the palm/sole. Mild constitutional symptoms may precede onset of rash. In adults, the rash is often atypical or absent, but polyarthropathy (arthralgia or arthritis) may occur. Arthropathy is uncommon in children but occurs in 50% of adults, more commonly in women; distribution is symmetric with involvement of small joints of hands and occasionally ankles, knees, and wrists. Arthropathy may last days to months but then resolves. Twenty-five percent or more of infections may be asymptomatic.

Differentiation from rubella, scarlet fever, dengue fever, and chikungunya fever is necessary. Usually the rash of erythema infectiosum (commonly called fifth disease) does not have raised maculopapular appearance unlike in these diseases. On dark skin the rash is very often missed on examination.

Complications are unusual, but persons with hemolytic anemias (e.g., sickle cell disease) may develop transient aplastic crisis, often even in the absence of a preceding rash. Intrauterine infection in the first half of pregnancy results in hydrops fetalis and fetal death in fewer than 10% of infections, and intrauterine infection infrequently results in fetal anemia that persists in the infant after birth. Immunosuppressed people may develop severe, chronic anemia. Red cell aplasia has been reported. Several diseases (e.g., rheumatoid arthritis, systemic vasculitis, fulminant hepatitis, and myocarditis) have been reported in association with erythema infectiosum, but no causal link has been established.

2. Causative agent—Human parvovirus B19, a 20- to 25-nm deoxyribonucleic acid (DNA) virus, belonging to the family *Parvoviridae,* genus *erythrovirus.* The virus replicates primarily in erythroid precursor cells. B19 is resistant to inactivation by various methods, including heating to 80°C (176°F) for 72 hours.

3. Diagnosis—Usually on clinical and epidemiological grounds. Can be confirmed by detection of parvovirus B19 specific immunoglobulin class M (IgM) antibodies or by a rise in immunoglobulin class G (IgG) antibody titers. IgM titers begin to decline 1-2 months after the onset of symptoms. Diagnosis of B19 infection is ideally made by detecting viral DNA by nucleic acid amplification by polymerase chain reaction (PCR), which is highly sensitive and specific, and will often remain positive during the first month of acute infection and for prolonged periods in some people, showing that the infection is chronic in some.

4. Occurrence—Worldwide, common in children; both sporadic and epidemic. In temperate zones, epidemics tend to occur in winter and spring, with a periodicity of 3-7 years in a given community.

5. Reservoir—Humans.

6. Incubation period—Variable; 4-20 days to development of rash or symptoms of aplastic crisis.

7. Transmission—Primarily through contact with respiratory secretions; also from mother to fetus, and through transfusion of blood and blood products. The child with disease is infectious starting from a few days before onset of rash until the rash has faded, usually a span of 1 week to 10 days. Those who have an aplastic crisis may be infectious longer. Those with chronic infection may remain infectious for longer periods of time; the immunosuppressed with chronic infection and severe anemia are infectious for months to years. Transmission as a result of transfusion is mostly from pooled blood components.

8. Risk groups—Universal susceptibility in persons with blood group P antigen, the receptor for B19 in erythroid cells. Attack rates among susceptibles can be high: 50% in household contacts and 10%-60% in the day care or school setting during a 2-6 month outbreak period. Those with preexisting anemia or immunodeficiency and pregnant women not immune to B19 are most at risk of serious complications.

9. Prevention—

1) As the disease is generally benign, prevention efforts should focus on preventing complications in those most likely to

develop them, who should avoid exposure to potentially infectious people in hospital or outbreak settings.

2) Susceptible women who are pregnant or who might become pregnant, and have continued close contact to people with B19 infection (e.g., at school, home, or in health care facilities), should be advised of the potential for acquiring infection and of the potential risk of complications to the fetus. Pregnant women with sick children at home are advised to keep reasonable physical distance, wash hands frequently, and avoid sharing eating utensils.

3) Health care workers should be advised of the importance of following good infection control measures. Rare nosocomial outbreaks have been reported. Strict handwashing is required after patient contact.

4) Plasma pools should be screened by PCR (nucleic acid amplification) and positive pools should be discarded.

11. Management of patient—

1) Cases of transient aplastic crisis in the hospital setting should be placed on droplet precautions. Although children with B19 infection are most infectious before onset of illness, it may be prudent to exclude them from school or day care attendance while fever or rash is present.

2) Treatment: intravenous immunoglobulin (IVIG) has been successfully used to treat chronic anemia in persistent infections, but relapses can occur and may require additional IVIG therapy.

12. Management of contacts and the immediate environment—

1) A recombinant B19 capsid vaccine is in development at time of writing.

2) Exposed pregnant women should be offered B19 IgG and IgM antibody testing to determine susceptibility, and to assist with counseling regarding risks to their fetuses.

13. Special considerations—

1) Reporting: any detected outbreak should be reported to the local health authority.

2) During outbreaks in school or day care settings, those with hemolytic anemia or immunodeficiency and pregnant women should be informed of the possible risk of acquiring and transmitting infection.

[T. J. John]

❖

EXANTHEMA SUBITUM

DISEASE	ICD-10 CODE
EXANTHEMA SUBITUM	ICD-10 B08.2

1. Clinical features—Exanthema subitum results from primary infection with a human herpesvirus, particularly the 6B strain (HHV-6B), in children younger than 2 years. It is unusual in children older than this and in adults, where primary infection causes a mild glandular fever-like illness in some individuals. Most infections with HHV are asymptomatic or cause a nonspecific fever. Exanthema subitum presents as an acute febrile illness, up to 41°C (106°F), which subsides in 3–5 days, followed a few days later by a maculopapular rash on the trunk and later on the remainder of the body, which then fades rapidly. Symptoms are generally mild, but febrile seizures and more severe illness, such as meningoencephalitis or hepatitis, occur in a small proportion.

Occasionally exanthema subitum is caused by other viruses, such as enteroviruses and adenoviruses. Also, it may clinically resemble other viral exanthems such as measles, rubella, and parvovirus B19 (erythema infectiosum) infection. However, the mild nature of the illness and the gap between resolution of the fever and onset of the rash are important diagnostic clues.

2. Causative agent—HHV-6 (subfamily betaherpesvirus, genus *Roseolovirus*) is the most common cause of exanthema subitum, particularly the HHV-6B strain, with occasional cases due to HHV-7. As with the other herpesviruses, primary infection is followed by lifelong latent infection, mainly in the salivary glands and monocyte/macrophages. Reactivations occur regularly and are usually asymptomatic. Immunosuppressed individuals may get severe disease due to both primary infection and reactivation, including fever, encephalitis, pneumonitis, hepatitis, and bone marrow suppression.

3. Diagnosis—Virus can be detected by polymerase chain reaction (PCR) in saliva, peripheral blood, urine, cervical secretions, and other sites during primary infection and reactivation, though titers are higher in primary infection. Peripheral blood PCR assays are usually reserved for immunosuppressed patients. Serologically, primary infection is indicated by immunoglobulin class G (IgG) seroconversion or a rise in IgG over the course of 7–14 days, with detectable immunoglobulin class M (IgM) appearing 1 week after onset and disappearing by 3–4 weeks. Reactivations are usually marked by a rapid rise in IgG with or without IgM.

4. Occurrence—Worldwide, the incidence peaks in 6–13 months of age, with 65%–100% seroprevalence by 2 years of age. Seroprevalence in women of childbearing age ranges from 80%-100% in most of the world, although rates as low as 20% have been observed in Morocco, and 49% in Malaysia. HHV-6 infections and exanthema subitum occur year round, though a seasonal predilection (late winter, early spring) has been described in Japan.

5. Reservoir—Latently infected humans are the only known reservoir of infection.

6. Incubation period—10 days, with a usual range of 5-15 days. For susceptible organ transplant recipients, onset of illness after primary infection is usually 2-4 weeks after transplantation.

7. Transmission—Infection is most likely acquired by direct or indirect contact with saliva from individuals with primary infection or reactivation, especially within household or day care settings. Transplacental transmission is well described but rarely causes adverse fetal outcomes, and the virus can also be transmitted by transfusion of blood or blood products. Organ transplant recipients may acquire infection from the transplant, though currently there is no standard recommendation for HHV-6 testing or matching of infected donors and recipients. Other potential modes of transmission, including breastfeeding and sexual contact, do not appear to be important.

8. Risk groups—Infection rates in infants younger than 6 months are low, possibly due to temporary protection from transplacentally acquired maternal antibodies, but increase rapidly thereafter. Most children are infected within the first 2 years of life so that disease is uncommon after that age. Immunosuppressed individuals, including those with organ transplants, are at increased risk of severe disease due to both primary infection and reactivation.

9. Prevention—Effective measures are not available, and screening before organ transplants is not routinely done.

10. Management of patient—There is no specific treatment for immunocompetent patients. Antiviral agents may be useful in immunosuppressed patients. No special precautions are recommended.

11. Management of contacts and the immediate environment—Investigation of contacts and source of infection is not recommended because of the high prevalence of asymptomatic shedders in the population.

12. Special considerations—None.

[D. Smith]

FASCIOLIASIS

DISEASE	ICD-10 CODE
FASCIOLIASIS	ICD-10 B66.3

1. Clinical features—A zoonotic disease caused by *Fasciola* parasites (liver flukes), which predominantly affect the hepatobiliary system. During the acute (early) phase of infection, immature *Fasciola* larvae migrate from the intestine through the abdominal cavity and liver, where they can cause parenchymal damage. The chronic phase begins when the larvae reach the bile ducts, where they mature into adult flukes and start to produce eggs (3–4 months after initial exposure), which are passed from the bile ducts into the intestine (thereafter into feces); the flukes may cause biliary colic or obstructive jaundice. During both phases, clinical features can include fever, malaise, abdominal symptoms (e.g., pain, anorexia, nausea, vomiting, diarrhea, weight loss), eosinophilia (especially during the acute phase), hepatomegaly, and abnormal liver function tests. Ectopic infection, especially by *Fasciola gigantica*, may produce transient or migrating areas of inflammation in the skin over the trunk or other areas of the body.

2. Causative agents—The trematodes *Fasciola hepatica* (also known as the common liver fluke) and *F. gigantica*.

3. Diagnosis—Based on finding eggs in feces or in biliary or duodenal aspirates during the chronic phase. Serologic testing (available through some centers) can be useful (i.e., positive results can provide supportive evidence of the diagnosis) during the acute phase, before eggs are produced; during the chronic phase, in cases with low-level production of eggs; and in cases of ectopic infection. False fascioliasis (pseudofascioliasis) refers to the presence of noninfective *Fasciola* eggs in feces after consumption of liver from an infected animal.

4. Occurrence—Human infection has been reported from more than 50 countries, on all continents except Antarctica, mainly in sheep- and cattle-raising areas; *F. hepatica* is more widespread than *F. gigantica*. In some areas (e.g., in the USA), only sporadic human cases of *Fasciola* infection have been documented, whereas human fascioliasis is hyperendemic in some regions (e.g., the Andean highlands of Bolivia and Peru). Outbreaks have occurred in multiple countries.

5. Reservoir—Maintained in a cycle between animals—mainly sheep, cattle, water buffalo, and other large herbivorous mammals—and freshwater snails of the family *Lymnaeidae*. Humans are considered accidental hosts; in some areas, environmental contamination by infected humans may lead to ongoing transmission.

6. Incubation period—Clinical manifestations, if any, during the acute phase of infection can start 4–7 days after the exposure and can last several weeks or months. Symptoms/signs, if any, during the chronic phase can start months to years after the exposure.

7. Transmission—Eggs passed in feces develop in freshwater; in about 2 weeks, a motile ciliated larva (miracidium) hatches. After entering a snail (lymnaeid), larvae develop to produce large numbers of free-swimming cercariae, which attach to aquatic plants and encyst; these encysted forms (metacercariae) resist drying. Infection is acquired by eating uncooked aquatic plants (such as watercress) that are contaminated with metacercariae, the infective stage; transmission also can occur by ingesting contaminated water. Infection is not transmitted directly from person to person.

8. Risk groups—Persons in endemic areas who eat uncooked watercress or other aquatic plants from grazing areas.

9. Prevention—

1) Educate the public in endemic areas to avoid eating uncooked watercress and other aquatic plants of wild or unknown origin (and to avoid drinking potentially contaminated water), especially from grazing areas or places where the disease is known to be endemic. Vegetables grown in fields that might have been irrigated with contaminated water should be thoroughly cooked.

2) Control the growth and sale of watercress and other edible water plants. For example, avoid using livestock feces to fertilize water plants.

3) Drain the land or use chemical molluscicides to eliminate mollusks in areas where this is technically and economically feasible. Of note, the appropriate measures for control programs depend on the setting.

10. Management of patient—Treatment: triclabendazole is the treatment of choice. Praziquantel typically is not active against *Fasciola* parasites. On the basis of limited data, nitazoxanide might be effective therapy for some patients.

11. Management of contacts and the immediate environment—Identification of the source(s) of infection may be useful in preventing/interrupting transmission. See Prevention in this chapter.

12. Special considerations—None.

[B. L. Herwaldt]

FASCIOLOPSIASIS

DISEASE	ICD-10 CODE
FASCIOLOPSIASIS	ICD-10 B66.5

1. **Clinical features**—A zoonotic trematode infection of the small intestine, particularly the duodenum. Symptoms result from local inflammation, ulceration of intestinal wall, and systemic toxic effects. Diarrhea usually alternates with constipation; vomiting and anorexia are frequent. Large numbers of flukes may produce acute intestinal obstruction. Patients may show edema of the face, abdominal wall, and legs within 20 days after massive infection; ascites is common. Eosinophilia is usual; secondary anemia may occur. Death is rare; light infections are usually asymptomatic.

2. **Causative agent**—*Fasciolopsis buski*, a large trematode, 2-4 cm long, but reaching lengths up to 7 cm.

3. **Diagnosis**—Through detection of the large flukes or characteristic eggs in stool or vomitus.

4. **Occurrence**—Widely distributed in rural southeastern Asia, especially central and south China, parts of India, and Thailand. Prevalence is often high in pig-rearing areas.

5. **Reservoir**—Swine and humans are definitive hosts and reservoirs of adult flukes; dogs less commonly.

6. **Incubation period**—Eggs appear in feces about 3 months after infection.

7. **Transmission**—Acquired by eating aquatic plants uncooked. Eggs passed in human and swine feces develop in water within 3-7 weeks under favorable conditions; miracidia hatch and penetrate planorbid snails as intermediate hosts; cercariae develop, are liberated, and encyst on aquatic plants to become infective metacercariae. In China, chief sources of infection are the nuts of the red water caltrop (*Tapa bicornis, Tapa natans*), grown in enclosed ponds, and tubers of the so-called water chestnut (*Eliocharis tuberosa*) and water bamboo (*Zizania aquatica*); infection frequently results when the hull or skin is peeled off with teeth and lips; less often from metacercaria in pond water. The period of communicability lasts as long as viable eggs are discharged in feces; without treatment, probably for 1 year. No direct person-to person transmission.

8. Risk groups—Risk for infection occurs in those who eat uncooked aquatic plants. In malnourished individuals, ill effects are pronounced; the number of worms influences severity of disease.

9. Prevention—

1) Educate the population at risk in endemic areas on the mode of transmission and life cycle of the parasite.
2) Sanitary disposal of human waste. Prevent human and pig fecal contamination of water where aquatic plants are grown.
3) Bar swine from contaminating areas where water plants are growing; do not feed water plants to pigs.
4) Dry suspected plants, or if plants are to be eaten fresh, dip them in boiling water for a few seconds; both methods kill metacercariae.

10. Management of patient—

1) Safe disposal of feces.
2) Treatment: praziquantel is the drug of choice.

11. Management of contacts and the immediate environment—Identify aquatic plants that harbor encysted metacercariae and are eaten fresh; identify infected snail species living in water with such plants; and prevent contamination of water with human and pig feces.

12. Special considerations—Reporting: case report to local health authority may be required in some endemic areas.

[J. Jones, M. Eberhard]

FILARIASIS

DISEASE	ICD-10 CODE
BANCROFTIAN FILARIASIS	ICD-10 B74.0
MALAYAN FILARIASIS	ICD-10 B74.1
TIMOREAN FILARIASIS	ICD-10 B74.2
DIROFILARIASIS	ICD-10 B74.8
OTHER NEMATODES PRODUCING MICROFILARIAE IN HUMANS	
MANSONELLOSIS	ICD-10 B74.4
Loiasis (see "Loiasis")	
Onchocerciasis (see "Onchocerciasis")	

The term filarias\is denotes infection with any of several nematodes belonging to the superfamily *Filarioidea*. However, as used here, the term refers only to the lymphatic-dwelling filariae listed later. For others, refer to the specific disease.

I. BANCROFTIAN FILARIASIS, MALAYAN FILARIASIS (Brugian filariasis), TIMOREAN FILARIASIS

1. **Clinical features**—Bancroftian filariasis occurs in 2 biologically different forms. In one, the microfilariae circulate in the peripheral blood at night (nocturnal periodicity) with greatest concentrations between 10 PM and 2 AM; in the other, microfilariae circulate continuously in the peripheral blood, but occur in greater concentration in the daytime (diurnal subperiodicity). Adult parasites primarily cause lymphatic damage; the subsequent lymphoedema and its progression are due to secondary bacterial infections. Clinical manifestations in regions of endemic filariasis include: (a) a symptomatic and parasitologically negative form; (b) asymptomatic microfilaremia; (c) filarial fevers manifested by high fever, acute recurrent lymphadenitis, and retrograde lymphangitis with or without microfilaremia; (d) lymphostasis associated with chronic signs, including hydrocele, chyluria, lymphoedema and elephantiasis of the limbs, breasts and genitalia, with low-level or undetectable microfilaremia; and (e) tropical pulmonary eosinophilic syndrome, manifested by paroxysmal nocturnal asthma, chronic interstitial lung disease, recurrent low-grade fever, profound eosinophilia, and degenerating microfilariae in lung tissues but not in the bloodstream (occult filariasis).

Brugian and Timorean filariasis have clinical manifestations similar to those of Bancroftian filariasis, except that the recurrent acute attacks of adenitis and retrograde lymphangitis associated with fever are more severe, while chyluria is uncommon and elephantiasis is usually confined to the distal extremities, most frequently to the legs below the knees. Hydrocele and breast lymphoedema are rarely if ever seen.

2. Causative agents—*Wuchereria bancrofti*, *Brugia malayi*, and *Brugia timori*; long threadlike worms.

3. Diagnosis—Microfilariae are best detected during periods of maximal microfilaremia. Live microfilariae can be seen under low power in a drop of peripheral blood (finger prick) on a slide or in hemolyzed blood in a counting chamber. Giemsa-stained thick and thin smears permit species identification. Microfilariae may be concentrated by filtration of anticoagulated blood through a Nuclepore filter (2-5 μm pore size), in a Swinnex adapter, or by the Knott technique (centrifugal sedimentation of 2 mL of anticoagulated blood mixed with 10 mL of 2% formalin). More sensitive techniques to detect circulating filarial antigen of *W. bancrofti* by enzyme-linked immunosorbent assay (ELISA) or immunochromatic test cards have recently become available commercially. The adult worms in nests can be visualized on ultrasound by the "filarial dance sign"—the random motion of echogenic particles in patients with filariasis caused by the typical movement of these filariae in dilated intrascrotal lymphatic vessels (little is known about the prevalent worm nest locations in women)—but the sensitivity of this technique is too low for routine diagnosis.

4. Occurrence—*W. bancrofti*, the most widespread of the 3 parasites responsible for 90% of the lymphatic filariases, is endemic in most of the warm humid regions of the world, including Latin America (scattered foci in Brazil, the Dominican Republic, Guyana, and Haiti), Africa, Asia, and the Pacific Islands. It is common in areas where conditions favor breeding of vector mosquitoes. In general, nocturnal subperiodicity in *Wuchereria*-infected areas of the Pacific is found West of 140°E longitude, and diurnal subperiodicity East of 180°E longitude. *B. malayi* is endemic in rural southwestern India and southeastern Asia. *B. timori* occurs in Timor-Leste and on the rural islands of Flores, Alor, and Roti in southeastern Indonesia.

5. Reservoir—Humans with microfilariae in the blood for *W. bancrofti*, periodic *B. malayi*, and *B. timori*. In Malaysia, southern Thailand, the Philippines, Timor-Leste, and Indonesia, cats, civets (*Viverra tangalunga*), and nonhuman primates serve as reservoirs for subperiodic *B. malayi*, but zoonotic transmission is thought to be of limited significance.

6. Incubation period—Microfilariae may not appear in the blood until after 3-6 months in *B. malayi* and 6-12 months in *W. bancrofti* infections.

7. Transmission—Through bite of a mosquito harboring infective larvae. *W. bancrofti* is transmitted by many species, the most important being *Culex quinquefasciatus*, *Anopheles gambiae*, *Anopheles funestus*, *Aedes polynesiensis*, *Aedes scapularis*, and *Aedes pseudoscutellaris*. *B.*

malayi is transmitted by various species of *Mansonia*, *Anopheles*, and *Aedes*. *B. timori* is transmitted by *Anopheles barbirostris*. In the female mosquito, ingested microfilariae penetrate the stomach wall and develop in the thoracic muscles into elongated, infective filariform larvae that migrate to the proboscis. When the mosquito feeds, the larvae emerge and enter the punctured skin following the mosquito bite. They travel via the lymphatics, where they molt twice before becoming adults.

Not directly transmitted from person to person. Humans may infect mosquitoes when microfilariae are present in the peripheral blood; microfilaremia may persist for 5-10 years or longer after initial infection. The mosquito becomes infective about 12-14 days after an infective blood meal. A large number of infected mosquito bites are required to initiate infection in the host.

8. Risk groups—Universal susceptibility to infection is probable; there is considerable geographic difference in the type and severity of disease. Repeated infections may occur in endemic regions.

9. Prevention—

1) Educate the inhabitants of endemic areas on the mode of transmission and methods of mosquito control.

2) Identify the vectors by detecting infective larvae in mosquitoes caught; identify times and places of mosquito biting, and locate breeding places. If indoor night biters are responsible, screen houses or use bed nets (preferably impregnated with synthetic pyrethroid) and insect repellents. Eliminate mosquito breeding places (e.g., standing water in open latrines, tires, coconut husks) and treat with polystyrene beads or larvicides. Where *Mansonia* species are vectors, clear ponds of vegetation (*Pistia*) that serve as sources of oxygen for the larvae.

3) Long-term vector control may involve changes in housing construction to include screening and environmental control in order to eliminate mosquito-breeding sites.

4) Mass treatment with diethylcarbamazine citrate (DEC) is effective in decreasing microfilariae and transmission, especially when followed by monthly treatment with a low dose of DEC for 1-2 years or the use of DEC-fortified cooking salt for 6 months to 2 years. However, DEC cannot be used in areas where onchocerciasis is coendemic due to possible adverse reactions. In areas co-endemic for onchocerciasis, ivermectin is used; albendazole in multiple and single doses also has antifilarial properties. In lymphatic filariasis where onchocerciasis is not endemic, WHO currently recommends mass drug administration as an annual single dose of combinations of DEC with albendazole for 4-6 years,

or the regular use of DEC-fortified salt for 1-2 years. In areas where onchocerciasis is coendemic, mass drug administration using ivermectin and albendazole is recommended. Certain groups of individuals, such as pregnant women, children younger than 2 years (DEC and albendazole coadministration), children with a height under 90 cm, and lactating women in the first week (ivermectin and albendazole coadministration), as well as severely ill persons, should not receive the drugs. Mass drug administration with either DEC or ivermectin is contraindicated at present in areas with concurrent loiasis, due to the risk of severe adverse reactions in patients with high-density Loa loa infections; WHO has recently recommended the use of albendazole mass drug administration in these areas.

10. **Management of patient**—Treatment: as described earlier, patients with microfilaremia should be treated with antifilarial drugs and protected from mosquitoes to reduce transmission. DEC is generally effective in destroying adult worms; ivermectin in combination with albendazole may not destroy all the adult worms. Low-level microfilaremia may reappear after treatment with any drug. Therefore, treatment must usually be repeated at yearly intervals. Low-level microfilaremia can be detected only by concentration techniques. Antigen or antibody testing may provide alternate tools for tracking therapeutic responses. DEC may cause acute generalized reactions during the first 24 hours of treatment because of death and degeneration of microfilariae; these reactions are mostly self-limiting and often controlled by paracetamol and antihistamines. Localized lymphadenitis and lymphangitis may follow the death of the adult worms and usually occurs 5-7 days after taking the drugs. Care of the skin to prevent entry lesions for bacteria and fungi; exercise; elevation of affected limbs; and use of topical anti-fungal or antibiotics for superinfection, all help prevent acute dermatoadenolymphangitis and subsequent progression to lymphoedema. Management of lymphoedema includes local limb care; surgical decompression may be required. Hydroceles can be surgically repaired.

11. **Management of contacts and the immediate environment**— None.

12. **Special considerations**—

1) Reporting: may be required in some endemic regions; reporting of cases with demonstrated microfilariae or circulating filarial antigen provides information on areas of transmission.
2) WHO has launched a global program for the elimination of lymphatic filariasis as a public health problem through an alliance of endemic countries and partners from the public and private sectors. Further information can be found at:

- http://www.filariasis.org
- http://www.cdc.gov/parasites/lymphaticfilariasis
- http://www.who.int/tdr/diseases/lymphfil/default.htm

II. DIROFILARIASIS (zoonotic filariasis)

Certain species of filariae commonly seen in wild or domestic animals occasionally infect humans, but microfilaremia occurs rarely. The genus *Dirofilaria* causes pulmonary and cutaneous disease in humans. Human infection with *Dirofilaria immitis*, the dog heartworm, has been reported from most parts of the world, including Australia, Europe, Canada, the USA, Japan, and other parts of Asia. Transmission to humans is by mosquito bite. The worm lodges in a pulmonary artery, where it may form the nidus of a thrombus; this can then lead to vascular occlusion, coagulation, necrosis, and fibrosis. Symptoms are chest pain, cough, and hemoptysis. Eosinophilia is infrequent. A fibrotic nodule, 1–3 cm in diameter, which is most commonly asymptomatic, is recognizable by X-ray as a "coin lesion."

Various species cause subcutaneous lesions, including *Dirofilaria tenuis*, a parasite of the raccoon in the USA; *Dirofilaria ursi*, a parasite of bears in Canada; and *Dirofilaria repens*, a parasite of dogs and cats in Europe, Africa, and Asia. The worms develop in or migrate to the conjunctivae and the subcutaneous tissues of the scrotum, breasts, arms, and legs, but microfilaremia is rare. Animal species of *Brugia* cause zoonotic infections, localize in lymph nodes, and have been reported from North and South America and Africa. Similarly, animal species of *Onchocerca* have increasingly been reported to cause zoonotic infections, typically localized in demarcated nodules, and have been reported from North America, Europe, Eurasia, North Africa, Japan, and the Arabian Peninsula. Diagnosis is usually made by the finding of worms in tissue sections of surgically excised lesions.

III. OTHER NEMATODES PRODUCING MICROFILARIAE IN HUMANS

Several other nematodes may infect humans and produce microfilariae. These include *Onchocerca volvulus* and *Loa loa*, which cause onchocerciasis and loiasis, respectively (see "Onchocerciasis" and "Loiasis").

Other infections are forms of mansonellosis: *Mansonella perstans* is widely distributed in western Africa and northeastern South America; the adult is found in the body cavities, and the unsheathed microfilariae circulate with no regular periodicity. Infection is usually asymptomatic, but eye infection from immature stages has been reported. In some countries of western and central Africa, infection with *Mansonella streptocerca* is common and is suspected of causing cutaneous edema and thickening of the skin, hypopigmented macules, pruritus, and papules. Adult worms and unsheathed microfilariae occur in the skin as in onchocerciasis. *Mansonella ozzardi* occurs from the Yucatan Peninsula in Mexico to northern Argentina, and in the West Indies; diagnosis is based on demonstration of the circulating unsheathed nonperiodic microfilariae. Infection is generally asymptomatic but may be associated with allergic manifestations such as arthralgia, pruritus, headaches, and lymphadenopathy.

Culicoides midges are the main vectors for *M. streptocerca*, *M. ozzardi*, and *M. perstans*; in the Caribbean area, blackflies also transmit *M. ozzardi*. *Mansonella rodhaini*, a parasite of chimpanzees, was found in 1.7% of skin snips taken from humans in Gabon. Diethylcarbamazine is effective against *M. streptocerca* and occasionally against *M. perstans* and *M. ozzardi*. Ivermectin is effective against *M. ozzardi*.

[M. Eberhard, P. Lammie]

FOODBORNE INTOXICATIONS

DISEASE	ICD-10 CODE
FOODBORNE STAPHYLOCOCCAL INTOXICATION	ICD-10 A05.0
FOODBORNE *CLOSTRIDIUM PERFRINGENS* INTOXICATION	ICD-10 A05.2
FOODBORNE *BACILLUS CEREUS* INTOXICATION	ICD-10 A05.4
SEAFOOD POISONING	
SCOMBROID FISH POISONING	ICD-10 T61.1
CIGUATERA FISH POISONING	ICD-10 T61.0
PARALYTIC SHELLFISH POISONING	ICD-10 T61.2
NEUROTOXIC SHELLFISH POISONING	
DIARRHETIC SHELLFISH POISONING	ICD-10 T61.2
AMNESIC SHELLFISH POISONING	ICD-10 T61.2
PUFFER FISH POISONING	ICD-10 T61.2
(TETRODOTOXIN)	ICD-10 T61.2
AZASPIRACID POISONING	ICD-10 T61.2

The frequent causes of foodborne illnesses are:

- Toxins elaborated by bacterial growth in the intestines (*Clostridium perfringens*) or in the food before consumption (*Clostridium botulinum*, *Staphylococcus aureus*, and *Bacillus cereus*). Scombroid fish poisoning is associated with elevated histamine levels, not a specific toxin.
- Bacterial, viral, or parasitic infections (amebiasis, brucellosis, *Campylobacter* enteritis, diarrhea caused by *Escherichia coli*, hepatitis A,

listeriosis, salmonellosis, shigellosis, toxoplasmosis, viral gastroenteritis, teniasis, trichinosis, and infection with vibrios).

- Toxins produced by harmful algal species (ciguatera fish poisoning; paralytic, neurotoxic, diarrhetic, or amnesic shellfish poisoning) or present in specific species (puffer fish poisoning, azaspiracid poisoning, [AZP]).

This chapter deals specifically with toxin-related foodborne illnesses (with the exception of botulism, elaborated in a separate chapter). foodborne illnesses associated with infection by specific agents are covered in chapters dealing with these agents.

Foodborne disease outbreaks are recognized by the occurrence of illness within a variable but usually short time period (a few hours to a few weeks) after a meal among individuals who have consumed foods in common. Prompt and thorough laboratory evaluation of cases and implicated foods is essential. Single cases of foodborne disease are difficult to identify unless, as in botulism, there is a distinctive clinical syndrome. Foodborne disease may be one of the most common causes of acute illness; many cases and outbreaks are unrecognized and unreported.

Prevention and control of these diseases, regardless of cause, are based on the same principles: avoiding food contamination, destroying or denaturing contaminants, and preventing further spread or multiplication of these contaminants. Specific problems and appropriate modes of intervention may vary from one country to another and depend on environmental, economic, political, technological, and sociocultural factors. Ultimately, prevention also depends on educating food handlers about proper practices in cooking and storage of food, and personal hygiene. To this end, the WHO Five Keys to Safer Food (http://www.who.int/fsf/Documents/5keys-ID-eng.pdf) sets out 5 steps to ensuring safer food:

1) Keep clean (including hands, utensils, surfaces).
2) Separate raw and cooked.
3) Cook thoroughly.
4) Keep food at safe temperatures.
5) Use safe water and raw materials.

I. FOODBORNE STAPHYLOCOCCAL INTOXICATION

1. Clinical features—An intoxication (not an infection) of abrupt and sometimes violent onset, with severe nausea, cramps, vomiting, and prostration, often accompanied by diarrhea and sometimes with subnormal temperature and lowered blood pressure. Deaths are rare. Illness commonly lasts only a day or 2, but can take longer in severe cases. In rare cases, the intensity of symptoms may require hospitalization; and unnecessary surgical exploration has sometimes been done in pursuit of a diagnosis.

2. Causative agent—Staphylococci multiply in food and produce the toxins even when water activity is too low for the growth of many other competing bacteria. However, the level of enterotoxin only reaches dangerous levels when a relatively high (e.g., >1,000/g) concentration of Staphylococci is reached in the food. Therefore low levels of Staphylococci are typically accepted in certain foods in national legislation. It should be noted that several enterotoxins of *Staphylococcus aureus* are stable at boiling point and resist some thermal processing procedures; therefore in outbreak investigations, detection of enterotoxin is more reliable than enumeration of staphylococci.

3. Diagnosis—Easier when a group of cases present with the characteristic acute, predominantly upper gastrointestinal symptoms and a short interval between eating a common food item and the onset of symptoms (usually within 4 hours). Differential diagnosis includes other recognized forms of food poisoning as well as chemical poisons.

In the outbreak setting, recovery of large numbers of staphylococci ($\geq 10^5$ organisms/g of food), or detection of enterotoxin from an epidemiologically implicated food item, confirms the diagnosis. In heat-treated food it may be possible to identify enterotoxin or thermonuclease in the food in the absence of viable organisms, but killed staphylococci can be detectable through Gram stain of food samples. Isolation of organisms of the same phage type from stools or vomitus of 2 or more ill persons confirms the diagnosis. Recovery of large numbers of enterotoxin-producing staphylococci from stool or vomitus from a single person supports the diagnosis. Phage typing and enterotoxin tests may help epidemiological investigations, but are not routinely available or indicated. In outbreak settings, pulsed field gel electrophoresis may be more useful in subtyping strains, as might whole genome sequencing.

4. Occurrence—Widespread and relatively frequent; one of the principal acute food intoxications worldwide.

5. Reservoir—Humans in most instances (~25% of healthy people are carriers of *Staphylococcus aureus*); occasionally cows with mastitis, as well as dogs and fowl.

6. Incubation period—Interval between eating the contaminated food and onset of symptoms is 30 minutes to 8 hours, usually 2-4 hours.

7. Transmission—Through ingestion of a food product containing staphylococcal enterotoxin, particularly those foods that come in contact with food handlers' hands, either without subsequent cooking or with inadequate heating or refrigeration. Pastries, custards, salad dressings, sandwiches, meat products, and sliced meat are at great risk of contamination. Toxins have also developed in inadequately cured ham and salami, and in unprocessed or inadequately processed cheese. When these foods remain at room temperature for several hours before being eaten, toxin-producing staphylococci can multiply and elaborate the heat-stable toxin at dangerous levels. Organisms may be of human origin from purulent discharges of an infected finger or eye, abscesses, acneiform facial eruptions, nasopharyngeal secretions, or apparently normal skin; or of bovine origin, from products originating from contaminated milk, especially cheese.

8. Risk groups—Most people are susceptible. To date there is no data suggesting specific at-risk groups, but it should be noted that the elderly, infants, and people suffering from underlying diseases are most susceptible to dehydration

9. Prevention—

1) Educate food handlers about strict food hygiene; sanitation and cleanliness of kitchens; proper temperature control; and hand washing and cleaning of fingernails. Also ensure awareness of the danger of contaminating food by working when there is exposed skin, nose, or eye infection and uncovered wounds.

2) Reduce food-handling time, from initial preparation to service, to a minimum—no more than 4 hours at ambient temperature. If perishable foods are to be stored for more than 2 hours, keep them hot (>60°C/140°F) or cold (<5°C/41°F), in shallow containers, and covered.

3) Temporarily exclude people with boils, abscesses, and other purulent lesions of hands, face, or nose from handling food until lesions are fully healed.

10. Management of patient—Fluid replacement when indicated.

11. Management of contacts and the immediate environment—Control is of outbreaks; single cases are rarely identified.

12. Special considerations—

1) Reporting: it is obligatory in some countries to report outbreaks of suspected or confirmed cases to the local health authority.

2) Epidemic measures:

- Review reported cases to determine time and place of exposure and population at risk; obtain a complete listing of the foods served and embargo, under refrigeration, all foods still available. The prominent clinical features, coupled with an estimate of the incubation period, provide useful leads to the most probable causal agent. Collect specimens of feces and vomitus for laboratory examination. Alert the laboratory to suspected causal agents. Conduct an epidemiological investigation, and if relevant a case-control study including interviews of ill and well persons, to determine the association of illness with consumption of a given food.

- Inquire about the origin of incriminated food and the manner of its preparation and storage before serving. Look for possible sources of contamination and periods of inadequate refrigeration and heating that would permit growth of staphylococci. Submit leftover suspected foods promptly for laboratory examination; failure to isolate staphylococci does not exclude the presence of the heat-resistant enterotoxin if the food has been heated.

- Identify food handlers with skin infections, particularly on the hands. Culture all purulent lesions and collect nasal swabs from all food handlers. Antibiograms and/or phage typing and/or whole genome sequencing of representative strains of enterotoxin-producing staphylococci isolated from foods and food handlers and from patient vomitus or feces may be helpful.

3) Disaster implications: a potential risk in situations involving mass feeding and lack of refrigeration facilities, including feeding during air travel.

WHO Collaborating Centres provide support as required. Further information can be found at: http://www.who.int/collaboratingcentres/database/en.

II. FOODBORNE *CLOSTRIDIUM PERFRINGENS* INTOXICATION (enteritis necroticans, pigbel)

1. **Clinical features**—An intestinal disorder characterized by sudden onset of colic followed by diarrhea; nausea is common, vomiting and fever are usually absent. Generally a mild disease of short duration—1 day or less—and rarely fatal in previously healthy people. Outbreaks of severe disease with high case-fatality rates associated with necrotizing enteritis have been documented in postwar Germany and in Papua New Guinea (pigbel).

2. **Causative agent**—Type A strains of *C. perfringens* cause typical food poisoning outbreaks through production of *C. perfringens* enterotoxin (CPE) in the ileum. Type C strains cause necrotizing enteritis through production of the beta toxin.

3. Diagnosis—In the outbreak setting, diagnosis is confirmed by demonstration of *C. perfringens* in semiquantitative anerobic cultures of food ($\geq10^5$/g) or patients' stool ($\geq10^6$/g), in addition to clinical and epidemiological evidence. Detection of CPE in patients' stool also confirms the diagnosis. Typing, including genomic typing, can help in comparing food and patient strains.

4. Occurrence—Widespread and relatively frequent in countries with cooking practices that favor multiplication of clostridia to high levels (discussed later).

5. Reservoir—Gastrointestinal tract of healthy people and animals (cattle, fish, pigs, and poultry); soil, where spores can survive for years.

6. Incubation period—From 6-24 hours, usually 10-12 hours.

7. Transmission—Through ingestion of food containing soil or feces and then held under conditions that permit multiplication of the organism. Almost all outbreaks are associated with inadequately heated or (especially) reheated meats. Spores survive normal cooking temperatures, germinate, and multiply during slow cooling, storage at ambient temperature, and/or inadequate reheating. Upon ingestion of large numbers ($>10^5$ cells/g food) of vegetative *C. perfringens* cells, they sporulate in the intestinal lumen and produce CPE. Outbreaks are usually traced to catering firms, restaurants, cafeterias, and schools with inadequate cooling and refrigeration facilities for large-scale service.

8. Risk groups—Most people are probably susceptible. In volunteer studies, no resistance to reinfection was observed after repeated exposures. Fatalities are rare but possible in elderly or debilitated patients.

9. Prevention—

1) Educate food handlers about the risks inherent in large-scale cooking, especially of meat dishes. Promote the WHO Five Keys to Safer Food (http://www.who.int/foodsafety/consumer/5keys/en).

2) Serve meat dishes hot ($>60°C/140°F$), as soon as cooked, or cool them rapidly in a properly designed chiller and refrigerate until serving time. Reheating, if necessary, should be rapid and thorough (internal temperature of $\geq70°C/158°F$). For more rapid cooling of cooked foods, divide stews and similar dishes prepared in bulk into many shallow containers, and place in a rapid chiller.

10. Management of patient; 11. Management of contacts and the immediate environment; 12. Special considerations— See Foodborne Staphylococcal Intoxication section in this chapter.

III. FOODBORNE *BACILLUS CEREUS* INTOXICATION

1. Clinical features—An intoxication characterized in some cases by sudden onset of nausea and vomiting, and in others by colic and diarrhea. Illness generally persists no longer than 24 hours and is rarely fatal. Very rare fatal cases seem to be related to liver failure.

2. Causative agent—*Bacillus cereus*, an aerobic spore former. Two enterotoxins have been identified: a heat-stable emetic toxin: cereulide causing vomiting is produced in food when *B. cereus* levels reach 10^5 colony-forming units per gram of food; and several heat-labile toxins, causing diarrhea, which are formed during vegetative growth of *B. cereus* in the small intestine of the patient.

3. Diagnosis—In outbreak settings, diagnosis is confirmed through quantitative cultures on selective media to estimate the number of organisms present in the suspected food (generally $>10^5$-10^6 organisms/g of the incriminated food are required). Isolation of organisms from the stool of 2 or more ill persons and not from stools of controls also confirms the diagnosis. Enterotoxin testing is valuable but may not be widely available.

4. Occurrence—A well-recognized cause of foodborne disease throughout the world.

5. Reservoir—A ubiquitous organism in soil and environment, commonly found at low levels in raw, dried, and processed foods.

6. Incubation period—From 1-6 hours in cases where vomiting is the predominant symptom; from 8-16 hours where diarrhea predominates.

7. Transmission—Through ingestion of food kept at ambient temperatures after cooking, with germination of spores surviving heat treatment and multiplication of vegetative forms of the organism. Outbreaks associated with vomiting have been most commonly associated with cooked rice held at ambient room temperatures before reheating. Various mishandled foods have been implicated in outbreaks associated with diarrhea. Not communicable from person to person.

8. Risk groups—Unknown.

9. Prevention—Foods should not remain at ambient temperature after cooking, since the ubiquitous *B. cereus* spores can survive boiling, germinate, and multiply rapidly at room temperature. The emetic toxin is also heat-resistant. Refrigerate leftover food promptly (toxin formation is unlikely at temperatures $<10°C/50°F$); reheat thoroughly and rapidly to avoid multiplication of microorganisms.

10. Management of patient; 11. Management of contacts and the immediate environment; 12. Special considerations—See Foodborne Staphylococcal Intoxication section in this chapter.

SEAFOOD POISONING

IV. SCOMBROID POISONING (histamine poisoning)

A syndrome of tingling and burning sensations around the mouth, facial flushing and sweating, nausea and vomiting, headache, palpitations, dizziness, and rash. Histamine poisoning (scombroid poisoning) is a worldwide problem that occurs after the consumption of food containing biogenic amines, particularly histamine at concentrations higher than 500 ppm. Symptoms occur within a few hours after eating food containing high levels of free histamine; biogenic amines are typically formed through microbial decarboxylation of amino acids in the food in question, and these substances are heat stable. Histamine poisoning is often caused by fish products, often from the Scombroidea fish group (e.g., mackerel and tuna), although cheese has also been implicated. Symptoms resolve spontaneously within 12 hours and there are no long-term sequelae. In severe cases, antihistamines, either through inhalators or intravenously, may be effective in relieving symptoms.

Occurrence is worldwide. Detection of histamine in epidemiologically implicated food confirms the diagnosis. Good hygiene and rapid refrigeration prevents microbial spoilage and decarboxylation. Symptoms may be markedly worse in patients taking isoniazid or other drugs interfering with histamine metabolism.

V. CIGUATERA FISH POISONING

A characteristic gastrointestinal and neurological syndrome may occur within 1 hour after eating tropical reef fish. Gastrointestinal symptoms (diarrhea, vomiting, abdominal pain) occur first, usually within 24 hours of consumption. In severe cases, patients may also become hypotensive, with a paradoxical bradycardia. Neurological symptoms, including pain and weakness in the lower extremities and circumoral and peripheral aresthesias, may occur at the same time as the acute symptoms or follow 1–2 days later; they may persist for weeks or months. Symptoms such as temperature reversal (ice cream tastes hot, hot coffee seems cold) and "aching teeth" are frequently reported. In very severe cases, neurological symptoms may progress to coma and respiratory arrest within the first 24 hours of illness. Most patients recover completely within a few weeks; intermittent recrudescence of symptoms can occur over a period of months to years.

This syndrome is caused by the presence in the fish of heat-stable toxins elaborated by the dinoflagellate *Gambierdiscus toxicus,* an algae growing on underwater reefs. Fish eating the algae become toxic, and the effect is magnified through the food chain so that large predatory fish become the most toxic; this occurs worldwide in tropical areas.

Ciguatera poisoning is the most commonly reported marine food poisoning. It is a significant cause of morbidity where consumption of reef fish is common. Ciguatera occurs in very localized, time-limited outbreaks, so it is very difficult to predict risk. Risk of ciguatera is higher after events that disturb coral reefs, like tsunamis. Incidence has been estimated at 500 cases per 100,000 population per year in the South Pacific, with rates 50 times higher reported for some island groups. More than 400 fish species may have the potential for becoming toxic. Worldwide 50,000 cases of ciguatera are estimated to occur per year. Evidence of ciguatoxin in epidemiologically implicated fish confirms the diagnosis.

The consumption of large reef fish should be avoided. It is especially important to avoid eating the heads, viscera, and roe of reef fish. Where assays for toxic fish are available, screening all large "high-risk" fish before consumption can reduce risk. The occurrence of toxic fish is sporadic, and not all fish of a given species or from a given locale will be toxic.

Intravenous infusion of mannitol has been suggested to have an effect on acute symptoms of ciguatera poisoning, but follow-up double-blind studies have not been able to confirm this.

VI. PARALYTIC SHELLFISH POISONING

Paralytic shellfish poisoning (PSP) is a characteristic syndrome, predominantly neurological, starting within minutes to several hours after eating bivalve mollusks. Initial symptoms can begin from 15 minutes to 10 hours after eating and include paresthesias of the mouth and extremities accompanied by gastrointestinal symptoms. In severe cases, ataxia, dysphonia, dysphagia, and muscle paralysis with respiratory arrest and death may occur within 12 hours. Symptoms usually resolve completely within hours to days after shellfish ingestion.

This syndrome is caused by the presence in shellfish of saxitoxins or other toxins produced by *Alexandrium* species and other dinoflagellates. Concentration of these toxins occurs during massive algal blooms known as "red tides," but also in the absence of recognizable algal bloom. PSP is common in shellfish harvested from colder waters above 30°N and below 30°S latitude, but may also occur in tropical waters. In North America, PSP is primarily a problem in northern latitudes. Blooms of the causative *Alexandrium* species occur several times each year, in the Northern hemisphere primarily from April through October. Shellfish remain toxic for several weeks after the bloom subsides. Most cases occur in individuals or small groups who gather shellfish for personal consumption. Detection of toxin in epidemiologically implicated food confirms the diagnosis.

PSP neurotoxins are heat-stable. Surveillance of high-risk harvest areas is routine in Canada, the EU, Japan, and the USA. When toxin levels in shellfish exceed 80 micrograms of saxitoxin equivalent per 100 grams, areas are closed to harvesting and warnings posted in shellfish-growing areas, on beaches, and in the media.

VII. NEUROTOXIC SHELLFISH POISONING

Neurotoxic shellfish poisoning is associated with algal blooms (red tides) of *Karenia brevis*, which produce brevetoxin. Red tides have long occurred along the Florida coast, where the syndrome has been most studied, with associated mortality in fish, seabirds, and marine mammals. Symptoms after eating toxic shellfish—including circumoral paresthesias and paresthesias of the extremities, dizziness and ataxia, myalgia, and gastrointestinal symptoms—tend to be mild and resolve quickly and completely. Respiratory and eye irritation can also occur, apparently through aerosolization of the toxin through wind and wave action.

VIII. DIARRHETIC SHELLFISH POISONING

Diarrhetic shellfish poisoning (DSP) results from eating mussels, scallops, or clams that have fed on *Dinophysis* spp. dinoflaggelates. These algae can produce okadaic acid and a number of derivative toxins. Symptoms include diarrhea, nausea, vomiting, and abdominal pain.

In scallops, the distribution of toxins was localized in the hepatopancreas (midgut gland), the elimination of which renders scallops safe to eat. Ordinary cooking such as boiling in water or steaming cannot reduce okadaic acids in this gland because of their chemical stability and lipophilic properties. Methods of detection of DSP in shellfish include mouse bioassay, enzyme-linked immunosorbent assay (ELISA), and liquid chromatography-mass spectrometry. The USA has established the action level for DSP at 0.2 ppm OA plus 35-methyl okadaic acid.

IX. AMNESIC SHELLFISH POISONING

Amnesic shellfish poisoning results from ingestion of shellfish containing domoic acid produced by the diatom *Pseudonitzschia pungens*. Cases were first reported in the Atlantic provinces of Canada in 1987, with vomiting, abdominal cramps, diarrhea, headache, and short-term memory loss. When tested several months after acute intoxication, patients show antegrade memory deficits with relative preservation of other cognitive functions together with clinical and electromyographical evidence of pure motor or sensorimotor neuropathy and axonopathy. Canadian authorities now analyze mussels and clams for domoic acid, and close shellfish beds to harvesting when levels exceed 20 ppm domoic acid. The clinical significance of ingestion of low levels of domoic acid (in persons eating shellfish and anchovies harvested from areas where *Pseudonitzschia* species are present) is unknown. European Community [EC]–directive 91/492/EEC and amendments for the safety of shellfish (Amendment 97/61/EC) state that: "total Amnesic Shellfish Poison (ASP) content in the edible part of mollusks (the entire body or any part edible separately) must not exceed 20 μm of domoic acid per gram using HPLC [high pressure liquid chromatography]."

X. PUFFER FISH POISONING (TETRODOTOXIN)

Puffer fish poisoning is characterized by onset of paresthesias, dizziness, gastrointestinal symptoms, and ataxia, often progressing to paralysis, including of the diaphragm muscles, leading to death within several hours after eating. Case-fatality rates from 10%-60% have been reported. The causative toxin is tetrodotoxin, a heat-stable, nonprotein neurotoxin, thought to be produced by bacteria in the gut, then concentrated in the skin and viscera of puffer fish, porcupine fish, ocean sunfish, and species of newts and salamanders. Most cases occur in Japan, where 912 cases in the period from 1980-1999 led to 106 deaths. Japan implements control measures such as species identification and adequate removal of toxic parts (e.g., ova, intestine) by qualified cooks.

XI. AZASPIRACID POISONING

Occurrence of azaspiracid poisoning (AZP) was first reported when mussels harvested in Ireland caused diarrhea in humans in the Netherlands in 1995. Since 1996 several AZP incidents have been identified in several European countries, and the toxin has been isolated from mussels in European waters as well as in North Africa and Canada. Symptoms occur 12-24 hours after consumption and persist for up to 5 days; they include severe diarrhea and vomiting with abdominal pain and occasional nausea, chills, headaches, and stomach cramps. Azaspiracid poisoning can cause necrosis in the intestine, thymus, and liver. A regulatory limit of 160 μg azaspiracids/kg whole shellfish flesh has been established by the EU.

[J. Schlundt]

FUNGAL DISEASES OF THE SKIN, HAIR, AND NAILS

(tinea, ringworm, dermatophytosis, dermatomycosis, epidermophytosis, trichophytosis, microsporosis)

DISEASE	ICD-10 CODE	CAUSATIVE AGENT	SITE	OCCURRENCE
TINEA BARBAE TINEA CAPITIS	ICD-10 B35.0	Various species of *Microsporum* and *Trichophyton*	Beard, scalp	Australia, UK, eastern USA, and Puerto Rico, as well as in many developing countries, Mexico, and western Africa
BLACK PIEDRA WHITE PIEDRA	ICD-10 B36.3	*Piedra hortae Trichosporon ovoides, Trichosporon inkin, Trichosporon asteroids, Trichosporon beigelii*	Hair shaft	Tropical areas of South America, southeastern Asia, and Africa
TINEA CRURIS TINEA CORPORIS	ICD-10 B35.6	Most species of *Microsporum* and *Trichophyton*; also *Epidermophyton floccosum*	Groin, perianal region	Worldwide and relatively frequent. Males are infected more often than females.
TINEA PEDIS	ICD-10 B35.3	*Trichophyton rubrum, Trichophyton mentagrophytes* var. *interdigitale,* and *Epidermophyton floccosum*	Feet	Common worldwide
ONYCHOMYCOSIS DUE TO DERMATOPHYTES	ICD-10 B35.1	Various species of *Trichophyton*; rarely, other dermatophytes	Nails	Common worldwide

I. TINEA BARBAE AND TINEA CAPITIS (ringworm of the beard and scalp, kerion, favus), BLACK PIEDRA, WHITE PIEDRA

1. **Clinical features**—A fungal disease that begins as a small area of erythema and/or scaling and spreads peripherally, leaving scaly patches of temporary baldness. Infected hairs become brittle and break off easily.

Occasionally, boggy, raised suppurative lesions develop, called kerions. Favus of the scalp, a variety of tinea capitis, is characterized by a mousy smell and by the formation of small, yellowish, cuplike crusts that amalgamate to form a pale or yellow visible mat on the scalp surface. Affected hairs of a favus do not break off but become grey and lusterless, eventually falling out and leaving baldness that may be permanent. Tinea capitis is easily distinguished from black piedra. Black piedra is characterized by black, hard "gritty" nodules on hair shafts, caused by *Piedraia hortai*. White piedra is caused by *Trichosporon* species, particularly *Trichosporon ovoides* or *Trichosporon inkin*, which produce white, soft, pasty nodules. Infections are usually seen on the scalp but may also be seen on armpit, facial, or pubic hair.

2. **Causative agents**—See the table in this chapter. Species and genus identification is important for epidemiological, prognostic, and therapeutic reasons.

3. **Diagnosis**—Examination of the scalp under ultraviolet (UV) light (Wood lamp) for yellow-green fluorescence is helpful in diagnosing tinea capitis caused by *Microsporum* species such as *Microsporum canis* and *Microsporum audouinii*; *Trichophyton* species do not fluoresce. In infections caused by *Microsporum* spp., microscopic examination of scales and hair in 10% potassium hydroxide or under UV microscopy of a calcofluor white preparation reveals characteristic nonpigmented ecto-thrix (outside the hair) arthrospores; many *Trichophyton* spp. present an endothrix (inside the hair) pattern of invasion; and *Trichophyton verrucosum*, the cause of cattle ringworm, produces large ectothrix spores. In black piedra, epilated hairs show hard black nodules on the shaft. Confirmation of the diagnosis requires culture of the fungus. Genetic identification methods and direct polymerase chain reaction (PCR) detection assays are a useful supplement to traditional morphology-based methods of identification.

4. **Occurrence**—Tinea capitis caused by *Trichophyton tonsurans* has been epidemic in urban areas in Australia, the UK, eastern USA, and Puerto Rico, as well as in Mexico and many developing countries. *M. canis* infections occur in rural and urban areas wherever infected cats and dogs are present. *M. audouinii* is endemic in western Africa and was formerly widespread in Europe and North America, particularly in urban areas; *T. verrucosum* and *Trichophyton mentagrophytes* var. *mentagro-phytes* infections occur primarily in rural areas where the disease exists in cattle, horses, rodents, and wild animals. Black piedra occurs in tropical areas of South America, southeastern Asia, and Africa.

5. **Reservoirs**—Humans for *T. tonsurans*, *Trichophyton schoenleinii*, and *M. audouinii*; animals, especially dogs, cats, and cattle, harbor the

other organisms noted above. Most cases of white piedra are endogenous in origin. The natural habitat of the black piedra agent other than human hair is not known.

6. Incubation period—Usually 10–14 days.

7. Transmission—Tinea barbae and tinea capitis are transmitted through direct skin-to-skin or indirect contact, especially from the backs of seats, barber clippers, toilet articles (combs, hairbrushes), clothing, and hats that are contaminated with hair from infected people or animals. Infected humans can generate considerable aerosols of infective arthrospores. Viable fungus and infective arthrospores may persist on contaminated materials for long periods. Black and white piedra are also spread by common use of combs, hairbrushes, and cosmetics; these agents are not transmitted directly from person to person.

8. Risk groups—Children below the age of puberty are highly susceptible to *M. canis*; all ages are subject to *Trichophyton* infections. Reinfections mainly occur for infections spread amongst humans.

9. Prevention—

1) Educate the public, especially parents, about the danger of acquiring infection from infected individuals, as well as from dogs, cats, and other animals.
2) In the presence of epidemics or in hyperendemic areas where non-*Trichophyton* species are prevalent, survey heads of young children by UV light (Wood lamp) before school entry.

10. Management of patient—

1) In mild cases, daily washing of scalp removes loose hair. Selenium sulfide or ketoconazole shampoos help remove scale. In severe cases, wash scalp daily and cover hair with a cap, which should be boiled after use.
2) Treatment: topical agents can be helpful in control, although relapse is common. Oral griseofulvin for at least 4 weeks is effective. Terbinafine and itraconazole are also effective. Terbinafine is more active than griseofulvin against agents such as *T. tonsurans*, but higher doses of this drug should be used in *Microsporum* infections. Systemic antibacterial agents are useful if lesions become secondarily infected by bacteria; in the case of kerions, also use an antiseptic cream and remove scaly crusts from the scalp by gentle soaking. Examine regularly and take cultures; when cultures become negative, complete recovery may be assumed.

11. Management of contacts and the immediate environment—
Study household contacts, pets, and farm animals for evidence of infection; treat if infected. Some animals, especially cats, may be inapparent carriers. With some agents (e.g., *T. tonsurans*), children may have mild infections accompanied by hair invasion; careful clinical examination of contacts is required.

12. Special considerations—

1) Reporting: report to local health authority of epidemics is obligatory in some countries. Outbreaks in schools should be reported to school authorities.
2) Epidemic measures: in school or other institutional epidemics, educate children and parents as to mode of spread, prevention, and personal hygiene. If more than 2 infected children are present in a class, examine the others. Enlist services of physicians and nurses for diagnosis; carry out follow-up surveys.

II. TINEA CRURIS (ringworm of groin and perianal region), TINEA CORPORIS (ringworm of the body)

1. Clinical features—A fungal disease of the skin other than of the scalp, bearded areas, and feet, characteristically appearing as flat, spreading, ring-shaped, or circular lesion with a characteristic raised edge around all or part of the lesion. This periphery is usually reddish, vesicular, or pustular, and may be dry and scaly or moist and crusted. As the lesion progresses peripherally, the central area often clears, leaving apparently normal skin. Differentiation from inguinal candidiasis, often distinguished by the presence of "satellite" pustules outside the lesion margins, is necessary, because treatment differs. Lesions are aggravated by friction and excessive perspiration in axillary and inguinal regions and when environmental temperatures and humidity are high. All ages are susceptible.

2. Infectious agents—See the table in this chapter.

3. Diagnosis—Presumptive diagnosis is made by taking scrapings from the advancing lesion margins, clearing in 10% potassium hydroxide, and examining microscopically or under UV microscopy of calcofluor white preparations for segmented, branched nonpigmented fungal filaments. Final identification is through culture or direct PCR analysis.

4. Occurrence—See the table in this chapter.

5. **Reservoirs**—Humans, farm animals, and soil.

6. **Incubation period**—Usually 4-10 days.

7. **Transmission**—Direct or indirect contact with skin and scalp lesions of infected people or lesions of animals, contaminated floors, shower stalls, benches, and similar articles. Communicable for as long as lesions are present and viable fungus persists on contaminated materials.

8. **Risk groups**—All humans are susceptible. Tinea cruris is seen mostly in men.

9. **Prevention**—Launder towels and clothing with hot water and/or fungicidal agent; general cleanliness in public showers and dressing rooms (repeated washing of benches; frequent hosing and rapid draining of shower rooms). A fungicidal agent such as cresol should be used to disinfect benches and floors.

10. **Management of patient**—

   1) While under treatment, infected persons should be excluded from swimming pools and activities likely to lead to exposure of others.
   2) Effective and frequent laundering of clothing.
   3) Treatment: thorough bathing with soap and water, removal of scabs and crusts, and application of an effective topical fungicide (miconazole, ketoconazole, clotrimazole, econazole, naftifine, terbinafine, tolnaftate, or ciclopirox) may suffice. Oral griseofulvin is effective, as are oral itraconazole and oral terbinafine.

11. **Management of contacts and the immediate environment**—Examine school and household contacts, household pets, and farm animals; treat infections as indicated.

12. **Special considerations**—

   1) Reporting: report to local health authority of epidemics is obligatory in some countries. Infections in children should be reported to school authorities.
   2) Epidemic measures: educate children and parents about the infection, its mode of spread, and the need to maintain good personal hygiene. Outbreaks are common amongst military personnel.

III. TINEA PEDIS (ringworm of the foot, athlete's foot)

1. Clinical features—Presents with characteristic scaling or cracking of the skin, especially between the toes (interdigital), diffuse scaling over the sole of the foot (dry type), or blisters containing a thin watery fluid; commonly called athlete's foot. In severe cases, vesicular lesions appear on various parts of the body, especially the hands; these dermatophytids do not contain the fungus but are an allergic reaction to fungus products. Itching is often a clue that dermatophyte fungi are present. *Scytalidium* can also cause similar dry lesions on the sole. Note that bacteria, including Gram-negative organisms and coryneforms, as well as *Candida* and *Scytalidium* species, may produce similar lesions.

2. Causative agents—See the table in this chapter.

3. Diagnosis—Presumptive diagnosis is verified by microscopic examination of potassium hydroxide- or calcofluor white-treated scrapings from lesions that reveal septate branching filaments. Clinical appearance is not diagnostic; final identification is through culture or direct PCR.

4. Occurrence—See the table in this chapter. Adults are more often affected than children, males more than females. Infections are more frequent and more severe in hot weather.

5. Reservoir—Humans.

6. Incubation period—Unknown.

7. Transmission—Direct or indirect contact with skin lesions of infected people or with contaminated floors, shower stalls, and other articles used by infected people. Communicable as long as lesions are present and viable spores persist on contaminated materials.

8. Risk groups—Common in industrial workers, school children, athletes, and military personnel who share shower or bathing facilities. Repeated attacks and chronic infections are frequent.

9. Prevention—See Tinea Corporis section in this chapter. Educate the public to maintain strict personal hygiene; take special care in drying between toes after bathing; regularly use a dusting powder or cream containing an effective antifungal on the feet, and particularly between the toes. Occlusive shoes may predispose to infection and disease.

10. Management of patient—

1) Launder socks of heavily infected individuals to prevent reinfection.

2) Treatment: topical antifungals (miconazole, clotrimazole, keto-conazole, terbinafine, ciclopirox, or tolnaftate). Expose feet to air by wearing sandals; use dusting powders. Oral terbinafine or itraconazole may be indicated in severe, extensive, or protracted disease; griseofulvin, although less active, is an alternative.

11. Management of contacts and the immediate environment— None.

12. Special considerations—

1) Reporting: obligatory report of epidemics in some countries (see "Reporting of Communicable Diseases Under the International Health Regulations"). Report high incidence in schools to school authorities.

2) Epidemic measures: thoroughly clean and wash floors of showers and similar sources of infection; disinfect with a fungicidal agent such as cresol. Educate the public about the mode of spread.

IV. ONYCHOMYCOSIS DUE TO DERMATOPHYTES
(tinea unguium, ringworm of the nails, onychomycosis)

1. Clinical features—A chronic fungal disease involving one or more nails of the hands or feet. The nail gradually becomes detached from the nail bed, thickens, and becomes discolored and brittle; an accumulation of soft keratinous material forms beneath the nail or the nail becomes chalky and disintegrates.

2. Causative agents—See the table in this chapter.

3. Diagnosis—By microscopic examination of potassium hydroxide preparations of the nail and of detritus beneath the nail for hyaline fungal elements. Etiology should be confirmed by culture. *Scytalidium dimidiatum* causes an almost identical disease (not strictly speaking a tinea infection), differentiated through culture on cycloheximide-free media.

4. Occurrence—See the table in this chapter.

5. Reservoir—Humans; rarely, animals or soil.

6. Incubation period—Unknown.

7. Transmission—Presumably through extension from skin infections acquired by direct contact with skin or nail lesions of infected people, or from indirect contact (contaminated floors and shower stalls). Low rate of transmission, even to close family associates. Communicable for as long as an infected lesion is present.

8. **Risk groups**—All humans are susceptible.

9. **Prevention**—Cleanliness and use of a fungicidal agent such as cresol for disinfecting floors in common use; frequent hosing and rapid draining of shower rooms.

10. **Management of patient**—Treatment: oral itraconazole and terbinafine are the drugs of choice. Oral griseofulvin is less effective. Treatment to be given until nails grow out (~3-6 months for fingernails, 12-18 months for toenails). At present there is no effective treatment for *Scytalidium* infections.

11. **Management of contacts and the immediate environment**—None.

12. **Special considerations**—None.

[M. Brandt]

GIARDIASIS
(*Giardia* enteritis)

DISEASE	ICD-10 CODE
GIARDIASIS	ICD-10 A07.1

1. **Clinical features**—A protozoan infection, principally of the upper small intestine; it can remain asymptomatic; cause acute diarrhea, self-limited in 2-4 weeks; lead to intestinal symptoms such as chronic diarrhea; steatorrhea; abdominal cramps; bloating; frequent loose and pale greasy stools; fatigue; malabsorption (of fats and fat-soluble vitamins); and weight loss. There is usually no extraintestinal invasion, but reactive arthritis and, in severe giardiasis, damage to duodenal and jejunal mucosal cells may occur.

2. **Causative agent**—*Giardia lamblia* (*Giardia intestinalis*, *Giardia duodenalis*), a flagellate protozoan.

3. **Diagnosis**—Identification of cysts or trophozoites in feces or duodenal fluid. To rule out the diagnosis at least 3 negative results are needed. Because *Giardia* infection is often asymptomatic, the presence of *G. lamblia* (in stool or duodenum) does not necessarily indicate that *Giardia* is the cause of illness. Tests using enzyme-linked immunosorbent assay (ELISA) or direct fluorescent antibody methods to detect antigens in

the stool, generally more sensitive than direct microscopy, are commercially available.

4. Occurrence—Worldwide. Children are infected more frequently than adults. Prevalence is higher in areas of poor sanitation and in institutions with children not toilet-trained, including day care centers. The prevalence of stool positivity in different areas may range between 1% and 30%, depending on the community and age group surveyed. Endemic infection in the temperate zone most commonly occurs in July through October among children aged younger than 5 years and adults aged 25–39 years.

5. Reservoir—Humans; wild and domestic animals such as cats, dogs, cattle, and beavers can carry the infection.

6. Incubation period—Usually 3–25 days or longer; median 7–10 days.

7. Transmission—Infection is associated with drinking water from unfiltered surface water sources or shallow wells, swimming in bodies of freshwater, and eating fecally contaminated food. Having a young family member in day care is a risk factor. Large community outbreaks have occurred from drinking treated but unfiltered water. Smaller outbreaks have resulted from contaminated food, person-to-person transmission in day care centers, and contaminated recreational waters (including swimming and wading pools).

Person-to-person transmission occurs by hand-to-mouth transfer of cysts from the feces of an infected individual, especially in institutions and day care centers; this is probably the principal mode of spread. Anal intercourse can also facilitate transmission.

Localized outbreaks may occur from ingestion of cysts in fecally contaminated drinking and recreational water more often than from fecally contaminated food. Concentrations of chlorine used in routine water treatment do not kill *Giardia* cysts, especially when the water is cold; unfiltered stream and lake waters open to contamination by human and animal feces are a source of infection. The disease is communicable for the entire period of infection, often months.

8. Risk groups—Persons with HIV infection may have more serious and prolonged giardiasis.

9. Prevention—

1) Educate families, personnel, and inmates of institutions—and especially adult personnel of day care centers—in personal hygiene, safe sexual practices, and the need for washing

hands before handling food, before eating, and after toilet use.
2) Dispose of feces in a sanitary manner.
3) Protect public water supplies against contamination with human and animal feces and filter supplies exposed to contamination.
4) Boil emergency drinking water supplies. Chemical treatment with hypochlorite or iodine is less reliable; use 0.1-0.2 ml (2-4 drops) of household bleach or 0.5 ml of 2% tincture of iodine per liter for 20 minutes (longer if water is cold or turbid).

10. Management of patient—

1) Enteric precautions.
2) Concurrent disinfection of feces and soiled articles. In communities with a modern and adequate sewage disposal system, feces can be discharged directly into sewers without preliminary disinfection. Terminal cleaning.
3) Treatment: metronidazole or tinidazole are the drugs of choice. Nitazoxanide may be effective; paromomycin, furazolidone, or quinacrine are alternatives. Furazolidone is available in pediatric suspension for young children and infants. Paromomycin can be used during pregnancy, but when disease is mild, delaying treatment until after delivery is recommended. Drug resistance and relapses may occur with any drug.

11. Management of contacts and the immediate environment—
Microscopic examination of feces of household members and other suspected contacts, especially if symptomatic.

12. Special considerations—

1) Reporting: case report to local health authority required in some areas.
2) Epidemic measures: institute an epidemiological investigation of clustered cases in an area or institution to determine source of infection and mode of transmission. A common vehicle, such as water, food, or association with a day care center or recreational area must be sought; institute applicable preventive or control measures. Control of person-to-person transmission requires special emphasis on personal cleanliness and sanitary disposal of feces.

[M. Eberhard, A. Gabrielli, A. Montresor, L. Savioli]

GONOCOCCAL INFECTIONS

DISEASE	ICD-10 CODE
GENITOURINARY GONOCOCCAL INFECTION	ICD-10 A54.0-A54.2
GONOCOCCAL OPHTHALMIA NEONATORUM	ICD-10 A54.3

GENITOURINARY GONOCOCCAL INFECTION (gonorrhea, gonococcal urethritis, gonococcal vulvovaginitis, gonococcal cervicitis, gonococcal bartholinitis, clap, strain, gleet, dose, GC)

1. **Clinical features**—A bacterial disease limited to noncornified columnar and cuboidal epithelium, which differs in males and females in course, severity, and ease of recognition. In males, gonococcal infection generally presents as an acute purulent discharge from the anterior urethra with dysuria within 2-7 days after exposure. A minority of gonococcal infections in males are asymptomatic. In females, infection is followed by the development of mucopurulent cervicitis, often asymptomatic, although some women with infection have abnormal vaginal discharge and vaginal bleeding after intercourse. In 10%-20%, there is uterine invasion, often timed with menstruation, with resultant endometritis, salpingitis, or pelvic peritonitis, and subsequent risk of infertility and ectopic pregnancy.

In females and men who have sex with men, pharyngeal and anorectal infections also occur. While infection of the pharynx and rectum often are asymptomatic, anorectal infections may cause pruritus, tenesmus, and discharge. Conjunctivitis occurs in newborns born to infected mothers with resultant blindness if not rapidly and adequately treated.

Septicemia (also known as disseminated gonococcal infection) may occur in 0.5%-3% of untreated gonococcal infections and can result in arthritis, skin lesions, and (rarely) endocarditis and meningitis. Arthritis can produce permanent joint damage if appropriate antibiotics are not used. Death is rare except among persons with endocarditis or underlying health conditions such as complement deficiency.

Nongonococcal urethritis (NGU) and mucopurulent cervicitis are caused by other sexually transmitted agents and seriously complicate the clinical diagnosis of gonorrhea; the organisms that cause these diseases often coexist with gonococcal infections. In many populations, the incidence of NGU exceeds that of gonorrhea. *Chlamydia trachomatis* (see "Chlamydial Infections") causes about 30%-40% of NGU in most industrialized countries.

2. **Causative agent**—*Neisseria gonorrhoeae*, the gonococcus.

3. **Diagnosis**—Made by Gram stain of discharge, bacteriological culture on selective media (e.g., modified Thayer-Martin agar), or tests that detect gonococcal nucleic acid. Typical Gram-negative intracellular diplococci can be considered diagnostic in male urethral smears, but Gram stain is not recommended to diagnose *N. gonorrhoeae* infection in women. Cultures on selective media, plus presumptive identification based on both macroscopic and microscopic examination and biochemical testing, are sensitive and specific, as are nucleic acid amplification tests. However, culture is highly dependent on adequate specimen collection, optimal transport conditions, and proficient laboratory procedures. Nucleic acid amplification tests (NAATs) are more sensitive than culture since viable bacteria are not required and additional specimen types can be utilized. In cases with potential legal implications, specimens should be cultured and isolates confirmed as *N. gonorrhoeae* by biochemical as well as enzymatic tests and preserved to enable additional or repeated testing. Because of decreased susceptibility to a number of antibiotics including third generation cephalosporins, intermittent regional (supranational) surveillance for antimicrobial susceptibility of *N. gonorrhoeae* should be undertaken.

4. **Occurrence**—Worldwide, the disease affects both men and women, especially sexually active adolescents and younger adults. Prevalence is highest in communities of lower socioeconomic status. In most industrialized countries, incidence has decreased for more than 20 years, but in recent years incidence has reached a plateau and is still at unacceptably high levels.

N. gonorrhoeae readily develops resistance to common antimicrobials, either through chromosomal mutations or acquisition of plasmids. Resistance to penicillin, tetracycline, and quinolones is widespread. For many regions there are inadequate susceptibility data available. Isolates resistant to azithromycin have been identified in many countries, and decreased susceptibility to azithromycin has become common in parts of Europe, South America, Asia, and the western Pacific. Resistance to spectinomycin has been documented but is rarely greater than 5% of tested isolates. Declining gonococcal susceptibility to third generation cephalosporins such as cefixime has been observed worldwide. Oral cephalosporin treatment failures associated with decreased in vitro susceptibility have been documented in Japan and several countries in Europe; isolates with high-level resistance to the injectable cephalosporin ceftriaxone have been identified in Japan and parts of Europe.

5. **Reservoir**—Humans.

6. **Incubation period**—Generally 1-14 days; can be longer.

7. Transmission—Through contact with exudates from mucous membranes of infected people, almost always as a result of sexual activity. Can be transmitted perinatally. Gonorrhea in children older than 1 year is considered indicative of sexual abuse. The disease may be communicable for months in untreated individuals. Effective treatment ends communicability within hours. Transmission by fomites is extremely rare.

8. Risk groups—Men who have sex with men, commercial sex workers, socioeconomically marginalized groups, and sexually active youth, especially when sexual contact is unprotected. Individuals deficient in complement components are uniquely susceptible to bacteremia. Infection with gonorrhea increases risk of both acquisition and transmission of HIV infection. Humoral and secretory antibodies have been demonstrated, but gonococcal strains are antigenically heterogeneous and reinfection is common.

9. Prevention—

1) Same as for syphilis (see "Syphilis"), except for measures that apply specifically to gonorrhea (i.e., those described later).

2) Prevention is based primarily on safer sexual practices; that is, consistent and correct use of condoms with all partners not known to be infection-free, avoiding multiple sexual encounters or anonymous/casual sex, and mutual monogamy with a noninfected partner.

3) Treatment: on clinical, laboratory, or epidemiological grounds (contacts of a diagnosed case), adequate treatment must be given as follows. In the USA and Europe, the only recommended treatment regimen for uncomplicated gonococcal infections of the cervix, rectum, and urethra in adults is dual treatment that includes ceftriaxone intramuscular (IM). In the USA, the recommended regimen is ceftriaxone 250 mg IM plus either oral azithromycin or oral doxycycline. In Europe, the recommended regimen is ceftriaxone 500 mg IM plus oral azithromycin. Dual treatment provides effective treatment for chlamydial coinfection, which is common among patients diagnosed with gonorrhea and may also inhibit the emergence of antimicrobial-resistant gonococci. When ceftriaxone is not readily available, oral cefixime may be used in the dual treatment regimen in lieu of ceftriaxone. Patients who cannot take cephalosporins may be treated with higher-dose oral azithromycin (2 g as a single dose) or spectinomycin IM as monotherapy, but spectinomycin is not available in many countries and has poor efficacy in eradicating infections of the pharynx. Gonococcal infections of the pharynx are more difficult to eliminate than infections of the urethra,

cervix, or rectum. Recommended treatment for this infection includes dual treatment with ceftriaxone IM and either oral azithromycin or oral doxycycline. Treatment failure following a ceftriaxone-based regimen is rare; however, if an alternative regimen is used, test of cure should be considered. If symptoms persist, reinfection is most likely, but specimens should be obtained for culture and antimicrobial susceptibility testing to rule out treatment failure. Retesting of high-risk patients after 3 months is advisable to detect asymptomatic infections.

4) Patients with gonococcal infections are at increased risk of HIV infection and should be offered confidential counseling and testing.

10. Management of patient—

1) Patients should refrain from sexual intercourse until antimicrobial therapy is completed and, to avoid reinfection, abstain from sex with previous sexual partners until these have been treated.
2) Contact precautions for all newborn infants and prepubertal children with gonococcal infection until effective parenteral antimicrobial therapy has been administered for 24 hours. Effective antibiotics in adequate dosage promptly render discharges noninfectious.
3) Care in disposal of discharges from lesions and contaminated articles.

11. Management of contacts and the immediate environment—

1) Interview patients and notify sexual partners. With uncooperative patients, trained interviewers obtain the best results, but clinicians can motivate most patients to help arrange treatment for their partners. Sexual contacts of cases should be examined, tested, and treated if their last sexual contact with the case was within 60 days before the onset of symptoms or diagnosis in the case. Even outside these time limits the most recent sexual partner should be examined, tested, and treated. For treatment, see Treatment in Prevention under Genitourinary Gonococcal Infection in this chapter.
2) All infants born to infected mothers must receive prophylactic treatment.

12. Special considerations—Reporting: case report to local health authority is required in many countries. Further information can be found at:

- http://www.cdc.gov/std/treatment
- http://www.iusti.org/sti-information/guidelines/default.htm
- http://www.who.int/topics/sexually_transmitted_infections/en

II. GONOCOCCAL OPHTHALMIA NEONATORUM

1. **Clinical features**—Acute redness and swelling of conjunctiva in one or both eyes, with mucopurulent or purulent discharge, typically occurring within 1-5 days of birth. Corneal ulcer, perforation, and blindness may occur if antimicrobial treatment is not given promptly. The gonococcus is the most serious but not the most frequent infectious cause of ophthalmia neonatorum. The most common infectious cause is *Chlamydia trachomatis*, which produces inclusion conjunctivitis that tends to be less acute than gonococcal conjunctivitis and usually appears 5-14 days after birth (see "Chlamydial Conjunctivitis"). Any purulent neonatal conjunctivitis should be considered gonococcal until proven otherwise.

2. **Causative agent**—*Neisseria gonorrhoeae*, the gonococcus.

3. **Diagnosis**—Gonococci may be identified by microscope, nucleic acid amplification test, or culture.

4. **Occurrence**—The disease is an important cause of blindness throughout the world. Occurrence varies widely according to prevalence of maternal infection, prenatal screening coverage, and use of infant eye prophylaxis at delivery.

5. **Reservoir**—Infection of the maternal cervix.

6. **Incubation period**—Usually 1-5 days.

7. **Transmission**—Contact with the infected birth canal during childbirth. It is communicable while discharge persists if untreated; for 24 hours following initiation of specific treatment.

8. **Risk groups**—Newborns whose mothers are infected with *N. gonorrhoeae*.

9. **Prevention**—

   1) Ocular prophylaxis of all infants at birth is warranted because it can prevent sight-threatening gonococcal ophthalmia and because it is safe, easy to administer, and inexpensive (see Use an Established Effective Preparation in Prevention under Gonococcal Ophthalmia Neonatorum section in this chapter).
   2) Prevent maternal infection (see Genitourinary Gonococcal Infection section in this chapter; see "Syphylis"). Diagnose gonorrhea in pregnant women and treat the woman and her sexual partners. Routine culture of the cervix and rectum for gonococci should be considered prenatally, especially in the third trimester in populations where infection is prevalent.

3) Use an established effective preparation for protection of babies' eyes within 1 hour of birth, regardless of whether they are delivered vaginally or by cesarean section. Erythromycin (0.5%) and tetracycline (1%) ophthalmic ointments are both effective options. Single-use tubes or ampoules are preferable to multiple-use tubes. Instillation of 1% silver nitrate aqueous solution is also effective and widely used but may be associated with an increased risk of chemical irritation. Prophylaxis with 2.5% ophthalmic solution of povidone-iodine has not yet been studied adequately.

4) Infants born to mothers who have untreated gonorrhea are at high risk for infection. The recommended regimen for such infants in the absence of signs of gonococcal infection is a single dose of ceftriaxone intravenous (IV) or IM.

10. **Management of patient—**

1) Prompt treatment on diagnosis or clinical suspicion of infection.
2) Contact isolation for the first 24 hours after administration of effective therapy. Bacterial cure after therapy should be confirmed by culture.
3) Care in disposal of conjunctival discharges and contaminated articles.
4) Treatment: a single dose of ceftriaxone (≤125 mg) IV or IM, is recommended for the treatment of uncomplicated ophthalmia neonatorum. Mother and infant should also be treated for chlamydial infection. Infants who have gonococcal ophthalmia should be hospitalized and evaluated for signs of disseminated infection (e.g., sepsis, arthritis, and meningitis). Treatment of disseminated gonococcal infection in the newborn should be with ceftriaxone (≤125 mg) IV or IM in a single daily dose for 7 days, with a duration of 10–14 days if meningitis is documented; *or* cefotaxime IV or IM every 12 hours for 7 days, with a duration of 10–14 days, if meningitis is documented.

11. **Management of contacts and the immediate environment—** Examination and treatment of mothers and their sexual partners.

12. **Special Considerations—**Reporting: case report to local health authority is required in many countries.

[S. Kidd]

GRANULOMA INGUINALE
(donovanosis)

DISEASE	ICD-10 CODE
GRANULOMA INGUINALE	ICD-10 A.58

1. **Clinical features**—A chronic and progressively destructive, but poorly communicable bacterial disease of the skin and mucous membranes of the external genitalia, inguinal, and anal regions. One or more indurated nodules or papules lead to slowly spreading, nontender, hypertrophic, granulomatous, ulcerative, or sclerotic lesions. The lesions are characteristically nonfriable, beefy red granulomas, and extend peripherally with characteristic rolled edges to eventually form fibrous tissue. Lesions occur most commonly on warm, moist surfaces, such as the folds between the thighs, the perianal area, the scrotum, or the vulvar labia and vagina. The genitalia are involved in close to 90% of cases, the inguinal region in close to 10%, the anal region in 5%–10%, and distant sites in 1%–5%. If neglected, the process may result in extensive destruction of genital organs and may spread by autoinoculation to other parts of the body.

2. **Causative agent**—The causal agent is *Klebsiella granulomatis* (*Donovania granulomatis*, *Calymmatobacterium granulomatis*), a Gram-negative bacillus.

3. **Diagnosis**—Laboratory diagnosis is based on demonstration of intracytoplasmic Gram-negative, rod-shaped organisms (Donovan bodies) in Wright- or Giemsa-stained smears of granulation tissue or biopsy specimens. The presence of large infected mononuclear cells filled with deeply staining Donovan bodies is pathognomonic. Culture is not routinely available. Serological tests are unreliable and polymerase chain reaction (PCR) is available only in research settings. *Haemophilus ducreyi* should be excluded by culture on appropriate selective media.

4. **Occurrence**—Rare in industrialized countries, but cluster outbreaks occasionally occur. Endemic in tropical and subtropical areas, such as central and northern Australia, southern India, Papua New Guinea, Guyana, and Viet Nam; occasionally in Latin America, the Caribbean islands, and central, eastern and southern Africa.

5. **Reservoir**—Humans.

6. **Incubation period**—Variable; probably between 1 and 16 weeks.

7. **Transmission**—Presumably by direct contact with lesions during vaginal and anal sexual activity (less commonly by oral sex); in various

studies only 20%–65% of sexual partners were infected. Donovanosis occurs in sexually inactive individuals and the very young, suggesting that some cases are transmitted nonsexually. The period of communicability is unknown but probably lasts for the duration of open lesions.

8. Risk groups—It is more frequently seen among males than females and among people of lower socioeconomic status; it is rare in children and predominantly seen at ages 20–40 years. Immunity does not appear to follow infection.

9. Prevention—Preventive measures should include barrier methods during sexual activity, particularly during vaginal or anal contact. Educational programs in endemic areas should stress the importance of early diagnosis and treatment.

10. Management of patient—

1) Avoid close personal contact until lesions are healed.
2) Care in disposal of discharges from lesions and soiled articles.
3) Treatment: the recommended adult treatment is a 3-week minimum course of doxycycline, unless the patient is pregnant or lactating. Alternatives include azithromycin, erythromycin, triemethoprim-sulfamethoxazole (TMP-SMX), and ciprofloxacin. Strains resistant to erythromycin, TMP-SMX, and doxycycline have been identified. Doxycycline, TMP-SMX, and ciprofloxacin should not be used in pregnant women, and the addition of an aminoglycoside may be warranted in refractory patients and in those with HIV or underlying malignancy. Recurrence after treatment can occur, and requires repeat treatment.

11. Management of contacts and the immediate environment— Examination of sexual contacts.

12. Special considerations—Reporting: a reportable disease in most states and countries.

Further information can be found at:

- http://www.cdc.gov/std/treatment
- http://www.who.int/topics/sexually_transmitted_infections/en

[M. M. Taylor]

HANTAVIRAL DISEASES

DISEASE	ICD-10 CODE
HEMORRHAGIC FEVER WITH RENAL SYNDROME	ICD-10 A98.5
HANTAVIRUS PULMONARY SYNDROME	ICD-10 B33.4

HEMORRHAGIC FEVER WITH RENAL SYNDROME (epidemic hemorrhagic fever, Korean hemorrhagic fever, Nephropathia epidemica, hemorrhagic nephroso-nephritis, HFRS), HANTAVIRUS PULMONARY SYNDROME (hantavirus adult respiratory distress syndrome, hantavirus cardiopulmonary syndrome, HPS, HCPS)

1. Clinical features—An acute zoonotic disease with two similar syndromes, which share febrile prodrome, thrombocytopenia, leukocytosis, and capillary leakage.

1) Hemorrhagic fever with renal syndrome (HFRS): characterized by abrupt onset of fever, lower back pain, varying degrees of hemorrhagic manifestations, and renal involvement. Severe illness is associated with Hantaan (primarily in Asia), Seoul, and Dobrava (in the Balkans) viruses. Disease is characterized by 5 clinical phases that frequently overlap: febrile, hypotensive, oliguric, diuretic, and convalescent.

The febrile phase, which lasts 3–7 days, is characterized by high fever, headache, malaise, and anorexia, followed by severe abdominal or lower back pain, often accompanied by nausea and vomiting, facial flushing, petechiae, and conjunctival injection. Most cases show an elevated hematocrit, thrombocytopenia, and elevated creatinine. The hypotensive phase lasts from several hours to 3 days and is characterized by defervescence and abrupt onset of hypotension, which may progress to shock and more apparent hemorrhagic manifestations. Blood pressure returns to normal or is high in the oliguric phase (3–7 days); nausea and vomiting may persist, severe hemorrhage may occur and urinary output falls dramatically.

The case-fatality rate ranges from 5%–15%, and the majority of deaths occur during the hypotensive and oliguric phases. Diuresis heralds the onset of recovery in most cases, with polyuria of 3–6 liters per day. Convalescence takes weeks to months. Infections caused by Seoul virus are clinically milder, although severe disease may occur with this strain. They show less clear distinction between clinical phases.

Less severe illnesses (case-fatality rate <1%) are caused by Puumala virus, referred to as nephropathia epidemica, and Saaremaa viruses.

2) Hantavirus pulmonary syndrome (HPS): characterized by fever, myalgias, and gastrointestinal complaints, followed by the abrupt onset of respiratory distress and hypotension. The illness progresses rapidly to severe respiratory failure and shock. Most cases show an elevated hematocrit, hypoalbuminemia, and thrombocytopenia. The fatality rate can be as high as 35%–50%. In survivors, recovery from acute illness is rapid, but full convalescence may require weeks to months. Restoration of normal lung function generally occurs, but pulmonary function abnormalities may persist in some individuals. Renal and hemorrhagic manifestations are usually absent, except in some severe cases. No unapparent infections have been documented, but milder infections without frank pulmonary edema have occurred and antibody prevalence studies have detected serological-positive people with no recollection of the typical disease.

2. Causative agents—Hantaviruses (a genus of the family *Bunyaviridae*: 3-segmented ribonucleic acid (RNA) viruses with spherical to oval particles, 95–110 nm in diameter). More than 25 antigenically distinguishable viral species exist, each associated primarily with a single rodent species. Very few virus isolates from humans or rodents exist, however.

1) HFRS: Hantaan, Dobrava, Puumala, Saaremaa, Seoul viruses.

2) HPS: Andes (Argentina, Chile), Laguna Negra (Bolivia, Paraguay), Juquitiba (Brazil), Choclo (Panama), Black Creek Canal and Bayou (southeastern USA), New York-1 and Monongahela (eastern USA), Sin Nombre (North America).

3. Diagnosis—Almost all patients have immunoglobulin class M (IgM) and most even immunoglobulin class G (IgG) antibodies (detectable by immunofluorescence assay [IFA] or enzyme-linked immunosorbent assay [ELISA], western blot, or strip immunoblot techniques for HPS) at the time of hospitalization, and virus levels have declined so virus isolation is not usually possible. In these cases conventional or real-time polymerase chain reaction (PCR) is the preferred approach (blood clot, autopsy, or biopsy tissues are better than serum). Immunohistochemistry on formalin-fixed tissues is the method of choice for diagnosis when other samples are unavailable in fatal human cases.

4. Occurrence—The availability of newer diagnostic techniques has led to increasing recognition of hantaviruses and hantaviral infections.

1) HFRS: the disease is considered a major public health problem in China and the Republic of Korea but is likely to occur more

widely. Occurrence is seasonal, with most cases occurring in late autumn and early winter, primarily among rural populations. In the Balkans, a severe form of the disease due to Dobrava virus, affects a few hundred people annually, with case-fatality rates at least as high as those in Asia (5%–15%). Most cases there are seen during spring and early summer. Nephropathia epidemica, due to Puumala virus, is found in most of Europe, including the Balkans, and Russia west of the Ural Mountains. It is often seen in summer and in the autumn and early winter. Saaremaa viruses are detected in rodents from Croatia to Estonia, but human cases have mostly been described in Estonia and western Russia. Among medical research personnel and animal handlers in Asia and Europe, the disease has been traced to laboratory rats infected with Seoul virus, which has been mostly identified in captured urban rats worldwide, including in Argentina, Brazil, Thailand, and the USA; only in Asia has it been regularly associated with human disease.

2) HPS: first recognized in the spring and summer of 1993 in southwestern USA populations, caused by Sin Nombre virus; cases have been confirmed in Canada and in many eastern and western regions of the USA. A large number of cases have been reported in South America (Argentina, Bolivia, Brazil, Chile, Panama, and Paraguay). The disease is not restricted to any age, gender, or ethnic groups. Incidence appears to coincide with the geographic distribution and population density of carrier rodents, and with their level of infection.

5. Reservoir—Each hantavirus species is generally associated with one rodent species, but there is evidence for host-switches without epidemiological implications. Recently, hantaviruses have been detected in several insectivore (order *Soricimorpha*) species, but without any evidence of human-associated diseases. Humans are accidental hosts.

1) HFRS: field rodents—*Apodemus* spp. for Hantaan, Dobrava, and Saaremaa viruses in Asia and the central European areas; *Myodes* (formerly *Clethrionomys*) spp. for Puumala in Western Europe and Scandinavia; *Rattus* spp. for Seoul virus (worldwide).

2) HPS: in North America, the major reservoir of Sin Nombre virus appears to be the deer mouse, *Peromyscus maniculatus*. Antibodies have also been found in other *Peromyscus* species, pack rats, chipmunks, and other rodents. In other regions, other hantavirus strains have been associated mainly with rodent species of the subfamily *Sigmodontinae*.

6. Incubation period—From a few days to nearly 2 months, usually 2–4 weeks for HFRS. For HPS, the incubation period is incompletely defined, but thought to be approximately 2 weeks, with a range of a few days to 6 weeks.

7. Transmission—The presumed route is through aerosol transmission from rodent excreta, although this does not explain all human cases or all forms of inter-rodent transmission. Virus occurs in urine, feces, and saliva of persistently infected asymptomatic rodents, with maximal virus concentration in the lungs. Indoor exposure in closed, poorly ventilated homes, vehicles, and outbuildings with visible rodent infestation is especially important. Seasonal occupational and recreational activities probably influence the risk of exposure to Puumala virus and other hantaviruses, as do climate and other ecological factors on rodent population densities. Nosocomial and household transmission of Andes virus has been documented in Argentina but is believed rare and associated with direct contact. In other settings no human-to-human transmission has been recorded. The protection and duration of immunity conferred by previous infection is unknown, but antibodies seem to persist for several years. Reinfection has never been shown to occur in confirmed recovered patients.

8. Risk groups—The main human groups at risk are persons in rural populations who come into contact with rodents as part of their occupation (forestry workers, farmers), and outdoor enthusiasts have been found to have elevated risk of hantavirus exposure; laboratory workers processing clinical specimens or working in research laboratories; and persons handling patients infected with Andes virus and handling their secretions or excretions.

9. Prevention—

1) Exclude rodents from houses and other buildings.
2) Store human and animal food in rodent-proof containers.
3) Minimize exposure to wild rodents and their excreta in enzootic areas.
4) Disinfect rodent-contaminated areas by spraying a disinfectant solution (e.g., diluted bleach) prior to cleaning. Do not sweep or vacuum rat-contaminated areas; use a wet mop or towels moistened with disinfectant. As far as possible, ventilate potentially rodent-infected buildings that have been closed for some time prior to entry; avoid inhalation of dust by using approved respirators when cleaning previously unoccupied areas. People working with potentially infected rodents during ecological studies should wear appropriate protective equipment (based on risk assessment).
5) Trap rodents and dispose of them using suitable precautions. Live trapping is not recommended.
6) Laboratory rodent colonies, particularly *Rattus norvegicus*, must be tested to ensure freedom from asymptomatic hantavirus infection.
7) Health care workers should always use universal protections when managing patients.
8) Vaccines are available in South Korea and China against Hantaan and Seoul viruses, and appear to have some preventive effect.

10. **Management of patient**—Treatment is mostly symptomatic.

   1) HFRS: bed rest and early hospitalization are critical. Jostling and the effect of lowered atmospheric pressures during airborne evacuation of cases can be deleterious to patients critically ill with hantavirus. Careful attention to fluid management is important in order to avoid overload and minimize the effects of shock and renal failure. Dialysis is often required. Early initiation of intravenous (IV) ribavirin during the first few days of illness has shown some benefit, although patients are usually admitted late.

   2) HPS: provide respiratory intensive care management. Carefully avoid over-hydration that might lead to exacerbation of pulmonary edema. Cardiotonic drugs and pressors given early under careful monitoring help prevent shock. Strictly avoid hypoxia, particularly if transfer is contemplated. Ribavirin treatment has shown no proven benefit. Extracorporeal membrane oxygenation has been used with some success.

11. Management of contacts and the immediate environment—The risk of human-to-human transmission is limited to Andes virus cases. Where feasible, exterminate rodents and exclude them from households.

12. Special considerations—Reporting: suspected cases should be reported to the local health authorities, and confirmed cases are notifiable in several countries. Hantaviruses are not listed as agents that must be assessed in terms of the potential to cause Public Health Emergencies of International Concern under the International Health Regulations (IHR).

[P. E. Rollin, B. Knust, S. Nichol]

HELICOBACTER PYLORI INFECTION

DISEASE	ICD-10 CODE
HELICOBACTER PYLORI INFECTION	ICD-10 K29

1. Clinical features—A bacterial infection by *Helicobacter pylori* causing acute and chronic gastritis, primarily in the antrum of the stomach, and peptic ulcer disease. *H. pylori* colonizes humans and is found to colonize more than 50% of the human population worldwide. Most of those infected with *H. pylori* remain asymptomatic, and without treatment infection is often lifelong. The key pathophysiological event in *H. pylori* infection is initiation and continuance of an inflammatory response. Development of atrophy and intestinal metaplasia of the gastric mucosa are strongly associated with *H. pylori* infection. Infection with *H. pylori* is epidemiologically associated with development of gastric adenocarcinoma and gastric mucosa-associated lymphoid tissue (MALT) type lymphoma. Oxidative and nitrosative stress in combination with inflammation plays an important role in gastric carcinogenesis. Thus *H. pylori* infection has been found to be the major risk factor for gastric carcinogenesis, with environmental factors (e.g., high saline- or nitrosamine-containing food) and genetic susceptibility being additional contributing risk factors for development of gastric cancer.

Dyspepsia is a common and complex condition consisting of chronic upper gastrointestinal symptoms. Patients with alarm symptoms should be referred for prompt endoscopy and without alarm symptoms can be tested for *H. pylori*, and if positive, treated.

2. Causative agent—*H. pylori* is a Gram-negative, curved bacteria, which is positive for catalase, oxidase, and urease.

3. Diagnosis—Diagnostic methods are categorized according to whether or not an endoscopy is necessary and whether the diagnosis is to be set before or after an eradication treatment. Biopsy-based tests include histological evaluation, culture, polymerase chain reaction (PCR), and the rapid urease test, all of which are performed on tissue obtained during endoscopy. Alternatively, the urea breath test, serology, and stool antigen test can be performed as noninvasive procedures.

Serum antibody tests may remain positive for months after treatment. The sensitivity and specificity of different tests depend on the age of the patients and the disease they present.

Testing for *H. pylori* infection is indicated in patients with dyspeptic symptoms, a past history of documented peptic ulcer disease, gastric cancer, or gastric MALT lymphoma.

4. Occurrence—*H. pylori* is estimated to infect more than half of the world population. Infection rates could reach 70% in developing countries and 20%–50% in industrialized countries. Only a minority of those infected develop duodenal ulcer disease. Although individuals infected with the organism always have histological evidence of gastritis, the vast majority are asymptomatic. *H. pylori* infection is usually acquired during childhood, and atrophy of the gastric mucosa progresses during aging. Cross-sectional serological studies demonstrate increasing prevalence with increasing age.

5. Reservoir—Mainly humans, though recently *H. pylori* has been found in other primates. Isolation of *H. pylori* from nongastric sites such as oral secretions and stool has been reported, but is infrequent.

6. Incubation period—Data collected from 2 volunteers who ingested 10^6–10^9 organisms indicate that the onset of gastritis occurred within 5–10 days. No other information about inoculum size or incubation period is available.

7. Transmission—The mode of transmission has not been clearly established, but infection is almost certainly a result of ingesting organisms. Transmission is presumed, but not yet confirmed, to be either oral-oral and/or fecal-oral or from inadequately treated drinking water. As infection may be lifelong, those infected are potentially infectious for life. It is not known whether acutely infected patients are more infectious than those with long-standing infection. There is some evidence that persons with low stomach acidity may be more infectious.

8. Risk groups—Low socioeconomic status, especially in childhood, is associated with infection. It is generally thought that a variety of cofactors may be required for the development of disease. No immunity is apparent after infection.

9. Prevention—Persons living in uncrowded, clean environments are less likely to acquire *H. pylori*. Socioeconomic factors seem to affect the prevalence of the bacterium in the population. Appropriate treatment of drinking water is important, as is proper disinfection of gastroscopes, pH electrodes, and other instruments entering the stomach.

Gastric cancer is one of the most common causes of cancer death worldwide, but while it is now generally accepted that *H. pylori* is one of the most important underlying causes, no general public health measures have yet been instituted to treat infected individuals in populations at risk.

10. Management of patient—

1) Treatment for asymptomatic infection remains controversial. In Europe it is recommended to treat patients with dyspepsia and *H. pylori* infection. *H. pylori* eradication as standard therapy in *H. pylori*-positive ulcers has been suggested, as this strategy could decrease the risk of ulcer relapse. A wide variety of treatment regimens are available for curing infections in individuals with symptoms of disease attributable to *H. pylori*, such as gastritis, peptic ulcer disease, or MALT lymphoma. Regimens for first- and second-line treatment include: combinations of proton-pump inhibitor drugs with clarithromycin and amoxicillin or metronidazole; or bismuth subsalicylate with tetracycline and metronidazole. Cure rates of up to 90% have been reported with these regimens, yet recent reports

show lower cure rates (80%) and that many patients receive multiple treatments with no effect. If infection persists, culture should be performed after the first treatment failure and isolates should be checked for resistance to the antibiotics.

A recent multicenter study showed that resistance rates in Europe for adults were 17.5% for clarithromycin, 14.1% for levofloxacin, and 34.9% for metronidazole, with rates higher in western/central and southern Europe than in northern Europe. A steady increase in clarithromycin resistance and almost doubling of levofloxacin resistance was noted, linked with an increase in outpatient antibiotic usage. Bismuth quadruple regimes are recommended as first- and second-line treatment options in areas of high clarithromycin resistance.

11. Management of contacts and the immediate environment—Prototype protein-based vaccines have shown promising results in animal models but have not cleared infection and/or prevented reinfection.

12. Special considerations—None.

[J. Schlundt]

HEPATITIS, VIRAL

DISEASE	ICD-10 CODE
HEPATITIS A	ICD-10 B15
HEPATITIS B	ICD-10 B16
HEPATITIS C	ICD-10 B17.1
HEPATITIS D	ICD-10 B17.0
HEPATITIS E	ICD-10 B17.2
HEPATOCELLULAR CARCINOMA	ICD-10 C22.0

Several distinct infections are grouped as the viral hepatitides; they are primarily hepatotrophic and have similar clinical presentations, but differ in etiology and in some epidemiological, immunological, clinical, and pathological characteristics. Their prevention and control vary greatly. Each is presented later in a separate section.

I. HEPATITIS A (infectious hepatitis, epidemic hepatitis, epidemic jaundice, catarrhal jaundice, type A hepatitis, HA)

1. Clinical features—The disease varies in clinical severity from asymptomatic illness to a severely disabling disease lasting several months. In most developing countries, infection manifests as an asymptomatic or mild illness in childhood. Onset of illness in adults in nonendemic areas is usually abrupt, with fever, malaise, anorexia, nausea, and abdominal discomfort, followed within a few days by jaundice. Prolonged, relapsing hepatitis for up to 1 year occurs in 15% of cases; no chronic infection is known to occur. Convalescence is often prolonged. In general, severity increases with age, but complete recovery without sequelae or recurrences is the rule. Reported case-fatality is normally low, 0.1–0.3%; it can reach 1.8% for adults older than 50 years.

2. Causative agent—Hepatitis A virus (HAV), a 27-nm picornavirus (positive-strand ribonucleic acid [RNA] virus). It has been classified as a member of the family *Picornaviridae*.

3. Diagnosis—Mild infections may be detectable only through laboratory tests of liver function. Demonstration of immunoglobulin class M (IgM) antibodies against hepatitis A virus (IgM anti-HAV) in the serum of acutely or recently ill patients establishes the diagnosis and become detectable 5–10 days after exposure. If laboratory tests are not available, epidemiological evidence may provide support for the diagnosis. HAV RNA can be detected in blood and stools of most persons during the acute phase of infection through nucleic acid amplification methods, but these are not generally used for diagnostic purposes.

4. Occurrence—Worldwide; geographic areas can be characterized by high, intermediate, or low levels of endemicity. In areas of high endemicity, environmental sanitation is generally poor, and infection is common and occurs at an early age. In some areas of Africa and Asia, more than 90% of the general population has serological evidence of prior HAV infection, versus a rate of 33% in industrialized countries. In these high endemicity areas, adults are usually immune, and outbreaks are uncommon. In many parts of the world that have formerly been highly endemic, improved sanitation has decreased the rate of HAV infection and endemicity has become intermediate. In these areas, young adults are susceptible, and the frequency of outbreaks is increasing. Regions of intermediate endemicity include China, countries in South America, Central and Southeast Asia, and the Middle East. In most industrialized countries endemicity is low and outbreaks rare.

5. Reservoir—Humans; rarely chimpanzees and other primates.

6. Incubation period—Average 28-30 days (range 15-50 days).

7. Transmission—Person-to-person by the fecal-oral route. Levels of endemicity are related to hygienic and sanitary conditions. The virus is found in feces, reaches peak levels a week or 2 before the onset of symptoms, and diminishes rapidly after liver dysfunction or symptoms appear, which is concurrent with the appearance of circulating antibodies to HAV. Because most children have asymptomatic or unrecognized infections, they play an important role in HAV transmission and serve as a source of infection for others.

Maximum infectivity is believed to occur during the latter half of the incubation period and continues for a few days after onset of jaundice (or during peak aminotransferase activity in anicteric cases). Most cases are probably noninfectious after the first week of jaundice, although prolonged viral excretion (≤6 months) has been documented in infants and children. Chronic shedding of HAV in feces does not occur.

8. Risk groups—

1) Children living in high endemicity areas.
2) Children and adults living in intermediate endemicity areas.
3) Susceptible persons traveling to, or working in, HAV-endemic countries.
4) Injection drug users.
5) Close personal contacts (e.g., household, sexual) of hepatitis A patients. Cases have resulted from contact with newly adopted children from HAV-endemic countries.
6) Those working with infected primates or with HAV in research laboratories.
7) Persons with chronic liver disease who have an elevated risk of death from fulminant hepatitis A.

Homologous immunity after infection probably lasts for life.

9. Prevention—

1) Educate the public about proper sanitation and personal hygiene, with special emphasis on careful handwashing and sanitary disposal of feces.
2) Provide proper water treatment and distribution systems and sewage disposal.
3) Preexposure immunization: both inactivated and live attenuated hepatitis A vaccines are highly immunogenic and generate long-lasting protection against hepatitis A in children and adults. Protection against clinical hepatitis A begins as soon as 14-21 days after a single dose of vaccine. A second dose is felt to be

necessary for long-term protection. Depending on the level of HAV endemicity, it may in some cases be cost-effective to screen for HAV antibody prior to immunization.

- Hepatitis A vaccination should be integrated into the national immunization schedule for children aged 12 months and older based on hepatitis A incidence, on a change from high to intermediate endemicity (i.e., transitional), or on consideration of cost-effectiveness. WHO does not, however, recommend its routine use in highly endemic countries where almost all persons are infected with HAV in childhood situations.
- Hepatitis A vaccine should be considered for use in other risk populations as well.
- All susceptible travelers to intermediate, or highly endemic areas, should be vaccinated prior to departure, possibly together with immune globulin (IG) if departure takes place in less than 1 week.

4) Raw oysters, clams and other shellfish are risky for a variety of infections including hepatitis. Preferably, these items should be heated to a temperature of 85°C–90°C (185°F–194°F) for 4 minutes or steamed for 90 seconds before eating. In endemic areas, travelers should take only boiled and still hot or bottled beverages and well-cooked food served hot.

5) Raw vegetables and fruits washed with contaminated water or prepared by an infectious food handler are also a risk. Raw vegetable and fruits should always be washed with clean water or peeled.

10. Management of Patient—For proven hepatitis A, use enteric precautions during the first 2 weeks of illness, but no more than 1 week after onset of jaundice; the exception is an outbreak in a neonatal intensive care setting, where prolonged enteric precautions must be considered. Feces, urine, and blood should be disposed of in a sanitary manner. There is no curative treatment for acute infection.

11. Management of contacts and the immediate environment—

1) Postexposure immunization: hepatitis A vaccine should be given as soon as possible, but no later than 2 weeks after exposure. As data regarding the postexposure efficacy of vaccine versus IG are limited for persons older than 40 years or those with underlying medical conditions, IG may be given for such persons, if available, but also within 2 weeks after exposure. Because hepatitis A cannot be reliably diagnosed on clinical presentation alone, serological confirmation of HAV infection in

index patients by IgM anti-HAV testing should be obtained before postexposure prophylaxis of contacts. Hepatitis A vaccine or IG is not indicated for contacts in the usual office, school, or factory settings. Hepatitis A vaccine (or IG, depending on age and presence of medical comorbidities) should be given to previously unimmunized persons in the situations listed:

- Close personal contacts, including household, sexual, drug using, and other close personal contacts.
- Attenders at day care centers if one or more cases of hepatitis A are recognized in children or employees, or if cases are recognized in 2 or more households of attenders—vaccine or IG may be given to classroom contacts of an index case.
- In a common source outbreak, if a food handler is diagnosed with hepatitis A, hepatitis A vaccine or IG should be administered to other food handlers in the same establishment. Hepatitis A vaccine or IG is usually not offered to patrons, but this may be considered if:

  ○ Food handlers were involved in the preparations of foods that were not heated.
  ○ Deficiencies in personal hygiene are noted or the food handler has had diarrhea.
  ○ The hepatitis A vaccine or IG can be given within 2 weeks after the most recent exposure.

- Use of hepatitis A vaccination in widespread outbreak situations depends on the epidemiology of hepatitis A in the community, and the feasibility of rapid implementation of a widespread vaccination program. The use of vaccine to control community-wide outbreaks has been most successful when vaccination is started early in the course of the outbreak and with high coverage of multiple-age cohorts.

2) Search for missed cases and maintain surveillance of contacts in the patient's household and the community; in a common-source outbreak, search among people exposed to the same risk.

12. **Special considerations—**

1) Reporting: report to local health authority is obligatory in some countries.
2) Epidemic measures:

- Determine mode of transmission (person-to-person or common vehicle) through epidemiological investigation; identify the population exposed. Eliminate common sources of infection.
- Make special efforts to improve sanitary and hygienic practices to eliminate fecal contamination of food and water.
- Outbreaks in institutions may warrant mass prophylaxis with hepatitis A vaccine or IG.

3) Disaster implications: hepatitis A is a potential problem in large collections of susceptible people with overcrowding, inadequate sanitation, and access to clean water; if cases occur, increase efforts to improve sanitation and safety of water supplies. Mass administration of hepatitis A vaccine, which should be carefully planned, is not a substitute for environmental measures.

II. HEPATITIS B (type B hepatitis, serum hepatitis, homologous serum jaundice, Australia antigen hepatitis, HB)

1. Clinical features—Fewer than 10% of children and 30%–50% of adults with acute hepatitis B virus (HBV) infection show icteric disease: disease is often milder and anicteric in children; in infants it is usually asymptomatic. In those with clinical illness, the onset is usually insidious, with anorexia, vague abdominal discomfort, nausea, and vomiting, sometimes arthralgia and rash, often progressing to jaundice. Fever may be absent or mild. Severity ranges from unapparent cases detectable only by liver function tests to fulminating, fatal cases of acute hepatic necrosis. The case-fatality rate is about 1%; higher in those older than 40 years of age. Fulminant HBV infection also may occur during pregnancy and among newborns of infected mothers.

After acute HBV infection, the risk of developing chronic infection varies inversely with age; chronic HBV infection occurs among about 90% of infants infected at birth, 20%–50% of children infected from ages 1 to 5 years, and 1%–10% of persons infected as older children and adults. Chronic HBV infection is also common in persons with immunodeficiency. Persons with chronic infection, may or may not, have a history of clinical hepatitis. Those with active chronic HBV infection have elevated aminotransferases; biopsy findings range from normal to severe necro-inflammatory hepatitis, with or without cirrhosis. An estimated 15%–25% of persons with chronic HBV infection die prematurely of either cirrhosis or hepatocellular carcinoma (HCC). Approximately 50% of HCC cases globally are attributable to chronic HBV infection.

2. Causative agent—HBV, a hepadnavirus, is a 42-nm partially double-stranded deoxyribonucleic acid (DNA) virus composed of a 27-nm nucleocapsid core (hepatis B core antigen [HBcAg]), surrounded by an outer lipoprotein coat containing the hepatitis B surface antigen (HBsAg). HBsAg is antigenically heterogeneous, with a common antigen (designated a) and 2 pairs of mutually exclusive antigens (d, y, w [including several subdeterminants], and r), resulting in 4 major subtypes: adw, ayw, adr, and ayr. The distribution of subtypes varies geographically; because of the common "a" determinant, protection against one subtype appears to confer protection against the other subtypes, and no differences in clinical features have been related to subtype. Genotype classification based on sequencing of genetic material has been introduced and is becoming the standard: HBV is currently classified into 8 main genotypes (A–H). HBV genotypes are associated with the modes of HBV transmission (vertical vs. horizontal) and with the risk of certain outcomes of chronic infection, such as cirrhosis and HCC. In the North American Arctic, HBV genotype F is associated with HCC in young children, as well as adults younger than 30 years. In Asia as well as the Arctic, HBV genotype C has also been associated with a significantly higher risk of HCC than other genotypes.

3. Diagnosis—Demonstration in serum of specific antigens and/or antibodies confirms diagnosis. Three clinically useful antigen-antibody systems are identified for hepatitis B:

- HBsAg and antibody to HBsAg (anti-HBs).
- HBcAg and antibody to HBcAg (anti-HBc).
- Hepatitis B e antigen (HBeAg) and antibody to HBeAg (anti-HBe).

Commercial kits are available for all markers except HBcAg. HBsAg can be detected in serum from several weeks before onset of symptoms to days, weeks, or months after onset; it is present in serum during acute infections and persists in chronic infections. The presence of HBsAg indicates that the person is infectious. Anti-HBc appears at the onset of illness and persists indefinitely. Demonstration of anti-HBc in serum indicates HBV infection, current or past; high titers of IgM anti-HBc occur during acute infection—IgM anti-HBc usually disappears within 6 months, but can persist in some cases of chronic hepatitis. The presence of HBeAg is associated with relatively high infectivity. Protective immunity follows infection if antibodies to HBsAg (anti-HBs) develop and HBsAg is negative.

4. Occurrence—Worldwide; endemic in many countries. WHO estimates that more than 2 billion persons have been infected with HBV globally (including 240 million chronically infected). Each year approximately 600,000 persons die as a result of HBV infection. In countries where HBV is highly endemic (HBsAg prevalence ≥8%), most infections occur during infancy and early childhood. Where HBV endemicity is intermediate (HBsAg prevalence from 2%-7%), infections occur commonly in all age groups, although the high rate of chronic infection is primarily maintained by transmission during infancy and early childhood. Where endemicity is low (HBsAg prevalence <2%), most infections occur in young adults, especially through sexual contact and injection drug use. Even in countries with low HBV endemicity, a high proportion of chronic infections may be acquired during childhood, because the development of chronic infection is age dependent. Almost all of these infections would be prevented by perinatal vaccination against hepatitis B of all newborns or infants.

5. Reservoir—Humans. Chimpanzees are susceptible, but an animal reservoir in nature has not been recognized. Closely related hepadnaviruses are found in woodchucks, ducks, ground squirrels, and other animals, such as snow leopards and German herons; none cause disease in humans.

6. Incubation period—Usually 45-180 days, average 60-90 days. As short as 2 weeks to the appearance of HBsAg, and rarely as long as 6-9 months; variation is related in part to amount of virus in the inoculum, mode of transmission, and host factors.

7. Transmission—Occurs by percutaneous and mucosal exposure to infective body fluids. Since HBV is stable on environmental surfaces for at least 7 days, indirect inoculation of HBV can occur via inanimate objects. Fecal-oral or vector-borne transmission has not been demonstrated.

Body substances capable of transmitting HBV include blood and blood products; saliva (although no outbreaks of HBV infection due to saliva alone have been documented); cerebrospinal fluid; peritoneal, pleural, pericardial, and synovial fluid; amniotic fluid; semen and vaginal secretions; any other body fluid containing blood; and unfixed tissues and organs. The presence of HBeAg or viral DNA (HBV DNA $>10^5$ copies/mL) indicates high virus titer and higher infectivity of these fluids.

Major modes of HBV transmission include sexual or close household contact with an infected person, perinatal mother-to-infant transmission, and injecting drug use (sharing syringes and needles either directly or through contamination of drug preparation equipment). Contaminated and inadequately sterilized syringes and needles have resulted in outbreaks of hepatitis B among patients; this risk has been decreased as a major mode of transmission worldwide with the introduction of auto-destructing needles and syringes. Nosocomial exposures, such as transfusion of blood or blood products, hemodialysis, use of meters and lancets for glucose monitoring, insulin pens, acupuncture, and needlestick or other "sharps" injuries sustained by hospital personnel, have all resulted in HBV transmission. Rare transmission to patients from HBsAg-positive health care workers has been documented. Outbreaks have been reported among patients in dialysis centers in many countries through failure to adhere to recommended infection control practices against transmission of HBV and other blood-borne pathogens in these settings. IG, heat-treated plasma protein fraction, albumin, and fibrinolysin are considered safe. In the past, outbreaks have been traced to tattoo parlors, acupuncturists, and barbers.

Perinatal transmission is common, especially when HBV-infected mothers are also HBeAg-positive (rate of transmission >70%) or if they are highly viremic.

All persons who are HBsAg-positive are potentially infectious. Blood from experimentally inoculated volunteers has been shown to be infective weeks before the onset of first symptoms and to remain infective through the acute clinical course of disease. The infectivity of chronically infected persons varies from high (HBeAg-positive, HBV-DNA $>10^5$ copies/mL) to modest (anti-HBe positive).

Any parenteral or mucosal exposure to infected blood represents a potential risk for acquisition of hepatitis B, and accounts for the 100 times more efficient transmission of HBV compared to HIV after needle-stick exposure.

8. **Risk groups—**

- Sexual partners and household contacts of HBsAg-positive persons, including men who have sex with men.
- Persons with a history of injection drug use.
- Hemodialysis patients.
- Inmates of juvenile detention facilities, prisons, and jails.
- Health care and public safety workers who perform tasks involving contact with blood or blood-contaminated body fluids.
- Clients and staff of institutions for the developmentally disabled who are bitten by patients.
- Those diagnosed as having recently acquired a sexually transmitted disease and those who have a history of sexual activity with more than one partner in the previous 6 months.
- International travelers who plan to spend more than 6 months in areas with intermediate-to-high rates of chronic HBV infection ($\geq$2%), and who will have close contact with the local population.
- Persons with diabetes who require blood glucose monitoring and other chronic conditions requiring frequent injections.

In the past, recipients of blood products were at high risk. In countries where pretransfusion screening of blood for HBsAg is performed and where pooled blood clotting factors (especially antihemophilic factor) are processed to destroy the virus, this risk has been virtually eliminated; however, it is still present in many developing countries.

9. **Prevention—**

1) Vaccination: effective hepatitis B vaccines are available. Vaccines licensed in different parts of the world may have varying dosages and schedules. Among persons vaccinated as children or adults, vaccine-induced immunity lasts for at least 20 years and may be lifelong. Vaccine-induced immunity among persons vaccinated at birth may be less sustained; however, booster injections are not recommended for immunocompetent persons vaccinated at any age. Several combined vaccines (e.g., hepatitis A & B and tetra and pentavalent vaccines) have been licensed and show comparable efficacy.

- The current WHO hepatitis B prevention strategy is routine universal newborn or infant immunization. The greatest fall in incidence and prevalence of hepatitis B is in countries with high vaccine coverage at birth or in infancy. Immunization of successive infant cohorts produces a highly immune population and suffices to interrupt transmission. Combined passive-active immunoprophylaxis with hepatitis B immune globulin (HBIG) and vaccine to prevent perinatal HBV transmission from HBsAg-positive mothers is preferred to vaccine alone in newly instituted routine vaccination programs, but is expensive and not available in all countries.

- In countries with high HBV endemicity, routine infant immunization rapidly eliminates transmission because virtually all chronic infections are acquired among young children. Where HBV endemicity is low or intermediate, immunizing infants alone will not substantially lower disease incidence for about 15 years because most infections occur among adolescents and young adults; vaccine strategies for older children, adolescents, and adults may be desirable. In addition, immunization strategies can be targeted to high-risk groups, which account for most cases among adolescents and adults.

- Testing to exclude adolescents or adults with preexisting anti-HBs or anti-HBc is not required prior to immunization but may be considered as a potential cost-saving method in countries or among high-risk populations where the level of preexisting infection is high and screening is less costly than vaccination.

- Persons at high risk should routinely receive preexposure hepatitis B immunization.
- Pregnancy is not a contraindication for receiving hepatitis B vaccine.

2) Single-use, disposable syringes and needles (including acupuncture needles), and lancets for finger puncture used whenever possible. Glucose monitoring equipment and insulin pens should not be shared. A sterile syringe and needle are essential for each individual receiving skin tests, parenteral inoculations, or venipuncture. Aseptic sanitary practices in tattoo parlors, including proper disposal of sharp or cutting tools, should be enforced and traditional tattooing and scarring practices should be discouraged.

3) Blood banks should test all donated blood for HBsAg with sensitive tests and reject as donors all persons with a history of viral hepatitis, those who have a history of injection drug use or show evidence of drug addiction, or those who have received a blood transfusion or tattoo within the preceding 6 months. Avoid using paid donors; limit administration of unscreened whole blood or potentially hazardous blood products to those in life-threatening need of such therapeutic measures.

4) Maintain surveillance for all cases of posttransfusion hepatitis; keep a register of all people who donated blood for each case. Notify blood banks of potential carriers so that future donations may be identified promptly.

5) HBV infection alone should not disqualify infected persons from the practice or study of medicine, dentistry, or allied health. Many countries have developed recommendations applicable to HBV-infected health care providers, and these should be consulted. For instance, in the USA, recent guidelines from the Advisory Committee on Immunization Practices (ACIP) recommend: no prenotification of patients of a health care provider's or student's HBV infection status; use of HBV DNA serum levels rather than hepatitis B e antigen status to monitor infectivity; and, for those health care professionals performing exposure-prone procedures such as certain types of surgery, counsel and advice from an expert review panel regarding in what circumstances—if any—they may continue to perform these procedures.

10. **Management of patient**—No specific treatment is available for acute hepatitis B. In fulminant hepatitis B, uncontrolled reports suggest some efficacy of lamivudine; therefore, it may be tried (as may any other

rapidly acting antiviral drug) if there is evidence of ongoing HBV replication.

Two major groups of antiviral treatment have been licensed for the treatment of chronic HBV infection in many countries. These include interferon alpha (or pegylated interferon alpha) and nucleoside or nucleotide analogues, such as lamivudine, adefovir, entecavir, telbivudine, and tenofovir. Many other drugs are being evaluated. Persons with chronic HBV infection are generally considered for treatment when they have HBV DNA levels above 2,000 IU/mL, serum alanine aminotransferase levels above the upper limit of normal and severity, or liver disease assessed by liver biopsy (or noninvasive markers once validated in HBV-infected patients) showing moderate to severe active necroinflammation and/or at least moderate fibrosis. The majority of patients require prolonged treatment in order to maintain suppression of viral replication and treatment costs are high. The efficacy of combination therapy is being studied and is likely to diminish the occurrence of virus mutants resistant to treatment. Medications have significant side effects that require careful monitoring.

11. **Management of contacts and the immediate environment—**

   1) Universal precautions to prevent exposures to blood and body fluids.
   2) Concurrent disinfection of equipment contaminated with blood or infectious body fluids.
   3) Immunization of contacts: products available for postexposure prophylaxis include hepatitis B vaccine and HBIG. Administer hepatitis B vaccine and, when indicated, HBIG as soon as possible after exposure.

      - Infants born to HBsAg positive mothers should receive a single dose of vaccine within 12 hours of birth and, where available and depending on the epidemiology, HBIG. The first dose of vaccine should be given concurrently with HBIG, but at a separate site; second and third doses of vaccine (without HBIG) 1-2 and 6 months later. The infant should be tested for HBsAg and anti-HBs at 9-15 months of age to monitor the success or failure of prophylaxis. Infants who are anti-HBs positive and HBsAg negative are protected and do not need further vaccine doses. Infants found to be anti-HBs negative and HBsAg negative should be re-immunized with a complete vaccine series.
      - After percutaneous (e.g., needle-stick) or mucous membrane exposures to blood that might contain HBV, a decision to provide postexposure prophylaxis must include considera-tion of: (a) whether the source of the blood is available for

testing, (b) what the HBsAg status of the source is, and (c) what the hepatitis B immunization status of the exposed person is. For previously unimmunized persons exposed to blood from an HBsAg positive source, a single dose of HBIG should be given as soon as possible, but at least within 24 hours of high-risk needle-stick exposure, and the hepatitis B vaccine series should be started. If active immunization cannot be given, another dose of HBIG should be given 1 month after the first. HBIG is not usually given for needle-stick exposure to blood that is not known, or highly suspected, to be positive for HBsAg, since the risk of infection in these instances is small; however, initiation of hepatitis B immunization is recommended if the person has not previously been immunized. For previously immunized persons exposed to an HBsAg positive source, postexposure prophylaxis is not needed in cases with a protective antibody response to immunization (anti-HBs titer of ≥10 milli-IUs/mL). For persons whose response to immunization is unknown, hepatitis B vaccine and/or HBIG should be administered.

- After sexual, percutaneous (e.g., needle-stick), or mucous membrane exposures to a person with acute or chronic HBV infection, hepatitis B vaccine together with a single dose of HBIG is recommended (in the case of sexual contact if it can be given within 14 days of the most recent contact).

12. Special considerations—

1) Reporting: official report obligatory in some countries.
2) Epidemic measures: institute strict aseptic techniques and universal precautions. When 2 or more cases occur in association with some common exposure, search for additional cases. Consider vaccination of susceptible persons at risk for exposure. If a plasma-derived product is implicated, withdraw the lot from use and trace all recipients of the same lot in a search for additional cases. Information on the investigation and management of hepatitis B outbreaks in particular settings can be found at: http://www.cdc.gov/hepatitis/Settings.

III. HEPATITIS C (type C hepatitis; non-A, non-B hepatitis)

1. Clinical features—Onset is usually insidious, with anorexia, vague abdominal discomfort, nausea, and vomiting; progression to jaundice is less frequent than with hepatitis B. While only 20%–30% of acute infections are symptomatic, 75%–85% of acute infections become chronic. Reinfection may occur among persons with previous, resolved infections, and among those with chronic infection. Of chronically infected persons, about 5–20% develop cirrhosis over a period of 20–30 years, and 1%–5% will die from the consequence of chronic infection (i.e., from cirrhosis and hepatocellular carcinoma).

2. Causative agent—The hepatitis C virus is an enveloped RNA virus classified as a separate genus (*Hepacivirus*) in the *Flaviviridae* family. At least 6 different genotypes and approximately 100 subtypes of hepatitis C virus (HCV) exist. Evidence is limited regarding differences in clinical features, disease outcome, or progression to cirrhosis or HCC among persons with different genotypes. However, differences do exist in responses to antiviral therapy according to HCV genotypes.

3. Diagnosis—Detection of antibody to the hepatitis C virus (anti-HCV) and HCV RNA. Tests that detect antibodies include the enzyme immunoassay (EIA), the enhanced chemiluminescence immunoassay, and the recombinant immunoblot assay. These tests do not distinguish between acute, chronic, or resolved infection. EIA tests are suitable for screening at-risk populations. A negative EIA test suffices to exclude a diagnosis of chronic HCV infection in immunocompetent patients. Immunoblot assays are sometimes used as a supplemental assay for persons screened in nonclinical settings and in persons with a positive EIA who test negative for HCV RNA.

Acute or chronic HCV infection in a patient with a positive EIA test should be confirmed by detection of the presence of HCV RNA in the serum using a sensitive assay. Target amplification techniques using polymerase chain reaction (PCR), transcription-mediated amplification, and signal amplification techniques (branched DNA) may be used to measure HCV RNA levels. Among persons with possible recent HCV exposure, a single positive qualitative assay for HCV RNA confirms active HCV replication, but a single negative assay does not exclude viremia and may reflect a transient decline in viral level below the level of detection of the assay. A follow-up HCV RNA detection should be performed to confirm the absence of active HCV replication in such persons. Among persons without suspicion of recent exposure who are undergoing routine screening, a single negative HCV RNA assay may be sufficient to exclude chronic infection. Quantitative determination of HCV RNA levels and of HCV genotype provides information on the likelihood of response to treatment among patients undergoing antiviral therapy. Liver biopsy can provide direct histological assessment of liver injury due to HCV, but cannot be used to diagnose HCV infection. Noninvasive serum markers (e.g., aspartate aminotransferase-to-platelet ratio index) may sometimes be used to provide an indirect histological assessment.

In some countries, HCV point-of-care assays have been licensed that can provide results in less than 1 hour, using venous and finger stick blood specimens.

4. Occurrence—Worldwide. HCV prevalence is directly related to the prevalence of persons who routinely share injection equipment and to the prevalence of unsafe parenteral practices in health care settings. WHO estimates that some 130–170 million people (~2%–3% of world population) are chronically infected with HCV globally, and more than 350,000 deaths are attributed to HCV infection annually. Approximately 25%–50% of global cases of cirrhosis and hepatocellular carcinoma cases are attributable to HCV infection. Most populations in Africa, the Americas, Western Europe, most of the Middle East, and South Asia have anti-HCV prevalence rates under 2.0%. Prevalence rates in Eastern Europe, most of Asia, and the Western Pacific regions average 2.0%–2.9%. In North and Saharan Africa, and the Middle East, the prevalence of anti-HCV ranges from 1% to more than 12%.

5. Reservoir—Humans; virus has been transmitted experimentally to chimpanzees.

6. Incubation period—Ranges from 2 weeks to 6 months; commonly 6–9 weeks. Chronic infection may persist for several decades before the onset of cirrhosis or hepatocellular carcinoma.

7. Transmission—HCV transmission is primarily parenteral including injection drug use; exposure to blood contaminating inadequately sterilized instruments and needles used in medical and dental procedures; unsterilized objects for rituals (e.g., circumcision, scarification), traditional medicine (e.g., blood-letting) or other activities that break the skin (e.g., tattooing, ear, or body piercing); and transfusion of blood or blood products from unscreened donors or blood products that have not undergone viral inactivation. Sexual transmission and mother-to-child transmission have been documented, but appear uncommon except for instances of HIV co-infection. The period of communicability is from one or more weeks before onset of the first symptoms and may persist indefinitely among persons with chronic infection. Peaks in virus concentration appear to correlate with peaks in alanine aminotransferase activity.

8. Risk groups—

1) Persons have received injections with nonsterilized needles and syringes in health care settings.
2) Present or past injection drug users.
3) Recipients of unscreened donated blood, blood products, and organs.

4) People who received a blood product for clotting problems made before 1987.
5) Hemodialysis patients or persons who spent many years on dialysis for kidney failure.
6) People who received body piercing or tattoos done with non-sterile instruments.
7) People with known exposures to the HCV, such as:

- Health care workers injured by needlesticks.
- Recipients of blood or organs from a donor who tested positive for the HCV.

8) HIV-infected men who have sex with men.
9) Children born to mothers infected with the HCV.

9. Prevention—General control measures are similar to those that apply to HBV infection (see Hepatitis B section in this chapter). A vaccine is not available and prophylactic IG is not effective. In blood bank operations, all donors should be routinely screened for anti-HCV, and all donor units with elevated liver enzyme levels should be discarded. Routine virus inactivation of plasma-derived products, risk-reduction counseling for persons uninfected but at high risk (e.g., injecting drug users, health care workers), and nosocomial control activities must be maintained.

10. Management of patient—Treatment decisions should be based on the severity of liver disease, the potential for side effects, the likelihood of response, presence of comorbid conditions, and the patient's readiness for treatment. If liver histology is available, treatment is indicated in those with bridging fibrosis or compensated cirrhosis. HCV RNA should be tested initially and at weeks 4, 8, and 12 of treatment. Genotype influences treatment and its duration. The optimal therapy for genotype 1 infection is boceprevir or telaprevir in combination with peg-interferon alpha and ribavirin. At present, all other genotypes are treated with peg-interferon plus ribavirin. All medications for the treatment of HCV infection have significant side effects that require careful monitoring. Ribavirin is a teratogen; thus pregnancy should be avoided during treatment. Corticosteroids and acyclovir have not been effective. Many new direct-acting antiviral agents are under development.

11. Management of contacts and the immediate environment—There is neither passive nor active immunization available to prevent HCV infection.

12. Special considerations—

1) Reporting: official report obligatory in some countries.

2) Epidemic measures: similar to hepatitis B. Information on the investigation and management of hepatitis C outbreaks in particular settings can be found at: http://www.cdc.gov/hepatitis/Settings.

3) International measures: ensure adequate virus inactivation for all internationally traded biological products.

IV. HEPATITIS D (viral hepatitis D, hepatitis delta virus, delta agent hepatitis, delta-associated hepatitis, HDV infection)

1. Clinical features—Onset is usually abrupt, with signs and symptoms resembling those of hepatitis B; may be severe and is always associated with a coexistent HBV infection, either as acute coinfection or as superinfection among persons with chronic HBV infection. In the former case the infection is usually self-limited; in the latter, it usually progresses to chronic hepatitis. Acute hepatitis D can be misdiagnosed as an exacerbation of chronic hepatitis B. As the outcome of hepatitis D virus (HDV) infection is associated with the host response to HBV, children with acute coinfection may have a severe clinical course with greater likelihood of progression to chronic hepatitis. In studies throughout Europe and the USA, 25%–50% of fulminant hepatitis cases thought to be caused by HBV were associated with concurrent HDV infection.

2. Causative agent—HDV is a virus-like particle of 35-37 nm consisting of a coat of HBsAg and a unique internal antigen, the delta antigen. Encapsulated with the delta antigen is the genome, a single-stranded RNA that can have a linear or circular conformation. HDV is unable to infect a cell by itself and requires coinfection with the HBV to undergo a complete replication cycle. Synthesis of HDV, in turn, results in temporary suppression of synthesis of HBV components. About 70%–90% of patients with HDV coinfection are HBeAg negative, and most have low serum HBV DNA. HDV is best considered a defective RNA virus that is related more to plant viroids than to other human pathogens. Eight genotypes (1–8) and 2 sub-genotypes (1a and 1b) of HDV have been identified.

3. Diagnosis—Through detection of total antibody to HDV (anti-HDV) by EIA; immunoglobulin class G (IgG) anti-HDV persists after HDV infection has cleared. A positive IgM titer indicates ongoing replication; reverse transcription PCR is the most sensitive assay for detecting HDV viremia.

4. Occurrence—Worldwide, but prevalence varies widely. An estimated 5% of the 240 million people infected with HBV globally have serologic evidence of exposure to HDV. HDV occurs epidemically or endemically among populations at high risk of HBV infection, in areas where hepatitis B is endemic (highest in Africa and South America, Romania, and parts of Russia). Severe epidemics have been observed in tropical South America (Brazil, Colombia, Venezuela), in the Central African Republic, and among injecting drug users in the USA. Since HDV requires a concomitant HBV infection, the recent decrease in prevalence of chronic HBsAg carriers in the general population in the Mediterranean area (Greece, Italy, Spain), and in many other parts of the world, has led to a rapid decline in both acute and chronic hepatitis D. Better sanitation and social standards may also have contributed. New foci of high HDV infection prevalence continue to appear in countries such as Albania, areas of China, northern India, and Japan (Okinawa).

5. Reservoir—Humans. Virus can be transmitted experimentally to chimpanzees and to woodchucks infected with HBV and woodchuck hepatitis virus, respectively.

6. Incubation period—Approximately 2–8 weeks.

7. Transmission—The mode of transmission is thought to be similar to that of HBV: exposure to infected blood and serous body fluids, contaminated needles, syringes, and plasma derivatives such as antihemophilic factor, and through sexual transmission. Blood is potentially infectious during all phases of active infection. Peak infectivity probably occurs just prior to onset of acute illness, when particles containing the delta antigen are readily detected in the blood. Following the onset of infection, viremia falls rapidly to low or undetectable levels; HDV has been transmitted to chimpanzees from the blood of chronically infected patients in whom particles containing the HDV antigen could not be detected.

8. Risk groups—All persons susceptible to HBV infection, or who have chronic HBV, can be infected with HDV. High-risk populations include injection drug users, hemophiliacs, and others who come in frequent contact with blood or blood products; among persons in institutions for the developmentally disabled; and among sexually active adults including men who have sex with men.

9. Prevention—For persons susceptible to HBV infection, same as for hepatitis B. Prevention of HBV infection with hepatitis B vaccine prevents infection with HDV. A vaccine for HDV infection is not available. Among persons with chronic HBV, the only effective measure is avoidance of exposure to any potential source of HDV. Studies suggest that measures decreasing sexual exposure and needle sharing are associated with a decline in the incidence of HDV infection.

10. Management of patient—Treatment: the only approved therapy for chronic hepatitis D is pegylated interferon every week for 48 weeks.

Treatment should be considered in patients with active replication of HDV RNA and histological evidence of disease injury.

11. **Management of contacts and the immediate environment—**

1) Universal precautions to prevent exposures to blood and body fluids.

2) Concurrent disinfection of equipment contaminated with blood or infectious body fluids.

3) Immunization of contacts susceptible to HBV infection for persons exposed simultaneously to HBV and HDV, using hepatitis B vaccine and HBIG as soon as possible after exposure. For persons with established chronic HBV infection, there are no products available to prevent HDV superinfection.

12. **Special considerations—**Epidemic measures: as for Hepatitis B.

V. HEPATITIS E (enterically transmitted non-A, non-B hepatitis [ET-NANB]; epidemic non-A, non-B hepatitis; fecal-oral non-A, non-B hepatitis)

1. **Clinical features—**Clinical course similar to that of hepatitis A, with a short prodromal phase, and a period of symptoms or jaundice lasting days to several weeks. Clinical and epidemiologic characteristics differ according to genotype. Infection with genotype 1 or 2 is common in developing countries and is associated with fecal-waterborne transmission, high rates of icteric disease, and a higher attack rate among adolescents and young adults. Mortality is high among pregnant women (20%). Development of chronic disease has not been reported.

In contrast, infection with genotypes 3 or 4 is associated with endemic disease in developed countries, foodborne transmission, a low rate of icteric disease, and high rates of illness and greater mortality among older adults. Neurologic complications and chronic disease among immunocompromised persons have been reported, and infections can become chronic.

2. **Causative agent—**The hepatitis E virus (HEV), the only known Hepevirus, is a spherical, nonenveloped, single-stranded RNA virus approximately 32–34 nm in diameter, classified in the *Hepeviridae* family. There are 4 HEV genotypes.

3. **Diagnosis—**Depends on clinical and epidemiological features and exclusion of other causes of hepatitis, especially hepatitis A, by serological means. Commercial assays are available in some countries. Viremia occurs during the incubation period and antibodies (IgM and IgG) appear just before elevations in serum aminotransferase levels and symptoms. Acute hepatitis E is diagnosed if IgM anti-HEV is present. Tests for HEV RNA in

serum and stool are confirmatory, but currently still experimental. Recovery is marked by viral clearance, and by increase in IgG (which may persist for years), and decrease in IgM levels (disappearance after 3–12 months).

4. Occurrence—HEV is the most common cause of acute hepatitis and jaundice in the world. In developing countries, hepatitis E occurs sporadically and as epidemic disease, and is largely due to genotype 1 (genotype 2 is more common in Mexico and parts of Africa); anti-HEV prevalence ranges from 30%–80%. Outbreaks often occur as waterborne epidemics, but sporadic cases and epidemics not clearly related to water have been reported. Outbreaks have been reported from: Algeria, Bangladesh, Chad, China, Côte d'Ivoire, Egypt, Ethiopia, Greece, India, Indonesia, the Islamic Republic of Iran, Jordan, Libya, Mexico, Myanmar, Nepal, Nigeria, Pakistan, southern areas of Russia, Somalia, Sudan and South Sudan, Uganda, and The Gambia.

Anti-HEV prevalence is lower in Europe and the USA than in Asia and Africa. Previous surveys in the USA (during 1988–1994) showed relatively high rates (21%) in the general population.

5. Reservoir—Humans are natural hosts for HEV; some nonhuman primates (e.g., chimpanzees, cynomolgus monkeys, rhesus monkeys, pigtail monkeys, owl monkeys, tamarins, and African green monkeys) are reported as susceptible to infection with HEV. HEV strains have been detected in domestic and wild pigs, deer, elk, sheep, cattle, rats, and rabbits. Thus, they are possibly sources of zoonotic infections of humans.

6. Incubation period—The range is 15–64 days; the mean incubation period has ranged from 26–42 days in various epidemics.

7. Transmission—Primarily by the fecal-oral route; fecally contaminated drinking water is the most commonly documented vehicle of transmission. Person-to-person transmission probably also occurs through the fecal-oral route; secondary spread among household cases has been described during outbreaks. Studies suggest that hepatitis E, may in fact, be a zoonotic infection with coincident introduction in areas of high human infection. The period of communicability is not known. HEV has been detected in stools 14 days after the onset of jaundice and approximately 4 weeks after oral ingestion of contaminated food or water, where it persists for about 2 weeks. Blood transfusion is a potential but rare route of HEV transmission.

8. Risk groups—Women in the third trimester of pregnancy are especially susceptible to fulminant disease and death (typically with genotype 1 or 2 infection). Among endemic cases, elderly adults appear particularly susceptible to infection with genotype 3 and 4. The occurrence of major epidemics among young adults in regions where other enteric viruses are highly endemic and most of the population acquires infection in infancy, remains unexplained.

9. **Prevention—**

1) Provide educational programs to stress sanitary disposal of feces and careful hand washing after defecation and before handling food; follow basic measures to prevent fecal-oral transmission.
2) Boiling and chlorination of water inactivates HEV.
3) Administration of immune globulin, though in endemic areas has not decreased infection rates during epidemics.
4) Thorough cooking of pork and avoidance of raw shellfish may be advisable.
5) No HEV vaccine is available.

10. **Management of Patient**—Feces, urine, and blood should be disposed of in a sanitary manner. Treatment is supportive during acute infection. Among those with chronic HEV infection, case series have reported viral clearance and sustained response in a high proportion of patients with peg-interferon and/or ribavirin.

11. **Management of contacts and the immediate environment—**

1) Immune globulin prepared from plasma collected in high-HEV endemic areas is not effective in preventing clinical disease during hepatitis E outbreaks. Prototype hepatitis E vaccines have been shown to prevent significant illness, but despite these successes in field trials, they are not yet marketed except in China.
2) Search for missed cases and maintain surveillance of contacts in the patient's household or, in a common source outbreak, among people exposed to the same risk.

12. **Special considerations—**

1) Reporting: report to local health authority is obligatory in some countries.
2) Epidemic measures: determine mode of transmission through epidemiological investigation; investigate water supply and identify populations at increased risk of infection; make special efforts to improve sanitary and hygienic practices in order to eliminate fecal contamination of foods and water.
3) A potential problem where there is mass crowding and inadequate sanitation and water supplies. If cases occur, increased effort should be exerted to improve sanitation and the safety of water supplies.

VI. HEPATOCELLULAR CARCINOMA (HCC, primary liver cancer, primary hepatocellular carcinoma, hepatoma)

1. **Clinical features**—A small proportion of persons with chronic HBV or HCV infection may eventually develop HCC. HCC rarely occurs before age 40 years and peaks at approximately age 70 years. Cirrhosis is present in 80%–90% of HCV-associated HCC cases (70%–80% of persons with HBV-associated HCC). The progression to cirrhosis is often clinically silent, and some patients are not known to have underlying viral hepatitis until they present with HCC. Symptoms, including anorexia, weight loss, right upper quadrant abdominal pain, or tenderness; ascites and jaundice commonly appear later in the course of the illness. Depending on lesion size and cancer stage at diagnosis, 5-year survival may be high (75%–90%) among persons with limited disease to very low (<10% 1-year survival) among persons with extrahepatic spread or vascular involvement.

2. **Causative agents**—Approximately 50% of cases of HCC are attributable to chronic HBV infection, a slightly lower percentage to chronic HCV infection, and a small proportion to noninfectious causes. Aflatoxin, alcohol, and nonalcoholic fatty liver disease (with or without obesity, metabolic syndrome, and type 2 diabetes) may serve as important cofactors in the development of HCC.

3. **Diagnosis**—Often made using noninvasive imaging tests, particularly with cirrhotic patients with focal hepatic masses greater than 2 cm in diameter and elevated alpha-fetoprotein levels. Image guided biopsy is reserved for focal masses with atypical imaging features.

4. **Occurrence**—HCC is the fifth most common cancer in men and the seventh most common in women worldwide, with an estimated one-half to one million new cases per year (~5% of all cancers worldwide). Most of the burden of disease (85%) occurs in developing countries; however, HCC related to infection with HCV has become the fastest-rising cause of cancer in the USA (where incidence has tripled in the last 20 years) and some other industrialized countries. HCC is one of the most common malignant neoplasms in many parts of Asia and Africa, and its occurrence correlates with rates of chronic HBV and HCV infection in the population. Thus, it occurs with high frequency in areas with high prevalence of HBV carriers, including most of Asia, Africa, the South Pacific, and part of the Middle East. Rates are intermediate on the Indian subcontinent and relatively low in North America and Western Europe. In industrialized countries, including Japan, and other countries such as Pakistan, Egypt, and Mongolia, HCV infection is considered the dominant viral etiology of HCC.

5. Reservoir—See Hepatitis B and Hepatitis C sections in this chapter.

6. Incubation period—The duration from infection with HBV or HCV to development of HCC, when it does occur, typically takes several decades, depending on the presence of cofactors (see Risk Groups under Hepatocellular Carcinoma section in this chapter). In the presence of cirrhosis, the 5-year cumulative risk of HCC ranges from 5%–30%.

7. Transmission—See Hepatitis B and Hepatitis C sections in this chapter.

8. Risk groups—Rates of HCC among men are 2–4 times higher than among women.

Among persons with chronic HBV infection, risk of HCC further increases by male sex, older age, infection of long duration, family history of HCC, coinfection with HIV or HDV, exposure to aflatoxin, use of alcohol or tobacco, high levels of HBV DNA, or infection with genotype C. Among persons with chronic HCV infection, risk of HCC increases by older age at time of infection, male sex, coinfection with HIV or HBV, alcohol, and probably diabetes or obesity.

9. Prevention—Vaccination to prevent HBV infection. There is moderately strong evidence that antiviral treatment that controls HBV replication among HBsAg-positive patients, and that eradicating HCV among persons with viremia, substantially reduces but does not eliminate the risk of HCC. Periodic screening of carriers of HBV for alpha-fetoprotein and ultrasound can, in some cases, detect the tumor at an early, resectable stage. Newer technologies, such as computerized tomography (CT) or magnetic resonance imaging (MRI) scanning, are being evaluated as screening strategies for hepatocellular carcinoma but currently are too costly for most populations.

10. Management of patient—Choice of treatment is determined by cancer stage; few randomized controlled trials have compared therapeutic approaches. Depending on stage, treatment options include surgical resection, liver transplantation, local ablation, transarterial chemo- or radioembolization, and chemotherapy.

11. Management of contacts and the immediate environment—See Hepatitis B and Hepatitis C sections in this chapter.

12. Special considerations—Hepatocellular cancer cases should be reported to a tumor registry according to standard cancer registration procedures.

[P. R. Spradling]

HERPESVIRUS DISEASE

DISEASE	ICD-CODE
HERPESVIRAL INFECTIONS	ICD-10 A60 (anogenital herpes viral infection), B00 (herpes viral infection), P35.2 (congenital herpes viral infection)
HERPESVIRAL ENCEPHALITIS, SIMIAN B	ICD-10 B00.4
KAPOSI'S SARCOMA	ICD-10 C46.0-C46.9

I. HERPESVIRAL INFECTIONS (herpes simplex, genital herpes, alphaherpesviral disease, herpesvirus hominis, human herpesviruses 1 and 2)

1. Clinical features—Infections with herpes simplex virus (HSV) type 1 (HSV-1) or type 2 (HSV-2) are characterized by neurovirulence, latency, and a tendency to localized recurrence. After primary infection, herpes viruses establish latency and persist for life. Reactivation of latent virus results in viral shedding, which may be accompanied by symptoms, but which is usually asymptomatic. When present, symptoms may be localized or systemic. The clinical syndrome and course of infection depends on the anatomic site of infection, age, and immune status of the host, and infecting viral type. However, either viral type may infect the genital tract or oral mucosa, or cause systemic disease. Severe and extensive spread of infection may occur in those who are immunodeficient or immunosuppressed and may result in fatal, generalized infections in newborn infants (neonatal herpes).

Oral herpes infection is usually caused by HSV-1; infection, may be mild and inapparent and often occurs in early childhood. Approximately 10% of newly acquired (primary) infections result in overt disease, with illness of varying severity, marked by fever and malaise lasting a week or more; it may be associated with gingivostomatitis accompanied by vesicular lesions in the oropharynx. HSV-1 can also cause severe keratoconjunctivitis, a generalized cutaneous eruption complicating chronic eczema, or encephalitis. HSV-1 causes about 2% of acute pharyngotonsillitis, usually as a primary infection. Symptomatic reactivations commonly result in herpes labialis (fever blisters, cold sores), manifested usually on the face or lips, by superficial clear vesicles on an erythematous base that crust and heal within days. Reactivation is precipitated by various forms of trauma, fever, physiological changes, or intercurrent disease and may also involve other body tissues; it occurs in the presence of circulating antibodies, which are seldom elevated by reactivation. Symptomatic reactivation is heralded by tingling prior to the onset of vesicles; if patients learn this sign, they can prevent or shorten the clinical course of the reactivated infection through the use of antivirals.

Central nervous system (CNS) involvement may appear in association with primary or recurrent disease with either HSV-1 or HSV-2 and may manifest as aseptic meningitis, transverse myelitis, sacral radiculopathy, or encephalitis. Findings in herpesviral encephalitis may include: fever, headache, leukocytosis, meningeal irritation, drowsiness, confusion, stupor, coma, and focal neurological signs, frequently referable to one or the other temporal region. The condition may be confused with other intracranial lesions, including brain abscess and tuberculous meningitis. Because antiviral therapy can reduce mortality, suspected encephalitis infections should be treated presumptively for herpes with antiviral therapy.

Genital herpes occurs mainly in adults. Newly acquired, symptomatic infections often include systemic symptoms such as fever and malaise and are classically characterized by bilateral vesiculopustular or ulcerative lesions on the cervix or external genitalia in women and on the external genitalia in men. Men or women engaging in anal sex may become infected at the anus and/or rectum. However, the classical findings are often absent, and the clinical diagnosis of genital herpes is both nonsensitive and nonspecific. Recurrent disease can involve areas other than the site of initial infection, typically in related dermatomes; such as the perineum, legs, and buttocks. Primary lesions may last 2–3 weeks. Recurrent disease is usually unilateral and has a much smaller area of involvement and shorter duration than that of primary infection. Many herpes-infected persons do not have recognized symptoms of genital herpes but still shed virus intermittently in the genital tract. Symptomatic primary infection with HSV-1 cannot be distinguished clinically from that caused by HSV-2; however, recurrences and subclinical shedding are less common with genital HSV-1 than with genital HSV-2 infection. Clinical manifestations of genital herpes may be more severe in immunocompromised persons.

Neonatal infections can be divided into 3 clinical presentations: disseminated infections involving multiple organs such as the liver; central nervous system infection; and infections limited to the skin, eyes, or mouth. The first two forms are often lethal and associated with significant morbidity. Because skin lesions are present in only 70%, and fever in only 40% of babies with HSV, clinicians must maintain a high index of suspicion for HSV infection, especially in the first month of life. Infections are due to either HSV-1 or HSV-2.

2. Causative agent—HSV, which is in the virus family *Herpesviridae*, subfamily *Alphaherpesvirinae*. Historically, genital herpes was caused by HSV-2 and oral herpes by HSV-1; however, HSV-1 is now a common cause of primary genital herpes in some populations and causes a substantial proportion of neonatal herpes infections.

3. **Diagnosis**—Can be confirmed by viral isolation, HSV deoxyribonucleic acid (DNA) detection by polymerase chain reaction (PCR), or HSV antigen detection by enzyme immunoassay (EIA) or direct fluorescent antibody (DFA). Cytologic detection of cellular changes (e.g., Tzanck preparation) is insensitive and nonspecific for diagnosis and should not be relied upon.

Viral culture isolates can be typed to determine whether HSV-1 or HSV-2 is the cause of infection. HSV types 1 and 2 can be differentiated immunologically (especially when type-specific or monoclonal antibodies are used) and differ with respect to their growth patterns in cell culture, embryonated eggs, and experimental animals.

HSV DNA PCR on spinal fluid is the test of choice for diagnosing CNS infection. Neuroimaging, preferably by magnetic resonance imaging (MRI), should be done early during the diagnostic workup. Brain biopsy may be considered in atypical cases when other diagnostic testing is not definitive. Accurate type-specific HSV serologic tests based on glycoprotein G are now available and can reliably distinguish HSV-1 and HSV-2 antibodies. Antibodies to HSV may take several weeks to develop after initial infection but then persist indefinitely; false negative serologic results may occur at early stages of infection. Herpes immunoglobulin class M (IgM) antibody tests are not reliable in determining whether infection is newly acquired. Neonates being evaluated for possible herpes infection should have "surface cultures" of the mouth, nasopharynx, conjunctivae, and anus, and culture or PCR of skin vesicles. Neonates should also have whole blood tested for alanine tranferase (ALT); elevated transaminase values can suggest HSV hepatitis, or disseminated infection, which may occur in an afebrile infant.

4. **Occurrence**—Worldwide; 50%–90% of adults possess circulating antibodies against HSV-1; initial, oral infection with HSV-1 usually occurs before the fifth year of life, but more primary infections in adults are now being reported. HSV-2 infection usually begins with sexual activity and is rare before adolescence, except in sexually abused children. HSV-2 antibody occurs in approximately 20% of adults in some developed countries. Seroprevalence increases with age and is higher among females, certain racial/ethnic groups, and persons with multiple sexual partners. The majority (≤90%) of persons infected with HSV-2 have not been diagnosed with genital herpes.

5. **Reservoir**—Humans.

6. **Incubation period**—From 2–12 days; may be longer for neonatal infections.

7. **Transmission**—Contact with HSV-1 or HSV-2 in saliva or genital secretions is the most important mode of spread. Both types 1 and 2 may

be transmitted to various sites by genital-genital, oral-genital, oral-anal, or anal-genital contact. Herpes transmission via a shared towel has not been documented. Ungloved health care personnel (e.g., dentists) may acquire infection on the hands (herpetic whitlow) from patients shedding HSV from the oral cavity. Transmission to the neonate usually (~85% of cases) occurs via the infected birth canal, less commonly in utero or postpartum. Most cases of neonatal herpes occur in infants born to women with no known history of genital herpes. Modes of postnatal transmission to neonates include direct orogenital suction during ritual Jewish circumcision.

Transmission of HSV can occur during asymptomatic periods. HSV may be shed intermittently from mucosal sites for years and possibly lifelong, in the presence or absence of clinical manifestations. Viral shedding can be detected by PCR on 18% of days HSV-2 seropositive people are swabbed in the genital area; viral shedding is more common among those with a history of symptomatic genital herpes (20%) than among those with no history of symptoms (10%), lasts longer with symptomatic reactivations than with subclinical reactivations, and is of shorter duration with recurrent compared to primary lesions.

8. Risk groups—Persons engaging in unprotected sexual intercourse, oral or anal sex with an infected partner, and neonates born to women with genital HSV infection. The risk of transmission to the neonate from an infected mother depends mainly on whether the maternal infection is primary or recurrent. The risk for transmission is high (30%–50%) among women who acquire infection in late pregnancy and is low (<1%) among women with histories of recurrent herpes at term or who acquire genital HSV infection during the first half of pregnancy, in part because maternal immunity confers a degree of protection. Persons with HSV-2 infection are at increased risk for acquiring HIV infection.

9. Prevention—

1) Health education and personal hygiene directed toward minimizing the transfer of infectious material.
2) Avoid contaminating the skin of eczematous patients with infectious material.
3) Health care personnel should wear gloves when in direct contact with mucous membranes or potentially infectious lesions.
4) Correct and consistent use of latex condoms in sexual practice may decrease the risk of genital infection. Persons with known genital herpes infection should disclose their infection status to sex partners.
5) For sexual partnerships in which one member is known to have genital herpes infection, type-specific serologic testing can be

used to determine whether the other partner is at risk for acquiring herpes infection.

6) Treatment with daily valacyclovir can decrease the rate of HSV-2 transmission in discordant, heterosexual couples in which the one partner has a history of genital HSV-2 infection. Sexual activity should be avoided when lesions are present.

7) When primary genital herpes infections occur in late pregnancy, caesarean section is often advised before the membranes rupture because risk of transmission to the neonate is high (30%–50%). However, some specialists recommend use of antiviral medications instead of, or in addition to, caesarean section in this situation. The risk of neonatal infection from women with a history of recurrent genital herpes infection is much lower (<1%), and caesarean section is advisable only when active lesions or prodromal symptoms are present at delivery. Suppressive antiviral therapy starting at 36 weeks gestation can reduce the need for caesarean delivery among women with active recurrent genital herpes but does not eliminate the risk for transmission to the neonate. Some specialists recommend type-specific HSV serologic testing for pregnant women and their sex partners to identify women at risk for acquiring herpes from a sex partner during pregnancy; however this approach needs further study.

8) In settings with access to viral culture and PCR and type-specific serologic testing, women delivering with active genital lesions should have lesions tested by PCR or culture with typing, and if there is no history of genital herpes before pregnancy, then type-specific serologic testing should be performed at the same time. Asymptomatic infants born by vaginal or cesarean delivery to women with active genital lesions should have HSV testing of surface swab specimens, blood, and cerebrospinal fluid (CSF) performed 24 hours after birth, with infant treatment with parenteral acyclovir starting immediately after specimen collection if the mother has no history of genital lesions before pregnancy. Decisions regarding the duration of the neonates treatment when mothers have no history of genital herpes hinge on the results of both infant and maternal test results. When mothers have a history of genital herpes, decisions on initiating treatment in the neonate hinge on the neonatal virologic test results. The risk for neonatal infection is much higher for infants born to women with a first time genital herpes infection during pregnancy.

10. **Management of patient—**

1) Contact isolation for neonatal and disseminated or primary severe lesions; for recurrent lesions, drainage and secretion precautions. Patients with herpetic lesions should have no contact with newborns, children with eczema or burns, or immunodeficient patients.

2) Persons with genital herpes should avoid sexual activity with uninfected partners when lesions or prodromal symptoms are present. Daily use of valacyclovir by persons with genital herpes can decrease the risk of HSV-2 sexual transmission to an uninfected partner.

3) Treatment: the acute manifestations of herpetic keratitis and early dendritic ulcers may be treated with antiviral ophthalmic ointments or solutions (e.g., trifluridine, acyclovir, ganciclovir, idoxuridine, or vidarabine). Interferon used in combination with nucleoside antivirals may facilitate early healing. Only an experienced ophthalmologist should administer corticosteroids for ocular involvement. Acyclovir used orally or intravenously has been shown to reduce shedding of virus, diminish pain, and accelerate healing time in primary and recurrent genital herpes, rectal herpes, stomatitis, and herpetic whitlow. Valacyclovir and famciclovir are more recently licensed congeners of acyclovir that are also efficacious. Oral preparations of these 3 antiviral drugs are most convenient to use and can provide benefit even with extensive anogenital infection. Prophylactic daily administration of these drugs (suppressive therapy) can reduce the frequency of both clinical and subclinical HSV recurrences in adults. Topical creams are not effective in genital herpes. Strains of herpes virus resistant to antivirals have been reported, though these are uncommon in infections of immunocompetent persons. Intravenous acyclovir should be provided for patients with severe HSV disease, disseminated infection, or CNS complications (e.g., meningitis or encephalitis). Neonatal infections should be treated with high-dose intravenous acyclovir; suppressive acyclovir therapy for 6 months after treatment reduces risk for skin recurrences and improves neurodevelopmental outcomes in neonates with central nervous system infection.

11. Management of contacts and the immediate environment—
In sexual partnerships with one member known to have genital herpes infection, type-specific serologic testing can be used to determine whether the other partner is at risk for acquiring herpes infection.

12. **Special considerations—**

1) Reporting: neonatal infections are reportable in some areas.
2) HIV-infected persons: HSV infection can be more severe and prolonged in persons with HIV infection; recommended treatment regimens differ. Treatment of HSV infection in HSV-HIV coinfected persons can reduce HIV viral load.

II. HERPESVIRAL ENCEPHALITIS, SIMIAN B (B virus, simian B disease, cercopithecine herpes virus 1)

1. Clinical features—A zoonotic CNS disease (encephalomyelitis) that is rare in humans and can present with lesions (vesicular or ulcerative), tingling, pain, or itching at exposure site and local lymphadenopathy, influenza-like illness with fever and myalgia or nausea and vomiting and CNS symptoms including headache. Infection ends in death in an estimated 80% of untreated cases, 1 day to 3 weeks after onset of symptoms. Occasional recoveries have been associated with considerable residual disability; a few cases, treated with acyclovir, have recovered completely.

2. Causative agent—Cercopithecine herpesvirus 1 (B virus), a zoonotic virus closely related to HSV.

3. Diagnosis—Culture, PCR, and serology for B virus can only be performed by certain reference laboratories.

4. Reservoir—Macaque monkeys; 30%-80% of rhesus monkeys (*Macaca mulatta*) are seropositive.

6. Incubation period—Between 3 days and 3 weeks.

7. Transmission—Human illness has been acquired through monkey bites and scratches or exposure of naked skin or mucous membrane to infected saliva or monkey cell cultures, exposure to tissue culture or autopsy material, needlestick injuries, cage scratches, and mucosal splash. On a given day, approximately 2% of seropositive rhesus monkeys shed B virus, but shedding increases during periods of stress (e.g., shipping and handling). The ocular, oral, and genital secretions; CNS tissues and CSF; and cell cultures from macaque monkeys are potentially infectious.

8. Risk groups—Veterinarians, laboratory workers, and others in close contact with macaque monkeys or their secretions or tissues.

9. Prevention—Depends on proper use of protective gauntlets, eyewear and masks, and care taken to minimize exposure to monkeys.

Those working with macaque monkeys need to be educated about the risk of exposure to infection.

10. Management of patient—

1) All bite or scratch wounds or other exposure to potentially infectious material from macaques or from cages possibly contaminated with macaque secretions and that result in bleeding must be immediately and thoroughly scrubbed and cleaned for at least 15 minutes. Eyes and mucous membranes should be flushed with sterile saline or water. Skin should be washed preferably with a solution containing detergent soap (e.g., chlorhexidine or povidone-iodine).

2) Prophylactic treatment with an antiviral agent such as valacyclovir or acyclovir is recommended when an animal handler sustains a deep, penetrating wound; a wound that was not adequately cleaned; a laceration of the head, neck, or torso; an exposure from a high-risk source (e.g., a macaque that is ill or objects contaminated with fluids likely to contain B virus); or when a postcleansing culture is positive for the virus. Prophylaxis should be considered for other exposures involving a mucosal splash, skin laceration, or puncture. It is not recommended for skin exposures in which the skin remains intact or for exposures from nonmacaque species.

3) The appearance of any skin lesions, itching, pain, or numbness near the site of the wound or neurological symptoms, calls for expert medical consultation for diagnosis and possible treatment.

11. Management of contacts and the immediate environment— The usefulness of B virus culture or serology of the monkeys to evaluate the virus status of the monkey and risk of infection is uncertain.

12. Special considerations—Because infection has occurred in macaque handlers who did not recall obvious exposures, such workers should report episodes of fever lasting more than 48 hours or symptoms compatible with B virus infection to appropriate health care personnel.

III. KAPOSI'S SARCOMA (idiopathic multiple pigmented hemorrhagic sarcoma)

Kaposi's sarcoma (KS) is an angioproliferative disorder that involves angiogenesis, inflammation, and spindle cell proliferation. It is characterized by solitary or multiple purplish, reddish-blue, or dark brown/black macules, plaques, and nodules of the skin which can occur anywhere but usually in the lower extremities and associated with lymphedema. Skin lesions vary in size (up to several centimeters in diameter) and may be unchanged for years or grow rapidly and disseminate within a few weeks. Mucous membranes of the mouth and gastrointestinal tract and regional lymph nodes may be affected; involvement of other organs (lung, liver, bone, bone marrow) is extremely rare.

There are 4 types of KS. The classical form occurs in older males of mainly Mediterranean or central/eastern European backgrounds. An endemic form occurs in all age groups in parts of equatorial Africa; neither is associated with immune deficiency. The remaining types—in recipients of organ transplants who undergo immunosuppressive treatment (iatrogenic form) or in HIV-infected persons (epidemic form)— are accompanied by immune impairment. Overall, males are predominantly afflicted. The epidemic form presents the most aggressive clinical course and is seen almost exclusively in HIV-infected individuals. Despite differences in clinical manifestations and serostatus, it is appropriate to consider all forms of KS as one entity, given the identical pathological stages in the progression of the lesions of KS (patch stage, plaque stage, and nodular stage) and the immunohistochemical features angiogenesis, inflammation, and the characteristic spindle cell of the tumor.

KS-associated herpesvirus (KSHV), or human herpesvirus-8, is believed to be the causal agent of KS. It is a human *Gammaherpesvirus* related to an oncogenic herpesvirus of monkeys, *Herpesvirus saimiri*. Evidence of viral infection is found in virtually all cases, and several lines of evidence point to a key etiologic role in this disease. HHV-8 infection precedes clinical sarcoma, is highly associated with increased risk in all populations studied thus far, and affects the endothelial (spindle) cell thought to be the prime determinant of tumorigenesis. HHV-8 has also been shown to infect primary endothelial cells.

Seroepidemiological analysis suggests that KSHV has a more limited distribution than any of the other 7 human herpesviruses. In North America, seroprevalence ranges from 0%–1% in blood donors to about 35% in HIV-infected individuals and up to 100% in KS patients with AIDS. In Milan, Italy, blood donors have a 4% seropositivity rate whereas seroprevalence in Sardinia was 35% and 19% for Italy overall. Data suggest even higher KSHV rates in central Africa, where 58% of persons aged 14–84 years were KSHV positive in one study and seroprevalence (similar in men and women) increased linearly with age.

Serological analyses also suggest that infection occurs primarily in sexually active people, particularly men who have sex with men. Differences in risk of KS for AIDS patients who acquired HIV via sexual transmission and those whose HIV infections derived from blood product exposure support the role of sexual transmission: only 1%–3% of hemophilia and transfusion-related AIDS patients develop Kaposi's sarcoma. Transplacental transmission of anti-KSHV antibody is almost certain, and the virus may also be transmitted transplacentally since children of KSHV-positive mothers are at increased risk of infection after the neonatal period. In Africa, the high seroprevalence among adolescents and the relatively linear increase in prevalence with age suggest that nonsexual modes of transmission for KSHV may also be important.

There is no consensus for treatment for KS. Cases should be reported to a tumor registry.

[H. Badaruddin, J. A. Schillinger]

HISTOPLASMOSIS

DISEASE	ICD-10 CODE
HISTOPLASMOSIS CAPSULATI	ICD-10 B39.4
HISTOPLASMOSIS DUBOISII	ICD-10 B39.5

Two clinically different mycoses are designated as histoplasmosis; the pathogens that cause them cannot be distinguished morphologically when grown on culture media as molds. Detailed information is given for the infection caused by *Histoplasma capsulatum* var. *capsulatum*, and a brief summary for that caused by *H. capsulatum* var. *duboisii*.

I. HISTOPLASMOSIS CAPSULATI (histoplasmosis due to *H. capsulatum* var. *capsulatum*, American histoplasmosis)

1. **Clinical features**—A systemic mycosis of varying severity ranging from symptom-free, or minor self-limited, to life-threatening illnesses. The primary lesion is usually in the lungs. While infection is common, overt clinical disease is not. Four clinical forms are recognized:

1) Acute respiratory: varies from a mild respiratory illness to temporary incapacity with general malaise, fever, chills, headache, myalgia, chest pains, and nonproductive cough; occasional erythema multiforme; and erythema nodosum. Multiple, small scattered calcifications in the lung, hilar lymph nodes, spleen, and liver may be late findings.

2) Acute disseminated histoplasmosis: with debilitating fever, gastrointestinal (GI) symptoms, evidence of bone marrow suppression, hepatosplenomegaly, lymphadenopathy, and a

rapid course; most frequent in infants and young children and immunocompromised patients, including those with HIV infection. Usually fatal unless treated.

3) Chronic disseminated disease: with low-grade intermittent fever, weight loss, weakness, hepatosplenomegaly, mild hematological abnormalities, and focal manifestations of disease (e.g., endocarditis, meningitis, mucosal ulcers of mouth, larynx, stomach or bowel, and Addison disease). Subacute course progressing over the course of 10–11 months and usually fatal unless treated.

4) Chronic pulmonary form: clinically and radiologically resembling chronic pulmonary tuberculosis with cavitation; occurs most often in middle-aged and elderly men with underlying emphysema. Progresses over months or years, with periods of quiescence and sometimes spontaneous cure.

2. Causative agent—*Histoplasma capsulatum* (*Ajellomyces capsulatus*), a dimorphic fungus growing as a mold in soil and as a yeast in animal and human tissue.

3. Diagnosis—Confirmed by culture, deoxyribonucleic acid (DNA) probe, or by visualizing the fungus in Giemsa- or Wright-stained smears of ulcer exudates, bone marrow, sputum or blood; demonstrating the fungus in biopsies of ulcers, liver, bone marrow, lymph nodes, or lung requires special stains. Serology is a vital instrument in diagnosis of infection. The immunodiffusion test is the most specific and reliable of available serological tests. A rise in complement fixation titers in paired sera may occur early in acute infection; a titer of 1:32 or greater is suggestive of active disease. Low levels of complement fixation (CF) antibodies are detected in approximately 10% of healthy individuals who reside in an endemic region. False-negative tests are common, particularly in HIV-infected patients, and negative serology does not exclude the diagnosis. Detection of antigen in serum, bronchial lavage fluids, or urine is useful in making the diagnosis and following the results of treatment for disseminated histoplasmosis; however, there is a high degree of crossreactivity with patients infected with *Histoplasma duboisii*, *Blastomyces dermatitidis*, *Paracoccidioides brasiliensis*, and *Penicillium marneffei*. Requires differentiation from penicilliosis in endemic regions. DNA-based direct detection assays for fluids and tissues are available on a research basis.

4. Occurrence—Commonly occurs in geographic foci over wide areas of the Americas, Africa, eastern Asia, and Australia; rare in Europe. Exposure is common in endemic pockets of the Americas, Africa, eastern and southeast Asia, and Australia; clinical disease is less frequent and severe progressive disease is rare. Prevalence increases from childhood to age 15 years; the chronic pulmonary form is more common in males. Outbreaks have occurred in endemic areas in families, students, and workers with exposure to bird, chicken, or bat droppings, or recently disturbed contaminated soil. Histoplasmosis occurs in many animals, often with a clinical picture comparable to that in humans.

5. Reservoir—Soil with high organic content and undisturbed bird and bat droppings, in particular that around and in old chicken houses, in bat caves, and around starling, blackbird, and pigeon roosts.

7. Transmission—Growth of the fungus in soil produces microconidia and tuberculate macroconidia; infection results from inhalation of airborne microconidia. Person-to-person transmission can occur only if infected tissue is inoculated into a healthy person.

6. Incubation period—Range 3–17 days, average 12–14 days; may be shorter with heavy exposure.

8. Risk groups—May be an opportunistic infection in those with compromised immunity. Susceptibility is general. Inapparent infections are common in endemic areas and usually result in increased resistance to infection.

9. Prevention—Minimize exposure to dust in a contaminated environment, such as chicken coops and surrounding soil. Spray with water or oil to reduce dust; use protective masks.

10. Management of patient—

1) Concurrent disinfection of sputum and soiled articles. Terminal cleaning.
2) Treatment: mild infection may be self-resolving. For patients with severe disease, induction with Amphotericin B followed by itraconazole is recommended; corticosteroids with Amphotericin B are indicated in patients with severe acute pulmonary disease. Itraconazole is the consolidation and maintenance drug of choice; patients with HIV infection should be maintained on itraconazole for life. Mild to moderate infections can be treated with itraconazole. Fluconazole is less effective and associated with relapse.

11. Management of contacts and the immediate environment—Investigate household and occupational contacts for evidence of infection from a common environmental source.

12. Special considerations—

1) Reporting: report to local health authority may be required in some endemic areas.

2) Occurrence of grouped cases of acute pulmonary disease in or outside of an endemic area, particularly with history of exposure to dust within a closed space (caves or construction sites), should arouse suspicion of histoplasmosis. Suspected sites such as attics, basements, caves, or construction sites with large amounts of bird droppings or bat guano must be investigated.

3) Possible hazard if large groups, especially from nonendemic areas, are forced to move through, live in, or disturb soil in areas where the mold is prevalent.

II. HISTOPLASMOSIS DUBOISII (histoplasmosis due to *H. capsulatum* var. *duboisii*, African histoplasmosis)

This usually presents as a subacute granuloma of skin or bone. Thus far, the disease has been recognized only in Africa and Madagascar. Infection, though usually localized, may be disseminated in the skin, subcutaneous tissue, lymph nodes, bones, joints, lungs, and abdominal viscera. Disease is more common in males and may occur at any age but especially in the second decade of life. Diagnosis is made through culture or demonstration of yeast cells of *H. capsulatum* var. *duboisii* in tissue by smear or biopsy. These cells are much larger than the yeast cells of *H. capsulatum* var. *capsulatum*. The true prevalence of *H. duboisii*, its reservoir, mode of transmission, and incubation period are unknown. It is not communicable from person to person. Treatment is the same as for histoplasmosis due to *H. capsulatum*.

[M. Brandt]

HIV INFECTION AND AIDS

DISEASE	ICD-10 CODE
HIV INFECTION AND AIDS	ICD-10 B20-B24

1. Clinical features—Acquired Immune Deficiency Syndrome, or AIDS, is the late clinical stage of infection with the human immunodeficiency virus (HIV). Within several weeks after infection with HIV, many individuals develop an acute self-limited mononucleosis-like illness lasting for a week or two. They may then be free of clinical signs or symptoms for years before other clinical manifestations develop, the result of HIV-related opportunistic infections or cancers. The frequency and severity of HIV-related opportunistic infections or cancers is, in general, directly correlated with the degree of immune system dysfunction.

2. Causative agent(s)—AIDS was first recognized in the early 1980s, and in 1983 a retrovirus, later named HIV, was first isolated. Two serologically and geographically distinct species, HIV-1 and HIV-2, have since been identified. This chapter refers to HIV-1 except where specified. Three groups of HIV-1 have been identified—M, N, and O. Group M is the most prevalent and is subdivided into 7 subtypes or clades.

3. Diagnosis—HIV infection is defined by laboratory criteria, usually based on detection of HIV-1/2 antibodies and/or HIV-1 p24 antigen, but molecular tests for HIV deoxyribonucleic acid (DNA) and/or ribonucleic acid (RNA) may also be included. For diagnostic purposes, a 3-test strategy is recommended in populations with an HIV prevalence rate less than 5%, whereby 3 sequential reactive results from 3 different assays are required to confirm HIV positivity. A 3-test strategy is also recommended for populations with prevalence greater than 5%, with the third assay used when the first and second assays are discrepant. Individuals with a reactive third assay result should not be considered positive but should be referred for follow-up testing. Selection of tests depends on such factors as performance characteristics (accuracy), potential for cross-reactivity, and local operational characteristics. DNA and RNA nucleic acid testing plays an important role in early infant HIV diagnosis because the presence of passively transferred maternal antibody can result in positive HIV serology results before 18 months of age in the absence of HIV infection. The WHO guidelines for assuring the accuracy and reliability of HIV rapid testing provide more detailed information and can be found at: http://whqlibdoc. who.int/publications/2005/9241593563_eng.pdf?ua=1.

4. Occurrence—An estimated 35 million persons worldwide were living with HIV at the end of 2013. Globally, there were an estimated 1.5 million AIDS-related deaths in 2013. The number of new HIV infections worldwide is declining, with an estimated 2.1 million new infections in 2013 compared with 3.2 million in 2001. At the end of 2013, 3.2 million children younger than 15 years were living with HIV. HIV-1 is the most prevalent HIV species throughout the world; HIV-2 has been found primarily in western Africa, with infections also in countries linked epidemiologically to western Africa. Sub-Saharan Africa is the most affected region accounting for 71% of people living with HIV worldwide. The Caribbean region is also heavily affected, especially the Dominican Republic and Haiti, which account for most infections in the Caribbean region.

Prevalence has stabilized or is decreasing in most countries, along with some evidence of decreasing risk behavior. The greatest declines in HIV incidence have been in sub-Saharan Africa, with 33% fewer new HIV infections in 2013 as compared with 2005. In Asia, prevalence is highest in South-East Asia Region, with considerable variation in trends—declining in some countries while continuing to grow in others. In Eastern Europe and central Asia, Russia and Ukraine account for most new HIV diagnoses, but rates are also rising in other countries.

In 2013, 16 million women aged 15 years and older were living with HIV, representing almost half of people living with HIV globally, but in sub-Saharan Africa the percentage is higher, where it is estimated that 58% of all infections are in women.

5. Reservoir—Humans. HIV-1 appears to have evolved from chimpanzee simian immunodeficiency viruses that crossed over to humans, presumably from blood exposure from hunting and butchering of bush meat. HIV-2 appears to have evolved from cross-species transmission events of sooty mangabey simian immunodeficiency viruses.

6. Incubation period—Variable. Although the time from infection to the development of detectable antibodies is generally less than 1 month, the time from HIV infection to diagnosis of AIDS has an observed range of less than 1 to 15 years or longer. The median time to development of AIDS in infected infants is shorter than in adults. There is some evidence that disease progression from HIV infection to AIDS is more rapid in developing countries than in other populations. The only factor that has been consistently shown to affect progression from HIV infection to AIDS is age at initial infection: adolescent and adults (males and females) who acquire HIV infection at an early age progress to AIDS more slowly than those infected at an older age. Disease progression may also vary by viral subtype.

7. Transmission—Person-to-person transmission through unprotected penile-vaginal or penile-anal intercourse; the use of HIV-contaminated injecting and skin-piercing equipment, including sharing of needles and syringes by people who inject drugs; vertical transmission from mother to infant during pregnancy, delivery, or breastfeeding; and transfusion of infected blood or its components. Heterosexual sexual transmission is the predominant mode of HIV transmission in sub-Saharan Africa as well as in the South-East Asia Region, with young women particularly vulnerable. However, most epidemics in the region are mixed with epidemics also occurring among populations at higher risk, including sex workers and men who have sex with men. Injection drug use is the major mode of transmission in Eastern Europe and central Asia. In Latin America, transmission occurs primarily in higher-risk populations such as sex workers and men who have sex with men. In North America, Western and Central Europe, Australia, and New Zealand, HIV continues to be transmitted mainly through unprotected sex between men and unsafe injection practices among people who inject drugs. Less common modes of transmission include contact of abraded skin or mucosa with infectious body secretions, the transplantation of HIV-infected tissues or organs, and tattooing or skin-piercing procedures with improperly sterilized needles. The risk of transmission from oral sex is not easily quantifiable but is presumed to be low. While the virus has occasionally been found in saliva, tears, urine, and bronchial secretions, transmission after contact with these secretions in the absence of blood has not been reported. No laboratory or epidemiological evidence suggests that biting insects have transmitted HIV infection. The period of communicability is not known precisely, begins early after onset of HIV infection, and presumably extends throughout life. Infectiousness is related to viral load. The risk of transmission may be high in the first months after infection when viral load is high, even before immune suppression has occurred, and while the high-risk behaviors that led to infection may still be ongoing. Viral load also increases in late symptomatic infection when immunosuppression is present. While use of antiretroviral drugs reduces HIV viral load in blood and genital secretions, there is a risk that individuals on treatment may still transmit HIV, and therefore they should use appropriate prevention interventions, including male and female condoms. Susceptibility is presumed to be general: race, gender, and pregnancy status do not appear to affect susceptibility to HIV infection or progression to AIDS. Male circumcision significantly reduces the risk of female-to-male transmission. The presence of other sexually transmitted infections (STIs), especially if ulcerative, increases risk of transmission and infection.

8. Risk groups—At the population level, the frequency of unprotected sex and injecting drug use, the mixing of sexual and drug-using networks, and concurrent sex partners (multiple partners in the same time period) are important determinants of HIV infection rates.

In the absence of prevention interventions, the transmission rate from infected mothers to their children is about 25% in the absence of breastfeeding and about 35% in breastfeeding populations.

In health care workers, after direct exposure to HIV-infected blood through injury with needles and other sharp objects, the rate of seroconversion is less than 0.5%, much lower than the risk of hepatitis B virus infection after similar exposures (~25%). The risk to health care workers after mucous membrane exposure has been estimated to be 0.09%; the risk after exposure of nonintact skin has not been quantified, but is estimated to be lower than for mucous membrane exposure.

HIV coinfection with *Mycobacterium tuberculosis* is of major public health importance. Persons with latent tuberculosis coinfected with HIV develop clinical tuberculosis at an increased rate, a lifetime risk of developing tuberculosis multiplied by a factor of 6–8. This increased risk and the resulting increased tuberculosis transmission have contributed to parallel epidemics of HIV and tuberculosis: in some urban sub-Saharan African populations where 10%–15% of the adult population have dual tuberculosis (TB)/HIV infections, annual incidence rates for tuberculosis increased 5- to 10-fold during the latter half of the 1990s. HIV infection may increase rates and severity of malarial infection, and antimalarial treatment may be less effective in HIV-infected individuals. Other common and significant opportunistic infections and coinfections with HIV include genital herpes, pneumococcal infection, nontyphi salmonellosis, visceral leishmaniasis, pneumocystis pneumonia, cyptococcosis, and viral hepatitis. Infections such as tuberculosis, malaria, and genital herpes may increase HIV viral load and the rate of decline of cluster of differentiation 4 glycoprotein + (CD4+) cells. However, the long-term clinical implications of these laboratory findings are less well understood.

9. Prevention—HIV prevention programs can be effective only with full community and political commitment to facilitate change and/or reduce HIV risk behaviors. Health education efforts should include both broad-based campaigns to raise awareness of risk, modes of transmission, and prevention measures; and targeted campaigns to reduce risk among high-risk groups such as sex workers, people who inject drugs, transgender people, and men who have sex with men. They should also strive to reduce stigmatization and discrimination.

1) Abstaining from sexual intercourse prevents sexual transmission. Engaging in sex with an uninfected, mutually monogamous partner is also effective, although ensuring mutual monogamy and absence of infection may be challenging. Correct and consistent use of male and female condoms is highly effective in preventing transmission.

2) Prevention of injection drug use and effective drug dependence treatment, especially the use of opioid substitution therapy for opioid users, reduces HIV transmission. Programs that provide clean injection equipment and risk-reduction counseling for people who inject drugs are very effective in preventing both HIV transmission and the transmission of other bloodborne infections, including viral hepatitis B and C.

3) Postexposure prophylaxis with combination antiretroviral drugs is available and recommended in some settings after exposure to HIV, such as occupational exposure, and after sexual assault. If indicated, treatment should begin within hours of exposure and is usually recommended to continue for 28 days.

4) HIV testing and counseling is important to identify individuals with HIV for referral for care and treatment and, for pregnant women, to prevent vertical transmission of HIV. HIV testing also provides a setting for condom distribution and delivery of prevention messages for HIV-negative persons. In many settings, the emphasis is on universal, opt-out testing for all individuals, especially in high-prevalence communities. All HIV testing must follow the 5 Cs principles: consent, confidentiality, counseling, correct test results, and linkage to care.

5) Mother-to-child transmission of HIV can be minimized through primary prevention of HIV infection in women of childbearing age, prevention of unintended pregnancy in women with HIV, and universal HIV screening of pregnant women. An additional HIV test in the third trimester of pregnancy may identify women who seroconverted during pregnancy. Vertical transmission rates can be reduced by 50%–90% or more with the use of maternal and infant antiretrovirals in accordance with national guidelines. WHO recommends that all HIV-infected pregnant and breastfeeding women be initiated on life-long triple antiretroviral therapy to prevent HIV transmission to their infants, and for their own health. If lifelong treatment is not provided, if breastfeeding, the mother should use antiretrovirals until 1 week after the complete cessation of breastfeeding, in association with the infant being provided with antiretroviral prophylaxis for the first 6 weeks of life. Replacement feeding should only be used where infant formula is acceptable, feasible, affordable, sustainable, and safe. Elective cesarean section may also play a role in resource-rich settings but is only recommended for obstetrical and other medical indications in resource-limited settings.

6) Blood donations should only be sought from unpaid, volunteer donors. The use of autologous transfusions should be encouraged when feasible. All donated units of blood must be tested for HIV antibody; only donations testing negative should be used. Organizations that collect plasma, blood, or other body fluids or organs should inform potential donors of this recommendation and test all donors. Testing for HIV antigen or nucleic acid can further reduce the risk of contamination. Patients, their sexual partners, and others who have engaged in behaviors that place them at increased risk of HIV infection should not donate plasma, blood, organs, tissue, or cells (including semen for artificial insemination). Although not widely recommended, some centers have reported safe impregnation of women by HIV-infected male partners through semen processing or viral suppression in the men with antiretroviral treatment. When possible, donations of sperm, milk, or bone should be frozen and stored for 3–6 months before use. Donors who test negative after that interval can be considered free of infection at the time of donation. Only clotting factor products that have been screened and treated to inactivate HIV should be used.

7) Only medically necessary injections should be given. Care must be taken in handling, using, and disposing of needles or other sharp instruments. Medical waste should be safely stored and destroyed. Health care workers should be provided with and

instructed on the proper use of latex gloves, eye protection, and other personal protective equipment as needed in order to avoid contact with blood or with fluids. Universal precautions must be taken in the care of all patients and in all laboratory procedures.

8) Universal precautions should be taken by services that provide tattooing and skin-piercing procedures, including the appropriate sterilizations of any equipment that is reused.

10. Management of patient—The proportion of HIV-infected people who, in the absence of anti-HIV treatment, will ultimately develop AIDS has been estimated at over 90%. In the absence of effective antiretroviral therapy, the AIDS case-fatality rate is high. Universal precautions apply to all hospitalized patients. Observe additional precautions appropriate for HIV and specific infections that occur in HIV patients and use bleach solution or germicides effective against HIV and *M. tuberculosis* to disinfect equipment contaminated with blood or body fluids and with excretions and secretions visibly contaminated with blood and body fluids.

Treatment: early diagnosis of infection and referral for medical evaluation are indicated. The absolute T-helper cell (CD4+) count or percentage is used most often to evaluate the progression of HIV infection and to help clinicians make treatment decisions. Viral load monitoring is becoming the preferred approach to monitor treatment success and diagnose antiretroviral treatment failure. Ongoing education and counseling to maintain the patient's health, adherence to treatment, and prevention of transmission are indicated. Nationally recommended doses should be used.

1) Prophylaxis of opportunistic infections: prophylactic use of oral cotrimoxazole is recommended to prevent pneumocystis pneumonia and other susceptible infections. Isoniazid preventive treatment for tuberculosis is given in some settings, with or without use of tuberculin skin tests. Other primary or secondary prophylactic medications may be recommended in specific situations.

2) HIV infection must be managed as a chronic condition. General HIV care and antiretroviral therapy, while complex, are becoming easier to manage for both patients and carers. Once the decision to initiate antiretroviral therapy has been made, treatment should be lifelong and aggressive with the goal of maximal viral suppression. Antiretroviral therapy involves treatment with a combination of at least 3 antiretrovirals. In general, the first-line treatment regimen should consist of 2 nucleoside reverse transcriptase inhibitors and a nonnucleoside reverse transcriptase inhibitor, preferably in a fixed-dose combination formulation. HIV drug resistance will rapidly appear if only 1 or 2 antiretroviral drugs are used, if treatment adherence is poor, or if there are interruptions in treatment. Despite the development of simpler, safer, and more

effective antiretroviral regimens, antiretroviral side effects and toxicities are common and may require substituting one antiretroviral for another. Successful treatment results in suppression of viral replication and allows for immune reconstitution, but does not result in a cure. Ideally, decisions to initiate or change antiretroviral treatment should be guided by the laboratory parameters of both plasma HIV ribonucleic acid (RNA) (viral load) and CD4+ T cell count where available and by assessing the clinical condition of the patient. Laboratory results provide important information on the virological and immunological status of the patient and the risk of progression to AIDS. Antiretroviral regimens should be harmonized across adults, adolescents, and pregnant women. Special considerations apply to treatment regimens for pediatric patients. Treatment schedules are widely available.

3) The concurrent/associated opportunistic infections/diseases should be managed according to national guidelines.

11. Management of contacts and the immediate environment—

1) Notification of contacts and source of infection: sexual and needle-sharing partners should be notified of their exposure. Notification may be done by the index patient or by health staff with strict confidentiality.

2) Sexual and needle-sharing partners should not donate blood, plasma, organs, tissues, cells, or breast milk.

12. Special considerations—

1) Reporting: reporting of AIDS cases is obligatory in most countries. Whether or not name-based reporting is the rule, care must be taken to protect patient confidentiality.

2) Requiring foreign travelers to undergo HIV testing or examinations prior to entry into a country is not recommended.

3) HIV-infected children can safely be given routine childhood immunizations, except for Bacillus Calmette-Guérin (BCG) vaccine.

4) For case definitions, refer to: http://www.who.int/hiv/pub/guidelines/HIVstaging150307.pdf?ua=1.

[A. Ball]

HOOKWORM
(ancylostomiasis, uncinariasis, necatoriasis)

DISEASE	ICD-10 CODE
HOOKWORM	ICD-10 B76

1. **Clinical features**—A common chronic helminth infection of the intestine that causes anemia with a variety of symptoms, usually in proportion to the degree of iron deficiency. In heavy infections, the bloodletting activity of the nematode leads to iron deficiency and hypochromic, microcytic anemia, the major cause of disability. Children with heavy long-term infection may have hypoproteinemia and may have retarded mental and physical development. Occasionally, severe acute pulmonary and gastrointestinal reactions follow exposure to infective larvae. Light hookworm infections generally produce few or no clinical effects. Some species of the causative helminth are unable to survive in the skin and do not cause intestinal infection.

2. **Causative agents**—*Ancylostoma duodenale*, *Ancylostoma ceylanicum*, *Ancylostoma braziliense*, *Ancylostoma caninum*, and *Necator americanus*.

3. **Diagnosis**—The standard method for diagnosis is by identifying hookworm eggs and larvae in a stool sample using microscopic techniques. The eggs of both species are ovoid or ellipsoidal, thin-shelled, and colorless. The eggs of *Ancylostoma* and *Necator* cannot be differentiated microscopically. Adult worms are rarely seen (except via endoscopy, surgery, or autopsy), but if found, allow for definitive species identification. Hookworm infection is usually diagnosed based on characteristic laboratory findings, such as eosinophilia, in combination with detection of eggs with a specific shape and appearance on stool microscopic examination.

4. **Occurrence**—Endemic in tropical and subtropical countries where facilities for sanitary disposal of human feces are not available and soil, moisture, and temperature conditions favor development of infective larvae. Also occurs in temperate climates under similar environmental conditions (e.g., mines). Both *Necator* and *Ancylostoma* occur in many parts of Asia (particularly southeastern Asia), the South Pacific, and eastern Africa. *N. americanus* is the prevailing species throughout southeastern Asia, most of tropical Africa, and America; *A. duodenale* prevails in North Africa, including the Nile Valley, northern India, northern parts of eastern Asia, and the Andean areas of South America. *Ancylostoma ceylanicum*

occurs in southeastern Asia, but is less common than either *N. americanus* or *A. duodenale*. *Ancylostoma caninum* has been described in Australia as a cause of eosinophilic enteritis syndrome.

5. Reservoir—Humans for *A. duodenale* and *N. americanus*; cats and dogs for *A. ceylanicum*, *A. braziliense*, and *A. caninum*.

6. Incubation period—A few weeks to many months, depending on intensity of infection and iron intake of the host. Pulmonary infiltration, cough, and tracheitis may occur early in infection during the lung migration phase, particularly in *Necator* infections. After entering the body, *A. duodenale* may become dormant for up to 8 months, after which development resumes, with evidence of infection (stools containing eggs) a month later.

7. Transmission—Eggs in feces are deposited on the ground, embryonate, and hatch; under favorable conditions of moisture, temperature, and soil type, larvae develop and become infective in 7-10 days. Human infection usually occurs when infective larvae penetrate the skin, usually of the foot; in so doing, they produce a characteristic dermatitis (ground itch). The larvae of *A. caninum* and *A. braziliense* die within the skin, having produced cutaneous larva migrans. Normally, the larvae of *Necator*, *A. duodenale*, *A. ceylanicum*, and other *Ancylostoma* enter the skin and pass via lymphatics and bloodstream to the lungs, enter the alveoli, migrate up the trachea to the pharynx, are swallowed and reach the small intestine, where they attach to the intestinal wall, developing to maturity in 6-7 weeks (3-4 weeks in the case of *A. ceylanicum*), and typically producing thousands of eggs per day. Infection with *Ancylostoma* may also be acquired by ingesting infective larvae; possible vertical transmission through breast milk has been reported. Infected people can contaminate soil for several years in the absence of treatment. Under favorable conditions, larvae remain infective in soil for several weeks.

8. Risk groups—People living in areas with warm and moist climates and where sanitation and hygiene are poor, and who walk barefoot or in other ways allow their skin to have direct contact with contaminated soil.

9. Prevention—

    1) Educate the public to the dangers of soil contamination by human, cat, or dog feces, and in preventive measures, including wearing shoes in endemic areas.

    2) Prevent soil contamination by installation of sanitary disposal systems for human feces, especially sanitary latrines in rural

areas. Night soil and sewage effluents are hazardous, especially where used as fertilizer.

3) Examine and treat people migrating from endemic to nonendemic areas, especially those who work barefoot in mines, construct dams, or work in the agricultural sector.

4) WHO recommends a "preventive chemotherapy" strategy, focused on mebendazole or albendazole treatment of high-risk groups at regular intervals for the control of morbidity due to the soil-transmitted helminths causing ascariasis, trichuriasis, and hookworm disease (http://www.who.int/neglected_diseases/preventive_chemotherapy/pct_manual/en). See "Ascariasis."

10. Management of patient—

1) Safe disposal of feces to prevent contamination of soil.

2) Treatment: single-dose albendazole, or mebendazole given either as a single dose or over 3 days (albendazole is not Food and Drug Administration [FDA]-approved for this application). On theoretical grounds, both drugs are contraindicated during the first trimester of pregnancy. Pregnant women in the second or third trimester may want to discuss the decision of whether to delay treatment with their health care provider. Three-day treatment with pyrantel pamoate is also effective. Adverse reactions are infrequent. Follow-up stool examination is indicated after 2 weeks, and treatment must be repeated if a heavy worm burden persists. Iron supplementation will correct the anemia and should be used in conjunction with deworming. Transfusion may be necessary for severe anemia.

11. Management of patients and the immediate environment— Investigate contacts and source of infection. Each infected contact is a potential, or actual, indirect spreader of infection.

12. Special considerations—Epidemic measures: prevalence survey in highly endemic areas: provide periodic mass treatment. Health education in environmental sanitation and personal hygiene, and provide facilities for excreta disposal. Prevent the use of human excreta as fertilizer.

[M. Deming, M. Eberhard]

HUMAN PAPILLOMAVIRUS INFECTION

DISEASE	ICD-10 CODE
WARTS	ICD-10 B07
GENITAL WARTS	ICD-10 A63
CERVICAL CANCER	ICD-10 C53
VULVAR CANCER	ICD-10 C51
VAGINAL CANCER	ICD-10 C52
PENILE CANCER	ICD-10 C60
ANAL CANCER	ICD-10 C21
OROPHARYNGEAL CANCER	ICD-10 C10

Clinical manifestations of infection with human papillomavirus (HPV) of the *Papillomaviridae* group of deoxyribonucleic acid (DNA) viruses (the human wart viruses) vary from warts (verruca) to cervical, anogenital, cutaneous, and oropharyngeal cancers. There are more than 100 HPV types, and more than 40 types can infect the anogenital tract in both males and females.

Most HPV infections are asymptomatic, subclinical, or unrecognized. There are 2 types of genital HPV, nononcogenic, or low-risk types, which are associated with genital warts, and oncogenic, or high-risk types, which are associated with cancers (see Cancer section in this chapter).

I. WARTS (verruca vulgaris, common wart, condyloma acuminatum, papilloma venereum, palmar wart, plantar wart, periungal wart)

1. Clinical features—A viral disease manifested by diverse skin and mucous membrane lesions characterized by growths or changes in the epithelium. These are commonly located on the genitals and skin, but can also be located in the throat, respiratory tract, mouth, and conjunctiva. When HPV causes warts in the throat or respiratory tract they are typically called recurrent respiratory papillomatosis. When located on the genitals (penis, anus, vagina, vulva, cervix, and scrotum) they are called condyloma accuminata or genital warts. Some examples of clinical types of warts include:

1) Hyperkeratotic: 2 mm to 1 cm, well circumscribed, rough-textured papules, often in groups, can be found anywhere on the mucocutaneous surface.
2) Filiform: elongated, pointed, delicate lesions that may reach 1 cm in length.

3) Flat: smooth and flat, may be hypopigmented or hyperpigmented, slightly elevated, usually multiple lesions varying in size from 1 mm to 1 cm.

4) Condyloma accuminata: verruca seen in the genital and perianal area can present clinically as hyperkeratotic, filiform or flat, or have a cauliflower-like appearance.

Although warts are generally benign, malignancy can occur in rare clinical settings. Immunosuppressed patients, particularly those with HIV, and those who are immunosuppressed following organ transplant, are at risk for squamous cell carcinoma developing in condyloma or other verruca. Malignant lesions may arise de novo or may develop from previously benign-appearing lesions. Several acquired and genetic forms of specific immunodeficiency, including epidermodysplasia verruciformis, can result in widespread mucocutaneous HPV infection. In patients with epidermodysplasia verruciformis, warts occur in childhood and squamous cell skin cancers develop early in life. Warts in the throat or respiratory tract (recurrent respiratory papillomatosis) is generally a benign condition, but it can recur and result in respiratory tract obstruction requiring interventions.

2. Causative agent—Common skin warts, or verruca vulgaris, are caused by a variety of HPV types. Genital warts are usually caused by non-oncogenic HPV types 6 or 11 (90% of genital warts); these types can also cause warts on the uterine cervix and on the vulva, vagina, penis, scrotum, anus, and rectum.

3. Diagnosis—Usually based on visual examination. If the lesion is atypical, pigmented, indurated, fixed, bleeding, or ulcerated, or the lesion does not respond to therapy, or worsens during therapy, particularly in immunocompromised patients, the lesion should be biopsied and examined histologically.

4. Occurrence—Worldwide.

5. Reservoir—Humans.

6. Incubation period—About 2–3 months; range is 1–20 months.

7. Transmission—Transmission of verruca vulgaris is usually by direct contact but may also be transmitted through fomites and other sources (razors). Genital warts are also transmitted by direct skin-to-skin contact, usually through sexual intercourse. Recurrent respiratory papillomatosis in children is likely transmitted from mother to child during delivery through the birth canal.

The period of communicability is unknown, but probably at least as long as visible lesions persist. HPV may still be transmitted after lesions are treated or no longer present or visible.

8. Risk groups—Verruca vulgaris are most frequently seen in children, and genital warts are commonly seen in sexually active young adults. The incidence of all types of mucocutaneous verruca is increased in immunosuppressed patients.

9. Prevention—Avoid direct contact with lesions on another person; however, because most HPV infections are asymptomatic or subclinical, most people with the infection will not have visible lesions. Condoms may decrease the sexual transmission of genital HPV. Vaccination with the quadrivalent (types 6, 11, 16, 18) HPV vaccine (Gardasil) prophylactically has been demonstrated to be highly efficacious in the prevention of genital warts in both males and females aged 9–26 years.

10. Management of patient—Treatment: treatment can be divided into provider-administered and patient-applied therapies, and it can also be divided into therapies that are locally destructive and those that are immunomodulating. Treatment may be initiated based on desire of the patient, burden of disease, or other factors. In immunocompetent patients, mucocutaneous verruca usually regress spontaneously within months to years. Treatment may take months and require several different combinations of therapy. Provider-administered therapy for cutaneous and genital verruca includes curettage, trichloroacetic acid, cryotherapy with liquid nitrogen, and surgical debulking for larger lesions. Patient-applied therapies for genital warts include imiquimod 5% or 3.75% cream and sinecatechins 15% ointment, both of which are immunomodulators, and various forms of podophyllotoxin (podofilox) 0.5%, which is cytotoxic and locally destructive. Patient-applied therapy for cutaneous verruca includes various forms of salicylic acid, which is also a destructive therapy. Other emerging therapies include intralesional and topical cidofovir and laser removal. Combinations of these therapies, with patients applying medication at home and also receiving regular in-office treatments, might result in a decrease in the number and size of lesions, or clearing of the lesions earlier than monotherapy. Some of these topical therapies may not be appropriate for pregnant women and the immunosuppressed. Surgical removal or laser treatment may be required to relieve airway obstruction resulting from recurrent respiratory papillomatosis. Caesarean section may be needed if there is vaginal outlet obstruction due to extensive genital warts.

11. Management of contacts and the immediate environment—
Sexual contacts of patients with genital warts may be examined for genital warts and other sexually transmitted diseases.

12. Special considerations—None.

Further information can be found at:

- http://www.cdc.gov/std/treatment
- http://www.who.int/topics/sexually_transmitted_infections/en

II. CERVICAL AND OTHER HPV-RELATED CANCERS (vulvar, vaginal, penile, anal, oropharyngeal)

HPV infection causes cervical cancer, with HPV 16 and 18 accounting for more than 70% of cancers. Oncogenic or high-risk HPV also causes a proportion of vulvar, vaginal, penile, anal, and oropharyngeal cancers. In most of these cancers, invasive cancer is preceded by a pre-invasive phase recognized histologically as intraepithelial neoplasia. Clinically, intraepithelial neoplasia can present as atypical warts or skin changes, with pigmentation, erythema, very large size, or warts that are fixed to, or show induration of, the underlying skin or mucosa. On the cervix, there are characteristic changes that are detected by pap test, which may lead to colposcopic evaluation and biopsy. In the past, clinical forms of mucocutaneous intraepithelial neoplasia have been called Bowen's disease, bowenoid papulomatosis, or erythroplasia of Queyrat; these terms have been recently replaced with the term vaginal intraepithelial neoplasia. Histologically, vaginal, vulvar, penile, anal, and cervical intraepithelial neoplasias are categorized by increasing severity or grades of dysplastic changes. Detection and treatment of pre-cancers detected through well organized cervical cancer screening programs dramatically reduced cervical cancer incidence and mortality in the United States. Many countries with the greatest burden of disease do not have cervical cancer programs in place, because the resources and infrastructure needed for these programs are substantial. In these settings, low-cost, rapid approaches to screening, such as visual inspection of the cervix with a colposcope and possible use of acetic acid, ("see and treat"), or a simplified HPV test, are being evaluated.

There are 2 HPV vaccines currently available, the quadrivalent and bivalent vaccine (Gardasil and Cervarix); both vaccines target HPV 16 and 18, and one also targets HPV 6 and 11 (Gardasil). Either vaccine is recommended routinely for girls aged 11 or 12 years, and 1 vaccine (Gardasil) is recommended routinely for boys aged 11 or 12 years. Vaccines should be given through age 26 years in females and age 21 years in males. Those with HIV, immunocompromised populations, and men who have sex with men should receive the vaccine through age 26 years. These vaccines have been demonstrated to have high efficacy for prevention of cervical precancers, and one of these vaccines (Gardasil) has demonstrated efficacy against vaginal, vulvar, and anal precancers, as well as genital warts.

[E. F. Dunne, C. E. Introcaso]

HUMAN T-LYMPHOTROPIC VIRUS TYPE-1 INFECTION

DISEASE	ICD-10 CODE
HUMAN T-LYMPHOTROPIC VIRUS TYPE-1 INFECTION (asymptomatic carrier)	ICD-10 Z22.6
ADULT T-CELL LYMPHOMA/LEUKEMIA (acute, chronic, lymphomatoid, smoldering)	ICD-10 C91.5
HUMAN T-LYMPHOTROPIC VIRUS TYPE-1 INFECTION ASSOCIATED MYELOPATHY/ TROPICAL SPASTIC PARAPARESIS	ICD-10 G04.1
POLYMYOSITIS	ICD-10 B97.3
UVEITIS	ICD-10 B97.3
INFECTIVE DERMATITIS	ICD-10 B97.3
BRONCHIECTASIS	ICD-10 B97.3

I. HUMAN T-LYMPHOTROPIC VIRUS TYPE-1

1. Clinical features—Human T-lymphotropic virus type-1 (HTLV-1) causes a lifelong infection that chiefly persists by driving mitotic proliferation of infected cluster of differentiation 4 glycoprotein + (CD4+) T-lymphocytes. HTLV-1 causes a number of manifestations in 5%–10% of HTLV-1 infected individuals while 90% remain lifelong healthy asymptomatic carriers. The 2 most common diseases are an aggressive T-cell malignancy known as adult T-cell lymphoma/leukemia (ATL), and HTLV-1 associated myelopathy (formerly known as tropical spastic paraplegia, HAM/TSP), which clinically resembles primary progressive multiple sclerosis. In addition, HTLV-1 may cause inflammatory diseases such as polymyositis, uveitis, and infective dermatitis. It is recognized that there is a high incidence of bronchiectasis among HTLV-1 carriers. The mechanisms by which HTLV-1 causes diverse manifestations are unknown, but since no viral genotype is associated with clinical disease and there is a strong antiviral immune response, the currently accepted hypothesis is that the efficiency of the host immune response is the main determinant of disease.

2. Causative agent—There are 3 genotypes of HTLV-1 (Melanesian, Central African, and Cosmopolitan types), but there is no clear association between the viral genotype and disease. HTLV-2, which targets CD8+ T-lymphocytes, is not associated with clinical disease.

3. Diagnosis—HTLV-1 antibody detection by enzyme immunoassay (EIA) or Western Blot. Since HTLV-1 and HTLV-2 antibodies cross-react, any positive results should be confirmed by a second assay that can distinguish HTLV-1 and HTLV-2. Polymerase chain reaction (PCR) can resolve untypable or indeterminate results. Quantitative real-time PCR (qPCR) to quantify the HTLV-1 proviral load—the proportion of HTLV-1 infected mononuclear cells, is important for determining risk of clinical disease (disease risk highest with proviral load >4% in Japan and >10% in the Caribbean). In ATL tumor cells, demonstration of monoclonal integration of HTLV-1 provirus by Southern blot or inverse/linker mediated PCR (to distinguish ATL from other incidental T-cell malignancies in asymptomatic HTLV-1 carriers).

4. Occurrence—Worldwide. Endemic within regions of southern Japan, sub-Saharan Africa, Caribbean, Brazil, Peru, and Iran.

5. Reservoir—Humans. A genotypically similar simian virus (STLV-1) is found in nonhuman primates (e.g., Japanese monkey), and historical transmission from nonhuman to human primates via animal bites is thought to be the origin of HTLV-1.

6. Incubation period—50–60 years for disease manifestations.

7. Transmission—In endemic countries mother-to-child transmission via prolonged breastfeeding is the major route (30%–40% risk of transmission). HTLV-1 can also be contracted through infected cellular blood product transfusions, sexual contact, and solid organ transplantation.

8. Risk groups—Since clinical disease occurs several decades following asymptomatic infection, the major risk group for ATL or HAM/TSP comprises those infected during infancy from breastfeeding and via sexual transmission in endemic regions. Several countries, including many wealthy nations, still do not routinely screen blood products or organs, increasing the risk of HTLV-1 infection within low-prevalence regions.

9. Prevention—Antibody screening of pregnant women and known HTLV-1 carriers to avoid breastfeeding; condoms to prevent sexual transmission; antibody screening of blood products and organs for transplantation. In established HTLV-1 infection, there are no means to prevent the onset of clinical disease.

10. Management of patient—There is no specific treatment for chronic asymptomatic HTLV-1 carriers and the virus cannot be eradicated in persons with infection. The only known predictor of development of clinical disease is the proviral load (risk increases with proviral load >4%–10%).

11. Management of contacts and the immediate environment— Since the major route of transmission is via breastfeeding, the mother, siblings, children, and sexual contacts of an infected individual should be screened for HTLV-1 antibody.

12. Special considerations—The risk of HTLV-1 transmission following a needle-stick injury to a health care worker is unknown. Immediate postexposure prophylaxis with antiretrovirals (e.g., raltegravir and zidovudine) to prevent integration of the provirus and chronic infection, should be considered.

II. ADULT T-CELL LYMPHOMA/LEUKEMIA

ATL is an aggressive CD4+ CD25+ T-cell malignancy with 4 distinct clinical subtypes (Shimoyama classification) defined according to absolute lymphocyte count, percentage of abnormal lymphocytes ("flower cells") on a blood smear, corrected calcium, lactate dehydrogenase (LDH), and presence of enlarged lymph nodes and organ infiltration. The acute and lymphoma subtypes are regarded as aggressive while chronic or smoldering subtypes are regarded as indolent, although transformation from indolent to aggressive subtypes is frequent.

For acute subtypes, lymphocyte count is at least 4×10^9/L, with at least 5% abnormal lymphocytes; LDH is typically high; corrected calcium is usually high, often with widespread lymphadenopathy (not essential) and organ infiltration (skin, lung, liver, spleen, central nervous system, bone, ascites, pleural effusions, gastrointestinal tract).

For lymphoma subtypes, histology has proven lymphadenopathy with no peripheral blood involvement (lymphocyte <4×10^9/L, ≤1% abnormal lymphocytes); LDH is typically high; corrected calcium is usually high, often with organ infiltration (skin, lung, liver, spleen, central nervous system [CNS], bone, ascites, pleural effusions, gastrointestinal tract).

For chronic subtypes, there is peripheral blood and/or lymph node involvement (lymphocyte ≥4×10^9/L, ≥5% abnormal lymphocytes) but with LDH less than 2 times upper limit normal and normal corrected calcium. Skin and lung may be involved but no CNS, gastrointestinal (GI) tract, or bone infiltration.

For smoldering subtypes, there is increased abnormal lymphocytes on peripheral blood smear (≥5%) but with a normal absolute lymphocyte count (<4×10^9/L); LDH is less than 1.5 times upper limit normal and normal corrected calcium. There is no associated lymphadenopathy, although skin and lung infiltration may be observed.

For aggressive ATL subtypes, the prognosis of aggressive ATL is extremely poor mainly due to tumor resistance to steroids and cytotoxic agents combined with significant immune suppression and susceptibility to opportunistic infection. In aggressive subtypes, the best clinical trial results to date using combination chemotherapy report complete response rates in only 25%–40% patients, with median progression-free survival of 5-7 months and overall survival of 13 months. In the few cases of acute ATL that do not involve lymph nodes, the disease can respond to treatment with zidovudine and interferon. More recently, the monoclonal antibody mogamulizumab, which targets C-C chemokine receptor type 4 widely expressed on ATL tumor cells, has been licensed in Japan for clinical use in salvage therapy. The only "curative" treatment is allogeneic bone marrow transplantation, but this is only an option for those who are young enough, fit enough, and have achieved a response to induction treatment.

For indolent ATL subtypes, untreated, the median survival of chronic ATL is approximately 5 years, with death due to transformation to aggressive disease or opportunistic infection. In the USA and Europe combination with zidovudine and interferon alpha is the standard of care for those patients who can tolerate the treatment.

III. HTLV-1 ASSOCIATED MYELOPATHY/TROPICAL SPASTIC PARAPARESIS

HAM/TSP is characterized by a gradual symmetric parparesis of the lower limbs with signs of pyramidal tract involvement, which slowly progresses without remissions. Early in the disease the symptoms are weakness of the lower limbs and lumbar pain. Patients frequently describe urinary and sexual problems. Dizziness is common (with normal clinical examination). The weakness in the lower limbs is associated with moderate-to-severe spasticity. As the disease progresses, the weakness and spasticity increase and gait deteriorates. Neuropathic pain becomes common and autonomic dysfunction of the bladder and bowel are a common cause of significant morbidity. There has been a lack of large clinical trials and treatment remains largely palliative although some patients respond to immune suppression with methotrexate or cyclosporine.

[L. B. M. Cook]

INFLUENZA

DISEASE	ICD-10 CODE
SEASONAL INFLUENZA	ICD-10 J10, J11
OTHER INFLUENZA	ICD-10 J09

I. SEASONAL INFLUENZA

1. Clinical features—An acute viral disease of the respiratory tract characterized by fever, cough (usually dry), headache, myalgia, prostration, coryza, and sore throat. Cough is often severe and can last 2 or more weeks; fever and other symptoms generally resolve in 5–7 days. Syndromes consistent with influenza include acute upper respiratory illness, croup, bronchiolitis, febrile seizures, and pneumonia. In children, gastrointestinal (GI) tract manifestations (nausea, vomiting, diarrhea) may accompany the respiratory phase and have been reported in up to 25% of children in school outbreaks of influenza A and B. GI manifestations are uncommon in adults. Infants may present with atypical symptoms or a sepsis-like syndrome. Geriatric patients may not present with typical influenza-like symptoms, but can present with exacerbation of underlying conditions such as congestive heart failure, and may not have an elevated temperature.

Complications of influenza include lower respiratory tract involvement such as bronchitis and pneumonitis; bacterial pneumonia caused by common community-acquired pneumonia pathogens such as *Streptococcus pneumoniae* and *Staphylococcus aureus* (associated with higher mortality and significant proportion being methicillin-resistant *S. aureus* [MRSA]); viral pneumonia; exacerbation of underlying chronic conditions; sinusitis; otitis media; febrile seizures; encephalitis/encephalopathy; rhabdomyolysis; myocarditis; myositis; and Reye syndrome in association with use of salicylates (aspirin). Although seasonal influenza deaths can occur in any age group, more than 90% of influenza deaths occur among those aged 65 years and older. Annual epidemics of influenza can be explosive and overwhelm health care services.

2. Causative agents—Three types of seasonal influenza virus are recognized: A, B, and C. Influenza A viruses are further divided into subtypes based on 2 viral surface glycoproteins: the hemagglutination and the neuraminidase. There are 18 different haemagglutinin subtypes and 11 different neuraminidase subtypes. The current subtypes of influenza A viruses circulating widely among humans are subtypes A (H1N1) and A (H3N2). Influenza B viruses are not divided into subtypes, but two antigenically and genetically distinct lineages of B viruses currently circulate among humans. Both influenza A and B viruses can cause seasonal epidemics and sporadic outbreaks. Influenza viruses are named based on their type, geographic site of detection, laboratory number, year of isolation, and subtype (e.g., A/New Caledonia/20/99 (H1N1), A/Brisbane/10/2007 (H3N2), B/Malaysia/2506/2004). Type C influenza is considered associated with sporadic cases of milder infection and minor localized outbreaks. Type C influenza imposes much less of a disease burden than influenza A and B. Levels of antibody against the haemagglutinin correlate reasonably well with protection against infection by human influenza viruses. The detailed role of antibody against the neuraminidase has been under study but is believed to contribute to the protection. Genes encoding these viral surface glycoproteins are continuously changing through mutations, a process termed "drift" that occurs during virus replication. The constant emergence of new influenza viruses through drift results in the need for the biannual review and when needed replacement of A (H1N1), A (H3N2), and B viruses that are contained in vaccines to be used in the northern and southern hemisphere influenza season. The constant emergence of drifted viruses is the main reason for yearly epidemics of seasonal influenza and why an individual can catch influenza illness multiple times over their lifetime.

In addition to antigenic drift, type A influenza viruses can also undergo dramatic change called antigenic shift, which often refers to a subtype influenza A virus bearing either a hemagglutination protein or a combination of hemagglutination and neuraminidase proteins that have not been in circulation among humans in recent years. The majority of the world's population will have no immunity against the new virus. If and when the new virus is capable of sustained human-to-human transmission, it means the start of a potential pandemic (see Other Influenza section in this chapter).

3. **Diagnosis**—Influenza may be clinically indistinguishable from disease caused by other respiratory viruses, such as rhinovirus, respiratory syncytial virus (RSV), parainfluenza, adenovirus, and other pathogens. In temperate climates, recognition of potential influenza is commonly based on clinical presentation during winter months with a syndrome consistent with influenza-like illness. Clinical diagnosis improves when influenza surveillance information is available to indicate influenza viruses are in circulation.

Laboratory confirmation of influenza infection can be done by a number of methods. Currently the primary test for the rapid detection of influenza viruses is reverse transcription polymerase chain reaction (RT-PCR) assay for the detection of virus-specific ribonucleic acid sequences from throat, nasal, and nasopharyngeal secretions or tracheal aspirate or washings. Other procedures include isolation of viruses from these specimens using cell culture or embryonated eggs; identification of viral antigens in nasopharyngeal cells and fluids (fluorescent antibody [FA] test or enzyme-linked immunosorbent assay [ELISA]). Demonstration of a 4-fold or greater rise in specific antibody titre between acute and convalescent sera using haemagglutination-inhibition or neutralization assays can also be used to confirm acute infection. A single serum specimen is not ideal for diagnosis of an acute infection. Ideally, respiratory specimens should be collected as early in the illness as possible. Virus shedding starts to wane by the third day of onset of symptoms, and in most cases virus is not detected after 5 days in adults, though virus shedding can occur longer in children and immunocompromised individuals.

Commercially available point-of-care tests have variable sensitivity (50%-70%) but good specificity (90%-95%). Thus, in the setting of a known influenza epidemic, negative results from patients with symptoms consistent with influenza must be interpreted cautiously. If excluding a false-negative result is important, then more sensitive testing should be considered (e.g., RT-PCR or viral culture).

4. Occurrence—Seasonal influenza results in yearly epidemics of varying severity, with sporadic cases or outbreaks occurring outside of typical seasonal patterns. Clinical attack rates during annual epidemics can range from 5%-20% in the general community to more than 50% in closed populations (e.g., nursing homes, schools). During yearly epidemics in industrialized countries, influenza illness often appears earliest among school-age children or young adults. The highest illness rates generally occur in children, with accompanying increases in school absences, physician visits, and pediatric hospital admissions. Influenza illness among adults is associated with increases in workplace absenteeism, adult hospital admissions, and mortality especially among the elderly. In temperate areas, local epidemics generally last from 8-10 weeks. One or more subtypes and/or types of influenza can circulate within a single influenza season in the same area. In temperate zones epidemics tend to occur in winter months. In tropical and subtropical countries, influenza transmission can occur year-round, often with 1 or 2 peaks per year, and peak influenza activities may occur at predictable time periods and are sometimes associated with the rainy season.

The severity and relative impact of epidemics and pandemics depend upon several factors, including natural or vaccine-induced levels of protective immunity in the population, the age and health condition of the population, and the property of the influenza viruses including antigenicity and pathogenicity, as well as transmissibility of novel influenza viruses.

5. Reservoir—The primary reservoir of the influenza viruses is aquatic birds. Recent findings indicate that bats constitute a potential and likely ancient reservoir for a diverse pool of influenza viruses. With the exception of H17N10 and H18N11, which were found in bats, all subtypes of influenza A have been found among birds. Influenza A viruses can also circulate among other animals including pigs, horses, seals, and others. In humans, currently only 3 type/subtype (A [H1N1], A [H3N2], and B) viruses are circulating, and for these 3 subtypes, humans are considered the reservoir.

6. Incubation period—Average 2 days (range 1–4).

7. Transmission—All routes of transmission (droplet, droplet nuclei, and contact) have a potential role. The relative significance depends on the set of circumstances acting at a given time. The virus, host, and environment dictate the process, and transmission can likely occur through multiple routes. In adults, virus shedding and communicability is greatest in the first 3–5 days of illness. In young children, virus shedding can occur for longer, 7–10 days, and may be even longer in immunocompromised persons.

Infection induces immunity to the virus and may provide protection against antigenically similar viruses. The duration and breadth of cross-immunity depend, in part, upon the degree of antigenic similarity between viruses inducing immunity and those causing disease. During seasonal epidemics, much of the population has partial protection, because of earlier infections from related viruses. Vaccine induced protection can cover infections associated with antigenically similar viruses to those contained in the vaccines.

8. Risk groups—Yearly seasonal influenza epidemics impose a substantial health burden on all age groups, but the highest risk of complications occur among children younger than 2 years, adults older than 64 years, and persons of any age with certain chronic medical conditions such as cardiovascular, pulmonary, renal, hepatic, hematologic, or metabolic disorders (e.g., diabetes); immunodeficiency; pregnancy; and neurologic/neuromuscular conditions that can compromise respiratory function or ability in handling of respiratory secretions. In the influenza A (H1N1) pandemic in 2009, obesity was identified as a possible risk factor for severe outcome of influenza infection. Reports of influenza outbreak investigations in Africa and Indonesia suggest malnutrition and poor access to health care are likely to contribute to higher rates of complications and death.

Age-specific attack rates during seasonal influenza epidemics reflect persisting immunity from past exposure to variant viruses related to the epidemic subtype, so that the incidence of infection is often highest in children who have fewer prior influenza infections and less preexisting antibody.

9. Prevention—Detailed recommendations for the prevention and control of seasonal influenza epidemics are provided by national health agencies and WHO.

1) Educate the public and health care personnel in basic personal hygiene, including hand hygiene, cough etiquette (especially transmission via unprotected coughs and sneezes), and from hand to mucous membranes.

2) Vaccination: immunization with recommended inactivated influenza vaccines (IIV) and live-attenuated influenza vaccines (LAIV) may provide reasonable protection in healthy adults when the vaccine viruses closely match the circulating viruses. LAIV has been used in Russia for many years for individuals aged 3 years and older, and a different LAIV has been licensed in the USA for individuals aged 2–49 years and used in many countries. LAIVs are applied intranasally while IIVs are injected intramuscularly. In the elderly, although influenza vaccines may be less effective in preventing illness, immunization with IIV may reduce severity of disease and incidence of complications and death. Influenza immunization should preferably be coupled with immunization against S. pneumoniae for individuals recommended to receive both vaccines (see "Pneumonia"). A single dose of IIV suffices for those who have received seasonal influenza vaccine before or who have had prior exposures to influenza A and B viruses. Two doses at least 4 weeks apart are essential for children younger than 9 years who have not previously been vaccinated against influenza. Routine immunization programs should focus efforts on vaccinating those at greatest risk of serious complications or death from influenza (see Risk Groups under Seasonal Influenza section in this chapter) and those who might spread influenza (health care personnel and household contacts of high-risk persons) to high-risk persons. Immunization of children on long-term salicylates treatment is also recommended to prevent development of Reye syndrome after influenza infection.

The vaccine should be given each year before influenza is expected in the community; the timing of immunization should be based on a country's seasonal patterns of influenza circulation (i.e., winter months in temperate zones, often rainy season in tropical regions). Biannual recommendations for vaccine virus are based on the viruses currently circulating, as determined by WHO through global surveillance.

Contraindications: allergic hypersensitivity to vaccine components (e.g., egg protein for egg-based flu vaccines) is a contraindication for that specific vaccine, but there are different options. During the swine influenza vaccine program in 1976, the USA reported an increased risk of developing Guillain-Barré syndrome within 6 weeks after vaccination. Subsequent vaccines produced from other viruses in other years have not been clearly associated with an increased risk of Guillain-Barré syndrome. However, prior Guillain-Barré syndrome is a contraindication for receiving an LAIV. The development of Guillain-Barré syndrome within the 6 weeks following a dose of IIV is considered a precaution for future IIV use.

3) Prophylaxis: antiviral agents are supplemental to vaccine when immediate maximal protection is desired in situations such as institutional outbreaks or household settings to protect persons at increased risk for complications due to influenza. Antiviral agents are effective at reducing transmission in facilities during outbreaks, such as among residents of nursing homes for the elderly. The drugs will not interfere with the response to inactivated influenza vaccine and should ideally be continued throughout the period of likely exposure to influenza. However, antivirals ideally should not be administered for 2 weeks after receipt of LAIV and should be stopped for 2 days prior to LAIV vaccination.

Inhibitors of influenza neuraminidase (oseltamivir and zanamivir) have been shown to be safe and effective for both prophylaxis and treatment of influenza A and B. Oseltamivir is an orally administered medicine; zanamivir is a powder administered via an inhaler. Oseltamivir may be used for persons of all ages and zanamivir is approved for treatment and prophylaxis for persons aged 5 years and older. Dosing is twice a day for 5 days for treatment and once a day for prophylaxis, with dosing for oseltamivir adjusted by body weight for children. Serious cases of bronchospasm have been reported with zanamivir use in patients with and without underlying airways disease. Zanamivir use should be administered carefully in patients with underlying lung disease or reactive airway disease.

Wherever available, clinicians should take local antiviral susceptibility information into account when prescribing antivirals.

10. **Management of patient—**

1) Isolation: ideally, all persons admitted to a hospital with a respiratory illness, including suspected influenza, should be placed in single patient rooms or, if this is not possible, placed in a room with patients with similar illness (cohorting). When cohorting is used, adequate spacing between beds should be provided for droplet precautions. For influenza, isolation should continue for the initial 5–7 days of illness and possibly longer for patients who are severely immunocompromised and may be infectious for longer periods. Both standard and droplet precautions are recommended.

2) Treatment: early administration of neuraminidase inhibitors, ideally within 48 hours of influenza symptom onset, reduces severe complications and death and recommended for persons at increased risk and progressive disease. When influenza virus infection is suspected in such populations, antiviral therapy should not wait for diagnostic confirmation but should start immediately. If signs and symptoms of ongoing viral replication persist, later stage antiviral administration is warranted (e.g., ≥ 5 days from the onset of disease). Patients should be observed for bacterial complications, including coinfection with MRSA and antibiotics prescribed accordingly. Because of the association with Reye syndrome, avoid salicylates in children with suspected influenza infection.

11. Management of contacts and the immediate environment—A specific role has been shown for antiviral chemoprophylaxis (see Prevention under Seasonal Influenza section in this chapter).

12. Special considerations—

1) Reporting: weekly reporting from influenza sentinel surveillance sites to monitor disease activity (influenza-like illness and severe respiratory disease). Severe respiratory infection, especially when involving health care workers, should be immediately notified and investigated. Unsubtypable or new subtypes of influenza infections should be further tested by qualified laboratories in the country or WHO Collaborating Centres of the WHO Global Influenza Surveillance and Response System. Meanwhile, immediately notify public health authorities.

2) Epidemic measures:

- The severe and often disruptive effects of epidemic seasonal influenza on community activities may be reduced in part by effective health planning and education, particularly locally organized immunization programs for high-risk patients, their close contacts, and health care providers. Community surveillance for influenza illness, use of outbreak control measures, adherence to infection control recommendations, and reporting of surveillance and outbreak findings to the community are all important.

- Closure of individual schools can be a useful intervention during influenza outbreaks, with the greatest benefits occurring among school-age children, when applied early in the course of the outbreak. The benefit has to be weighed against the cost of disruption.

- Hospital administrators should anticipate increased demand for medical care during epidemic periods and possible absenteeism of health care personnel as a result of influenza. Health care personnel should be immunized annually to minimize absenteeism and transmission of seasonal influenza from health care personnel to patients.
- Maintaining adequate supplies of appropriate antiviral drugs would be desirable to treat high-risk patients, persons hospitalized with influenza, and essential personnel in the event of the emergence of a new pandemic virus for which no suitable vaccine is available in time for the initial wave.

3) Disaster implications: aggregations of people in emergency shelters will favor outbreaks of influenza if the virus is introduced into the group by infected individuals.

4) International measures: influenza is a disease under global surveillance coordinated by WHO. The following are recommended:

- Report regularly epidemiological and virological information to WHO electronic platforms (http://www.who.int/influenza/surveillance_monitoring/fluid/en, http://www.who.int/influenza/gisrs_laboratory/flunet/en).
- Respiratory specimens, throat and nasal swabs, nasopharyngeal swabs or aspirates, and paired blood samples may be sent to any WHO-recognized National Influenza Center (http://www.who.int/influenza/gisrs_laboratory/national_influenza_centres/list/en/index.html). Identify the causative virus in reports, and submit prototype virus to one of the WHO Centers for Reference and Research on Influenza in Atlanta, Beijing, London, Melbourne, or Tokyo (http://www.who.int/influenza/gisrs_laboratory/collaborating_centres/en).
- Conduct epidemiological studies; promptly identify and report viruses to national and international health agencies.
- Ensure sufficient commercial and/or governmental facilities to provide rapid production of adequate quantities of vaccine and antiviral drugs, and maintain programs for vaccine and antiviral drug administration to high-risk persons and essential personnel.

II. OTHER INFLUENZA

Humans can also be infected with influenza viruses that are circulating in animals, such as avian influenza virus subtypes A (H5N1), A (H7N9), and A

(H9N2) and swine influenza virus subtypes A (H1N1) and (H3N2). Other species including horses and dogs also have their own varieties of influenza viruses. Even though these viruses may be named as the same subtype as viruses found in humans, all of these animal viruses are distinct from human influenza viruses and do not easily transmit between humans. Some may occasionally infect humans, however, and may cause disease ranging from mild upper respiratory infection or conjunctivitis to severe pneumonia and even death. Usually these human infections of zoonotic influenza are acquired through direct contact with infected animals or contaminated environments and do not spread very far among humans. If such a virus acquired the capacity to spread easily among people either through adaptation or acquisition of certain genes from human viruses, it could start an epidemic or a pandemic. Pandemic viruses in the past have spread globally within weeks of detection. Modern air travel has facilitated the spread of a new pandemic virus leaving little time for vaccine development, manufacturing, or administration to the world's population. Planning for responses to pandemics ahead of actual pandemics is therefore critical for preparedness. Of the animal influenza virus infections of humans, avian influenza A (H5N1) has been the most studied; thus this chapter will focus mostly on H5N1.

1. **Clinical features**—Suspicion of a human infection with a zoonotic influenza A infection is heightened if illness has occurred after exposure to birds, pigs, or other animals that may be infected with influenza or exposure to their environments.

Human H5N1 illness, usually occurring after exposure to infected chickens or their environments, typically manifests as severe pneumonia. Common initial symptoms are fever (usually >38°C) and cough, plus signs and symptoms of lower respiratory tract involvement including dyspnea. Upper respiratory tract symptoms such as sore throat and coryza are present only sometimes. Gastrointestinal symptoms were frequently reported in cases in Thailand and Vietnam in 2004, but less frequently since 2005. Severe lower respiratory tract manifestations often develop early in the course of illness, and clinically apparent pneumonia with radiological changes has usually been found at presentation. The disease progresses rapidly, and often to an acute respiratory distress syndrome. Median times of 4 days from the onset of illness to hospitalization and 9-10 days from onset until death in fatal cases have been reported. Atypical presentations have included fever and diarrhea without pneumonia as well as fever with diarrhea and seizures progressing to coma. Common laboratory findings include leukopenia, lymphopenia, mild-to-moderate thrombocytopenia, and elevated levels of aminotransferases. Lymphopenia and increased levels of lactate dehydrogenase at presentation have been associated with a poor prognosis. Other reported abnormalities include elevated levels of creatine phosphokinase, hypoalbuminemia, and increased D-dimer levels and changes indicative of disseminated intravascular coagulopathy. Mild illnesses such as upper respiratory illnesses without clinical or radiological signs of pneumonia have been reported more frequently in children. Seroepidemiologic studies conducted since 2004 suggest that subclinical infection is uncommon.

The mortality among reported cases of zoonotic infection has been high (60% for A [H5N1]), but with differences between countries and over time. Potential explanation for the differences in mortality rates could be the differences in patient behaviors, types of exposure, time before case recognition, access to health care and/or clinical management, or differences in surveillance. The median age of patients with influenza A (H5N1) infection is approximately 18 years with 90% of patients aged 40 years or younger.

In most zoonotic influenza infections—with exception of A (H5N1)—symptoms presented are similar to those for seasonal influenza infections. Until 2013, reported human infections with avian H7 influenza virus have mostly been subclinical; or with conjunctivitis, and mild respiratory tract symptoms with one fatal exception in the Netherlands. However, recent human infections with H7 influenza virus— influenza A (H7N9) virus in China—have caused severe disease and deaths.

2. Causative agents—New subtypes of influenza A can emerge among humans through direct transmission of an animal influenza virus to humans, or through reassortment of genes derived from an animal influenza virus and a human influenza virus. Such genetic reassortment can create a new virus that combines human and animal influenza properties.

Animal influenza A virus subtypes that have infected humans include H5N1, H7N2, H7N3, H7N7, H9N2, H10N7, H7N9, and swine and avian H1 viruses, which are antigenically distinct from human H1 viruses. The current situation of widespread outbreaks of highly pathogenic avian influenza A (H5N1) virus infection among poultry is of great concern because the A (H5N1) virus is now endemic in poultry in some countries, causes high rates of death among infected poultry, and causes high case fatality in humans (60% of reported human cases have been fatal). Although human-to-human transmission of this A (H5N1) virus is currently limited and unsustained, continued vigilance is needed to detect changes in A (H5N1) viruses that might signal a pandemic.

As a result of the drift of the hemagglutination gene, A (H5N1) viruses can be divided into distinct clades and subclades, based on phylogenetic analysis of viral genome, that are antigenically distinguishable. Updated information on the clades of A (H5N1) can be found at: http://www.who.int/influenza/gisrs_laboratory/h5n1_nomenclature/en/index.html. The influenza A (H5N1) viruses that have infected humans so far have contained only avian influenza virus genes and generally have been similar to viruses circulating among poultry and wild birds in the same general geographical location.

3. Diagnosis—The first laboratory suggestion of a novel influenza A infection from animal source is the inability of available tests to subtype the detected influenza A viruses. Diagnosis of animal influenza viruses often requires specialized laboratories, since these viruses cannot be typed by reagents used for seasonal influenza viruses. Detection of viral ribonucleic acid (RNA) in respiratory and other clinical specimens by means of conventional or real-time RT-PCR remains the best method for the initial presumptive diagnosis, to be confirmed by other methods such as virus isolation. Infection can also be confirmed by demonstration of seroconversion based upon a rise in antibody titre between an acute and a convalescent serum. Commercially available point-of-care rapid testing (also sometimes called "rapid tests") used for human influenza viruses have shown variable sensitivities for animal influenza viruses. It may be useful to support clinical judgment for antiviral treatment during outbreak situations where access to specialized laboratories is limited. However, rapid methods are generally not recommended for definitive diagnosis. If an animal influenza virus infection is suspected, a negative test result by a point-of-care test does not exclude the presence of the virus infection.

4. **Occurrence**—In 1997, the first avian influenza A (H5N1) outbreak among chickens with spillover to humans occurred in Hong Kong. Since 2003, there has been a resurgence of H5N1 outbreaks, first among poultry in Southeast Asia, with subsequent spread to other parts of the world. The viruses are now endemically circulating in poultry populations in parts of Eurasia, Africa, and the Middle East. Avian influenza A (H5N1) virus infections have been associated with high levels of animal mortality among poultry farms and result in substantial economic losses. In 2005, outbreaks in migratory birds in China preceded spread of A (H5N1) through Mongolia and Russia to many European, Middle Eastern, and African countries.

In association with panzootic spread in poultry, sporadic cases and clusters of human infection have been reported. By the end of December 2013, more than 640 cases of human infection with highly pathogenic avian influenza A (H5N1) virus had been reported from Azerbaijan, Bangladesh, Cambodia, China, Djibouti, Egypt, Indonesia, Iraq, Lao People's Democratic Republic, Myanmar, Nigeria, Pakistan, Thailand, Turkey, and Viet Nam. Regular updates on case counts are available at: http://www.who.int/influenza/human_animal_interface/en.

Sporadic human infection with avian influenza A (H7) viruses associated with outbreaks in poultry have been reported, such as influenza A (H7N3) in Canada, Italy, the UK, and Mexico; influenza A (H7N2) in the USA and the UK; influenza A (H7N7) in the UK and the Netherlands; and influenza A (H7N9) in China. In addition, human infection with avian influenza A (H9N2) has been reported in Hong Kong and Bangladesh. In 2013, more than 140 sporadic human infections with influenza A (H7N9) were reported from China. Swine influenza viruses have also caused illness in humans. Earlier, in 1976, the A/New Jersey/76 (Hsw1N1) influenza virus of swine origin caused severe respiratory illness in 13 soldiers, including 1 death, at Fort Dix, New Jersey, but did not spread beyond Fort Dix. In 2012, the USA reported 309 cases of human influenza infection with a nonseasonal variant of A (H3N2) virus (designated A [H3N2]v) that was circulating in swine in the USA, mostly associated with swine exposure in agricultural fairs. Other human infections with swine influenza viruses have been sporadically identified.

5. Reservoir—Aquatic birds are natural reservoirs of influenza A subtypes. For some avian influenza viruses, and particularly A (H5N1), the range of mammals that can be infected with avian influenza viruses from aquatic birds has been wide (including pigs, whales, seals, horses, ferrets, cats, dogs, and tigers). Domestic poultry can also be infected and are likely the main source of human infections. Swine influenza viruses are endemic in pigs. Influenza infections are also known to occur in other animals besides birds and pigs, including horses and dogs, but with the exception of pigs, influenza viruses have not been shown to transmit from these mammals to humans.

6. Incubation period—For A (H5N1) infection associated with poultry exposure, incubation can be 7 days or less, and mostly 2–5 days. For infections with influenza viruses normally circulating in swine, an incubation of 2–7 days has been reported.

7. Transmission—Most human infections by animal influenza viruses are thought to result from direct contact with infected animals. Migratory birds may sometimes spread A (H5N1) viruses to new geographic regions, but their importance as a vector for spread is uncertain. For A (H5N1) virus infection, the exact mode and sites of the viral entry are incompletely understood. Possibilities include inhalation of small particles into the lower respiratory tract, contamination of facial mucus membranes by self-inoculation or by droplet contact, or ingestion. In about one quarter of patients, the source of exposure is unclear and infection arising from exposure to contaminated environments remains possible. Visiting live-poultry markets is a recognized risk factor. Human-to-human transmission is thought to have occurred in some instances when there had been very close and prolonged contact between a very sick patient and caregivers who have usually been family members. This observation suggests near-distance aerosol, droplet, or direct contact may have been routes of transmission. However, the potential contribution of each route has not been demonstrated. No evidence to support long-distance airborne transmission has been reported to date.

For swine influenza virus infections in humans, close proximity to ill pigs or visiting a place where pigs are exhibited has been reported for most cases, but some human-to-human transmission has occurred, such as among soldiers in the 1976 Fort Dix outbreak and more recently during the outbreak of influenza A (H3N2) in the USA in 2012. Serologic studies show increased prevalence of swine influenza antibody among persons occupationally exposed to pigs compared to controls.

For H5N1 disease, limited data suggest that patients may remain infectious as long as 3 weeks, and perhaps even longer in immunosuppressed patients (e.g., those using corticosteroids). The longest documented period has been 27 days after the onset of illness, based upon detection of virus antigen in a patient's respiratory specimens.

8. Risk groups—Groups considered at high risk of exposure to A (H5N1) infected birds include poultry workers, persons involved in mass culling operations, live animal market workers and customers, and children and adults in households with backyard poultry. A (H5N1) illness occurs in all age groups, and limited serological studies demonstrate negligible preexisting immunity in the subjects. Of 6 infected pregnant women, 4 have died, and the 2 survivors had spontaneous abortion.

Duration of protection from immunity generated by previous infection or immunization by an investigational A (H5N1) vaccine is unknown. Familial clustering as well as the relative absence of nonfamilial clusters suggests the existence of a host genetic influence on susceptibility to severe infection. The majority of human cases with other zoonotic influenza virus infection have had a history of contact with infected animals. Human infection with influenza A (H3N2) in the USA in 2012 was mainly associated with animal fairs.

9. Prevention—

1) Preventing human exposure to infected animals or contaminated environments and controlling spread of infection among domesticated animal populations are critical elements for protecting humans from animal influenza virus infections. Guidelines for controlling outbreaks in domesticated animals have been issued by relevant national and international agencies (e.g., the Food and Agriculture Organization of the United Nations and the World Organisation for Animal Health [OIE]).

2) Rapid information sharing between animal and/or agricultural sectors and human health authorities is essential for timely implementation of public health actions. Social mobilization and risk communication targeting high-risk populations in affected areas are important measures for raising disease awareness and initiating protective behavioral changes.

3) Use of appropriate personal protective equipment (PPEs) and proper training is recommended for those at high risk of exposure to infected birds. Following a probable exposure, asymptomatic persons should be followed for signs of illness for at least 1 week,

while symptomatic persons should be tested for infection, administered antiviral medicines, and monitored closely.

4) Immunization: inactivated and LAIV for A (H5N1) for human use have been developed based on WHO recommended candidate vaccine viruses and licensed in several countries. Some countries are stockpiling these vaccines as part of their pandemic preparedness measures. Although immunogenic at higher antigenic concentrations, the effectiveness of these vaccines in preventing A (H5N1) infection or ability to reduce disease severity is unknown. Use of seasonal influenza vaccination in certain high-risk occupational groups with animal exposure is recommended in some countries for reducing influenza-like illness caused by seasonal influenza viruses. Such vaccines will not provide direct protection against animal influenza virus infections but may prevent seasonal and animal influenza coinfections that may lead to reassortment, which may generate potential viruses with pandemic potential. Updates on available candidate vaccine viruses and potency reagents for nonseasonal influenza viruses infecting humans can be found at: http://www.who.int/influenza/vaccines/virus/candidates_reagents/home/en/index.html.

10. **Management of patient—**

1) Isolation: when possible, suspected or confirmed cases with H5N1 and other nonhuman influenza virus infections should be treated using well-ventilated single isolation rooms with implementation of Standard and Droplet Precautions. Use of higher-level precautions such as airborne precautions may be considered when aerosol-generating procedures (e.g., sampling respiratory specimens, suction, use of nebulizers, intubation, and mechanical ventilation) are to be performed.

2) Regular surface cleaning and disinfection with a commonly used detergent or hospital disinfectant is desirable during hospitalization and after removal of a patient from the room. Environmental disinfection should follow guidelines published by relevant agencies (e.g., Food and Agriculture Organization of the United Nations, World Organization for Animal Health).

3) Treatment: for H5N1 disease and other zoonotic influenza virus infection, particularly for those with increased risk of severe influenza-associated complications and progressive disease, early treatment with oseltamivir is recommended using the standard regimen indicated for treatment of seasonal influenza. For H5N1 disease, there is an accumulated evidence suggesting the antiviral treatment improves survival, although the optimal dose and

duration of therapy are uncertain. Based on in vitro and animal studies suggesting improved outcomes, physicians may consider using higher doses of oseltamivir therapy, longer durations of treatment, intravenous (IV) formulation of neuraminidase inhibitors where available, or combination therapy (triple combination of antiviral drugs: oseltamivir + amantadine + ribavirin). During oseltamivir therapy, the emergence of highly resistant H5N1 variants was observed in Vietnamese patients, with fatal outcomes. Infection by viruses partially resistant to oseltamivir, before treatment, was reported in 2 Egyptian patients who died.

Treatment of H5N1-associated acute respiratory distress syndrome (ARDS) and sepsis should follow published national or international guidelines. In principle, early intervention by intermittent positive pressure ventilation using low tidal volumes and low-pressure ventilation (lung-protective ventilation strategy) and conservative fluid management are recommended. Systemic high-dose corticosteroid therapy should not be used as this can result in serious adverse events in patients with severe acute respiratory illness, including opportunistic infection, avascular necrosis, new health care–associated bacterial infection and possibly prolonged viral replication. Therefore, corticosteroids should be avoided unless they are indicated for another reason, such as exacerbation of asthma or chronic obstructive lung disease or vasopressor-refractory shock. A limited number of studies suggest other immunomodulators such as serotherapy and statins may be useful, which warrants further clinical trial.

11. **Management of contacts and the immediate environment—**

1) Quarantine: in large-scale outbreak settings, voluntary home quarantine, and daily temperature recording of contacts may be used. Symptomatic contacts with mild illness that do not require hospitalization should be placed in isolation and provided with antiviral treatment.

2) Protection of contacts: postexposure prophylaxis may be considered for the high-risk exposure contacts with treatment regimen for seasonal influenza (i.e., oseltamivir 75 mg twice daily for 5 days). Optimal dose and duration of neuraminidase inhibitors for prophylactic use is uncertain and underdosing may result in emergence of drug resistance hence presumptive treatment may be preferred. Careful health observation of such contacts and initiation of neuraminidase inhibitor treatment upon illness onset is a reasonable option.

3) Investigation of contacts and source of infection: when an influenza infection with H5N1 is suspected, clinical samples

(e.g., throat swab and other respiratory specimens) should be collected and tested to confirm infection. Virus isolation or PCR testing will allow further genetic characterization of the virus. When concomitant animal outbreaks are ongoing, coordination with the animal and/or agricultural sectors is essential. Epidemiological field investigations should identify the source of infection, identify situation-specific control measures, and determine whether human-to-human transmission has occurred. If a novel influenza virus is associated with efficient spread among people, large-scale operations should be started/ considered to limit and prevent further spread.

12. **Special considerations—**

1) Reporting: laboratory-confirmed human infection with a novel subtype of influenza A virus, or influenza A infection where the virus cannot be subtyped, should be reported immediately to the national authority and then to WHO. Reporting to WHO is mandatory under the International Health Regulations (IHR).

   Under the IHR, human influenza caused by a new subtype is considered as an event that may constitute a public health emergency of international concern.

2) Any specimen from a patient suspected of novel influenza A virus infection, including H5N1, should be immediately tested and forwarded to a national reference laboratory or WHO Collaborating Centre/Reference Laboratories for confirmatory testing. WHO Collaborating Centres provide technical support for influenza surveillance, preparedness, and response. More information on the Centres can be found at: http://www.who.int/ influenza/gisrs_laboratory/collaborating_centres/en.

3) Continued viral and disease surveillance is critical for identifying human infections caused by influenza viruses of animal origin, including H5N1, and determining their ability to transmit efficiently among humans.

4) Epidemic measures:

   - Clinicians and local public health officers should be aware that human infections may occur in countries with outbreaks of influenza A (H5N1) among poultry. The clinical presentation of influenza A (H5N1) disease is nonspecific and has often resulted in an initial misdiagnosis, especially in circumstances in tropical countries where endemic acute febrile diseases are common. Influenza A (H5N1) virus infection should be considered in the differential diagnosis for patients who present with fever, rapidly progressing atypical pneumonia, and epidemiologic risk factors.

- Develop or use a case definition and undertake active surveillance in the appropriate epidemiological setting for early detection of human cases. If an infection occurs or is strongly suspected, family members and close contacts should be placed under medical observation with daily temperature monitoring and tested when developing symptoms.
- Establish a mechanism for rapidly obtaining reliable laboratory testing results. Characterization of the virus and its susceptibility to antivirals are important factors for disease control.
- Establish good communication between human and animal health sectors.
- Provide information about the disease and preventive measures to at-risk population. Social mobilization including sensitization campaigns may be required for effective message penetration. Timely provision of information to the public is essential.
- Collect epidemiological, clinical, and other information to assess the situation. If efficient human-to-human transmission is observed, a large-scale operation should be considered to stop or limit further spread of the infection.

5) Disaster implications: the emergence of an animal virus with the capacity to transmit and spread easily among humans could result in a pandemic.

6) Pandemic influenza: the response to an influenza pandemic must be planned at the local, national, and international levels; guidance is provided on the WHO website at: http://www.who.int/influenza/preparedness/pandemic/en/index.html. Similar information is available on the websites of many governments, including that of the USA at: www.pandemicflu.gov.

[C. B. Bridges, A. Mounts, T. Besselaar, J. Fitzner, K. Vandemaele, N. Shindo, J. S. Tam]

JAPANESE ENCEPHALITIS

DISEASE	ICD-10 CODE
JAPANESE ENCEPHALITIS	ICD-10 A83.0

1. Clinical features—The majority of human infections with Japanese encephalitis (JE) virus are asymptomatic; fewer than 1% of people infected develop clinical disease. Acute encephalitis is the most commonly recognized clinical presentation. Milder forms of disease such as aseptic meningitis or undifferentiated febrile illness also occur.

Among persons who develop clinical disease, initial symptoms are usually nonspecific and may include fever, diarrhea, headache, and vomiting. Subsequently, mental status changes, generalized weakness, focal neurologic deficits (e.g., paresis and cranial nerve palsies), and/or movement disorders might occur. Seizures are very common, especially among children, sometimes manifesting as subtle clinical findings (e.g., twitching of a digit, eye deviation, or irregular breathing).

A distinctive clinical presentation is a Parkinsonian syndrome resulting from extrapyramidal system involvement; findings include a flat, mask-like face with wide unblinking eyes, tremor, cogwheel rigidity, and choreoathetoid movements. In some patients, JE virus infection may result in a poliomyelitis-like acute flaccid paralysis due to anterior horn cell damage, without any alteration in consciousness. After a brief febrile illness, flaccid paralysis occurs in one or more limbs, usually asymmetric and more common in the lower than upper limbs. About 30% of these patients subsequently develop encephalitis. Abnormal behavior or acute psychosis may also be the initial clinical presentation in some patients. JE has a case-fatality ratio of approximately 20%–30%. About 30%–50% of survivors have long-term neurologic or psychiatric sequelae. JE virus infection should be considered in the differential diagnosis of acute neurologic or febrile illnesses in persons who have been in areas where JE virus transmission occurs. The differential diagnosis is broad and includes many infectious and noninfectious causes.

2. Causative agent—Japanese encephalitis virus, of the family *Flaviviridae* and genus *Flavivirus*.

3. Diagnosis—Confirmed most frequently by detection of virus-specific antibody in cerebrospinal fluid (CSF) or serum. Acute-phase specimens should be tested for JE virus-specific immunoglobulin class M (IgM) antibodies using an enzyme-linked immunosorbent assay (ELISA). JE IgM antibodies can be measured in CSF of most patients by 4 days after onset of symptoms and in serum by 7 days after onset. If JE is suspected and acute specimens collected within 10 days of illness onset lack detectable IgM, a convalescent specimen should be collected and tested. Detection of JE IgM in CSF is diagnostic of neuroinvasive disease and can help distinguish clinical disease attributable to JE virus infection from recent vaccination.

Plaque reduction neutralization tests can be performed to measure virus-specific neutralizing antibodies and to discriminate between cross-reacting antibodies in primary flavivirus infections. A 4-fold or greater rise in virus-specific neutralizing antibodies between acute- and convalescent-phase serum specimens collected 2–3 weeks apart may be used to confirm evidence of recent infection. Vaccination history, date of symptom onset, and information regarding other flaviviruses known to circulate in the geographic area that might cross-react in serologic assays should be considered when interpreting results. In patients who have been immunized against or infected with another flavivirus in the past (i.e., who have secondary flavivirus infections), cross-reactive antibodies in both ELISA and neutralization assays may make it difficult to identify which flavivirus is causing the patient's illness. Virus isolation or detection of viral ribonucleic acid (RNA) with a nucleic acid amplification test can be used to confirm JE virus infection, but positive results from blood or CSF are rare. Humans usually have low or undetectable levels of viremia by the time distinctive clinical symptoms are recognized, so these tests are insensitive and are not routinely recommended for diagnosis of JE virus infection.

4. Occurrence—Occurs throughout most of Asia and parts of the western Pacific. An estimated 67,900 cases occur annually in JE-endemic countries. Among travelers to these countries from nonendemic areas, the estimated incidence is less than 1 case per 1 million travelers. There are 2 general seasonal patterns of JE virus transmission. In temperate areas of Asia, most cases occur over a period of several months when the weather is warmest. Large, explosive outbreaks can occur. In the tropics and subtropics, transmission can occur year-round but often intensifies during the rainy season.

5. Reservoir—JE virus is transmitted in an enzootic cycle between mosquitoes and vertebrate amplifying hosts, primarily pigs and wading birds. Domestic pigs are the most important source of infection for mosquitoes that transmit JE virus to humans because they have high viremia levels and rapid population turnover with a large number of susceptible offspring. Humans are incidental and "dead-end" hosts in the JE virus transmission cycle, as concentrations of the virus in blood are generally not high enough to infect feeding mosquitoes. Infection is usually asymptomatic in pigs, but gestational infection can result in abortions and stillbirths. In horses, fatal encephalitis can occur, but horses are also considered "dead-end" hosts. Many other animals can be infected with JE virus, but there is little evidence for other animals playing a significant role in the transmission cycle.

6. Incubation period—5-15 days.

7. Transmission—Transmitted to humans through the bites of infected mosquitoes. *Culex* mosquitoes, especially *Cx. tritaeniorhynchus*, are the main vectors for both human and zoonotic JE virus transmission. *Cx. tritaeniorhynchus* commonly breeds in rice fields, marshes, and other shallow pools of water. It is an evening- and nighttime-biting mosquito and mainly feeds outdoors, preferentially on large animals and birds and only infrequently on humans.

Direct person-to-person spread of JE virus does not occur, except rarely through intrauterine transmission. Based on experience with other flaviviruses, blood transfusion and organ transplantation are possible modes of transmission. Laboratory-acquired JE virus infections have been reported. In a laboratory setting, JE virus might be transmitted through needlesticks, and theoretically, through mucosal or inhalational exposures.

8. Risk groups—The risk for JE virus infection is related to exposure to infected mosquitoes and is highest in rural agricultural areas, often those where rice production is common. In endemic areas, the majority of JE cases occur in children younger than 15 years. However, in areas with childhood JE immunization programs, a shift in age distribution occurs with similar numbers of cases observed in children and adults. In unvaccinated, nonimmune travelers, JE infection can occur at any age. Infection generally results in lifelong immunity.

9. Prevention—

1) Vector prevention measures (see "Arboviral Encephalitides").
2) Vaccine: Several inactivated and live attenuated JE vaccines are available worldwide. JE immunization is considered the most effective JE prevention strategy in endemic regions, and JE vaccine is a routine childhood vaccine in many countries in Asia. JE vaccine may be advised for those traveling to endemic areas. Recommendations should be based on evaluation of an individual traveler's risk of exposure taking into account the person's planned itinerary, trip duration, activities, and season. More detailed recommendations can be found at: http://www.cdc.gov/mmwr/pdf/rr/rr5901.pdf. Vaccine is recommended for laboratory workers with a potential for exposure to infectious JE virus.
3) Other prevention measures: To prevent laboratory infections, precautions should be taken when handling viruses in the laboratory at the appropriate biosafety level (http://www.cdc.gov/biosafety/publications/bmbl5/BMBL5_sect_VIII_f.pdf).

10. Management of patient—JE treatment consists of supportive care including control of intracranial pressure, management of seizures, and prevention of secondary complications. No antiviral or other medication is available to mitigate the effects of infection. Standard blood and body substance precautions are sufficient.

11. Management of contacts and the immediate environment—In endemic areas, raise awareness that JE virus transmission is occurring and, if available, encourage vaccination for unvaccinated persons in appropriate age groups. No additional interventions are generally required.

12. Special considerations—Reporting: local health authority may be required to report cases in residents in endemic areas or in travelers from nonendemic countries.

[S. L. Hills, M. Fischer]

KAWASAKI SYNDROME
(Kawasaki disease, mucocutaneous lymph node syndrome, acute febrile mucocutaneous lymph node syndrome)

DISEASE	ICD-10 CODE
KAWASAKI SYNDROME	ICD-10 M30.3

1. Clinical features—An acute febrile, mostly self-limited, systemic vasculitis of early childhood, presumably of infectious origin. Clinically characterized by a high, spiking fever, unresponsive to antibiotics, associated with pronounced irritability and mood change; usually solitary and frequently unilateral nonsuppurative cervical lymphadenopathy; bilateral nonexudative bulbar conjunctival injection; and an enanthem consisting of a "strawberry tongue," injected oropharynx, or dry fissured or erythematous lips. Also present are limb changes consisting of edema, erythema, or periungual/generalized desquamation and a generalized polymorphous erythematous exanthem that can be truncal or perineal and which ranges from morbilliform maculopapular rash to urticarial rash or vasculitic exanthem. Typically there are 3 phases:

1) Acute febrile phase of about 10 days, characterized by high, spiking fever, rash, adenopathy, peripheral erythema or edema, conjunctival injection, and enanthem.

2) Subacute phase lasting about 2 weeks, with thrombocytosis, desquamation, and resolution of fever.

3) Lengthy convalescent phase, during which clinical signs fade.

The case-fatality rate is approximately 0.1%; half the deaths occur within 2 months of illness. Coronary artery vasculitis leading to lumen dilatation and aneurysm are serious complications.

2. Causative agent—Unknown. Postulated to be a virus or a super-antigen bacterial toxin secreted by *Staphylococcus aureus* or group A streptococci, but this has neither been confirmed nor generally accepted.

3. Diagnosis—There is no pathognomonic laboratory test for Kawasaki syndrome, but an elevated erythrocyte sedimentation rate, C-reactive protein, and platelet counts above $450,000/mm^3$ (SI units 450,109/L) are common laboratory features. The following 6 principal clinical signs are part of the diagnostic criteria for Kawasaki syndrome:

1) Fever persisting 5 days or more (including cases in whom the fever has subsided before the fifth day in response to treatment).

2) Bilateral conjunctival redness.

3) Changes of lips and oral cavity: reddening of lips, strawberry tongue, and diffuse injection of oral and pharyngeal mucosa.

4) Polymorphous exanthema.

5) Changes of peripheral extremities: reddening of palms and soles, indurative edema in the initial stage, and membranous desquamation from fingertips in the convalescent stage.

6) Acute nonpurulent cervical lymphadenopathy.

In the USA, the presence of fever and at least 4 of the remaining 5 clinical signs are required for the diagnosis of Kawasaki syndrome. In contrast, the Japan Kawasaki Disease Research Committee recommends the presence of at least 5 of the 6 principal clinical signs to diagnose the illness; fever is not a required criterion. When evidence of coronary artery aneurysm or dilatation is present, Kawasaki syndrome can be diagnosed with fewer clinical signs.

4. Occurrence—Worldwide; the reported incidence per 100,000 children younger than 5 years is highest in Japan (>200 during 2007–2008) followed by South Korea (113 during 2006–2008), Taiwan (69 during 2003–2006), and Beijing, China (55 during 2004). The incidence in Japan has shown a steady increase since the 1970s; it has more than doubled during the last 2 decades. In the USA, the incidence appears to be stable at around 20 cases per 100,000 children younger than 5 years. European countries generally have much lower incidence than the United States. Cases are more frequent in the winter and spring.

5. **Reservoir**—Unknown, perhaps humans.

6. **Incubation period**—Unknown.

7. **Transmission**—Mode of transmission is unknown; there is no firm evidence of person-to-person transmission, even within families. Seasonal variation, limitation to the pediatric age group and outbreak occurrence in communities are all consistent with an infectious etiology.

8. **Risk groups**—Children younger than 5 years, male sex, and Asian ancestry seem to be risk factors for Kawasaki syndrome. In the USA, the incidence is highest among children of Asian origin, followed by African Americans and then whites. Recurrences appear infrequent (<3% of reported patients).

9. **Prevention**—Unknown.

10. **Management of patient**—Treatment: high-dose intravenous immunoglobulin (IVIG; 2 g/kg as a single dose given over a period of 10-12 hours) within the first 10 days of onset can reduce fever and inflammatory signs and reduce the frequency of aneurysm formation and other cardiac complications. Treatment should be considered even if the duration of fever exceeds 10 days. In addition, high-dose aspirin is recommended during the acute phase, followed by low dose for at least 2 months. Up to 15% of patients may not respond to initial IVIG treatment and may require retreatment. Measles and/or varicella vaccination should usually be deferred following receipt of IVIG. If the child's risk of measles or varicella is high, the child should be vaccinated and then revaccinated at least 11 months after IVIG administration. To reduce the risk of Reye syndrome, the child and household contacts should be vaccinated for influenza according to seasonal recommendations.

11. **Management of contacts and the immediate environment**—None.

12. **Special considerations**—

1) Reporting: clusters and epidemics should be reported immediately to the local health authority.
2) Investigate outbreaks and clusters to elucidate etiology and risk factors.

[E. Belay]

❖

LARVA MIGRANS

DISEASE	ICD-10 CODE
VISCERAL LARVA MIGRANS	ICD-10 B83.0
GNATHOSTOMIASIS	ICD-10 B83.1
CREEPING ERUPTION	ICD-10 B76.0
CUTANEOUS LARVA MIGRANS	ICD-10 B76.9

I. VISCERAL LARVA MIGRANS (larva migrans visceralis, visceral larva migrans, ocular larva migrans, *Toxocara* [*canis*] [*cati*] infection)

1. Clinical features—Usually a chronic infection and mild disease, predominantly of young children but increasingly recognized in adults, caused by migration of larval forms of nematodes in several organs and tissues, including the eye (in this case the term ocular larva migrans [OLM] is used). *Toxocara* species (*Toxocara canis* and *Toxocara cati*) are the most common causes of visceral larva migrans (VLM) and OLM. While infection with few larvae is usually asymptomatic, both VLM and OLM result from high-intensity infections.

VLM is characterized by hypereosinophilia of variable duration, hepatomegaly, hyperglobulinemia, pulmonary symptoms, and fever. With an acute and heavy infection, the white blood cell count may reach 100,000/mm^3 or more (SI units >100 × 10^9/L), with 50%–90% eosinophils. Symptoms may persist for a year or longer; symptomatology is related to total parasite load. Pneumonitis, chronic abdominal pain, a generalized rash, and focal neurological disturbances may occur.

Larvae may also enter the eye, thus causing an endophthalmitis that can result in loss of vision in the affected eye (OLM). This usually occurs in older children.

VLM is rarely fatal; differential diagnosis includes larval ascariasis (which has a shorter duration) and strongyloidiasis (longer duration). OLM should be distinguished from retinoblastoma and toxoplasmosis.

2. Causative agents—The nematode helminths *T. canis* and *T. cati*, predominantly the former; *Baylisascaris*, predominately *Baylisascaris procyonis*, is a rarer cause of VLM and OLM but is associated with a more severe syndrome. VLM and OLM might also be caused by *Ancylostoma suum* (pigs are the main reservoir), *Ancylostoma equorum* (horses), *Neoscaris vitulorum* (cattle), and others.

3. Diagnosis—Exposure to the reservoir host's feces (mainly canids in the case of toxocariasis), a history of pica, and suggestive laboratory findings orient the diagnosis, which is confirmed by serology. Enzyme-linked immunosorbent assay (ELISA) is the test of choice: testing with larval-stage antigens is highly sensitive and specific in both VLM and OLM. Western blotting procedures can be used to increase specificity of the ELISA screening test. Other tests are also available.

4. Occurrence—Worldwide. Severe disease occurs sporadically and affects mainly children aged 14–40 months, but also older children. Siblings often have eosinophilia or other evidence of light or residual infection. Serological studies in asymptomatic children have shown a wide range of prevalence in different populations. Internationally, seroprevalence ranges from lows of 0%–4% in Germany and urban Spain (Madrid) to 83% in some Caribbean subpopulations. Adults are less often acutely infected. *Baylisascaris* has been reported in humans in North America and occurs in raccoons in Europe, Japan, and elsewhere.

5. Reservoir—Dogs and cats, for *T. canis* and *T. cati*, respectively, raccoons for *B. procyonis*, and a wide range of other animals for the less common causative agents. Puppies are infected by transplacental and transmammary migration of larvae and pass eggs in their stools by the time they are 3 weeks old. Infection among bitches may end or become dormant with sexual maturity; with pregnancy, however, *T. canis* larvae become active. Similar though less marked differences apply for cats; older animals are less susceptible than young ones.

6. Incubation period—In children, weeks or months, depending on intensity of infection, reinfection, and sensitivity of the patient. Ocular manifestations may occur as late as 4–10 years after initial infection. In infections through ingestion of raw liver, very short incubation periods (hours or days) have been reported.

7. Transmission—For most infections in children, by transmission of infective *Toxocara* eggs from contaminated soil to the mouth, directly by contact with infected soil or indirectly by eating unwashed raw vegetables. Some infections may occur through ingestion of larvae in raw liver from infected chickens, cattle, and sheep.

Dog and cat feces are also a source of human infection: up to 30% of soil samples from certain parks in the UK and the USA contained eggs; in certain parks in Japan, up to 75% of sandboxes contained eggs. Eggs require 1–3 weeks' incubation to become infective but can remain infective in soil for more than a year; they are adversely affected by desiccation.

After ingestion, embryonated eggs hatch in the intestine; larvae penetrate the wall and migrate to the liver and other tissues via the lymphatic and circulatory systems. From the liver, larvae spread to other tissues, particularly the lungs and abdominal organs (VLM) or the eyes (OLM), and induce granulomatous lesions. The parasites cannot replicate in the human or other end-stage hosts; viable larvae may remain in tissues for years, usually in the absence of symptomatic disease. *Baylisascaris* is similar to *Toxocara*, except that larvae of *Baylisascaris* can grow in the human host to more than 1 mm in length. No direct person-to-person transmission.

8. Risk groups—Children playing in areas with soil or sand contaminated by dog or cat feces. Lower incidence in older children and adults relating mainly to lesser exposure. Reinfection can occur.

9. Prevention—

1) Educate the public, especially pet owners, concerning sources and origin of the infection; the need for removal of pet feces from public areas such as parks and beaches and proper collection and disposal of pet feces in the immediate vicinity of the house; the particular danger of pica; the danger of exposure to areas contaminated with feces of untreated puppies; and the danger of ingestion of raw or undercooked liver from animals exposed to dogs or cats. Parents of toddlers should be made aware of the risk associated with pets in the household and how to minimize them.

2) Prevent contamination of soil and sand by dog and cat feces in areas immediately adjacent to houses and children's play areas, especially in urban areas and multiple housing projects. Encourage cat and dog owners to practice responsible pet ownership, including prompt removal of pets' feces from areas of public access, particularly play areas. Children's sandboxes/sandpits offer an attractive site for defecating cats; cover when not in use. Control stray dogs and cats; ensure that raccoons do not live in close proximity to human dwellings.

3) Deworm dogs and cats, beginning at 3 weeks of age, repeated 3 times at 2-week intervals, and every 6 months thereafter. Also treat lactating bitches. Dispose of feces passed as a result of treatment, as well as other stools, in a sanitary manner.

4) Always wash hands after handling soil and sand and before eating.

5) Teach children not to put dirty objects into their mouths.

10. Management of patient—

1) Treatment of asymptomatic, ELISA positive individuals is not indicated; treatment may be considered for those with hypereosinophilia.

2) Treatment: diethylcarbamazine is the drug of choice. To reduce the intensity of allergic reactions induced by dying larvae, dosage is commonly raised progressively for 10-21 days. Alternative drugs are: albendazole, mebendazole, and thiabendazole, even though their effectiveness might be limited. For *Baylisascaris*, no drug has

been demonstrated effective, although albendazole, started as soon as possible, may prevent clinical disease and is recommended for children with known exposure. Mebendazole, levamisole, or ivermectin could be tried if albendazole is not available. Steroid therapy may be helpful, especially in ocular or central nervous system (CNS) infection.

11. Management of contacts and the immediate environment— Search for geographic site of infection of index case; identify others exposed. Intensify preventive measures.

12. Special considerations—None.

II. GNATHOSTOMIASIS (larva migrans profundus)

1. Clinical features—Transient inflammatory lesions or abscesses in various parts of the body, including the subcutaneous tissue, with a typical painless, migrating, intermittent edema. Larvae may also invade the brain, producing focal cerebral lesions associated with eosinophilic pleocytosis.

2. Causative agent—A nematode helminth parasite, *Gnathostoma spinigerum* is the causative agent in the vast majority of cases; other species include *Gnathostoma hispidum*, *Gnathostoma nipponicum*, and *Gnathostoma doloresi*. Epidemiology and clinical features of all species overlap significantly.

3. Diagnosis—Suggested by a history of eating raw poultry and fish (such as "sashimi" in Japan, "somfak" in Thailand, or "ceviche" in Central and South America) and by clinical and laboratory findings (eosinophilia); diagnosis is confirmed by ELISA test.

4. Occurrence—Common in Thailand and elsewhere in southeastern Asia; present in other tropical countries, especially in Central and South America.

5. Reservoir—Dogs, cats, and large carnivores, such as tigers and leopards.

6. Incubation period—3-4 weeks.

7. Transmission—Through ingestion of undercooked fish, frogs, poultry, or snakes containing third-stage larvae.

8. Risk groups—Habitual consumers of raw food.

9. Prevention—Thoroughly cooked poultry and fish.

10. Management of patient—Treatment: although no clear recommendation is available, albendazole and ivermectin have produced good cure rates. Mebendazole has also been shown to have some effect.

11. Management of contacts and the immediate environment—Search for geographic site of infection of index case; identify others exposed. Intensify preventive measures.

12. Special considerations—None.

III. CREEPING ERUPTION/CUTANEOUS LARVA MIGRANS

1. Clinical features—A dermatitis in which each larva causes a serpiginous, reddish track, advancing several millimeters to a few centimeters a day, with intense itching, especially at night. Most common locations include feet and buttocks. The disease is self-limited, with spontaneous cure after weeks or months. *Ancylostoma caninum* larvae may migrate to the small intestine where they cause eosinophilic enteritis.

2. Causative agents—Infective larvae of dog and cat hookworms *A. caninum* and *Ancylostoma braziliense* (nematode helminths), hatched in the soil from eggs shed in the feces of infected dogs (*A. caninum* and *A. braziliense*) and cats (*A. braziliense* only).

3. Diagnosis—Based on the clinical picture and on a history of exposure to soil or sand, especially in areas where dogs are common. Laboratory tests have a role in excluding other possible causes of larva migrans.

4. Occurrence—Most tropical and subtropical countries across the world.

5. Reservoir—Dogs and cats.

6. Incubation period—Creeping eruption usually appears a few days after skin penetration by larvae.

7. Transmission—Follows contact of the skin with soil or sand harboring infective larvae. The larvae enter the skin and migrate intracutaneously for long periods; eventually they may penetrate to deeper tissues. No person-to-person transmission.

8. Risk groups—Utility workers, gardeners, children, sea-bathers, and others who come in contact with damp sandy soil or sand contaminated with dog and cat feces.

9. Prevention—Reduce contact with soil or sand by wearing shoes and appropriate clothing.

10. Management of patient—Freezing the affected area with ethyl chloride spray can kill individual larvae. Thiabendazole is effective as a topical ointment; a single dose of albendazole or a single dose of ivermectin is effective systemically. A 7-day course of albendazole prevents recurrence. Eosinophilic enteritis responds to treatment with pyrantelpamoate, mebendazole, or albendazole.

11. Management of contacts and the immediate environment—Search for geographic site of infection of index case; identify others exposed. Intensify preventive measures.

12. Special considerations—None.

[M. Eberhard, A. Gabrielli, A. Montresor, L. Savioli]

LEGIONELLOSIS

DISEASE	ICD-10 CODE
LEGIONNAIRES' DISEASE	ICD-10 A48.1
PONTIAC FEVER	ICD-10 A48.2

1. Clinical features—Two distinct clinical manifestations: Legionnaires' disease and Pontiac fever. Both conditions present with anorexia, malaise, myalgia, headache, and fever. Abdominal pain and diarrhea are also common.

1) Legionnaires' disease: characterized by pneumonia and a non-productive cough. Chest imaging findings are variable and may show patchy or focal areas of consolidation or bilateral involvement. The illness can be quite severe and may ultimately progress to respiratory failure. Despite improvements in diagnostics and treatment, case-fatality rates remain at approximately 15%.

2) Pontiac fever: a self-limited febrile illness, usually accompanied by cough, which does not progress to pneumonia or death. Patients recover spontaneously in 2–5 days without treatment. This clinical syndrome may represent reaction to inhaled *Legionella* antigen rather than bacterial invasion.

2. Causative agents—*Legionellae,* Gram-negative bacilli. Of the 18 serogroups of *Legionellae pneumophila* currently recognized, *L. pneumophila* serogroup 1 is most commonly associated with disease. Related organisms, including *Legionellae micdadei*, *Legionellae bozemanii*, *Legionellae longbeachae*, and *Legionellae dumoffii* have been isolated, predominantly from immunosuppressed patients with pneumonia. Currently, 48 species of *Legionella* and at least 70 distinct serogroups are recognized.

3. **Diagnosis—**

1) Legionnaires' disease: isolate the causative organism from a lower respiratory specimen using selective media (buffered charcoal yeast extract); detect *L. pneumophila* serogroup 1 antigens in the urine; or measure a 4-fold rise in immunofluorescent antibody titer to *L. pneumophila* serogroup 1 between acute phase serum and serum drawn 3-6 weeks later. Urine antigen and some serologic tests only detect *L. pneumophila* serogroup 1, so disease due to other serogroups or species will be missed, emphasizing the importance of culture. Direct immunofluorescent antibody stain of involved tissue or respiratory secretions may be used, but sensitivity and specificity are highly variable and dependent upon the experience of laboratory personnel.

2) Pontiac fever: usually diagnosed by identifying symptoms consistent with the disease in the appropriate epidemiologic setting. If disease is due to *L. pneumophila* serogroup 1, urine antigen and serologic testing can be used to confirm the diagnosis, but test sensitivity is lower for Pontiac fever than for Legionnaires' disease.

4. **Occurrence**—The disease has been identified in North America, Asia, Africa, Australia, Europe, and South America. Although cases occur throughout the year, both sporadic cases and outbreaks are recognized more commonly in summer and autumn. In the few locations studied, antibodies to *L. pneumophila* serogroup 1 occur at a titer of 1:128 or greater in 1%-20% of the general population. The proportion of community-acquired pneumonia cases that are due to *Legionella* ranges between 0.5% and 5.0%. Outbreaks of Legionnaires' disease may be difficult to detect due to low attack rates (0.1-5%). Epidemic Pontiac fever tends to have an explosive presentation; attack rates as high as 95% have been documented.

5. **Reservoir**—Legionellosis is a waterborne disease. Man-made water supplies that aerosolize water, such as potable water systems (showers), air conditioning cooling towers, whirlpool spas, and decorative fountains, are the common sources for transmission. Conditions that are conducive to *Legionella* growth include warm water temperatures (25°C–42°C), stagnation, scale and sediment, and low biocide levels.

6. **Incubation period**—For Legionnaires' disease, 2–10 days, most often 5-6 days; For Pontiac fever 5-72 hours, most often 24-48 hours.

7. **Transmission**—Epidemiological evidence supports airborne transmission; other modes are possible, including aspiration of water. Person-to-person transmission has not been documented.

8. **Risk groups**—Risk factors include increasing age (most cases are >50 years of age), cigarette smoking, diabetes mellitus, chronic lung disease, renal disease, malignancy, and compromised immunity, particularly organ transplant recipients and patients receiving corticosteroids. The male-to-female ratio is about 2.5:1. Outbreaks are most commonly recognized among travelers and hospitalized patients.

9. **Prevention**—Avoid conditions known to enhance *Legionella* growth. Proper maintenance and disinfection of whirlpool spas, cooling towers, and drinking-water supplies are the most effective measures for preventing outbreaks. Cooling towers should be drained when not in use and mechanically cleaned periodically to remove scale and sediment. Appropriate biocides should be used to limit the growth of *Legionella* and the formation of protective biofilms. Maintaining hot water system temperatures at 50°C or higher may reduce the risk of transmission. Point-of-use water filtration (0.2 um) has been used under some circumstances to prevent healthcare-associated legionellosis in immunosuppressed patients. Tap water should not be used in respiratory therapy devices.

10. **Management of patient**—

   1) Legionnaires' disease: the recommended treatment Legionnaires' disease is either a respiratory fluoroquinolone, such as levofloxacin, or a macrolide (azithromycin). Observational studies suggest that levofloxacin may be more effective than macrolides, especially in severe cases.
   2) Pontiac fever: self-limited and does not require antimicrobial therapy.

11. **Management of contacts and the immediate environment**—

   1) Consider additional case finding to identify if there are other cases with the same exposures as the index case.
   2) Two or more cases of legionellosis occurring among travelers to the same destination during a 1-year period or a single case of laboratory-confirmed health care-associated Legionnaires' disease should trigger additional case finding measures and an environmental assessment.

12. **Special considerations**—The threshold for initiating environmental sampling and remediation varies among published guidelines. During an outbreak, identify common exposures and review maintenance logs for water systems that are potential sources of infection. *Legionella*

culture of water and biofilm swabs collected from the potential source(s) may be necessary to determine the cause for the outbreak, and should be considered for any cluster of health care–associated legionellosis. To optimize detection, at least 250 mL of water should be collected from each site. Remediation usually requires biocide disinfection of the implicated water system.

[L. Hicks]

LEISHMANIASIS

DISEASE	ICD-10 CODE
CUTANEOUS LEISHMANIASIS	ICD-10 B55.1
MUCOSAL LEISHMANIASIS	ICD-10 B55.2
VISCERAL LEISHMANIASIS	ICD-10 B55.0

I. CUTANEOUS AND MUCOSAL LEISHMANIASIS
(Aleppo evil, Baghdad boil, Delhi boil, chiclero ulcer, oriental sore, espundia)

1. Clinical features—A polymorphic disease of skin and mucous membranes that starts with a macule, then a papular or nodular lesion that enlarges and typically becomes an indolent ulcer in the absence of bacterial infection. The lesions can develop on any part of the body where the inoculation of the parasite has occurred. However, lesions usually appear on exposed surfaces of the body such as the face, arms, and legs. Lesions may be single or multiple, occasionally nonulcerative and diffuse. Lesions may heal spontaneously within weeks to months or last for a year or more. Recurrence of cutaneous lesions after apparent cure may occur as ulcers, papules, or nodules at or near the healed original ulcer.

In some individuals, certain strains (mainly from the western hemisphere) can disseminate to cause mucosal lesions (espundia), even years after the primary cutaneous lesion has healed. In the eastern hemisphere, a chronic granulomatous lesion occurs, following anthroponotic cutaneous leishmaniasis due to *Leishmania tropica* called the recidivans form. These sequelae, which involve nasopharyngeal tissues, are characterized by progressive tissue destruction and often scanty presence of parasites and can be severely disfiguring if left untreated.

Eventual spontaneous healing occurs in most cases, but the rate of healing varies by species. A small proportion of patients infected with *Leishmania amazonensis* or *Leishmania aethiopica* may develop diffuse parasite-rich cutaneous lesions that do not heal without treatment. Metastatic mucosal lesions may develop months or years later in a small proportion of infections with parasites of the *Leishmania braziliensis* complex.

2. **Causative agents**—*Leishmania* protozoa. These are obligate intracellular parasites in humans and other mammals. Eastern hemisphere: *L. tropica*, *Leishmania major*, *L. aethiopica*, *Leishmania infantum*, and *Leishmania donovani*. *L. tropica* is the usual cause of "leishmaniasis recidivans" cutaneous lesions. Western hemisphere: *L. braziliensis* and *Leishmania mexicana* complexes. Members of the *L. braziliensis* complex are more likely to produce mucosal lesions; members of *L. donovani* complex usually cause visceral disease in the eastern hemisphere; in the western hemisphere the responsible organism is *L. infantum/chagasi.* Both may cause cutaneous leishmaniasis without concomitant visceral involvement. Post–Kala-azar dermal leishmaniasis is a condition characterized by hypopigmented or erythematous macules, papules, or nodules that develops usually after apparent cure of visceral leishmaniasis. Post–Kala-azar dermal leishmaniasis cases are considered to be residual reservoirs for the maintenance and dissemination of the parasite.

3. **Diagnosis**—Through microscope identification of the nonmotile, intracellular form (amastigote) in stained specimens from lesions and through culture of the motile, extracellular form (promastigote) on suitable media. An intradermal (Montenegro) test with leishmanin, an antigen derived from promastigotes, is usually positive in established disease; it is not helpful with very early lesions, anergic disease, or immunosuppressed patients. Serological (immunofluorescence assay [IFA] or enzyme-linked immunosorbent assay [ELISA]) testing can be done, but antibody levels are typically low or undetectable; this may not be helpful in diagnosis (except for mucosal leishmaniasis).

Species identification is based on biological (development in sandflies, culture media, and animals), immunological (monoclonal antibodies), molecular (deoxyribonucleic acid [DNA] techniques), and biochemical (isoenzyme analysis) criteria.

4. **Occurrence**—China; India; Pakistan; southwestern Asia, including Afghanistan and Iran; southern regions of the former Soviet Union; the Mediterranean littoral; the sub-Saharan African savanna; Sudan; the highlands of Ethiopia and Kenya; Namibia; the Dominican Republic, Mexico (especially Yucatan); south central Texas; all of Central America; and every country of South America except Chile and Uruguay. About 1 million new cases are diagnosed per year.

A nonulcerative, keloid-like form due to *L. infantum/chagasi* (atypical cutaneous leishmaniasis) has been observed with increasing frequency in Central America, especially Honduras and Nicaragua. In some areas in the eastern hemisphere, urban population groups, including children, are at risk for anthroponotic cutaneous leishmaniasis due to *L. tropica*. In rural areas, people are at risk for zoonotic cutaneous leishmaniasis due to *L. major*. In the western hemisphere, disease is usually restricted to special groups, such as those working in forested areas, those whose homes are in or next to a forest, and visitors to such areas from nonendemic countries. Cutaneous leishmaniasis is generally more common in rural than urban areas, with the exception of *L. tropica*, which can cause large urban outbreaks—such as that in Kabul, Afghanistan, in the late 1990s and mid-2000s.

5. Reservoir—Locally variable; humans (in anthroponotic cutaneous leishmaniasis); wild rodents (gerbils); hyraxes; edentates (sloths); marsupials; and domestic dogs (considered victims more than reservoirs except for *L. infantum*). Unknown hosts in many areas.

6. Incubation period—At least a week, up to many months.

7. Transmission—In zoonotic foci, from the animal reservoir through the bite of infective female sandflies (phlebotomines). Motile promastigotes develop and multiply in the gut of the sandfly after it has fed on an infected mammalian host; in 8–20 days, infective parasites develop and are injected during biting. In humans and other mammals, the organisms are taken up by macrophages and transform into amastigote forms, which multiply within the macrophages until the cells rupture, enabling spread to other macrophages. In anthroponotic foci, indirect person-to-person transmission occurs through sandfly bites as long as parasites remain in lesions in untreated cases, usually a few months to 2 years. Person-to-person transmission can occur, very rarely, through blood transfusion.

8. Risk groups—Factors responsible for late mutilating disease are still poorly understood, although nutritional and immunogenetic factors have been implicated; occult infections may be activated years after the primary infection. Lifelong immunity may be present after lesions due to *L. tropica* or *L. major* heal but may not protect against other leishmanial species.

9. Prevention—No vaccine is currently available, although candidate vaccines are in development. Control measures vary according to the habits of mammalian hosts and phlebotomine vectors and include the following:

　　1) Vector control: apply residual insecticides periodically at the beginning of the active season for sandflies. Phlebotomine sandflies have a relatively short flight range and are highly susceptible to control by systematic spraying with residual insecticides. Spraying must cover exteriors and interiors of

doorways and other openings if transmission occurs in dwellings. Possible breeding places of eastern hemisphere sandflies, such as stone walls, animal houses, and refuse heaps, must be sprayed. Exclude vectors by screening with a fine mesh screen (10–12 holes/linear cm or 25–30 holes/linear in, with an aperture of ≤0.89 mm or 0.035 in). Insecticide-treated bed nets are additional vector control measures and should be promoted especially in anthroponotic foci.

2) Eliminate refuse heaps and other breeding places for eastern hemisphere phlebotomines.

3) Destroy gerbils (and their burrows) implicated as reservoirs in local areas by deep plowing and removal of the plants they feed on (chenopods).

4) In the western hemisphere, avoid sandfly-infested and thickly forested areas, particularly after sundown; use insect repellents and protective clothing if exposure to sandflies is unavoidable.

5) Apply appropriate environmental management and forest clearance.

10. **Management of patient—**

1) Detect cases systematically and treat rapidly. This applies to all forms of leishmaniasis and is an important measure in preventing development of destructive mucosal lesions in the western hemisphere and recidivans forms in the eastern hemisphere, particularly where the reservoir is largely or solely human.

2) Treatment: mainly pentavalent antimonials: either sodium stibogluconate or meglumine antimonate. The imidazoles, ketoconazole and itraconazole, may have moderate antileishmanial activity against some leishmanial species. Liposomal or conventional amphotericin B may be required in South American mucosal disease if it does not respond to antimonial therapy. Miltefosine, an alkylphospholipid and the first oral drug active against visceral leishmaniasis, has had variable efficacy for New World cutaneous leishmaniasis in clinical trials; its efficacy may be dependent on the leishmanial species. Topical formulations of 15% aminosidine (paromomycin) plus 10% urea have reduced the time to healing in cases due to *L. major*. Although spontaneous healing of simple cutaneous lesions occurs, infections acquired in geographic regions where mucosal disease has been reported should be treated promptly.

11. **Management of contacts and the immediate environment—** Interrupt the local transmission cycle in the most practical fashion.

12. **Special considerations—**

1) The WHO operational case definition is "a person showing clinical signs [of leishmaniasis] with parasitological confirmation and/or, for mucosal leishmaniasis only, serological diagnosis."

2) Epidemic measures: in areas of high incidence, use intensive efforts to control the disease by provision of diagnostic facilities and appropriate measures directed against phlebotomine sand-flies and the mammalian reservoir hosts.

II. VISCERAL LEISHMANIASIS (Kala-azar)

1. **Clinical features—**A systemic disease caused by intracellular protozoa of the genus *Leishmania*. The disease is characterized by fever, hepatosplenomegaly, lymphadenopathy, anemia, leukopenia, thrombocy-topenia, and progressive emaciation and weakness. Untreated clinically evident disease is usually fatal. Evidence indicates that asymptomatic and subclinical infections are common. Only very few progress to develop full-blown disease. However, the role of asymptomatic infections in transmis-sion is yet to be elucidated. Fever may have gradual or sudden onset, is persistent and irregular, and may alternate with periods of apyrexia or low-grade fever. Post–Kala-azar dermal leishmaniasis consists of macular, papular, and/or nodular skin lesions that occur weeks to years after apparent cure of systemic disease. Post–Kala-azar dermal leishmaniasis occurs in up to 50% of visceral leishmaniasis cases in Sudan and 10%–20% of cases in the Indian subcontinent. *Leishmania*/HIV coinfection is a serious form of the disease in southern Europe, eastern Africa, and southeast Asia.

2. **Causative agents—**Typically *L. donovani*, *L. infantum* (in eastern hemisphere) and *L. infantum/chagasi* (in western hemisphere).

3. **Diagnosis—**Parasitological diagnosis, based on invasive methods, is demonstration of intracellular amastigotes in stained smears from bone marrow, spleen, liver, and lymph nodes aspirates. The polymerase chain reaction (PCR) technique is the most sensitive but remains expensive. Serological diagnosis has traditionally been based on IFA and ELISA, tests that are expensive and difficult to decentralize. Recently, inexpensive, reliable rapid tests, such as the recombinant k39 immunochromatographic strip test, have become available for first-line diagnosis and field use, becoming the primary diagnostic modality for uncomplicated cases. An antigen detection test in urine has shown good specificity but low-to-moderate sensitivity. Serologic testing has poor sensitivity in HIV-coinfected patients; parasitolog-ical diagnosis is recommended.

4. **Occurrence—**Visceral leishmaniasis occurs in 62 countries, with an estimated annual incidence of 300,000 cases and a population at risk of

120 million. It is usually a rural disease, occurring in foci in Asia, Africa, and the Americas. More than 90% of the global disease burden occurs in India, Bangladesh, Sudan, South Sudan, Brazil, and Ethiopia. In Brazil, many cases now occur in periurban areas. Foci also occur in China, Pakistan, southern regions of eastern Europe, the Middle East including Turkey, the Mediterranean basin, Mexico, Central and South America, and in Kenya, Uganda, and sub-Saharan savanna parts of Africa. In many affected areas, the disease occurs as scattered cases among infants, children, and adolescents but occasionally in epidemic waves. Incidence is modified by the use of antimalarial insecticides. Where zoonotic transmission was predominant and dog populations have been drastically reduced (e.g., China), human disease has also been reduced.

5. Reservoir—Known or presumed reservoirs include humans, wild *Canidae* (foxes and jackals), and domestic dogs. Humans are the only known reservoir in Bangladesh, India, and Nepal.

6. Incubation period—Generally 2–6 months; range is 10 days to years.

7. Transmission—Through the bite of infected phlebotomine sandflies. In foci of anthroponotic visceral leishmaniasis, humans with visceral leishmaniasis or post–Kala-azar dermal leishmaniasis (especially the highly infectious nodular form) are the sole reservoir, and transmission occurs from person to person through the sandfly bite. In foci of zoonotic visceral leishmaniasis, dogs constitute the main source of infection for sandflies. Person-to-person transmission has been reported in *Leishmania*/HIV-coinfected intravenous drug users through exchange of syringes. HIV-coinfected patients are highly infectious to sandflies, acting as human reservoirs even in zoonotic foci.

Infectivity for phlebotomines may persist after clinical recovery of human patients.

8. Risk groups—Evidence indicates that malnutrition and HIV infection increases the likelihood of progression to clinical disease. Manifest disease occurs among AIDS patients, presumably as reactivation of latent infections. Kala-azar apparently induces lasting homologous immunity.

9. Prevention—See Cutaneous and Mucosal Leishmaniasis section in this chapter. Infection in dogs should be monitored and infected dogs should be treated or managed according to locally acceptable measures. In industrialized countries, dogs are usually treated, but they often relapse. In many developing countries, massive culling of infected dogs has failed, except in China. Insecticide-impregnated collars have proved effective in the Islamic Republic of Iran and southern Europe, reducing incidence of canine and human visceral leishmaniasis.

10. **Management of patient—**

1) Blood and body fluid precautions.
2) Treatment: the most effective drug is liposomal amphotericin B, but its high cost has generally restricted its use to industrialized countries. However, recently introduced preferential pricing for public sectors and nonprofit organizations in developing countries has increased its use. Pentavalent antimonials (sodium stibogluconate and meglumine antimonate) remain the first-line treatment in most countries. Combination treatment with pentavalent antimonials and paromomycin are found to be effective and recommended as first-line treatment in East Africa. Cases that do not respond to antimony may be treated with liposomal amphotericin B or amphotericin B deoxycholate. Liposomal amphotericin B is the safest antileishmanial medicine at present.

    Due to a high level of primary resistance to antimonials in southeast Asia and better efficacy of miltefosine and its suitability for the elimination program as the only oral drug, it was recommended as first-line treatment in this region. However, recent studies indicated high treatment failure in Nepal. Liposomal amphotericin B is currently recommended in southeast Asia as first-line treatment for visceral leishmaniasis. Studies are underway to determine the safety and efficacy of various combinations and to prevent development of resistance.

11. **Management of contacts and the immediate environment—** Control measures to interrupt the local transmission cycle in the most practical way.

12. **Special considerations—**

1) Reporting: report to local health authority is required in most endemic areas.
2) Epidemic measures: effective control must include an understanding of the local ecology and transmission cycle, followed by adoption of practical measures to reduce mortality, stop transmission, and avoid geographic extension of the epidemic, especially in anthroponotic foci. Active case detection and treatment of patients should reduce transmission rate. Institute coordinated programs of control among neighboring countries where the disease is endemic.

WHO Collaborating Centres provide support as required. More information can be found at: http://www.who.int/collaboratingcentres/database/en. Further information can be found at:

- http://www.who.int/leishmaniasis/en
- http://www.who.int/tdr/diseases-topics/leishmaniasis/en/index.html

[D. A. Dagne, J. Jannin]

LEPROSY
(Hansen's disease)

DISEASE	ICD-10 CODE
LEPROSY	ICD-10 A30

1. Clinical features—A chronic infectious disease of the skin and peripheral nerves whose clinical manifestations reflect a continuum between 2 forms of disease, tuberculoid and lepromatous. Under WHO classification, tuberculoid leprosy is termed paucibacillary and exhibits 1-5 hypopigmented or reddish anesthetic lesions, generally characterized as large, flat plaques with irregular borders and asymmetric distribution. Lepromatus leprosy is termed multibacillary under WHO classification and the lesions are more numerous, typically symmetric, and consist of small, smooth hyperpigmented papules and plaques which may or may not exhibit loss of sensation. In addition, enlargement of superficial nerves (e.g., auricular, ulnar, median, radial, superficial peroneal, posterior tibial nerves) may be seen. Nerve involvement may occur together or separately as sensory, motor, and/or autonomic neuropathies.

Clinical manifestations can include 2 acute adverse events: reversal reactions and erythema nodosum leprosum (ENL). The former is characterized by edema and erythema of existing skin lesions, formation of new skin lesions, neuritis, additional sensory and motor loss, and/or edema of hands, feet, and face. ENL is characterized by appearance of tender, erythematous subcutaneous nodules on apparently normal skin and is often accompanied by systemic symptoms such as fever, malaise, anorexia, arthralgia, and edema. Both are considered medical emergencies. Differential diagnosis of leprosy includes psoriasis, vitiligo, tinea versicolor, pityriasis alba, sarcoidosis, syphilis, mycosis fungoides, miliaria profunda, and streptocerciasis, as well as other mycobacterial infections and infiltrative skin diseases.

2. Causative agent—*Mycobacterium leprae*. This bacterium cannot be grown in bacteriological media or cell cultures.

3. Diagnosis—Clinical diagnosis is based on complete skin examination.

1) Identification of one or more chronic skin lesions that have not responded to treatment for other diagnoses, often with reduction or loss of sensation within the lesion.
2) Search for signs of peripheral nerve involvement (hypoesthesia, anesthesia, paralysis, muscle wasting, and/or trophic ulcers).
3) Conduct bilateral palpation of peripheral nerves (great auricular nerve, ulnar nerve at the elbow, radial cutaneous nerve and median nerve at wrist, peroneal nerve at the head of the fibula, and the posterior tibial nerve at the medial malleolus) for enlargement and tenderness.
4) Test skin lesions for sensation (light touch, pinprick, and temperature discrimination).
5) Test for motor weakness and sensory loss (see WHO Eye, Hand, and Foot Examination and Scoring [section 7.3] at: http://apps.who.int/iris/bitstream/10665/37409/1/WHO_TRS_768.pdf?us=1).

Laboratory diagnosis is through identification of the presence of alcohol-acid-fast bacilli in slit skin smears (incision-scrape method) or by full thickness skin biopsy (preferable). In practice, laboratory studies are not essential for the diagnosis of leprosy; however, confirmation by skin biopsy is recommended if at all possible. The immunological lepromin test, used in the past to classify patients, is not diagnostic and should be reserved only for research activities.

4. Occurrence—Though changes in data reporting make trend analysis difficult, the incidence of leprosy appears to be declining in most countries. Declines are attributable to a combination of socioeconomic development, effective treatment of cases, and widespread Bacillus Calmette–Guérin (BCG) vaccination. During 2011, approximately 219,000 persons were reported to have been diagnosed with leprosy, more than three-quarters of them in India, Brazil, and Indonesia.

WHO has targeted the disease for elimination (defined as registered prevalence of <1 case/10,000 population). By 2010 this had been achieved in all but 3 of the 122 countries where the disease was considered a public health problem by WHO in 1985: Brazil, Sudan, and Liberia; however, the highest prevalence rates in the world are currently found in the Republic of the Marshall Islands, the Federated States of Micronesia, and Kiribati.

5. Reservoir—Humans and armadillos are the only proven reservoirs.

6. Incubation period—Incubation has been reported from as short as a few weeks to 30 years; however, the average incubation period is between 3 and 10 years.

7. Transmission—*M. leprae* transmission is favored by close contact. The bacterium may be transmitted from nasal mucosa, possibly through respiratory secretions, but the exact mechanism of transmission is not clearly understood. Indirect transmission is unlikely, although the bacillus can survive up to 7 days in dried nasal secretions.

Clinical and laboratory evidence suggest that infectiousness is lost in most instances within a day of beginning treatment with multidrug therapy (MDT).

8. Risk groups—Persons at highest risk are those living in endemic areas in close contact with multibacillary cases. The disease is rarely seen in children younger than 3 years (however, cases have been identified in children <1 year). There is accumulating evidence that genetic factors play a major part in determining risk of disease, leading to varying estimates of the percentage of population with innate immunity, the maximum estimate being up to 95% of individuals of northern European descent. Leprosy reactions may be masked in patients with advanced HIV disease and patients may be at risk for reversal reactions after immune reconstitution while under antiretroviral treatment.

9. Prevention—

1) Early detection and prompt MDT of cases.
2) Evaluation and treatment of infected household contacts.

10. Management of patient—The availability of effective and time-limited treatment, with rapid elimination of infectiousness, has changed the management of the leprosy patient from societal isolation to ambulatory treatment.

1) Health education and counseling of patients and relatives must stress that effective MDT is available, that patients under continuous treatment are not infectious, and that physical and social disabilities can be prevented.
2) Isolation is unnecessary and can lead to stigmatization. No restrictions in employment or attendance at school are indicated.
3) Hospitalization should be limited to those in need of procedures such as surgical correction of deformities and treatment of trophic ulcers.
4) Treatment: combined chemotherapy regimens are essential and drugs are available free of charge to most countries from WHO or through national health programs.

The number of skin lesions is taken as an indicator of bacillary load and is used to guide treatment. The standard WHO regimens are:

- Adults with more than 5 skin lesions—a 12-month oral course of rifampicin, dapsone, and clofazimine.
- Adults with 1-5 skin lesions—a 6-month oral course of rifampicin and dapsone.

Patients must be advised to complete the full course of treatment and to seek care in the event of drug side effects and leprosy reactions. Serious side effects from MDT include pruritic skin rashes, urticaria, jaundice, and renal failure. Patients under treatment should be monitored for complications and may need to be treated in a referral center.

Corticosteroids are the mainstay of management of acute reactions associated with neuritis (both reversal reactions and ENL). Thalidomide is also very effective in treating ENL; however, teratogenicity is a major side effect limiting its use. Clofazimine is not useful in managing acute ENL but may be of value in treating chronic cases as well as in the prevention of ENL reactions.

11. Management of contacts and the immediate environment—
Examination and follow-up of close contacts is recommended.

12. Special considerations—

1) Continuity of care in patients is critical in order to assure completion of treatment and thus minimize risk of recurrent disease and disability. This is especially true for patients who move from one country to another, and they should be advised, prior to moving, to contact the public health service in their new country when they arrive.
2) Leprosy reactions can occur prior to, during, or after completion of treatment; this does not indicate inadequate treatment, but rather immune reaction to antigens of *M. leprae*. As these reactions may result in disability, follow up with patients should continue for several years after completion of treatment.

Further information can be found at: http://www.who.int/lep and http://www.who.int/tdr/diseases/leprosy/en. Information about The National Hansen's Disease Program (providing free services for the USA at 1-800-642-2477) can be found at: http://www.hrsa.gov/hansensdisease.

[T. Doker, D. Blaney]

❖

LEPTOSPIROSIS
(Weil's disease, canicola fever, hemorrhagic jaundice, mud fever, canefield fever, swineherd disease, rat urine disease)

DISEASE	ICD-10 CODE
LEPTOSPIROSIS	ICD-10 A27

1. Clinical features—A bacterial zoonotic disease that is self-limiting and often clinically inapparent in the majority of cases but can cause fulminant fatal disease. The disease typically presents as one of the following 4 clinical categories:

1) mild, influenza-like illness
2) Weil's syndrome characterized by jaundice, renal failure, hemorrhage, and myocarditis with arrhythmias
3) meningitis or meningoencephalitis
4) pulmonary hemorrhage with respiratory failure (Leptospirosis Associated Pulmonary Haemorrhage Syndrome)

Clinical illness lasts from a few days to 3 weeks or longer. Generally, there are 2 phases in the illness. The acute, or leptospiremic, phase occurs during the first week of illness and is characterized by the abrupt onset of high fever, myalgias (calves and lumbar region), and headache (retro-orbital and frontal). Other acute manifestations can include nausea, vomiting, abdominal pain, diarrhea, cough, photophobia, and a truncal or pretibial rash. About 30% or more of patients also have conjunctival suffusion (redness of the conjunctiva)—a pathognomonic finding of leptospirosis when observed with scleral icterus. The second, or immune, phase occurs in conjunction with the development of the antibody response and is characterized by prolonged fever and systemic complications, such as jaundice, renal failure, bleeding, respiratory insufficiency with or without hemoptysis, hypotension, myocarditis, meningitis, mental confusion, and depression. The 2 phases can be separated by a 3- to 4-day abatement of fever. However, the distinction between the phases might not be apparent, and patients sometimes present only in the second phase. Recovery of untreated cases can take several months.

It is estimated that between 5% and 10% of clinical infections progress to severe illness. The icteric form (Weil's disease) is associated with severe hepatic dysfunction and hemorrhage, cardiac, pulmonary and neurological involvement, and high mortality. However, severe complications can also occur in patients without jaundice. Prognostic predictors for death include age older than 40 years, oliguria, respiratory insufficiency, pulmonary hemorrhage, cardiac arrhythmias, and altered mental status. Deaths are mainly due to renal failure, cardiopulmonary failure, widespread hemor-rhage, and, rarely, liver failure. Case-fatality rates are estimated to be from 5%–15% in patients with severe illness, to more than 50% in those with pulmonary hemorrhage syndrome, characterized by massive pulmonary bleeding and acute respiratory distress.

In countries where leptospirosis is endemic, it appears to be a significant cause of undiagnosed aseptic meningitis (between 5% and 40% of cases). Late sequelae can occur including chronic fatigue; neuropsychiatric symptoms (paresis, depression); and unilateral or bilateral uveitis, characterized by iritis, iridocyclitis, and chorioretinitis, which can develop up to 18 months after acute illness and persist for years.

Cases are often under-recognized or misdiagnosed as dengue, malaria, aseptic meningitis, encephalitis, and influenza due to the nonspecific manifestations of acute leptospirosis. Severe leptospirosis must be differentiated from other causes of acute jaundice and renal failure, such as rickettsial disease, hantaviral infection, enteric fevers, viral hepatitis, and Gram-negative sepsis. During pregnancy infection can result in fetal death, abortion, stillbirth, or congenital infection.

2. Causative agents—Organisms from the genus *Leptospira* are classified into 20 named pathogenic and nonpathogenic genomospecies as determined by deoxyribonucleic acid (DNA)–DNA hybridization. They are subdivided into nearly 300 antigenically defined serovars, which are grouped into 26 serogroups based on serologic relatedness. Serologic classification continues to provide useful epidemiologic information, since serogroups and serovars are often associated with specific animal reservoirs. The severity of illness tends to vary with the infecting serovar.

3. Diagnosis—Clinical diagnosis is by isolation of leptospires from blood or cerebrospinal fluid during the first 7–10 days of acute illness, or from urine beginning in the second week of illness.

Immunoglobulin class G (IgG) assays, enzyme-linked immunosorbent assay [ELISA] assays, and antiwhole *Leptospira* immunoglobulin class M (IgM) detection kits in enzyme-linked immunosorbent assay or rapid formats, are used to provide presumptive confirmation for leptospirosis. However, sensitivity is low (39%–72%) during acute-phase illness (first 7 days). Immunofluorescence, immunohistochemical, and nucleic acid detection techniques are used for the demonstration of leptospires in clinical and autopsy specimens.

Polymerase chain reaction (PCR) assays for detection of leptospire DNA have been developed for use on clinical samples, such as blood or urine, and can be used for diagnostic testing on whole blood during the first 4 days of clinical illness, and on urine after the first week of illness. These tests are available in reference and research laboratories. Direct examination of blood or urine using dark-field microscopy has poor sensitivity and specificity. Inoculation of experimental animals, such as golden hamsters, guinea pigs, or gerbils, can also confirm diagnosis but is rarely used. Where laboratory capacity is not well established, a positive test by 2 different rapid diagnostic tests could be considered as a laboratory confirmed case.

Diagnosis is most frequently confirmed by seroconversion, from a negative to a positive value, or is demonstrated by 4-fold or greater increase in serum agglutination titer on the microscopic agglutination test (MAT)— the confirmatory serologic test, using acute and convalescent specimens obtained at least 10 days apart. Seroconversion can occur as early as 5–7 days after disease onset but might not develop until after 10 days or longer, especially if antimicrobial therapy is initiated. Patients can develop cross-reactive antibodies to several serovars during acute infection; these gradually decrease weeks to months later. Different serovars of leptospires can occur in different regions. Therefore, the MAT preferably uses a panel of locally occurring leptospire serovars. However, antibody titer increase can be delayed or absent in some patients, and seroconversion can occur asymptomatically, especially in endemic areas. IgM-class antibodies can remain detectable for months to years at low titers.

Culture and isolation can be very difficult, requiring special media and incubation for up to 16 weeks, and the sensitivity of culture for diagnosis is low.

4. Occurrence—Worldwide, except polar regions. The disease is most prevalent in tropical and subtropical regions, with the highest incidence reported in island countries or low-lying countries with frequent flooding. Leptospirosis is an endemic disease in rural subsistence farming areas and urban slum settlements in tropical regions because of the high density of domestic and wild reservoirs and poor sanitation. Rodent-borne leptospirosis exposure appears to be increasing in urban areas, especially during floods.

Outbreaks can occur following excessive rainfall or flooding, especially in endemic areas. They also occur among those exposed to fresh river, stream, canal, and lake water contaminated by the urine of domestic and wild animals and to the urine, body fluids, and tissues of infected animals. In recent years, large outbreaks have been reported in Asia, Europe, Australia, and the Americas. Affluent populations are increasingly affected following travel, recreation, and water sports in contaminated waters, especially after immersion or swallowing water.

5. Reservoir—Approximately half of the pathogenic serovars belong to *Leptospira interrogans* or *Leptospira borgpetersenii*. Pathogenic leptospires are naturally carried in the renal tubules and genital tract of wild and domestic animals, which serve as natural maintenance hosts and can remain asymptomatic shedders for years or even for life. Serovars are adapted to one or more reservoir animal species, such as rats (*L. interrogans* serovars Copenhageni and Icterohaemorrhagiae), swine (*L. interrogans* serovar Pomona), cattle (*L. borgpetersenii* serovar Hardjo), dogs (*L. interrogans* serovar Canicola), and raccoons (*L. interrogans* serovar Autumnalis). The leptospires can be shed in infected urine, amniotic fluid, or placental tissue and contaminate soil and water. They can remain viable for weeks or months under favorable conditions in moist soil or water, especially where temperatures are 28°C-32°C.

A high proportion of both stray and domestic dogs in some urban and suburban areas show evidence of infection and shed leptospires in the urine. Other animal hosts, some with a shorter carrier state, include feral rodents, badgers, deer, squirrels, foxes, skunks, raccoons, and opossums. Reptiles and frogs have been found to carry pathogenic leptospires but are unlikely to play an important epidemiological role.

6. Incubation period—Usually 5-14 days, with a range of 2-30 days.

7. Transmission—Contact of the skin (especially if abraded or after prolonged immersion) or mucous membranes with:

1) moist soil or vegetation contaminated with the urine of infected animals
2) contaminated waters (e.g., through swimming, wading in flood-waters, accidental immersion, or occupational abrasion)
3) urine, fluids, or tissues of infected animals

Occasionally, transmission can be by consuming water or food contaminated with urine of infected animals (often rats), or through inhalation of droplet aerosols of contaminated fluids.

Direct person-to-person transmission is rare. Leptospires can be excreted in the urine—usually for 1 month, although leptospiruria has been observed in humans for months, even years, after acute illness.

8. Risk groups—Children and adults in areas where infection is endemic in animal reservoirs. An occupational hazard for agricultural workers such as rice and sugarcane field workers; fish workers; miners; veterinarians; workers in animal husbandry, dairies, and abattoirs; sewer workers; and military troops.

9. Prevention—

1) Educate the public on modes of transmission, avoidance of swimming or wading in potentially contaminated waters.
2) Protect workers in hazardous occupations by providing protective clothing and equipment such as boots, gloves, and aprons. Covering wounds with waterproof dressings could reduce the risk of infection in persons with occupational or recreational exposure.
3) Recognize potentially contaminated waters and soil; drain such waters and when possible create physical barriers, such as closing open sewers, to prevent exposures to potential sources.

Small environmental areas, such as human habitations that become contaminated, can be cleaned and disinfected; leptospires are rapidly killed by disinfectants and desiccation.

4) Control rodents and reservoir wildlife populations (e.g., raccoons, opossums) in human habitations, urban or rural, and recreational areas. Refuse removal and improved sanitation can also reduce rodent infestation. Management of sugarcane fields, such as through controlled preharvest burning, reduces risks in harvesting.

5) Segregate infected domestic animals. Humans living, working, or playing in potentially contaminated areas must avoid direct or indirect contact with the urine of infected animals. Maintain hygienic measures during care and handling of animals, and avoid contact with urine or other bodily fluids.

6) Immunization of farm and pet animals prevents illness from serovars contained within the vaccine, but not necessarily from infection and renal shedding. Any vaccine must contain the dominant local strains.

7) Immunization of people has been carried out against occupational exposures to specific serovars with varying degrees of success, but is not available in most countries at present. Serovar-specific immunity follows infection or immunization occasionally, but may not protect against infection with a different serovar.

8) Doxycycline 200 mg stat dose and then weekly for the duration of exposure might provide effective prophylaxis against clinical disease. It could be considered for preventing leptospirosis among high-risk groups with short-term exposure.

10. Management of patient—

1) Blood and body fluid standard precautions.

2) Concurrent disinfection of articles soiled with urine.

3) Treatment: treatment with antimicrobial agents should be given as soon as possible. Penicillin G and doxycycline are effective in reducing morbidity. Penicillin G is recommended for the treatment of severe leptospirosis. Third-generation cephalosporins (ceftriaxone, cefotaxime) are an alternative to penicillin. Doxycycline, ampicillin, or amoxicillin can be used as oral regimens for the treatment of mild leptospirosis. Although their efficacy is not proven, fluoroquinolone agents, azithromycin, and clarithromycin are inhibitory in vitro and have been shown to be effective in animal models and can be considered in patients with a history of adverse reactions to penicillin.

Jarisch-Herxheimer reactions can occur following initiation of antimicrobial therapy. Prompt triage of high-risk patients and aggressive treatment is required for hypotension, hemorrhage, and renal and respiratory distress associated with severe leptospirosis. Timely initiation of dialysis and mechanical ventilation are essential to preventing mortality from oliguric renal insufficiency and pulmonary hemorrhage syndrome, respectively.

11. Management of contacts and the immediate environment— Search for exposure to infected animals. Recognize potentially contaminated waters, post risk of danger, and/or drain if possible.

12. Special considerations—

1) Reporting: obligatory case report in many countries.
2) Epidemic measures: search for source of infection, such as sewers, contaminated wells and swimming areas, or other contaminated water sources; eliminate the contamination or prohibit use. Investigate industrial and occupational sources, including potential animal exposures.
3) A potential problem in endemic areas following disasters such as heavy rainfall, monsoons, and extreme climactic events (e.g., hurricanes, flooding). Outbreaks can be confused with, or occur concurrently with, outbreaks of dengue or other viral hemorrhagic diseases, typhoid, rickettsial infection, malaria, or other febrile illnesses. Difficulties in diagnosis can compromise disease control and result in increased severity and elevated mortality.
4) Surveillance case definitions: the WHO-recommended case definition for leptospirosis can be found at: www.who.int/zoonoses/diseases/Leptospirosissurveillance.pdf. The Pan American Health Organization (PAHO)–recommended case definition for leptospirosis is found at: http://www1.paho.org/English/SHA/be_v21n2-cases.htm.

[R. Galloway, M. Guerra, S. Shadomy]

LISTERIOSIS

DISEASE	ICD-10 CODE
LISTERIOSIS	ICD-10 A32

1. Clinical features—A bacterial infection that typically causes invasive disease. In older adults and persons with certain immunocompromising conditions, invasive disease usually presents as septicemia or meningitis. The onset of meningitis can be sudden—with fever, intense headache, nausea, vomiting, and signs of meningeal irritation—or subacute meningoencephalitis or rhomboencephalitis can occur. Delirium and coma may appear early; occasionally there is collapse and shock. Endocarditis, granulomatous lesions in the liver and other organs, localized internal or external abscesses, septic arthritis or osteomyelitis, and pustular or papular cutaneous lesions may occur on rare occasions. Surveillance data from the USA indicate that the case-fatality rate among nonpregnant adults with invasive listeriosis is 18%. In otherwise healthy people, *Listeria* infection is often asymptomatic but may cause an acute febrile gastroenteritis.

In pregnant women, symptoms may be mild and nonspecific—fever, headache, myalgia, or gastrointestinal symptoms—or absent. However, placental invasion can lead to fetal infection resulting in stillbirth, preterm delivery, or neonatal infection. Neonatal infection typically presents as septicemia or meningitis; meningitis is more common with late onset of symptoms (>1 week of age). *Listeria* can also cause spontaneous abortions, although the incidence is difficult to estimate since bacterial cultures are not routinely obtained. Listeriosis has not been associated with recurrent pregnancy loss. The case-fatality rate is 20%–30% in infected newborns and approaches 50% when onset occurs in the first 4 days after birth.

2. Causative agent—*Listeria monocytogenes*, a Gram-positive rod-shaped bacterium. Most human infections (95%) are caused by serotypes 1/2a, 1/2b, and 4b.

3. Diagnosis—For symptomatic patients, diagnosis is confirmed only after isolation of *L. monocytogenes* from a normally sterile site, such as blood, cerebrospinal fluid (in the setting of nervous system involvement), or from amniotic fluid/placental or fetal tissue (in the setting of pregnancy). Stool samples are of limited use and are not recommended. *L. monocytogenes* can be isolated readily on routine media, but care must be taken to distinguish this organism from other Gram-positive rods, particularly diphtheroids. Selective enrichment media improve rates of isolation from contaminated specimens. The cultures can be expected to take 1–2 days to grow. Importantly, a negative culture does not rule out infection in the presence of strong clinical suspicion. Serological tests are unreliable and not recommended at the present time.

4. Occurrence—Worldwide, but uncommonly diagnosed and reported in many regions. *Listeria* infections account for a small fraction of all foodborne illnesses. However, listeriosis is an important cause of severe illness, and causes a disproportionately high number of hospitalizations and deaths compared with other foodborne pathogens, such as *Salmonella*. Most infections are sporadic, but numerous outbreaks have been reported.

Less than 20% of clinical cases are associated with pregnancy. In non-pregnant adults, infections occur mainly after 40 years of age. Outbreaks in health care settings have been reported. Asymptomatic infections probably occur at all ages, although they are only clinically important during pregnancy because of the risk of fetal loss.

5. Reservoir—Animal reservoirs include domestic and wild mammals, fowl, and humans. *Listeria monocytogenes* can be detected in soil, water, mud, forage, livestock food, and silage. The seasonal use of silage as fodder is frequently followed by an increased incidence of listeriosis in animals.

Unlike most other foodborne pathogens, *Listeria* can multiply in refrigerated foods. *Listeria* can grow and survive in biofilms in production facilities, enabling attachment (e.g., to stainless steel surfaces) and transfer to food products. Bacteria in biofilms can show increased resistance to sanitizers, disinfectants, and antimicrobial agents.

6. Incubation period—Typically, 2 or 3 weeks. However, cases have occurred up to 70 days after a single exposure to a contaminated product. Data from some outbreak investigations suggest that the median incubation period is longer among pregnant women than nonpregnant adults.

7. Transmission—Nearly all cases result from foodborne transmission. Outbreaks have been reported in association with dairy products, especially soft cheeses made from raw (unpasteurized) milk, processed and ready-to-eat meats (e.g., hot dogs, pâté, and deli meats), raw vegetables, and cantaloupe melon.

In neonatal infections, *L. monocytogenes* is almost always transmitted from mother to fetus—most likely transplacentally, during passage through the birth canal, or perhaps from ascending infection from vaginal colonization. Neonatal clusters in nursery settings have been reported, including one attributed to a fomite source (mineral oil).

Asymptomatic fecal carriage is common, even without a known exposure. Carriage rate estimates vary (point prevalence 1%-21%) and can be much higher among slaughterhouse workers, laboratory workers who work with *L. monocytogenes* cultures, and in asymptomatic house-hold contacts of persons with invasive listeriosis. Infected individuals can shed the organisms in their stools for several months.

Determination of the infectious dose has been elusive. Newer risk assessment modeling has enabled the preparation of dose-response curves that indicate that the probability of infection varies markedly, depending on the dose and strain ingested and on the susceptibility of the host.

8. Risk groups—There is a strong association between decreased immunity (particularly cell-mediated) and invasive listeriosis. The population groups at increased risk include pregnant women, persons with debilitating illnesses or conditions, such as malignancy, organ and bone marrow transplantation, diabetes, cirrhosis, renal disease, heart disease, and HIV infection, and persons who take corticosteroids. The normal immunosuppression of pregnancy may account for the higher risk of invasive disease in this population. Among older adults, risk increases with advancing age because of immunosenescence and the higher prevalence of underlying illnesses. There is no evidence of acquired immunity.

9. Prevention—Preventing listeriosis requires many actions that are similar to those for preventing other foodborne illnesses. However, additional actions to ensure food safety, including avoidance of certain foods and proper preparation and storage, are especially important for groups at higher risk for invasive listeriosis (pregnant women, older adults, and immunocompromised individuals).

1) Higher risk groups should not consume unpasteurized milk or soft cheeses made with unpasteurized milk. They should not eat ready-to-eat meats, hot dogs, other processed meats, or leftover foods unless heated until steaming hot. These groups should not eat refrigerated smoked seafood, unless it is part of a dish that is cooked and hot, such as a casserole, or unless it is a canned or shelf-stable product.

2) Thoroughly wash raw vegetables before eating, and keep them separate from raw food from animal sources (e.g., beef, pork, or poultry). Thoroughly cook raw food from animal sources. Wash hands, knives, and cutting boards after handling uncooked foods.

3) Use a thermometer to ensure the refrigerator is 4.4°C (40°F) or colder, and the freezer is −17.8°C (0°F) or colder.

4) Manufacturers should ensure the safety of all foods of animal origin. Pasteurize all dairy products, and irradiate soft cheeses after ripening. Use microbial growth inhibitors in processed meats where possible. Apply Hazard Analysis Critical Control Points systems and process monitoring (e.g., environmental culturing).

5) Processed, ready-to-eat, and raw foods found to be contaminated by *L. monocytogenes* (e.g., during routine bacteriological surveillance) should be recalled.

6) Avoid the use of untreated manure on vegetable crops.

7) Veterinarians and farmers must take proper precautions in handling aborted fetuses and sick or dead animals, especially sheep that died of encephalitis. Higher risk groups should avoid contact with possibly infectious materials.

10. Management of patient—

1) Enteric precautions.
2) Treatment: intravenous penicillin or ampicillin alone or together with an aminoglycoside. For penicillin-allergic patients, trimethoprim-sulfamethoxazole or erythromycin is preferred. Cephalosporins, including third-generation cephalosporins, are not effective. Tetracycline resistance has been observed.

11. Management of contacts and the immediate environment—

1) Relatively low incidence and long incubation periods can make identifying *Listeria* outbreaks difficult. Therefore, prompt and thorough investigation of all cases is important.
2) For rapid outbreak identification, case surveillance data—especially strain characteristics (e.g., pulsed-field gel electrophoresis subtyping)—should be analyzed frequently (weekly) for possible clustering. Patients in all suspected clusters should be interviewed promptly to identify common source exposures.

12. Special considerations—

1) Reporting: obligatory case report required in many countries. In others, report of clusters required.
2) WHO Risk assessment of *Listeria monocytogenes* in ready-to-eat food: http://www.who.int/foodsafety/publications/micro/en/mra4.pdf.

[B. Silk, B. Mahon]

LIVER FLUKE DISEASE

DISEASE	ICD-10 CODE
CLONORCHIASIS	ICD-10 B66.1
OPISTHORCHIASIS	ICD-10 B66.0
CHOLANGIOCARCINOMA	ICD-10 C22.1

I. CLONORCHIASIS AND OPISTHORCHIASIS

1. Clinical features—A trematode disease of the bile ducts. Clinical complaints may be slight or absent in light infections; and in heavy infections (>10,000 eggs/g of stool) abdominal symptoms occur in about 10% of patients. These result from local irritation of bile ducts by the flukes. Loss of appetite, diarrhea, and a sensation of abdominal pressure are common early symptoms. Rarely, bile duct obstruction producing jaundice may be followed by cirrhosis, enlargement, and tenderness of the liver, with progressive ascites and edema. Eggs in the gall bladder increase risk of gallstones. Liver fluke disease can become chronic, sometimes lasting 30 years or longer, but is rarely a direct or contributing cause of death, and it is often completely asymptomatic. However, it is a significant risk factor (≤15-fold increase) for the development of cholangiocarcinoma.

2. Causative agents—*Clonorchis sinensis* for clonorchiasis; *Opisthorchis felineus* and *Opisthorchis viverrini* for Opisthorchiasis. These worms are the leading cause of cholangiocarcinoma throughout the world.

3. Diagnosis—Demonstration of the characteristic eggs in feces or duodenal/bile drainage fluid. Eggs cannot be easily distinguished between these worms. Serological diagnosis by enzyme-linked immunosorbent assay (ELISA) can be performed but is not always specific. Immunoblot assays based on antigens have variable sensitivities. Polymerase chain reaction (PCR) for detection of eggs in stools has been reported to be sensitive for heavier infections and less so in light infections. Imaging, such as ultrasound, computerized tomography (CT), and magnetic resonance imaging (MRI) scans may be used as adjunct diagnostic tools.

4. Occurrence—Clonorchiasis is present throughout China (including Taiwan), except in northwestern areas, and is highly endemic in southeastern China and eastern Russia. It also occurs in Japan (rarely), the Republic of Korea, and in the Mekong River delta region of Viet Nam, and probably Cambodia and Lao People's Democratic Republic. In other parts of the world, imported cases may be recognized in immigrants from Asia. Opisthorchiasis occurs in Europe and Asia, especially in Russia and the former USSR republics, with prevalence rates of 40%–95% in some areas;

O. viverrini is endemic in southeastern Asia, with prevalence rates of between 24% and 80% in some areas, especially in Thailand, Lao People's Democratic Republic, and possibly Viet Nam.

It is estimated that the number of people infected with liver fluke are as many as 25 million, with 15 million for *C. sinensis*, 10 million for *O. viverrini*, and about 1 million for *O. felineus*. Up to 700 million people worldwide are at risk of infection.

5. Reservoirs—Humans, cats, dogs, swine, rats, and other animals for clonorchiasis; cats and some other fish-eating mammals for opisthorchiasis.

6. Incubation period—Unpredictable, as it varies with the number of worms present; flukes reach maturity within 1 month after encysted larvae are ingested.

7. Transmission—Acquired by eating raw or undercooked fresh-water fish containing encysted larvae. During digestion, larvae are freed from cysts and migrate via the common bile duct to biliary radicles. Eggs deposited in the bile passages are excreted in feces. Eggs in feces contain fully developed miracidia; when ingested by a susceptible operculate snail (e.g., *Parafossarulus*), they hatch in its intestine, penetrate the tissues, and asexually generate larvae (*cercariae*) that emerge into the water. On contact with a second intermediate host (~110 species of freshwater fish belonging mostly to the family *Cyprinidae*), *cercariae* penetrate the host fish and encyst (*metacercariae*), usually in muscle, occasionally on the underside of scales. The complete life cycle, from person to snail to fish to person, requires at least 3 months. Infected individuals may pass viable eggs for as long as 30 years; infection is not directly transmitted from person to person.

8. Risk groups—In most endemic areas, the highest prevalence is among adults older than 30 years.

9. Prevention—

1) Thoroughly cook or irradiate all freshwater fish, or freeze at −10°C (14°F) for at least 5 days. Storage of fish for several weeks in a saturated salt solution has been recommended, but effectiveness remains unproven.

2) In endemic areas, educate the public to the dangers of eating raw or improperly treated fish and the necessity of sanitary disposal of feces to avoid contaminating sources of food fish.

10. Management of patient—

1) Sanitary disposal of feces.

2) Treatment: the drug of choice is praziquantel. Albendazole, mebendazole, and tribendimidine are possible alternatives in clonorchiasis.

11. Management of contacts and the immediate environment— Prohibit disposal of night soil and animal waste (excreta) in fishponds.

12. Special considerations—Epidemic measures: locate source of infected fish. Shipments of dried or pickled fish are the likely source in non-endemic areas, as are fresh or chilled freshwater fish brought from endemic areas. Control fish or fish products imported from endemic areas.

II. CHOLANGIOCARCINOMA

Cholangiocarcinoma is malignancy of the biliary duct system. Incidence is low in western countries, but notably high in Asia where the prevalence of liver fluke infections is high. It can be divided into 2 types, intrahepatic and extrahepatic, depending on which bile ducts are affected.

The incidence of cholangiocarcinoma, especially of the intrahepatic type, is the highest in the world in the northeastern part of Thailand (78/100,000 population in males and 33/100,000 population in females) and has been associated with high prevalence of *O. viverrini* infection. Consumption of fermented food containing high levels of N-nitrosocompound and nitrosamines also accelerates carcinomatous changes of the epithelial cells in the bile duct.

Cholangiocarcinoma related to liver fluke infection may appear early in the fourth decade of life. Persons infected with liver flukes may have been carrying infection from as early as 1 year old. Cholangiocarcinoma can manifest as malignant obstructive jaundice or as a nonjaundice type with liver mass. Cholangitis is a common complication.

Alkaline phosphatase level is very high in both types. Tumor marker levels (e.g., CA 19-9, CA 125, and carcinoembryonic antigen) are high, but the alpha-fetoprotein tumor marker is normal. Ultrasonography of the liver may show single or multiple masses, with localized dilatation of bile ducts in peripheral type, or diffuse intrahepatic/extrahepatic bile duct dilatation. CT scan or MRI/magnetic resonance cholangiopancreatography is useful for staging of the disease and planning surgical intervention. Cholangiography has been replaced with magnetic resonance cholangiopancreatography where available. Surgical resection of the tumor mass can cure the disease in the early stages only. In late cases, palliative biliary bypass with stent using endoscopy, or surgery, can relieve the symptoms but does not affect survival. Results of chemotherapy are not good.

High levels of alkaline phosphatase in people with a history of liver fluke infection may be an early indication of cholangiocarcinoma and should be followed up with an ultrasonography of the liver. After confirming diagnosis, cases should be reported to a tumor registry and the patient should be managed by specialists.

[V. J. Lee, M. Ho]

LOIASIS
(*Loa loa* infection, eyeworm disease of Africa, Calabar swelling)

DISEASE	ICD-10 CODE
LOIASIS	ICD-10 B74.3

1. Clinical features—A chronic filarial disease characterized by migration of the adult worm through subcutaneous or deeper tissues of the body, causing transient swellings several centimeters in diameter, which can be located on any body part. These swellings may be preceded by localized pain with pruritus. A major symptom is pruritus localized on arms, thorax, face, and shoulders. Migration of the adult worm under the bulbar conjunctivae may be accompanied by pain and edema. Allergic reactions with giant urticaria (large urticaria with severe edema of the skin) and fever may occur occasionally.

2. Causative agent—*Loa loa*, a filarial nematode helminth.

3. Diagnosis—Larvae (microfilariae) are present in peripheral blood during the daytime and can be demonstrated in stained thick blood smears, stained sediment of blood where erythrocytes and hemoglobin have been separated (laking), or through membrane filtration. Eosinophilia is frequent. *Loa loa*-specific deoxyribonucleic acid (DNA) can be detected in blood from asymptomatic infected individuals. A travel history is essential for diagnosis in non-Africans.

Infections with other filariae, such as *Wuchereria bancrofti*, *Onchocerca volvulus*, *Mansonella (Dipetalonema) perstans*, and *Mansonella streptocerca* (common in areas where *Loa loa* is endemic) should be considered in the differential diagnosis.

4. Occurrence—Widely distributed in African rain forests, especially in central Africa. In the Congo River basin, up to 90% of indigenous inhabitants of some villages are infected.

5. Reservoir—Humans. Primate *Loa loa* occurs, but the 2 have different transmission complexes, and therefore the infection is not zoonotic.

6. Incubation period—Symptoms usually appear several years after infection but may occur as early as 4 months. Microfilariae may appear in the peripheral blood as early as 6 months after infection.

7. Transmission—Transmitted by *Chrysops* deer fly. *Chrysops dimidiata*, *Chrysops silacea*, and other species ingest blood that contains microfilariae. The larvae develop to their infectious stage within 10-12 days in the fly and migrate to the proboscis, from where they are transferred to a human host by the bite of the infective fly. The adult worm may persist in humans, shedding microfilariae into the blood for up to 17 years. In the fly, "communicability" starts from 10-12 days after its infection until all infective larvae have been released, or until the fly dies.

8. Risk groups—Susceptibility is universal. Immunity has not been demonstrated with repeated infections.

9. Prevention—

1) Diethyltoluamide or dimethyl phthalate applied to exposed skin are effective fly repellents.
2) Wear protective clothing (long sleeves and trousers) and apply screens to windows and doors of houses.
3) For temporary residents of endemic areas whose risk of exposure is high or prolonged, a weekly dose of diethylcarbamazine citrate (DEC) can be taken as prophylaxis.
4) Measures directed against the fly larvae are effective but have not proven practical, because the moist, muddy breeding areas are usually too extensive.

10. Management of patient—

1) As far as possible, patients with microfilaraemia should be protected from deer fly (*Chrysops*) bites to reduce transmission.
2) Treatment: DEC for 21 days eradicates microfilariae and may kill the adult worm and cure the infection. During treatment, hypersensitivity reactions (sometimes severe) are common.

   Ivermectin also reduces microfilaraemia, and adverse reactions may be milder than with DEC. However, when microfilaraemia is heavy (>2,000/mL blood), there is a risk of meningoencephalitis with ivermectin, and the advantages of treatment must be weighed against the risk of life-threatening encephalopathy.

   Treatment with either drug must be individualized and closely supervised. Corticosteroid and antihistamine cover should also be provided for the first 2-3 days, and treatment should be stopped at the first sign of cerebral involvement. Surgical removal of the migrating adult worm under the bulbar conjunctivae is indicated when feasible.

3) Specific recommendations exist for conduction of mass drug administration of ivermectin alone, albendazole alone, and ivermectin + albendazole in areas coendemic for loiasis and onchocerciasis, for loiasis and lymphatic filariasis, and for loiasis, onchocerciasis, and lymphatic filariasis respectively. As *Loa loa* encephalopathy has been reported following large-scale administration of ivermectin, enhanced community awareness and education on severe adverse events should be implemented prior to any such intervention.

11. Management of contacts and the immediate environment— No; a community problem.

12. Special considerations—None.

[A. Gabrielli, K. Ichimori, L. Savioli]

LYME DISEASE
(Lyme borreliosis, tickborne meningopolyneuritis)

DISEASE	ICD-10 CODE
LYME DISEASE	ICD-10 A69.2, L90.4

1. Clinical features—A tickborne, spirochetal, zoonotic disease. It is characterized by a distinctive skin lesion, systemic flu-like symptoms, and neurologic, rheumatologic, and cardiac involvement, occurring in varying combinations over months to years.

Early symptoms can vary. The first manifestation in 70%–80% of patients is a red macule, or papule, that expands slowly in an annular manner, often with central clearing. This lesion is called *erythema migrans* (formerly "erythema chronicum migrans"). *Erythema migrans* may be single or multiple. To be considered significant for case surveillance purposes, the *erythema migrans* lesion must reach at least 5 cm in diameter. With or without *erythema migrans*, early systemic manifestations may include malaise, fatigue, fever, headache, stiff neck, myalgia, migratory arthralgias, or lymphadenopathy, all of which may last several weeks in untreated patients.

Within weeks to months following infection, patients may develop neurological abnormalities, such as aseptic meningitis and cranial neuritis—including facial palsy, chorea, cerebellar ataxia, motor or sensory radiculoneuritis, myelitis, or encephalitis. Symptoms fluctuate and may become chronic. Cardiac abnormalities (including atrioventricular block and, rarely, acute myopericarditis or cardiomegaly) may occur within weeks following infection.

Weeks to years after onset (mean 6 months), patients may develop intermittent episodes of swelling and pain in large joints (especially the knees), leading to chronic arthritis; this may recur for several years. Antibiotic-refractory Lyme arthritis is a rare complication that was previously hypothesized to be linked to cross-reactivity between the borrelial outer surface protein A and the human leukocyte function associated antigen-1. This hypothesis is now considered unlikely. Chronic neurologic manifestations may rarely occur and include encephalopathy, polyneuropathy, or leukoencephalitis; in these patients the cerebrospinal fluid often shows lymphocytic pleocytosis and elevated protein levels, while the electromyogram is usually abnormal. In one published case series from Europe, which included patients of all infection stages, 89% had erythema migrans alone, 5% presented with arthritis, 3% with early neurologic manifestations, 2% with lymphocytoma, 1% with acrodermatitis chronica atrophicans, and less than 1% with cardiac manifestations. Similar observations on clinical presentation have been reported in the USA.

2. Causative agents—The spirochete that causes Lyme disease in North America is *Borrelia burgdorferi* sensu stricto, which was identified in 1982. Five other Lyme borrelia have been associated with human disease in Europe or Asia. These include *Borrelia afzelii*, *Borrelia bavariensis*, *B. burgdorferi*, *Borrelia garinii*, and *Borrelia spielmanii*. Three additional species, *Borrelia bissettii*, *Borrelia lusitaniae*, and *Borrelia valaisiana*, have been detected in patients, but their importance as human pathogens is not clear.

3. Diagnosis—In a Lyme disease endemic region, diagnosis can be made in patients presenting with an *erythema migrans* rash, with or without the knowledge of a tick bite. Similarly, patients with symptoms of later stages of illness, such as arthritis or Bell's palsy, can be clinically diagnosed and treated. In later stages of illness, however, diagnosis should be supported by 2-tiered serologic testing, typically an enzyme immunoassay (EIA), or rarely, an immunofluorescence assay (IFA), followed by Western immunoblotting in patients with a positive or equivocal EIA or IFA result. Serological tests in the early stages of illness should be interpreted with caution, however, because they are insensitive during the first weeks of infection and may remain negative in people treated early with antibiotics. In patients who have been symptomatic for less than 30 days, an immunoglobulin class M (IgM) Western blot may be helpful for diagnosis. VlsE (Vls locus expression site), or C6 recombinant antigens, increase the sensitivity of immunoglobulin class G (IgG) immunoblot. Test sensitivity increases in patients who have progressed to later stages of illness. Cross-reacting IFA and enzyme-linked immunosorbent assay (ELISA) antibodies may cause false-positive reactions in patients with syphilis, relapsing fever, leptospirosis, HIV infection, Rocky Mountain spotted fever, infectious mononucleosis, lupus, or rheumatoid arthritis.

Diagnosis of neuroborreliosis in Europe is typically accomplished through serologic testing for borrelial antibodies in cerebrospinal fluid.

4. Occurrence—USA, Canada, Europe, Russia, China, and Japan. In the USA, the vast majority of all Lyme disease cases are acquired from the northeastern and upper midwestern regions of the country, where the disease is considered to be enzootic in ticks and small rodent reservoir hosts. In Canada, the areas of risk include southern parts of Manitoba, Ontario, and Quebec; in some parts of New Brunswick and Nova Scotia; and in southern British Columbia. In Europe, Lyme disease risk extends from Portugal and the British Isles, east to Turkey, and north into Scandinavia and Russia. In Asia, disease distribution reaches across Eurasia, extending from Japan to the western part of Russia.

Disease more frequently occurs when nymphal ticks are most active in late spring or in the summer, peaking in June and July, but may occur throughout the year, depending on the seasonal abundance of local tick vectors. Dogs, cattle, and horses develop systemic disease that may include the articular and cardiac manifestations seen in human patients. The explosive repopulation of the eastern USA by white-tailed deer, on which adult ticks feed, has been linked to the spread of Lyme disease in this region.

5. Reservoir—The disease is maintained in an enzootic transmission cycle that involves ixodid ticks and wild rodents. A broad range of small rodents, and possibly birds, may serve as reservoir hosts. Of particular importance, however, are *Peromyscus* spp. in the northeastern and midwestern USA, and *Neotoma* spp. and gray squirrels in the western USA. Ixodid ticks become infected as larvae or nymphs when they feed on an infected reservoir host, and they remain infected for life. Deer serve as important mammalian maintenance hosts for vector tick species, but are refractory to infection with the Lyme borrelia. Larval and nymphal ticks feed on small mammals, and adult ticks feed primarily on deer. The majority of human Lyme disease cases result from bites by infected nymphs. Research in Europe supports the possible role of birds in dispersing *B. garinii* and *B. valaisiana*. Other studies support a relationship between *B. afzelii* and European rodents, notably *Clethrionomys* voles.

6. Incubation period—For *erythema migrans*, 3-32 days after tick exposure (mean 7-10 days). Early stages of the illness may be unapparent and the patient may present with later manifestations.

7. Transmission—Tickborne; in experimental animals, transmission by *Ixodes scapularis* and *Ixodes pacificus* usually does not occur until the tick has been attached for 36 hours or more; this is likely the case in humans as well. Shorter attachment times may be seen with *Ixodes ricinus*, however. *Borrelia* can potentially be transmitted through blood transfusion. Although no such cases have been reported, patients undergoing

Lyme treatment should refrain from donating blood. There is no evidence of natural person-to-person transmission. Despite rare case reports of congenital transmission, epidemiological studies have not shown a link between maternal Lyme disease and adverse outcomes of pregnancy.

8. Risk groups—All persons are probably susceptible. Reinfection has occurred in those treated with antibiotics for early-stage disease.

9. Prevention—

1) *Borrelia* live in blood products: no blood donation should be accepted from people suspected to have Lyme disease.
2) Educate the public about the mode of tick transmission and the means for personal protection.
3) Avoid tick-infested areas (wooded areas, or areas with high grass or leaf litter) when feasible. To minimize exposure, wear light-colored clothing that covers legs and arms, so that ticks may be more easily seen, and apply tick repellents such as N,N-diethyl-meta-toluamide (DEET) to the skin, and/or permethrin (repellent and contact acaricide) to sleeves and trouser legs.
4) If working or playing in an infested area, shower soon after being outdoors. Check for ticks daily, examining the total body area. Do not neglect hairy areas. Remove ticks promptly; these may be very small, especially nymphs. Remove ticks by using gentle, steady traction with forceps (tweezers) applied close to the skin, so as to avoid leaving mouth parts in the skin. Protect hands with gloves, cloth, or tissue when removing ticks. Following removal, clean the attachment site with soap and water.
5) Measures designed to reduce tick populations on residential properties (host management, habitat modification, chemical control) are usually impractical on a large scale.

10. Management of patient—

1) Carefully remove all ticks from patients.
2) Treatment: for adults, the *erythema migrans* stage can usually be treated effectively with amoxicillin or doxycycline. For localized *erythema migrans*, 2 weeks of treatment is usually sufficient; for early disseminated infection, 3–4 weeks. Children younger than 9 years can be treated with amoxicillin for the same period of time as adults. Cefuroxime axetil or erythromycin can be used in those allergic to penicillin or who cannot receive tetracyclines.
3) Lyme arthritis can usually be treated successfully with a 4-week course of the oral agents. However, objective neurological abnormalities, with the possible exception of isolated facial palsy, are

best treated with intravenous (IV) ceftriaxone or IV penicillin for 3–4 weeks. Treatment failures may occasionally occur with any of these regimens and retreatment may be necessary.

11. Management of contacts and the environment—Determine source of infection when cases occur outside a recognized endemic focus.

12. Special considerations—

1) Reporting: case report obligatory in some countries.
2) Epidemic measures: in hyperendemic and infested areas, identify tick species involved, if possible. See Prevention in this chapter.

[C. B. Beard]

LYMPHOCYTIC CHORIOMENINGITIS
(LCM, benign [or serous] lymphocytic meningitis)

DISEASE	ICD-10 CODE
LYMPHOCYTIC CHORIOMENINGITIS	ICD-10 A87.2

1. Clinical features—A viral infection of rodents—especially mice—transmissible to humans, in whom it produces diverse clinical manifestations. There may be influenza-like symptoms, with myalgia, retro-orbital headache, leukopenia, and thrombocytopenia, followed by complete recovery. In some cases, the illness may begin with meningeal or meningo encephalomyelitic symptoms, or these symptoms may appear after a brief remission. Orchitis, parotitis, arthritis, myocarditis, and rash occur occasionally. The acute course is usually short, very rarely fatal, and even with severe manifestations (e.g., coma with meningoencephalitis), prognosis for recovery without sequelae is usually good—although convalescence with fatigue and vasomotor instability may be prolonged. The cerebrospinal fluid (CSF) in cases with neurological involvement typically shows a lymphocytic pleocytosis and, at times, a low glucose level. The primary pathological finding in the rare human fatality is diffuse meningoencephalitis. Fatal cases of hemorrhagic fever-like disease have been reported in immunosuppressed patients after organ transplantation from lymphocytic choriomeningitis virus (LCMV)-infected donor. Transplacental infection of the fetus leading to hydrocephalus and chorioretinitis occurs, and such cases should be tested for LCMV.

2. Causative agent—LCM virus is an enveloped ambisense ribonucleic acid (RNA) virus in the genus *Arenavirus*, family *Arenaviridae*. Among viruses in the *Arenavirus* genus, LCM virus is the prototype of the Old World arenaviruses, which include Lassa and Lujo viruses.

3. Diagnosis—Laboratory methods include detection of virus RNA by conventional or real-time polymerase chain reaction (PCR) or isolation of the virus by inoculation of cell cultures with CSF collected early in the course of illness. Specific immunoglobulin class M (IgM) in serum or CSF, as evidenced by IgM capture enzyme-linked immunosorbent assay (ELISA), or rising antibody titers by immunofluorescence assay (IFA) in paired sera, are considered diagnostic. LCM requires differentiation from other aseptic meningitides and viral encephalitides in young adults or differentiation from other TORCH (toxoplasmosis, other [e.g., HIV, syphilis], rubella, cytomegalovirus, herpes simplex virus) etiologies in neonatal hydrocephalus and chorioretinitis.

4. Occurrence—Underdiagnosed, but not uncommon in Europe and the Americas. Antibody prevalence of 5%–10% has been reported among adults from the USA, Argentina, and endemic areas of Germany. Loci of infection among feral mice often persist over long periods and cause sporadic clinical disease. Outbreaks have occurred from exposure to infected laboratory animals, and infected breeding colonies of mice and hamsters for the pet industry.

5. Reservoir—The house mouse *Mus musculus* is the natural reservoir. Infected females transmit infection to their offspring, which become asymptomatic persistent viral shedders. Infection is present in some mouse and hamster colonies and transplantable tumor lines.

6. Incubation period—Thought to be 8–21 days.

7. Transmission—Virus is excreted in urine, saliva, and feces of infected animals. Transmission to humans is usually from mice, and probably through oral or respiratory contact with excreta, food or dust, or through contamination of skin lesions or cuts. Handling articles contaminated by infected mice may place individuals at a high risk of infection. Person-to-person transmission between immune-competent individuals has not been demonstrated and is unlikely. Several clusters of transmission through organ transplants have been described with severe, often fatal, clinical outcome in immunosuppressed recipients. Recovery from the disease probably indicates long-term immunity.

8. Risk groups—Individuals of all ages who come into contact with urine, feces, saliva, or blood of the house mouse are potentially at risk for infection. Laboratory workers who work with the virus or handle infected animals are also at risk as well as personnel working in breeding colonies of mice or hamsters for laboratory or pet production. Owners of pet mice or hamsters may be at risk for infection if these animals originate from colonies that have become contaminated with LCMV or if the animals become infected from other wild mice or hamsters. Human fetuses are at risk of acquiring infection vertically.

9. Prevention—Keep home and work environments clean. Eliminate wild mice and understand that rodent pets, such as hamsters and mice, could be infected. Wash hands after handling or changing animal bedding and food. Keep foods in closed containers. Pathogens monitoring of commercial rodent breeding establishments, especially those producing hamsters and mice, is helpful. Colony managers should take measures to ensure that laboratory mice do not come into contact with wild mice and that, within animal facilities, personnel handling mice follow strict biosecurity procedures to prevent transmission from infected animals. Pregnant women and immunosuppressed individuals should avoid rodent exposure.

10. Management of patient—No specific treatment. In case of severe disease in immunosuppressed people, treatment with ribavirin has been proposed. Although there is no human-to-human transmission, standard precautions are recommended.

11. Management of contacts and the immediate environment—Search home and work place for house mice, or sick or potentially infected rodent pets. Search for other people potentially exposed, especially among pregnant women or immunosuppressed people, and test them. Depopulation and surface disinfection of LCM-infected animal facilities and equipment by trained and protected personnel is recommended.

12. Special considerations—Reporting: report to local health authority may be required in some areas.

[P. E. Rollin, B. Knust, S. Nichol]

LYMPHOGRANULOMA VENEREUM
(lymphogranuloma inguinale, climatic or tropical bubo, LGV)

DISEASE	ICD-10 CODE
LYMPHOGRANULOMA VENEREUM	ICD-10 A55

1. Clinical features—A sexually acquired chlamydial infection, which, in its classic form, consists of 3 stages. The first stage is characterized by a small, painless, self-limited papule or ulcer at the site of inoculation (e.g., on the penis or within the urethra in men, or on the vulva, vaginal wall, or cervix in women), which has often resolved by the time the patient seeks care. The second stage involves extension to the regional lymph nodes draining the area of the primary lesion, where suppuration may occur. In men, inguinal and/or femoral buboes (inflamed or purulent lymph nodes) are seen that may become adherent to the skin, fluctuate, and result in sinus formation. In women, these external nodes are less frequently affected and involvement is mainly of the pelvic nodes with extension to the rectum and rectovaginal septum. This stage can be associated with fever and other systemic symptoms. If untreated, some patients progress to a chronic inflammatory stage that can be prolonged and debilitating, with fibrosis and lymphatic obstruction that can lead to formation of colorectal strictures, fistulas, lymphedema, and genital elephantiasis.

Rectal exposure in women or men who have sex with men can result in proctocolitis, with mucoid and/or hemorrhagic rectal discharge, anal pain, constipation, fever, and/or tenesmus. This syndrome may be difficult to distinguish clinically or histologically from other conditions such as inflammatory bowel disease, colorectal cancer, and lymphoma; if untreated, it can lead to chronic colorectal fistulas and strictures.

2. Causative agent—The invasive *Chlamydia trachomatis*, genotypes L-1, L-2, and L-3. These are related to, but distinct from, those chlamydial genotypes that cause ocular (trachoma) and nonlymphogranuloma (non-LGV or genital) infections.

3. Diagnosis—Direct detection of chlamydial organisms in swabs from lesions or bubo aspirates by direct immunofluorescence, nucleic acid detection, or culture is suggestive of lymphogranuloma venereum (LGV) since non-LGV chlamydial infections rarely result in lesion formation or lymphadenopathy. However, most tests are not specific for LGV, and positive specimens may need additional testing to differentiate LGV from non-LGV chlamydial infections. LGV-specific tests include serotyping, genotyping, and LGV-specific polymerase chain reaction (PCR). Serologic tests, such as complement fixation (CF) and microimmunofluorescence (MIF), can be used in conjunction with clinical presentation to support the diagnosis (single titer of $\geq 1{:}64$ and $1{:}256$, in the CF and MIF tests respectively). However, these tests have not been validated for proctitis presentation.

4. Occurrence—LGV occurs worldwide, especially in tropical and subtropical areas. It is endemic in parts of Africa, India, Southeast Asia, Latin America, and the Caribbean. Acute LGV is reported much more frequently in men than in women, whereas late complications, such as hypertrophy of the genitalia and rectal strictures, are reported to be more frequent in women.

Since 2003, LGV infection has been increasingly reported in developed countries, predominantly presenting as proctitis among HIV-infected men who have sex with men.

5. Reservoir—Humans.

6. Incubation period—Variable, with a range of 3-30 days for a primary lesion. If a bubo is the first manifestation, incubation ranges from 10-30 days to several months.

7. Transmission—Transmitted through anal, vaginal, or oral sex. Neonatal infection can be acquired during passage through an infected birth canal. The period of communicability is variable, from weeks to years.

8. Risk groups—In tropical or subtropical climates: sexually active persons. In temperate climates: men who have sex with men, especially those who are HIV-infected and have had unprotected receptive anal intercourse.

9. Prevention—Except for measures that are specific for syphilis, preventive measures are those for sexually transmitted diseases. See "Syphilis" and "Granuloma Inguinale."

10. Management of patient—

1) Refrain from sexual contact until treatment of active infection is completed and all lesions are healed.
2) Careful disposal of discharges from lesions and of soiled articles.
3) Treatment: doxycycline or erythromycin, orally for 21 days. Pregnant and lactating women should be treated with erythromycin. Although clinical data are lacking, azithromycin weekly for 3 weeks may be effective, based on chlamydial antimicrobial activity. Fluctuant buboes may require needle-and-syringe aspiration to prevent rupture.
4) In the absence of specific LGV testing, patients with a clinical syndrome consistent with LGV, including proctocolitis or genital ulcer disease with lymphadenopathy, should be treated for LGV.

11. Management of contacts and the immediate environment—Search for, test, and treat recent (e.g., past 60 days) sexual contacts of confirmed or suspected active cases.

12. Special considerations—

1) Reporting: few countries require official notification of LGV cases.
2) International measures: see "Syphilis."

Further information can be found at:

- http://www.cdc.gov/std/treatment
- http://www.who.int/topics/sexually_transmitted_infections/en

[R. Gorwitz, J. Papp]

MALARIA

DISEASE	ICD-10 CODE
MALARIA	ICD-10 B50-B54

1. **Clinical features**—Malaria is an acute febrile illness. The clinical syndrome initially resembles that in early stages of many other febrile illnesses due to bacterial, viral, or parasitic causes and is similar enough among *Plasmodium* species to make differentiation impossible without laboratory studies. Malaria should be part of the differential diagnosis in all cases of fever starting at any time between 7 days after the first possible exposure to malaria and 3 months (or, rarely, later) after the last possible exposure. It is imperative to ask for a travel history. The diagnosis must be considered in all febrile patients who have traveled to or live(d) in malaria-endemic areas during the preceding 12 months or who have received blood products, tissues, or organs from persons who have been to such areas.

Persons infected with *Plasmodium falciparum* may present with variable clinical features including fever, chills, headache, muscular aching and weakness, vomiting, cough, diarrhea, and abdominal pain. In a young child there may be irritability, refusal to eat, and vomiting. If treatment is delayed after the onset of clinical symptoms, severe malaria may develop and death may result. This is especially so for malaria due to *P. falciparum*. Clinical features of severe falciparum malaria include impaired consciousness (including coma), prostration (inability to walk or sit without assistance), multiple convulsions (>2/24 hours), deep breathing and respiratory distress (acidotic breathing), acute pulmonary edema and respiratory distress syndrome, circulatory collapse and shock, acute kidney failure, clinical jaundice plus evidence of other vital organ dysfunction, and coagulation defects. Severe falciparum malaria should be considered as a possible cause of coma and/or other central nervous system (CNS) symptoms in any person living in or recently returned from an endemic area. Case-fatality rates of children and nonimmunes with uncomplicated falciparum malaria are about 0.3%. This increases to 15%–20% once complications appear. Untreated severe falciparum malaria is almost always fatal.

The other human malarias (vivax, ovale, and malariae) are not usually considered life-threatening, although there are increasing reports of severe vivax malaria. Illness generally begins with malaise and fever for several days, followed by shaking chills and rapidly rising temperature, accompanied by headache and nausea, followed by profuse sweating with defervescence. After a fever-free interval, the cycle of chills, fever, and sweating recurs daily, every other day, or every third day. An untreated primary infection may last from a week to a month or longer and be accompanied by prostration, anemia, and splenomegaly. True relapses following periods with no parasitemia can occur in vivax and ovale infections at irregular intervals for up to 4 years due to a relapsing parasite stage sequestered in the liver (hypnozoites).

Persons who have grown up in endemic areas and acquired partial immunity, or nonimmune persons who have been taking prophylactic antimalarial drugs, may show an atypical clinical picture of malaria and a prolonged incubation period.

2. Causative agent(s)—The protozoan parasites *P. falciparum*, *Plasmodium vivax*, *Plasmodium ovale*, and *Plasmodium malariae*. Mixed species infections are frequent in endemic areas. *P. falciparum* and *P. vivax* infections are the most common species worldwide. *P. falciparum* infection represents a serious public health problem because of its tendency toward severe and fatal disease. Humans occasionally become infected with *Plasmodium* species that normally only infect nonhuman primates, such as *Plasmodium knowlesi*.

3. Diagnosis—WHO recommends that every suspected case of malaria receive a diagnostic test. Several diagnostic methods exist, including microscopy, lateral flow immunochromatographic antigen detection assays (widely known as "rapid diagnostic tests," or RDTs), polymerase chain reaction (PCR)-based assays, and serological tests. Direct microscopic examination of intracellular parasites on stained blood films allows identification of species, detection of gametocytes, and quantification of parasite density. High quality RDTs that detect malaria parasite antigens (histidine-rich protein 2 [HRP2], parasite lactate dehydrogenase [pLDH], aldolase) have comparable sensitivity and specificity to quality-assured microscopy and are useful for the initial diagnosis of malaria when quality microscopy is not available. RDTs may target one or more *Plasmodium* species. Combination RDTs can distinguish between falciparum and nonfalciparum infections and some are specific for both *P. falciparum* and *P. vivax*. HRP2-detecting RDTs may remain positive for a few weeks after parasite clearance.

Serological tests may not detect current infection. They generally determine past exposure and are therefore not useful in the acute management of individual patients. Current molecular methods of diagnosis are very sensitive but not usually affordable or practical for routine use in malaria endemic areas.

In nonimmune persons, such as travelers, early diagnosis by microscopy or RDTs and effective treatment can be lifesaving. In nearly all cases examination of the thick and thin blood film by a competent microscopist will reveal malaria parasites. If the initial test is negative, a series of blood films should be examined at 6–12 hour intervals. Malaria RDTs should be used if malaria microscopy is not available or not reliable, and HRP2-detecting RDTs can be useful for persons receiving antimalarials and in whom blood films can be transiently negative. If both the slide examination and the RDTs results are negative, malaria is extremely unlikely and other causes of illness should be sought and treated.

4. Occurrence—In 2010, 99 countries reported ongoing malaria transmission, causing an estimated 219 million cases (range 154–289 million) and 660,000 deaths (range 490,000–836,000), mostly in young children in Africa. Endemic malaria no longer occurs in most temperate-zone countries, nor in many areas of subtropical countries. Vivax malaria has the broadest geographical distribution. High falciparum transmission areas occur throughout tropical Africa, in the southwestern Pacific, in forested areas of South America (e.g., Brazil, Guyana), in southeastern Asia, and in parts of the Indian subcontinent. Malariae malaria has a similar distribution but is rare. Ovale malaria occurs at a low frequency mainly in sub-Saharan Africa, where vivax malaria occurs much less frequently in comparison.

5. Reservoir(s)—Humans are the most important reservoir of human malaria, except for *P. malariae*, which is common to man, the African apes, and probably some South American monkeys. Nonhuman primates have their own malaria parasite species, some of which are closely related to the human malarias and natural transmission occurs sporadically. *P. knowlesi* has been documented as a cause of hundreds of human infections and some fatalities in forest fringe areas in Asia where the natural monkey hosts and mosquito vector of this species occur. The species has a 24-hour life cycle, causing daily fever spikes 9–12 days after human infection. Prevention is the same as for falciparum malaria; chloroquine is effective for treatment.

6. Incubation period—Approximately 9–14 days for *P. falciparum*; 12–18 days for *P. vivax* and *P. ovale*; and 18–40 days for *P. malariae*. Some *P. vivax* strains in temperate areas have an incubation period of 6–12 months. Use of chemoprophylaxis does not prevent late-onset *P. vivax*. The incubation periods of infections acquired through blood transfusion depend on the number of parasites infused and are usually short, but may range up to 2 months. With *P. malariae*, low levels of erythrocytic parasites may persist for years before being activated to a level that may result again in clinical illness.

7. Transmission—Malaria is transmitted by the bite of an infective female *Anopheles* sp. mosquito. Most species feed at night; some important vectors also bite at dusk or in the early morning. Malaria infection begins when an infective female mosquito injects *Plasmodium* sp. sporozoites contained in her saliva into the bloodstream while feeding. A mosquito that feeds on an infected human can ingest gametocytes (the sexual stage of the parasite) circulating in the blood, and is then able to pass on the infection during her subsequent blood meals after the parasite has matured and released sporozoites into the mosquito's salivary glands.

Induced malaria refers to infection that is passed directly from one individual to another through contaminated blood or blood products, injection equipment, or organ transplant. Transfusional transmission may occur as long as asexual forms remain in the circulating blood (with *P. malariae*, ≤40 years or longer). Stored blood can remain infective for at least a month. Because there is no liver stage with transfusion-transmitted malaria, vivax or ovale relapses cannot occur. Congenital malaria refers to infection passed from mother to infant in utero.

Humans may infect mosquitoes as long as infective gametocytes are present in the blood; this varies with parasite species and with response to therapy. Untreated or insufficiently treated patients may be a source of mosquito infection for several decades in malariae, up to 5 years in vivax, and generally not more than 1 year in falciparum malaria.

8. Risk groups—Susceptibility is universal except in humans with specific genetic traits (see next 2 paragraphs in this section). Nonimmune persons, and especially young children, pregnant women, people who are immunosuppressed, and the elderly, are at risk of severe disease when infected with falciparum malaria. Clinical disease is present but often attenuated in adults in highly endemic communities who have acquired partial immunity following repeated exposure to infected anophelines over many years.

Most indigenous populations of West Africa show a natural resistance to infection with *P. vivax* because of the absence of the Duffy antigen on their erythrocytes, which is required for cell invasion and therefore infection. Persons with the inherited sickle cell trait (heterozygotes) show relatively low parasitemia when infected with *P. falciparum*, and thus are relatively protected from severe disease. Homozygotes suffering from sickle cell disease are at increased risk of severe and fatal falciparum malaria. Other genetic traits that may modify disease expression include other hemoglobinopathies (HbC, HbE), thalassemias, and glucose-6-phosphate dehydrogenase (G6PD) deficiency. The latter also affects treatment options, as primaquine causes hemolysis in G6PD-deficient persons. Immunosuppressed persons living in endemic areas are at increased risk of more frequent and higher density infections; people living with HIV/AIDS may be at increased risk of antimalarial treatment failure.

Pregnant women in endemic areas, especially primi- and secundigravidae, are at increased risk of the adverse effects of infection, especially with *P. falciparum*. In areas of intense transmission, *P. falciparum* may infect the placenta and contribute to low birth weight as well as maternal anemia. In low transmission areas, pregnant women are at high risk of severe falciparum malaria, miscarriage, and premature delivery. Vivax malaria in pregnancy in these areas has been associated with maternal anemia and low birthweight.

9. **Prevention—**

A. **Personal preventive measures for international travelers**—all people who visit an endemic area during the transmission season and who are exposed to mosquito bites (generally between dusk and dawn) are at risk of becoming infected with *Plasmodium* and developing clinical malaria. Because of the severity of malaria, the risks for nonimmune travelers and the large number of such travelers who visit endemic regions, personal protective measures taken by travelers are of utmost importance and are presented in detail. Depending on the malaria risk in the area visited, the recommended prevention method may be mosquito bite prevention only or mosquito bite prevention in combination with chemoprophylaxis or standby emergency treatment. Chemoprophylaxis should not automatically be prescribed: the choice of malaria prevention will depend on the destination, season, duration and conditions of travel, individual factors, and so forth.

1) People who may be exposed to mosquitoes in malarious areas should know the 4 principles—the ABCD—of malaria protection:

   - Be **A**ware of the risk, the incubation period, the possibility of delayed onset, and the main symptoms.
   - Avoid being **B**itten by mosquitoes, especially between dusk and dawn. Protection from biting mosquitoes is of paramount importance.
   - Take antimalarial drugs (**C**hemoprophylaxis) when appropriate to prevent infection developing into clinical disease. Antimalarial prophylactic regimens cannot give complete protection, but good adherence to the recommended drug regimen significantly reduces the risk of infection and fatal disease.
   - Immediately seek **D**iagnosis and treatment if a fever develops 1 week or more after entering an area where there is a malaria risk and up to 3 months (or, rarely, later) after departure from a risk area. Travelers to remote locations where medical care is not readily available may be counseled to carry standby emergency treatment.

   Malaria risk varies among countries and among different areas of each country. Further information, including recommended preventive measures, can be found in WHO's annually updated publication (see the country list) at: http://www.who.int/ith.

2) Reduce the risk of mosquito bites as much as possible, adapting to local circumstances:

   - Avoid being outdoors between dusk and dawn when anopheline mosquitoes commonly bite. Wear long-sleeved clothing and long trousers when going out at night. The thickness of the material used for protective clothing is critical.

- Systematically use insect repellent on exposed skin as well as clothing (especially socks and trousers). Choose a repellent containing N,N-diethyl-3-methyl-benzamide (DEET), IR3535 (3-[N-acetyl-N-butyl]-aminopropionic acid ethyl ester), or Icaridin (1-piperidinecarboxylic acid, 2-[2-hydroxyethyl]-1-methylpropylester). Apply in accordance with the manufacturers' instructions without exceeding the dosage.

- Stay in well-constructed, air-conditioned buildings in the most developed part of town if possible. Use screens over doors and windows; if no screens are available, close windows and doors at night.

- Sleep under an insecticide-treated mosquito net (ITN) or long-lasting insecticidal net (LLIN) with edges tucked in under the mattress; ensure that the net is not torn and that there are no mosquitoes inside it; sleep in the middle of the bed, avoiding contact between body and net.

- Use antimosquito sprays or insecticide dispensers that contain tablets impregnated with pyrethroids in bedrooms at night (or mosquito coils if there is no electricity).

    Protective measures should be used in combination, especially when staying in areas where there is intense malaria transmission.

3) Chemoprophylaxis: before travel, the most appropriate prophylactic antimalarial drug(s) (if any) for the destination(s) should be prescribed in the correct dosages.

- In areas with only very limited risk of malaria transmission, chemoprophylaxis may not be indicated, as the risk of side effects may outweigh the potential benefits. Travelers should, however, always be aware of the possibility of malaria if they develop a febrile disease.

- In areas where only *P. vivax* malaria occurs, and those rare places where *P. falciparum* remains fully sensitive to chloroquine, chemoprophylaxis with chloroquine can be used. Chloroquine combined with proguanil used to be a chemoprophylaxis option for mixed vivax–falciparum areas with emerging chloroquine resistance; however, this combination is now obsolete and should not be recommended.

- In areas with high risk of *P. falciparum* and reported antimalarial drug resistance, the chemoprophylaxis choices are atovaquone–proguanil, doxycycline, or mefloquine. This choice also applies to areas with moderate/low *P. falciparum* risk and high levels of drug resistance. The selection depends on the reported resistance pattern in the area to be visited, the contraindications of the various drugs, and personal preferences.

- Antimalarials that have to be taken daily (atovaquone-proguanil, chloroquine, doxycycline, proguanil) should be started the day before arrival in the risk area. Weekly chloroquine should be started 1 week before arrival. Mefloquine should preferably be started 2-3 weeks before departure, to achieve higher pretravel blood levels and to allow side effects to be detected before travel so that possible alternatives can be considered.

- All prophylactic drugs should be taken with unfailing regularity for the duration of the stay in the malaria risk area and should be continued for 4 weeks after the last possible exposure to infection, since parasites may still emerge from the liver during this period. The single exception is atovaquone-proguanil, which has an effect on early liver-stage parasites and can be stopped 1 week after return. Premature interruption of the daily atovaquone-proguanil regimen may lead to loss of this causal prophylactic effect, in which case it should also be continued for 4 weeks upon return.

- All antimalarial drugs have specific contraindications and possible side effects. Serious adverse events—defined as constituting an apparent threat to life, requiring or prolonging hospitalization, or resulting in persistent or significant disability or incapacity—are rare, and normally only identified in postmarketing surveillance once a drug has been in use for some time. Severe neuropsychiatric disturbances (seizures, psychosis, encephalopathy) occur in approximately 1 in 10,000 travelers receiving mefloquine prophylaxis and have also been reported for chloroquine at a similar rate. The risk of serious adverse reactions can be reduced by carefully observing the contraindications for each drug. A traveler who develops severe side effects to an antimalarial should stop taking it and seek immediate medical attention.

4) Standby emergency treatment (SBET): early diagnosis and immediate treatment determine the survival of patients with falciparum malaria. A minority of travelers will be exposed to a high risk of disease while more than 12 hours travel away from competent medical attention. WHO recommends that prescribers issue antimalarial medicines to be carried for self-administration by persons who may be in such exposed situations. Also, in light of the spread of counterfeit medicines,

some travelers may opt to buy antimalarial treatment before departure so that they can be confident of drug quality should they become ill. Persons prescribed SBET must receive precise written instructions on recognition of symptoms, when and how to take the treatment, possible side effects, and action to be taken in the event of drug failure. They must understand that SBET is a temporary measure and medical advice is to be sought as soon as possible for complete evaluation and to exclude other serious causes of fever. If several people travel together, the individual dosages for SBET should be specified. Weight-based dosages for children need to be clearly indicated. The drug options for SBET are in principle the same as for treatment of uncomplicated malaria, however quinine is less suitable for SBET because of the long and cumbersome treatment regimen and the dose-dependent side effects. Quinine is still needed for SBET during pregnancy. The choice of SBET will depend on the type of malaria in the area visited and the chemoprophylaxis regimen taken. Artemether–lumefantrine has been registered in some European countries for use as SBET for travelers.

5) Pregnant travelers:

- Malaria during pregnancy increases the risk of maternal death, miscarriage, stillbirth, low birth weight, and neonatal death. Pregnant travelers should not visit malarious areas unless this is absolutely necessary.

- Pregnant women have been shown to be particularly susceptible to mosquito bites. Extra diligence is needed in using protective measures, including ITN/LLIN and insect repellents, without exceeding the recommended repellent usage.

- Chemoprophylaxis with chloroquine (and proguanil) is safe, including during the first trimester, but is of very limited use. Mefloquine prophylaxis may be given during the second and third trimesters, but information on its safety during the first trimester is limited. Doxycycline is contraindicated during pregnancy. Atovaquone–proguanil has not been sufficiently investigated to be prescribed during pregnancy. In light of the danger of malaria to mother and fetus, experts increasingly agree that travel of pregnant women to a chloroquine-resistant *P. falciparum* area during the first trimester of pregnancy should be avoided or delayed at all costs; if this is impossible, good preventive measures should be taken, including prophylaxis with mefloquine where this is indicated. There is no prophylactic or SBET regimen that is effective and safe for pregnant women in areas of multidrug-resistant malaria.

- Competent medical help should be sought immediately if malaria is suspected, and SBET may need to be started as an interim first-aid measure when there are any delays.
- Women of childbearing age should preferably avoid pregnancy until 3 months after they have stopped mefloquine prophylaxis, for 1 week after doxycycline, and 3 weeks after atovaquone–proguanil. If pregnancy occurs during antimalarial prophylaxis, this is not considered to be an indication for pregnancy termination.

6) Young children:

- Falciparum malaria in a young child may be rapidly fatal. Early symptoms are atypical and difficult to recognize, and life-threatening complications can occur within hours of the initial symptoms. In infants, fever may be absent.
- Babies and young children should not be taken to areas with risk of falciparum malaria. If travel cannot be avoided, children must be very carefully protected with preventive measures.
- Keep infants between dusk and dawn as much as possible under an ITN/LLIN. Follow manufacturer's instructions on the use of insect repellents diligently, without exceeding the recommended dosage.
- Chemoprophylaxis dosage schedules for children should be based on body weight. Long-term travelers and expatriates should adjust the chemoprophylaxis dosage according to the increasing weight of the growing child. Chloroquine and proguanil are safe but of very limited use. Mefloquine may be given to infants of more than 5 kg body weight. Atovaquone–proguanil (in pediatric tablets) is used by several European and North American countries for prophylaxis in infants of more than 5 kg body weight.
- All antimalarial drugs should be kept out of the reach of children and stored in childproof containers: chloroquine is particularly toxic in case of overdose.

7) Blood donations: induced malaria is always of concern to blood transfusion services in endemic countries, and increasingly also in nonendemic countries. Blood donors should be questioned for a history of malaria or a history of travel to, or residence in, a malarious area. In many countries, travelers who have not taken antimalarial drugs and who have been free of symptoms may donate blood 6 months after return from an endemic area.

Sometimes travelers are deferred from donating blood for 1 year after their return, former residents of malaria-risk areas are deferred for 3 years, and persons diagnosed with malaria cannot donate blood for 3 years after treatment, during which time they must have remained free of symptoms of malaria. In virtually all cases, the deferral of risk individuals for a period of 6 months from the date of the last potential exposure combined with malarial antibody testing will prevent the transmission of malaria. Immigrants or visitors from areas where *P. malariae* malaria is or has been endemic may be a source of transfusion-induced infection for many years. Further information can be found at: http://www.who.int/topics/blood_safety/en.

B. Local community preventive measures in endemic areas—

1) Vector control for malaria prevention has 2 goals: protect individual people against infective mosquito bites, and reduce the intensity of transmission at community level. The most powerful and broadly applied interventions are LLIN and indoor residual spraying with insecticides (IRS), which in a few specific settings and circumstances may be complemented by other methods such as larval control and insect repellents.

- The insecticide of an LLIN kills the mosquitoes that are attracted by the person sleeping under it. LLINs protect the persons sleeping under the net and result in a mass effect on transmission when used by the vast majority of the population. WHO recommends universal coverage with LLINs, that is, full coverage of all people at risk of malaria in the areas targeted with the intervention. Information on WHO-recommended LLINs (13 products at present) can be found at: http://www.who.int/whopes/en. In order to obtain the best benefit of this highly cost-effective intervention, information on how nets should be used and maintained must be communicated to the people who will be using them.

- IRS involves the application of residual insecticides to the inner surfaces of dwellings where many anopheline vector species tend to rest after taking a blood meal. IRS has no individual protective effect but can rapidly reduce transmission when used as a community public health intervention by treatment of more than 80% of houses and animal shelters in the target area. The main constraints are operational: IRS requires a complex logistical effort involving teams of sprayers that move from community to community, and a certain number of households must be covered in a given time period. Depending on the insecticide chosen and the transmission pattern, indoor residual spraying with insecticides (IRS) may need to be carried out up to twice a year. There are currently 12 insecticides belonging to 4 chemical classes recommended by WHO Pesticide Evaluation Scheme for IRS. The choice of insecticide is made in a given area based on insecticide resistance, residual efficacy of the insecticide, the type of surface to be sprayed, safety, and costs. Dichlorodiphenyltrichloroethane (DDT) is still needed and used for IRS in some countries. Its use is closely monitored in the context of the Stockholm Convention on Persistent Organic Pollutants, which bans the use of DDT except for public health purposes. Further information can be found at: http://www.who.int/malaria/publications/atoz/who_htm_gmp_2011/en.

- In a few specific settings—where vector breeding sites are few, fixed, findable and easy to identify, map, and treat—larval control may be a useful complementary intervention. Examples of larval control include filling and draining breeding sites, increasing the speed of water flow in channels, and chemical and biological control methods (bacterial larvicides, larvivorous fish) applied to water bodies. It is carried out as part of a comprehensive strategy to control malaria or maintain low receptivity in areas where malaria elimination has been achieved. (see http://www.who.int/malaria/publications/atoz/larviciding_position_statement/en/index.html.)

2) Preventive chemotherapy, applied intermittently or seasonally, provides full antimalarial treatment to a specific high-risk target population (regardless of parasitaemia) to reduce malaria morbidity and mortality in this population. WHO presently recommends 2 strategies:

- Intermittent preventive treatment with sulfadoxine-pyrimethamine (SP) at specified time points during pregnancy (IPTp) and infancy (IPTi).

  ○ IPTp is recommended in areas of moderate-to-high malaria transmission and given at each scheduled antenatal care after the first trimester. The first IPTp dose is administered as early as possible during the second trimester of pregnancy, with subsequent doses given at least 1 month apart up to the time of delivery.

  ○ IPTi is recommended to all infants at risk of *P. falciparum* infection in countries in sub-Saharan Africa with moderate to high malaria transmission and given through the routine immunization program as 3 doses of SP along with the DPT2 (diphtheria, pertussis, and tetanus), DPT3, and measles vaccines.

- Seasonal malaria chemoprevention (SMC) is recommended across the Sahel subregion of Africa for areas of highly seasonal malaria transmission where more than 60% of clinical malaria cases occur within a maximum of 4 months. SMC is intermittent treatment with amodiaquine plus SP during the malaria season for children aged 3–59 months and is given monthly from the start of the transmission season and up to a maximum of 4 doses during the season.

3) Epidemic prevention and early detection is based on weekly reporting of surveillance data combined with monitoring of locally important factors regarding the genesis of epidemics, such as meteorological and environmental conditions and human population movements.

4) Vaccine: there are currently no licensed malaria vaccines. More than 20 vaccine projects are in clinical trials. Of these, the most advanced vaccine, known as RTS,S/AS01 is being evaluated in a large Phase 3 clinical trial at 11 sites in 7 sub-Saharan African countries. The clinical testing of RTS,S is at least 5–10 years ahead of other candidate malaria vaccines. RTS,S/AS01 is a vaccine against *P. falciparum*, with no protection expected against *P. vivax* malaria. Preliminary results have demonstrated efficacy among children aged 5–17 months in all 11 settings. If further trials confirm this, the vaccine could receive European regulatory approval as early as 2015 and would be considered as an addition to—and not a replacement for—existing malaria preventive measures.

10. Management of patient—Prompt treatment of falciparum malaria is essential, even in mild cases, since irreversible complications may rapidly appear. Infections with *P. knowlesi* may also progress rapidly into severe disease. *P. malariae* and *P. ovale* are not usually life-threatening. Cases of severe *P. vivax* malaria have been reported among populations living in (sub)tropical endemic areas.

1) For hospitalized patients, observe blood precautions. In nonendemic receptive areas, patients should be in mosquito-proof areas from dusk to dawn until microscopy shows that they have no gametocytes in the blood.

2) Antimalarial drug resistance: the development and spread of antimalarial drug resistance in *P. falciparum* threatens malaria

control. Chloroquine-resistance is widespread, with a few exceptional areas where chloroquine appears to remain effective (Central America west of the Panama Canal, Haiti, and the Dominican Republic). *P. falciparum* resistance has affected all the other antimalarial drugs to different degrees. Multidrug-resistant malaria (chloroquine, SP, mefloquine/quinine) has been reported from southeast Asia (Cambodia, Myanmar, Thailand, Viet Nam) and the Amazon basin of South America (parts of Brazil, French Guiana, and Suriname). Parasite resistance to artemisinins has been detected in 4 countries of the Greater Mekong subregion: Cambodia, Myanmar, Thailand, and Viet Nam.

Most *P. vivax* malaria infections remain sensitive to chloroquine. Focal chloroquine resistance or prophylactic and/or treatment failure has been observed in 21 dispersed countries in Africa, the Americas, and Asia. The relapsing hepatic stages of some *P. vivax* strains may be relatively tolerant to primaquine. A daily dose of 30 mg over the course of 14 days is generally required for infections acquired in the southwestern Pacific and for some strains from southeast Asia. Chloroquine-resistant *P. malariae* has been reported from Indonesia.

Current information on drug-resistant malaria can be found at: http://www.who.int/malaria.

3) Treatment of all forms of malaria:

- Severe malaria is a medical emergency. It is most commonly caused by infection with *P. falciparum*, although *P. vivax* (in [sub]tropical endemic areas) and *P. knowlesi* can also cause severe disease. After rapid clinical assessment and confirmation of the diagnosis, full doses of parenteral antimalarial treatment should be started without delay. Admit the patient to an acute illness room under close observation, or an intensive care unit if available (and in all cases of severe malaria in travelers).

- Treatment for severe malaria (all forms, in adults and children): artesunate 2.4 mg/kg body weight intravenous (IV) or intramuscular (IM), given on admission (time = 0), then at 12 hours and 24 hours, then once a day until the patient is able to take oral medication. Acceptable alternative if parenteral artesunate is not available are artemether 3.2 mg/kg body weight IM on admission then 1.6 mg/kg body weight per day, or quinine dihydrochloride 20 mg salt/kg body weight on admission (IV infusion or divided IM injection—in children in the anterior thigh and not the buttock), then 10 mg/kg body weight every 8 hours;

infusion rate should not exceed 5 mg salt/kg body weight per hour. If none of these medicines are available, use parenteral quinidine with careful electrocardiographic monitoring and frequent assessment of vital signs.

Complete the treatment by giving a full course of an effective artemisinin-based combination therapy (ACT) once the patient can take oral medication and after at least 24 hours of parenteral treatment.

Pregnant women with severe malaria should be given parenteral antimalarial agents in full doses without delay, at any stage of pregnancy. The rate of mortality from severe malaria in pregnancy is approximately 50% and higher than in nonpregnant women. Artesunate is the drug of choice. If this is not available, artemether is preferable to quinine in later pregnancy because quinine is associated with a 50% risk for hypoglycemia.

Prereferral treatment with suppositories containing artesunate (10 mg/kg body weight single dose) or any artemisinin is indicated for a severely ill or unconscious child if parenteral injection is not possible and referral is likely to be delayed.

Further information can be found at: http://apps.who.int/iris/bitstream/10665/79317/1/9789241548526_eng.pdf.

- For uncomplicated falciparum malaria most endemic countries now use ACTs as first line treatment. ACTs provide a greater than 90% cure rate in almost all situations. There are 5 ACT regimens currently recommended by WHO for treatment of uncomplicated falciparum malaria (listed in alphabetical order in next list) and the choice depends on the efficacy of the nonartemisinin partner medicine in that particular area or country:

  ○ Artemether-lumefantrine (adult dose: 4 tablets twice a day for 3 days, taken at 0, 8, 12, 24, 36, 48, and 60 hour[s]. Pediatric dosage by weight: 5–14 kg, 1 tablet at same time intervals; 15–24 kg, 2 tablets at same time intervals; 25–34 kg, 3 tablets at same time intervals; >34 kg adult regimen).

  ○ Artesunate plus amodiaquine (4 mg/kg body weight of artesunate plus 10 mg base/kg body weight of amodiaquine, given once a day for 3 days).

  ○ Artesunate plus mefloquine (4 mg/kg body weight of artesunate given once a day for 3 days plus 25 mg base/kg body weight of mefloquine usually split over 2 or 3 days).

  ○ Artesunate plus sulfadoxine-pyrimethamine (4 mg/kg body weight of artesunate given once a day for 3 days plus a single administration of SP [25/1.25 mg base/kg body weight] on day 1).

○ Dihydroartemisinin plus piperaquine (4 mg/kg body weight of dihydroartemisinin plus 18 mg/kg body weight of piperaquine, given once a day for 3 days)

In addition to improving efficacy, the use of combination therapy will help delay the emergence of drug resistance to both the artemisinin and the nonartemisinin partner medicine in the combination. Adding a single dose of primaquine renders the gametocytes of *P. falciparum* noninfectious and is recommended in settings of (pre)elimination as well as areas with identified resistance to artemisinins (http://www.who.int/entity/malaria/pq_updated_policy_recommendation_en_102012.pdf).

Alternatives to ACTs for the oral treatment of uncomplicated falciparum malaria would be a combination of quinine (10 mg salt/kg body weight 3 times daily for 7 days) together with either doxycycline (adults >50 kg: 800 mg salt over 7 days, taken as 2 tablets [100 mg salt each] 12 hours apart on day 1, followed by 1 tablet daily for 6 days. Children ≥8 years: 25-35 kg: 0.5 tablet per dose; 36-50 kg: 0.75 tablet per dose, >50 kg: 1 tablet per dose) or tetracycline (5 mg/kg/dose, maximal 250 mg/dose, 4 times a day for 7 days) or clindamycin (<60 kg: 5 mg base/kg 4 times daily for 5 days; ≥60 kg: 300 mg base per dose). If the patient is pregnant or younger than 8 years, quinine should be given with clindamycin. Atovaquone-proguanil (15/6 mg/kg body weight [adult dose: 4 tablets] once a day for 3 days) is used for treatment of uncomplicated falciparum malaria in travelers on return to countries or areas of no risk.

Acutely ill children with falciparum malaria require careful clinical monitoring as their condition may deteriorate rapidly. Every effort should be made to give oral treatment and ensure that it is retained. ACT as per national policy may be used as first-line treatment while in endemic areas. Oral treatment options for SBET and returning travelers are artemether-lumefantrine (not recommended for children weighing <5 kg because of lack of data), atovaquone-proguanil (apparently safe in children weighing ≥5 kg, but data are limited), dihydroartemisinin-piperaquine (considered safe in infants >6 months and weighing ≥5 kg), and quinine plus clindamycin (safe, but data on clindamycin are limited). Quinine + doxycycline is an option for children in some instances. Parenteral treatment and admission to hospital are indicated for very young children who cannot swallow antimalarials reliably.

Pregnant women with uncomplicated malaria can be treated in the first trimester with quinine + clindamycin (or artesunate + clindamycin if this treatment fails); ACT can be used if this is the only treatment immediately available, or if treatment with 7-day quinine + clindamycin fails, or if there is uncertainty about patient compliance with a 7-day treatment. In the second and third trimester, an effective ACT or artesunate + clindamycin or quinine + clindamycin can be given. Lactating mothers should receive the recommended antimalarial treatment (including ACTs), except for primaquine and tetracycline.

- For *P. vivax* and *P. ovale* infections, the recommended treatment is 3 days chloroquine, combined with 14 days primaquine against possible hypnozoites. Primaquine can produce hemolysis, especially in those with G6PD deficiency; patients should be tested for G6PD deficiency before primaquine is given. In moderate G6PD deficiency, prima-quine may be given spread out as weekly doses over a period of 8 weeks. Primaquine should not be administered during pregnancy, in young infants, and in severe G6PD deficiency. In areas where *P. vivax* resistance to chloroquine has been documented, an appropriate ACT (not artesunate plus SP) should be used, with quinine as a possible alternative. There is little benefit in giving primaquine antirelapse treatment in areas where reinfection is very frequent. Antirelapse treat-ment is not needed for induced infections (e.g., transfusion).
- *P. malariae* infections can be treated with chloroquine.

WHO recommendations, products, treatment doses, and drug policies can be found at: http://www.who.int/malaria. USA guidelines may differ (http://www.cdc.gov/malaria).

11. Management of contacts and the immediate environment— Determine history of previous infection or of possible exposure. If there is a history of sharing needles, investigate and treat all persons who shared the equipment. In transfusion-induced malaria, all donors must be located and their blood examined for malaria parasites and for antimalarial antibodies; parasite-positive donors must receive treatment. Malaria cases in nonendemic areas are usually imported, but some cases with no travel history have been reported in recent years. Some of these events are believed to have been caused by infected mosquitoes air-transported from an endemic area. In other situations, infected migrants and seasonal laborers from endemic areas to nonmalarious areas have been the source for outbreaks of local transmission. If the area is receptive to malaria (competent vectors present in suitable climatic conditions), persons living in the same community as well as health services should be advised about the risk of malaria; people developing malaria-like symptoms must be tested by rapid diagnostic test or microscopic examination of a blood film. The flight range of anopheline mosquitoes may reach 2 km, but in most cases it is only a few hundred meters. Vector control should be considered if several locally acquired cases occur in a small area.

12. **Special considerations—**

1) Reporting: in nonendemic areas, malaria cases should be reported to the local health authority. Outbreaks of falciparum malaria in a normally malaria-free country should be reported to WHO immediately. Ministries of Health in endemic countries report to WHO on their malaria situation, control/elimination program activities, and malaria risk areas in the context of the annually updated publications, *World Malaria Report* and *International Travel and Health*. WHO recommended surveillance standards can be found at: http://www.who.int/malaria.

Other international measures include the following:

- Disinsectization of aircraft before take-off from malaria endemic areas, using insecticide aerosols.
- Disinsectization of aircraft, ships, and other vehicles on arrival if the health authority at the place of arrival has reason to suspect importation of malaria vectors.
- Enforcing and maintaining rigid antimosquito sanitation within the mosquito flight range of all ports and airports.
- In special circumstances, screening and treatment of potentially infected migrants, refugees, seasonal workers, and other population groups, before arrival in an area receptive for malaria where transmission has been interrupted. Arrange housing of such populations as much as possible in areas nonreceptive to malaria, and/or in well constructed, screened housing that prevents mosquito entry.

2) Epidemic measures: malaria epidemics must be controlled through rapid and vigorous action and effective treatment of all cases. In confirmed *P. falciparum* epidemics where a large part of the population is infected, treatment based only on clinical grounds (fever) without laboratory confirmation of diagnosis may be necessary to cope with the patient load. As soon as possible, and before the peak of the epidemic, full coverage vector control measures should be instituted. Usually, IRS is preferred because of its rapid effect; this may be followed by the use of LLINs and antilarval measures as appropriate.

3) Disaster implications: disasters in endemic areas may lead to malaria epidemics as a result of population movements, ecological changes favoring vector breeding, breakdown of health services, crowding of people in poorly constructed housing, and/or the existence of large numbers of people without adequate housing, creating high-risk, high-exposure situations. In humanitarian emergencies in Africa, malaria has presented with an epidemic pattern, taking an extraordinarily high toll among children, and often adults. In complex emergencies antimalarial medicines with highest efficacy and safety profile are recommended for use as first-line medicine. Control priorities are early effective treatment and vector control; the latter is usually only possible after the acute emergency is over, and focuses on personal protection with LLINs, combined with IRS where feasible. In areas of intense transmission in Africa, IPTp and IPTi should be provided as soon as antenatal care and vaccination services have been (re)established. In areas of seasonal transmission in the Sahel subregion of Africa, SMC programs should be initiated as soon as is operationally feasible. Health education, as in any context, is required to support these interventions and promote better malaria control. Further information can be found at: http://www.who.int/malaria/publications/atoz/9789241548656/en/index.html.

[A. E. C. Rietveld, R. D. Newman]

MEASLES

(rubeola, hard measles, red measles, morbilli)

DISEASE	ICD-10 CODE
MEASLES	ICD-10 B05

1. **Clinical features**—An acute, highly communicable viral disease with prodromal fever, conjunctivitis, coryza, cough, and small spots with white or bluish-white centers on an erythematous base on the buccal mucosa (Koplik spots). A characteristic red blotchy rash appears on the face on the third to seventh day, becomes generalized, lasts 4-7 days, and sometimes ends in brawny desquamation. Leukopenia is common and serum vitamin A levels are often decreased. Complications, resulting from direct viral replication or bacterial superinfection, may occur up to 4 weeks after rash

and include otitis media, pneumonia, laryngotracheobronchitis (croup), diarrhea, febrile seizures, and encephalitis. In malnourished children measles may be associated with hemorrhagic rash, protein-losing enteropathy, otitis media, oral sores, dehydration, diarrhea, blindness, and severe skin infections. Persons with deficiencies of cell-mediated immunity may lack the characteristic rash and may have a progressive measles inclusion-body encephalitis. Very rarely (in ~4-11/100,000 cases), subacute sclerosing panencephalitis develops several years after infection; more than 50% of subacute sclerosing panencephalitis cases had measles diagnosed in the first 2 years of life. In adults hepatitis, hypocalcemia, and elevated creatinine phosphokinase levels are also seen.

The case-fatality rate is estimated to be less than 1% in developed countries but can be 3%-5% in developing countries, reaching 10%-30% in some localities. Both acute and delayed mortality in infants and children have been documented.

2. Causative agent—Measles virus, a member of the genus *Morbillivirus* of the family Paramyxoviridae.

3. Diagnosis—The WHO clinical case definition for measles is any person with fever, maculopapular rash and cough, coryza, or conjunctivitis. Confirmation by laboratory testing or epidemiological linkage is recommended in all cases. Laboratory confirmation is usually by detecting measles-specific immunoglobulin class M (IgM) antibodies or a significant (>4-fold) rise in immunoglobulin class G (IgG) antibody concentrations between acute and convalescent sera. Reverse transcription polymerase chain reaction (RT-PCR) is often used to confirm the presence of measles ribonucleic acid (RNA) in urine, blood, or nasopharyngeal mucus and can provide important genotype information. Less commonly used techniques include identification of viral antigen in nasopharyngeal mucosal swabs by fluorescent antibody (FA) techniques, or virus isolation in cell culture from blood or nasopharyngeal swabs collected before day 4 of rash, or from urine specimens before day 8 of rash. In low-incidence settings IgM serology may give false-positive results, often making correlation with epidemiologic data and culture or RT-PCR results necessary. Other causes of febrile rash illness include rubella, dengue, chikungunya, scarlet fever, toxoplasmosis, roseola infantum, erythema infectiosum, mononucleosis, meningococcemia, Kawasaki syndrome, and other viral exanthems.

4. Occurrence—Prior to widespread immunization, measles was common in childhood, with more than 90% of people infected by age 20 and an estimated 100 million cases and 6 million measles deaths occurring each year. Measles, endemic in large metropolitan communities, attained epidemic proportions about every second or third year. In smaller communities and areas, outbreaks tended to be more widely spaced and somewhat more severe. With longer intervals between outbreaks, as in the Arctic and some islands, measles outbreaks often involved a large proportion of the population, with a high case-fatality rate. In temperate climates, measles occurs primarily in the late winter and early spring. In tropical climates, measles occurs primarily in the dry season in the African Sahel and during the cooler rainy season in equatorial areas.

With effective childhood immunization programs, measles cases in many industrialized countries have dropped by up to 99% and generally occur in young unimmunized children or older children, adolescents, or young adults who received only 1 dose of vaccine and have a median age between 20 and 30 years. The countries of the Pan American Health Organization (PAHO) have reached the regional goal of elimination of indigenous measles transmission by providing measles vaccine through routine services to at least 95% of children, a second opportunity for measles immunization for all children at an older age, and careful measles surveillance. The second opportunity is designed to immunize children who escaped routine immunization and those who failed to respond immunologically to the first vaccine. The strategy started with a "catch-up" campaign targeting all children aged 9 months to 14 years regardless of disease history or previous vaccination status, and continued with "follow-up" campaigns conducted every 3–4 years, targeting all children aged 9 months to 4 years. In Canada and the USA, a second dose of measles vaccine is provided through routine immunization services, generally at school entry. Though the last indigenous case in the PAHO countries was in 2002, importations continue to occur and require maintenance of very high population immunity through vaccination. Measles elimination goals have been established in countries in the other 5 WHO regions—the Western Pacific region by 2012, the European and Eastern Mediterranean regions by 2015, and the African and South-East Asia region by 2020. Achievement of these goals is a key indicator of progress in the Global Vaccine Action Plan for the Decade of Vaccines.

Despite the existence of a safe, effective, and inexpensive measles vaccine for the past 50 years, measles remains a leading vaccine-preventable killer of children worldwide. After decreasing from 853,480 reported cases in 2000 to 278,417 in 2008, reported measles cases increased to 354,922 in 2011. Much of the increase is due to large outbreaks in Africa, Asia, and Europe in areas with low vaccination coverage, often combined with suboptimal or delayed campaigns. Outbreaks also revealed areas where high coverage masked the accumulation of susceptible adolescents and adults or the presence of groups with limited access to health services or reluctant to vaccinate their children. WHO estimates that 157,700 children died of measles in 2011, a 71% decrease from the estimated 548,300 deaths in 2000, with 99% of the deaths in Asia and Africa.

5. Reservoir—Humans.

6. Incubation period—From exposure to rash onset averages 14 days with a range of 7–21 days. Immune globulin given for passive protection early in the incubation period may extend the incubation period.

7. Transmission—Airborne by droplet spread, direct contact with nasal or throat secretions of infected persons; less commonly by articles freshly soiled with nose and throat secretions. Measles is one of the most highly communicable infectious diseases. The period of communicability extends from 4 days before rash onset to 4 days after rash appearance. It is minimal after the second day of rash. The vaccine virus has not been shown to be communicable.

8. Risk groups—All persons who have not had the disease or been successfully immunized are susceptible. Acquired immunity after illness is permanent. Successful immunization usually requires 2 doses of vaccine. Those receiving the first dose before 12 months of age without a second dose and those receiving only 1 dose at any time may still be susceptible. Infants born to mothers who have had measles are protected against disease for the first 6–9 months or more, depending on maternal measles antibody levels at the time of pregnancy and the rate of antibody degradation. Children born to mothers with vaccine-induced immunity receive less passive antibody and may become susceptible to measles at an earlier age. Persons at higher risk of complications with measles include children younger than 5 years, adults, pregnant women, and persons with clinical or subclinical vitamin A deficiency, malnutrition, congenital or acquired deficiencies of cellular immunity, including HIV infection and immunosuppressive therapy. Children living in more crowded conditions may also be at higher risk of complications. In children with borderline nutritional status, measles often precipitates acute kwashiorkor and exacerbates vitamin A deficiency, sometimes to the point of blindness.

9. Prevention (see also Management of Contacts and the Immediate Environment in this chapter)—

1) Public education by health departments and private physicians should encourage 2 doses of measles vaccine for all susceptible infants, children, adolescents, and young adults.

2) Immunization: live attenuated measles vaccine is the vaccine of choice. All persons not immune to measles should receive 2 doses of vaccine unless specifically contraindicated (see contraindications later in this section). Live measles vaccine, often combined with other live vaccines (mumps, rubella, varicella), can be administered concurrently with other inactivated vaccines or toxoids. Maternal antibody interferes with response to the vaccine in the infant. Vaccination at 12–15 months induces immunity in 94%–98% of recipients and reimmunization increases immunity levels to 99%.

About 5%–15% of nonimmune vaccinees may develop malaise and fever to 39.5°C (103°F) within 5–12 days after immunization; this reaction lasts 1–2 days, with little disability. Rash, coryza, mild cough, and Koplik spots may occasionally occur. Febrile seizures occur infrequently and without sequelae; the highest incidence is in children with a history of previous febrile seizures or seizures in parents or siblings. Encephalitis and encephalopathy occur in less than 1 case per million measles immunizations; since this rate is lower than the background rate, it is therefore possible that measles vaccine-associated encephalitis and encephalopathy events may not have been caused by the vaccine. Adverse events after administration of combined vaccines may also involve events associated with the other vaccines (mumps, rubella, varicella).

WHO recommends that all countries vaccinate children with 2 doses of measles vaccine. In countries with ongoing transmission in which the risk of measles mortality among infants remains high, the first dose should be administered at age 9 months and the routine second dose should be given at age 15–18 months with an interval between the first and second dose of at least 1 month. In countries with low rates of measles transmission (i.e., those that are near elimination) and a low risk of measles infection among infants, the first dose may be administered at age 12 months. The optimal age for delivering routine second dose is based on programmatic considerations that achieve the highest coverage of the second dose and, hence, the highest population immunity. Administration of the second dose at age 15–18 months ensures early protection of the individual, slows accumulation of susceptible young children, and may correspond with other routine immunizations (e.g., a diphtheria/tetanus and whole-cell pertussis vaccine [DTP] booster). If first dose coverage is high (>90%) and school enrolment is high (>95%), administration of the second dose at school entry may prove an effective strategy for achieving high coverage and preventing outbreaks in schools.

In countries where health systems are moderately or weakly functioning, conducting regular measles campaigns is a highly effective strategy for providing a second dose and protecting children who do not have access to routine health services. Because the risk of measles outbreaks is determined by the rate of accumulation of susceptible people in the population, data on vaccination coverage should be used to monitor the accumulation of susceptible people and follow-up campaigns should be conducted before the number of susceptible children of preschool age reaches the size of a birth cohort.

During community outbreaks, the recommended age for immunization using monovalent vaccine can be lowered to 6 months. Children vaccinated in these situations should still receive 2 additional doses when aged 9 months and older according to the routine schedule.

- Vaccine shipment and storage: immunization may not produce protection if the vaccine has been improperly handled or stored. Prior to reconstitution, freeze-dried measles vaccine is relatively stable and can be safely stored for over a year in a freezer or at 2°–8°C (35.6°–46.4°F). Reconstituted vaccine must be kept at 2°–8°C and discarded after 8 hours; both freeze-dried and reconstituted vaccine must be protected from prolonged exposure to ultraviolet light, which may inactivate the virus.

- Malnutrition: malnourished children are at higher risk of complications and should be a priority group for measles vaccination. Seroconversion rates after vaccination have been found in several studies to be similar in well-nourished and malnourished children.

- Revaccinations: in many industrialized countries, measles revaccination is offered at entry to high school and to universities or other institutions and to international travelers and health care workers, unless they have a documented history of measles disease or immunization with 2 doses of vaccine, or serological evidence of measles immunity. In those who have received only inactivated vaccine (available in the late 1960s), revaccination may produce reactions such as local edema and induration, lymphadenopathy, and fever but will protect against the atypical measles syndrome that has been associated with the use of inactivated measles vaccine. Children with HIV on stable highly active antiretroviral therapy should be revaccinated after achieving adequate cluster of differentiation 4 glycoprotein (CD4) levels.

- Contraindications to the use of live virus vaccines:

  ○ Patients with primary immune deficiency diseases affecting T-cell function or acquired immune deficiency due to leukemia, lymphoma, or generalized malignancy, or those undergoing therapy with corticosteroids, irradiation, alkylating drugs, or antimetabolites, should not receive live virus vaccines. Infection with HIV is not an absolute contraindication: unless severely immunocompromised, WHO recommends measles immunization of HIV-infected infants at 6 months of age followed by an additional dose at 9 months followed by a second dose after at least a 1-month interval. Many industrialized countries recommend measles vaccination only in asymptomatic HIV-positive individuals;

low CD4 counts are a contraindication to measles vaccine because of the risk of viral pneumonia.

○ In persons with severe acute illness with or without fever, immunization should be deferred until recovery from the acute phase; minor febrile illnesses such as diarrhea or upper respiratory infections are not a contraindication.

○ Persons with anaphylactic hypersensitivity to a previous dose of measles vaccine, gelatin, or neomycin should not receive measles vaccine. Egg allergy, even if anaphylactic, is no longer considered a contraindication.

○ Purely on theoretical grounds, vaccine should not be given to pregnant women; mothers should be advised of the theoretical risk of fetal damage if they become pregnant within 1 month after receipt of measles-containing vaccine.

○ Vaccine should be given at least 14 days before immune globulin (IG) or blood transfusion. IG can interfere with the response to measles vaccine for varying periods depending on the dose. The usual dose administered for hepatitis A prevention can interfere for 3 months; very large doses of intravenous IG can interfere for up to 11 months. Other IG containing blood products can also interfere.

10. **Management of patient—**

1) If practicable, children with measles should be kept out of school for 4 days after appearance of the rash. In hospitals, respiratory isolation from onset of catarrhal stage of the prodromal period up to and including the fourth day of rash reduces the exposure of other patients at high risk.

2) Quarantine of institutions, wards, or dormitories can sometimes be of value; strict segregation of infants if measles occurs in an institution.

3) Treatment: none for measles, though complications should be appropriately managed. During measles infection, vitamin A reserves fall rapidly (especially in malnourished children), which further weakens immunity. Vitamin A supplementation at the time of measles diagnosis replaces body reserves, prevents blindness due to corneal ulceration and keratomalacia, and significantly reduces measles fatality. The following Vitamin A schedule is recommended:

Age	Immediately	Next Day
<6 months	50,000 IU	50,000 IU
6-11 months	100,000 IU	100,000 IU
12 months	200,000 IU	200,000 IU

A third dose of vitamin A should be given 2–4 weeks later if at the initial diagnosis of measles signs of vitamin A deficiency (night blindness, Bitot spots, conjunctival or corneal dryness, corneal clouding, or ulceration) were present.

11. **Management of contacts and the immediate environment—**

1) Postexposure prophylaxis of contacts: household or other close contacts of persons with measles, particularly those less than 1 year of age, pregnant women, persons with immunodeficiencies, or those for whom vaccine is contraindicated, may be partially or completely protected by IG given within 6 days after exposure. Live measles vaccine should be given 5-6 months later to those for whom vaccine is not contraindicated. Measles vaccination within 72 hours of exposure may also confer some protection.

2) Investigation of contacts and source of infection: search and immunize exposed susceptible contacts to limit the spread of disease. Healthy carrier state does not occur.

12. **Special considerations—**

1) Reporting: obligatory case report in most countries. Early reporting (≤24 hours) provides opportunity for better outbreak control.

2) Epidemic measures:

- All potential outbreaks should be rapidly investigated and confirmed with an assessment of the risk of spread and mortality.
- Prompt reporting (≤24 hours) of suspected cases and comprehensive programs to immunize all susceptibles are needed to limit spread.
- All children 9-59 months of age presenting to any health facility who lack prior vaccination should be vaccinated against measles.
- If measles attack rates are high in children younger than 9 months, consideration should be given to temporarily recommend that children be vaccinated beginning at 6 months of age. Children vaccinated when younger than 9 months should be revaccinated when 9 months or older according to the routine immunization schedule.
- In day care, school, and university or other institutional outbreaks, all persons without documentation of 2 doses of live virus vaccine at least 1 month apart on or after the first birthday should be immunized unless they have documentation of prior physician-diagnosed measles or laboratory evidence of immunity. In other institutional outbreaks (e.g.,

military barracks, hospitals), new admissions should receive vaccine or IG.

- If the risk assessment indicates a high risk of a large outbreak, then a nonselective vaccination campaign should be considered. The campaign target population should be based on the susceptibility profile of the population, as determined by the age distribution of cases, and target areas should include outbreak-affected and adjacent areas where the risk assessment shows a high risk of spread.
- Effective communication to the public and to government authorities is critical to the success of outbreak response efforts.

3) Disaster/conflict implications: introduction of measles into refugee populations with a high proportion of susceptibles can result in devastating epidemics with high fatality rates. Providing measles vaccine to displaced persons living in camp settings within a week of entry is a public health priority.

4) Persons traveling to measles-endemic areas should ensure that they are immune to measles, ideally through receipt of 2 doses of measles vaccine given at least 1 month apart.

[R. Perry]

MELIOIDOSIS
(Whitmore disease)

DISEASE	ICD-10 CODE
MELIOIDOSIS	ICD-10 A24.1–A24.4
GLANDERS	ICD-10 A24.0

1. **Clinical features**—Clinical manifestations range from subclinical infection to localized acute or chronic cutaneous or visceral abscesses, necrotizing pneumonia, and/or a rapidly fatal septicemia. Melioidosis may simulate typhoid fever or tuberculosis, with pulmonary cavitation, empyema, chronic abscesses, and osteomyelitis. Overwhelming infection can occur, resulting in death from septic shock within 48 hours of generalized symptoms. Infection can become persistent and result in latent, recurrent, and recrudescing infections. A specific syndrome of meningoencephalitis with flaccid paraparesis or peripheral motor weakness occurs in 5% of cases in northern Australia. Cerebral abscess is

occasionally reported. Mortality ranges from 15%-40% despite use of appropriate antimicrobial therapy.

In humans, signs and symptoms of glanders—a highly communicable disease of horses, mules, and donkeys—are similar to melioidosis. Human glanders is associated with contact with sick animals, contaminated fomites, tissues, or bacterial cultures, and it no longer occurs in the western hemisphere.

2. Causative agent—*Burkholderia pseudomallei* is the causative agent for melioidosis; *Burkholderia mallei* for glanders. *Burkholderia pseudomallei* is a saprophytic Gram-negative motile rod; *Burkholderia mallei* is a Gram-negative nonmotile rod and is an obligate mammalian zoonotic pathogen, which can survive for only a short period in the environment.

3. Diagnosis—Depends on isolation of the causative agent from clinical specimens (blood, urine, sputum, skin lesions, and throat swab); a rising antibody titer in serological tests in conjunction with clinical signs and symptoms is highly suggestive. In some highly endemic areas, more than 50% of individuals have demonstrable antibodies but no history of overt disease. Direct immunofluorescent microscopy is 98% specific, but only about 70% sensitive compared with culture. The possibility of melioidosis must be kept in mind in any unexplained suppurative disease and sepsis, especially cavitating pulmonary disease, in patients living in or returned from endemic areas; disease has become manifest as long as 62 years after exposure.

Infection with *B. pseudomallei* cannot be differentiated serologically from infection with *B. mallei*; characterization of the isolated organism alone can lead to specific diagnosis.

4. Occurrence—Disease occurrence varies depending on location; northeast Thailand and northern Australia are considered to be highly endemic, with annual incidence rates of up to 50 cases per 100,000 people. In Thailand, it is considered to be primarily a disease of rice farmers and is a common cause of death from infectious disease in the northeast region of that country. As a result of increased recognition and availability of diagnostics, melioidosis is emerging as a significant cause of community-acquired sepsis in the tropics. Although it may manifest with a variety of clinical presentations, 50% of patients present with acute pneumonia. Cases have been recorded in many tropical and subtropical areas of Asia, Australia/Pacific Islands, and India, and less commonly in the Middle East, South and Central America, and the Caribbean; sporadic cases have been reported in Africa as well, but the extent of disease on that continent remains to be determined. Increasing numbers of imported cases in travelers visiting endemic countries are being seen in the USA and Europe. The disease is reported to be highly seasonal, with 75%-85% of cases presenting during the rainy season when exposure to the organism is believed to be greatest. Following the tsunami of 2004, an increase in the number of melioidosis cases was observed, mainly among repatriated tourists.

Glanders has been eliminated from most areas of the world, although enzootic foci are believed to exist in Asia and some eastern Mediterranean countries.

5. Reservoir—In endemic areas, *B. pseudomallei* is found in soil and water. Various animals, including sheep, goats, horses, swine, monkeys, and rodents can become infected, without evidence that they are important reservoirs, except in the transfer of the agent to new foci. *B. mallei* is zoonotic in nature, with equids serving as the primary reservoir.

6. Incubation period—Usual range is from 1–21 days with a mean of 9 days and can be as short as a few hours with high inoculum. However, for melioidosis, years may elapse between presumed exposure and appearance of clinical disease.

7. Transmission—For melioidosis, transmission usually occurs through contact with contaminated soil or water through overt or inapparent skin wounds, inhalation of soil dust, and aspiration or ingestion of contaminated water. Person-to-person transmission is extremely rare but has occurred through direct or sexual contact in 3 reported cases. Transmission has also been reported in utero and through breastfeeding in mothers with mastitis. Rare nosocomial transmission through contaminated needles has also been reported. Direct zoonotic transmission from animals to humans is not known to occur. Glanders, in contrast, is a zoonotic disease, with humans acquiring disease from direct contact with infected animals.

8. Risk groups—Up to 80% of adult cases have a predisposing medical condition such as diabetes, cirrhosis, alcoholism, or chronic renal disease, which may precipitate disease or recrudescence in asymptomatic infected individuals. Other risk factors for disease include chronic lung disease (such as that associated with cystic fibrosis and chronic obstructive pulmonary disease), thalassemia, and malignancy and glucocorticoid treatment or other non-HIV-related immune suppression; HIV infection is not associated with higher risk for disease. Fatality rate is also greater in persons with underlying predisposing disease risk. Highest risk for melioidosis exists for persons living in endemic areas, as well as military service personnel who have served in areas with endemic disease, adventure travelers, ecotourists, construction and resource extraction workers, and persons such as rice farmers, whose contact to contaminated soil and water may expose them to the infectious agent. Laboratory workers who work with isolates of *B. pseudomallei* are also at risk of infection if proper biosafety procedures are not followed. Disease in humans is more common than previously thought, especially among people in endemic areas who have close contact with soil or water containing the infectious agent, but is still thought to be underdiagnosed in most endemic areas.

Rare and sporadic human glanders infections are reported almost exclusively in those whose occupations involve contact with animals or work in laboratories (e.g., veterinarians, equine butchers, pathologists).

9. **Prevention—**

1) Persons with predisposing medical conditions, including diabetes, and those with traumatic wounds, should avoid exposure to soil or water in endemic areas.
2) In endemic areas, skin lacerations, abrasions, or burns that have been contaminated with soil or surface water should be immediately and thoroughly cleaned.
3) Use of boots and gloves is recommended for occupations that involve contact with soil and water, such as work in rice fields.
4) Prevention of glanders depends on control of glanders in equine species and care in handling causative organisms.

10. **Management of patient—**

1) Isolation: contact precautions. Standard blood and body fluid precautions should be taken.
2) Safe disposal of sputum and wound discharges.
3) Treatment: melioidosis requires long courses of antimicrobial therapy. Initial treatment consists of supportive measures and 10–14 days or more of intensive-phase therapy with intravenous ceftazidime, imipenem, or meropenem. Following intensive-phase therapy, treatment is ambulatory eradication phase therapy with 3–6 months of oral trimethoprim-sulfamethoxazole. The infection may be slow to respond to treatment, and even with 20 weeks of treatment, 10% of cases relapse. Treatment for an inadequate length of time leads to a high probability of relapse. Abscesses unresponsive to antimicrobial therapy should be drained if possible.

11. **Management of contacts and the immediate environment—** Human carriers are not known.

12. **Special considerations—**

1) Epidemic measures: usually a sporadic disease. Outbreaks should be investigated to determine if there is a point source.
2) Deliberate use: *B. pseudomallei* is a potential agent for deliberate use that is moderately easy to disseminate and has a high case fatality rate among symptomatic cases. In the unlikely event of the intentional release of *B. pseudomallei*, the value of prophylactic medication is unproven but may be efficacious. In

the event that postexposure prophylaxis is indicated, treatment with trimethoprim-sulfamethoxazole (co-trimoxazole) is recommended. *Burkholderia mallei* is also a potential agent for deliberate use, with the same recommendation for postexposure prophylaxis as *B. pseudomallei*.

[D. Blaney]

MENINGITIS

DISEASE	ICD-10 CODE
VIRAL MENINGITIS	ICD-10 A87
NONPYOGENIC MENINGITIS	ICD-10 G03.0
BACTERIAL MENINGITIS	ICD-10 G00
MENINGOCOCCAL MENINGITIS	ICD-10 A39.0
HEMOPHILUS MENINGITIS	ICD-10 G00.0
PNEUMOCOCCAL MENINGITIS	ICD-10 G00.1
NEONATAL MENINGITIS	ICD-10 P37.8, P35-P37, G00, G03

Meningitis is caused by inflammation of the meninges that covers the brain and spinal cord, and it can be caused by a variety of organisms that include bacteria, fungi, or viruses. It is a serious condition that can be life-threatening.

I. VIRAL MENINGITIS (aseptic meningitis, nonbacterial meningitis)

1. Clinical features—A relatively common but rarely serious clinical syndrome with multiple viral etiologies, characterized by sudden onset of febrile illness with signs and symptoms of headache with meningeal involvement. Cerebrospinal fluid (CSF) findings are pleocytosis (usually mononuclear, occasionally polymorphonuclear in early stages), increased protein, normal sugar, and absence of bacteria. A rubella-like rash characterizes certain types caused by enteroviruses, including coxsackie-viruses, echoviruses, and the more recently identified numbered enteroviruses (e.g., EV68-EV115), and excluding the rhinoviruses. Vesicular and petechial rashes may also occur. Active illness seldom exceeds 10 days. Transient paresis and encephalitic manifestations may occur; paralysis is unusual. Residual signs lasting a year or more may include weakness, muscle spasm, insomnia, and personality changes. Recovery is usually complete. Gastrointestinal and respiratory symptoms may be associated with enterovirus infection.

Various diseases caused by nonviral infectious agents may mimic viral meningitis. These include inadequately treated pyogenic meningitis; tuberculous and cryptococcal meningitis; meningitis caused by other fungi; cerebrovascular syphilis; and lymphogranuloma venereum. Post-infectious and postvaccinal reactions require differentiation from sequelae to measles, mumps, varicella, and immunization against rabies and smallpox; these syndromes are usually encephalitic in type. Leptospirosis, listeriosis, syphilis, lymphocytic choriomeningitis, viral hepatitis, infectious mononucleosis, influenza, and other diseases may produce the same clinical syndrome.

Infection by enteroviruses (excluding rhinoviruses) transmitted from the mother is a frequent cause of neonatal fever with neurological signs. In polio-free countries, the most prevalent infectious agent causing flaccid paralysis is enterovirus 71, responsible for outbreaks of meningitis and paralysis in many countries. Children and adults with B cell deficiencies are subject to chronic relapsing meningitis, usually caused by enteroviruses.

2. Causative agents—A wide variety of causative agents exist, many associated with other specific diseases. Predominant causative agents can vary by geographic location and season. Several viruses can produce meningeal features. The causative agent may not be identified in a large proportion of viral meningitis cases (e.g., 50%). In epidemic periods, mumps may be responsible for more than 25% of cases of established etiology in nonimmunized populations. In developed countries, enteroviruses (coxsackieviruses, echoviruses, and the numbered enteroviruses) cause many epidemics/outbreaks of known etiology. Arboviruses, measles, herpes simplex and varicella viruses, lymphocytic choriomeningitis virus, adenovirus, enterovirus, and others may cause sporadic cases. Incidence of specific types varies with geographic location and time. *Leptospira* may cause up to 20% of cases of aseptic meningitis in various areas (see "Leptospirosis"), and this bacterial infection should be included in the differential diagnosis of viral meningitis.

3. Diagnosis—Epidemiologic patterns, patient characteristics (e.g., age, clinical findings, vaccination history) and laboratory information should be used to make a diagnosis and identify the causative agent. Under optimal conditions, specific identification is possible in about half of all viral meningitis cases, through molecular diagnostic, serological, and isolation techniques. Molecular diagnostic methods often yield a more rapid diagnosis and are available for the detection and characterization of most viruses. Viral agents may be detected in early stages from nasopharyngeal and oropharyngeal swabs and stool, CSF, and blood/serum. Other specimens, such as pathologic specimens may also be useful in some instances.

4. **Occurrence**—Worldwide, as epidemics and sporadic cases; true incidence is unknown. Seasonal increases in late summer and early autumn are due mainly to arboviruses and enteroviruses, while late winter outbreaks may be due primarily to mumps.

5. **Reservoir; 6. Incubation period; 7. Transmission; 8. Risk groups; 9. Prevention**—Varies according to the causative agent (see specific disease chapters).

10. **Management of patient**—

1) Diagnosis depends on laboratory data not usually available until after recovery. Therefore, enteric precautions are indicated for 7 days after onset of illness, unless a nonenteroviral diagnosis is established.
2) Treatment: treatment is often supportive. Specific treatment is available depending on the causative agent (e.g., acyclovir may be given for herpes simplex meningitis). No antiviral therapy is presently available for enterovirus infections.

11. **Management of contacts and the immediate environment**—

1) Immunization of contacts: depends on causative agent.
2) Investigation of contacts and source of infection are not usually indicated.
3) Risk of acquiring infection can be lowered if good personal hygiene (e.g., handwashing), disinfection of environmental surfaces/items, enteric precautions, and avoiding close contact with an infected person are maintained.

12. **Special considerations**—

1) Reporting: depends on causative agent.
2) Epidemic measures: refer to the chapter relevant to the causative agent.

II. BACTERIAL MENINGITIS

Neisseria meningitidis, *Streptococcus pneumoniae* and *Haemophilus in-fluenzae* type b (Hib) are thought to cause more than 75% of all bacterial meningitis, and 90% of bacterial meningitis in children. Meningitis due to Hib, previously the most common cause of bacterial meningitis, has largely been eliminated in many industrialized countries through immunization programs. Meningococcal disease is unique among the major causes of bacterial meningitis in that it causes both endemic disease and large epidemics. The less common bacterial causes of meningitis, such as staphylococci, enteric bacteria, group B streptococci and *Listeria*, occur in susceptible persons (such as neonates and patients with impaired immunity) or as the consequence of head trauma.

A. MENINGOCOCCAL MENINGITIS (cerebrospinal fever)

1. Clinical features—An acute bacterial meningitis, characterized by sudden onset of fever, intense headache, nausea and often vomiting, stiff neck, and photophobia. A petechial rash with pink macules or occasionally vesicles may be observed in Europe and North America, but rarely in Africa. Even with antibiotics, case-fatality remains high at 8%–15%. In addition, 10%–20% of survivors will suffer long-term sequelae, including neurologic deficits, hearing loss, and limb loss. Invasive disease is characterized by one or more clinical syndromes including meningitis (the most common presentation), bacteremia, and sepsis. Meningococcemia, or meningococcal sepsis, is the most severe form of infection, with petechial rash, hypotension, disseminated intravascular coagulation, and multiorgan failure. Other forms of meningococcal disease, such as pneumonia, purulent arthritis, and pericarditis, are less common.

2. Causative agents—*N. meningitidis*, also called meningococcus, is a Gram-negative, aerobic diplococcus. *Neisseria* are divided into serogroups according to the immunological reactivity of their capsular polysaccharide. Groups A, B, and C account for at least 90% of cases worldwide, although the proportion of groups W, X, and Y is increasing. In most European and many Latin American countries, serogroups B and C cause the majority of disease, while A is the main cause in Africa and Asia. Serogroup Y causes about one-third of disease in the USA, but less in other countries. As countries introduce meningococcal conjugate vaccine programs against the most common circulating serogroups (serogroup C in Europe, serogroup A in Africa), the proportion of disease caused by serogroup B is increasing.

3. Diagnosis—The gold standard for diagnosis is recovery of meningococci from a sterile site, primarily CSF or blood. However, the sensitivity of culture, especially in patients who have received antibiotics, may be low. In culture-negative cases, identification of group-specific meningococcal polysaccharides in CSF by latex agglutination can help but false-negative results are common, especially for serogroup B. Polymerase chain reaction (PCR) offers the advantage of detecting meningococcal deoxyribonucleic acid (DNA) in CSF or plasma and does not require live organisms, but it is not yet widely available in many countries. Microscopic examination of gram-stained smears from petechiae may show *Neisseria*.

4. Occurrence—In Europe and North America the incidence of meningococcal disease is higher during winter and spring; in sub-Saharan Africa the disease classically peaks during the dry season.

The highest burden of the disease lies in the African meningitis belt, a large area that stretches from Senegal to Ethiopia and affects all or part of 21 countries. In this region, high rates of sporadic infections (1–20 cases/

100,000 population) occur in annual cycles, with periodical super-imposition of large-scale epidemics (usually caused by serogroup A, occasionally C, and more recently W-135). In the countries of the African meningitis belt, epidemics with incidence rates as high as 1,000 cases per 100,000 population have occurred every 8–12 years over the course of at least the past 50 years. In addition, major epidemics have occurred in adjacent countries not usually considered part of the African meningitis belt (such as Kenya and the United Republic of Tanzania).

5. Reservoir—Humans.

6. Incubation period—2–10 days, commonly 3–4 days.

7. Transmission—Through direct contact, including respiratory droplets from the nose and throat, although this usually causes only a subclinical mucosal infection. Up to 5%–10% of people may be asymptomatic carriers with nasopharyngeal colonization by *N. meningitidis*. Carrier rates of up to 25% have been documented in some populations in the absence of any cases of meningococcal disease. Less than 1% of those colonized will progress to invasive disease. In contrast, during some meningococcal outbreaks in industrialized countries, no carriers of the "outbreak stain" have been identified. Fomite transmission is insignificant.

Communicability continues until live meningococci are no longer present in discharges from nose and mouth. Meningococci usually disappear from the nasopharynx within 24 hours after institution of antimicrobial treatment to which the organisms are sensitive, and with substantial concentrations, in oronasopharyngeal secretions. Penicillin will temporarily suppress the organisms but does not usually eradicate them from the oronasopharynx.

8. Risk groups—Travelers to countries where disease is epidemic, Hajj pilgrims, military groups, and individuals with underlying immune dysfunctions, such as asplenia, properdin deficiency, and a deficiency of terminal complement components. Crowding, low socioeconomic status, active or passive exposure to tobacco smoke, and concurrent upper respiratory tract infections also increase the risk of meningococcal disease. Infants are at highest risk but rates decrease after infancy and then increase in adolescence and young adulthood. Group-specific immunity of unknown duration follows even subclinical infections.

9. Prevention—

1) Several meningococcal polysaccharide conjugate vaccines are available. Different serogroup compositions are licensed in different countries, usually determined by the epidemiology of disease in those countries. In many European countries, Serogroup C and and quadrivalent (serogroups A, C, Y, and W)

conjugate vaccines are licensed. In the USA, 2 quadrivalent vaccines, and one bivalent meningococcal conjugate vaccine, are licensed. In Africa, a serogroup A conjugate vaccine is licensed. Routine recommendations for targeted age groups have been implemented in many countries. In the meningitis belt in Africa, countries have implemented mass vaccination campaigns with conjugate meningitis A vaccine of persons aged 1–29 years being a strategy to eliminate serogroup A epidemic meningitis.

2) Vaccines are licensed against serogroup B meningococcal disease in certain countries where they are used against specific epidemic clones (i.e., New Zealand, Cuba). In serogroup B outbreaks, increasing public awareness and reducing overcrowding may prevent spread of disease.

10. Management of patient—

1) Respiratory isolation for 24 hours after start of chemotreatment.
2) Concurrent disinfection of discharges from the nose and throat and articles soiled therewith. Terminal cleaning.
3) Treatment: Ceftriaxone or penicillin given parenterally in adequate doses is the drug of choice for proven meningococcal disease; ampicillin and chloramphenicol are also effective. Penicillin-resistant strains have been reported in many countries, including Spain, the UK, and the USA; strains resistant to chloramphenicol have been reported in France and Viet Nam. Treatment should start as soon as the presumptive clinical diagnosis is made, even before meningococci have been identified. In children, until the specific agent has been identified, the drug chosen must be effective against Hib as well as *S. pneumoniae*. While ampicillin is the drug of choice for both as long as the organisms are ampicillin-sensitive, it should be combined with a third-generation cephalosporin, or chloramphenicol or vancomycin should be substituted in the many places where ampicillin-resistant *H. influenzae* or penicillin-resistant *S. pneumoniae* strains are known to occur. Patients with meningococcal or Hib disease should receive rifampicin or ciprofloxacin prior to discharge if neither a third-generation cephalosporin nor ciprofloxacin was given as treatment, to ensure elimination of the organism from the nasopharynx.

11. Management of contacts and the immediate environment—

1) Close surveillance of household, day care and other intimate contacts for early signs of illness, especially fever. Initiate appropriate therapy without delay.

2) Prophylaxis of close contacts: throat or nasopharyngeal cultures are of no value in deciding who should receive prophylaxis, since nasal carriage is variable and there is no consistent relationship between that found in the normal population and that found in an epidemic.

Effective prophylactic treatment should be given to intimate contacts, such as household contacts; military personnel sharing the same sleeping space; and people socially close enough to have shared eating utensils (e.g., close friends at school but not the whole class). Younger children in day care centers, even if not close friends, should all be given prophylaxis after an index case is identified.

Rifampicin, ceftriaxone, and ciprofloxacin are equally effective prophylactic agents. Rifampicin should not be given to pregnant women and may reduce the effectiveness of oral contraceptives. Health care personnel are rarely at risk even when caring for infected patients; only intimate exposure to nasopharyngeal secretions (e.g., as in mouth-to-mouth resuscitation) warrants prophylaxis.

Persons who have been vaccinated with meningococcal conjugate vaccine should also receive chemoprophylaxis, and it should be given immediately, even before the result of the serogroup testing is available.

12. Special considerations—

1) Reporting: case report is obligatory in most countries.
2) Epidemic measures: outbreaks may develop in situations of forced crowding. When an outbreak occurs, major emphasis must be placed on surveillance, early diagnosis and identification of serogroup, vaccination if caused by a vaccine-preventable serogroup and immediate treatment of suspected cases. A high index of suspicion is necessary. A threshold approach tailored to the epidemiology of the country is used in many countries to differentiate endemic disease from outbreaks. When thresholds are passed and the serogroup causing the outbreak is vaccine-preventable, immunization campaigns should be considered.

- Thresholds for a country with high rates of endemic disease (African meningitis belt):

  ○ Alert threshold: 5 cases per 100,000 population **or** increase in relation to previous nonepidemic years. Once alert threshold is reached: mandatory investigation, confirmation of agent, reinforcing of surveillance, enhancing of preparedness, and treatment of patients.

○ Epidemic threshold: 10 cases per 100,000 population and alert threshold crossed early in meningitis season *or* weekly doubling of cases each week during a 3-week period *or* 15 cases per 100,000 population *or* 2 cases at a mass gathering or among refugees or displaced persons. Once epidemic threshold is reached: mass vaccination, provision of drugs to health units, treatment of cases, and public education.

● Steps used in some industrialized countries:

○ Determine whether the outbreak is organization-based (e.g., school, university, prison) or community-based (town, city, county).

○ Investigate links between cases, because secondary or coprimary cases are excluded from calculations.

○ Calculate attack rates with the outbreak strain among the population at risk.

○ Subtype *N. meningitidis* isolates, if available, from cases of disease, using molecular typing methods.

If at least 3 cases have occurred during a 3-month period, the attack rate exceeds 10 cases per 100,000 in the population at risk, and the strain is vaccine-preventable (serogroup A, C, Y, or W), immunization of those in the group at risk should be considered.

Reduce overcrowding and ventilate living and sleeping quarters for all people exposed to infection because of living conditions (e.g., soldiers, miners, and prisoners).

Mass chemoprophylaxis is not usually effective in controlling outbreaks. In outbreaks involving small populations (e.g., a single school), consider chemoprophylaxis to all members of the community, especially if the outbreak is caused by a serogroup not included in the available vaccine. If undertaken, chemoprophylaxis should be administered to all members at the same time. Intimate contacts should all be considered for prophylaxis, regardless of whether the entire small population is treated.

Vaccination in all age groups affected is strongly recommended if an outbreak occurs in a large institutional or community setting in which the cases are due to groups A, C, W-135, or Y. Meningococcal vaccine has been very effective in halting epidemics due to A and C serogroups.

In countries where large-scale epidemics occur, mass vaccination of the entire population in affected areas should be considered when vaccine supply and administrative facilities allow. Geographical distribution of cases, age-specific attack rates, and available resources all must be considered in estimating the target population. Decisions about vaccination should consider where the intervention is likely to have the largest impact in preventing disease and death.

3) Although the disease is not covered by the International Health Regulations, some countries may require a valid certificate of immunization against meningococcal meningitis as a condition of entry (e.g., Saudi Arabia for Hajj pilgrims). Further information can be found at: http://www.who.int/topics/meningitis/en.

B. HEMOPHILUS MENINGITIS (meningitis due to Haemophilus influenzae)

1. Clinical features—In industrialized countries, before widespread use of Hib conjugate vaccines, Hib most commonly presented as meningitis. Epiglottitis and bacteremia without focus were the next most common presentations. In developing countries, the primary manifestation of Hib is lower respiratory tract infection. It may account for 5%–8% of all pneumonia in children in these areas, and causes an estimated 480,000 pneumonia deaths each year among children younger than 5 years.

Infection is usually associated with bacteremia. Onset can be subacute but is usually sudden, including fever, vomiting, lethargy, and meningeal irritation, with bulging fontanelle in infants or stiff neck and back in older children. Progressive stupor or coma is common. Occasionally, there is a low-grade fever for several days, with subtler central nervous system symptoms. Overall mortality rate for Hib meningitis is 5%; 6% of the survivors have permanent sensorineural hearing loss; 25% have significant disability of some type.

2. Causative agent—H. influenzae are Gram-negative coccobacilli that are divided into unencapsulated (nontypeable) and encapsulated strains. The encapsulated strains are further classified into serotypes a through f, based on the antigenic characteristics of their polysaccharide capsules. Hib is the most pathogenic.

3. Diagnosis—May be made through isolation of organisms from blood or cerebrospinal fluid. Specific capsular polysaccharide may be identified by slide agglutination or latex agglutination techniques. Polymerase chain reaction offers the advantage of detecting meningococcal DNA in CSF or plasma and does not require live organisms, but it is not yet widely available in many countries.

4. **Occurrence**—Worldwide. Most prevalent among children aged 2 months to 3 years; unusual in those older than 5 years. In developing countries, peak incidence is in children younger than 6 months; in industrialized countries, it is generally in children aged 6-12 months. As of the late 2000s, with widespread vaccination in early childhood, Hib meningitis has virtually disappeared in industrialized countries and in developing countries that have introduced Hib vaccine. Secondary cases in families and day care centers are rare.

5. **Reservoir**—Humans.

6. **Incubation period**—Unknown; probably 2-4 days.

7. **Transmission**—Through droplet infection and discharges from nose and throat during the infectious period. The portal of entry is most commonly the nasopharynx. The period of communicability lasts as long as organisms are present, which may be for a prolonged period even without nasal discharge. Transmission stops within 24-48 hours of starting effective antimicrobial therapy.

8. **Risk groups**—Susceptibility is assumed to be universal. Immunity is associated with the presence of circulating bactericidal and/or anti-capsular antibodies, acquired transplacentally, from prior infection, or through immunization.

9. **Prevention**—Routine childhood immunization. Several protein polysaccharide conjugate vaccines have been shown to prevent Hib meningitis in children older than 2 months and are licensed in many countries, both individually and combined with other vaccines. Immunization is recommended, starting at 2 months of age, followed by additional doses after an interval of 2 months; dosages vary with the vaccine in use. All vaccines require boosters at 12-15 months of age. Immunization is not routinely recommended for children older than 5 years.

Hib conjugate vaccines have been available since the 1980s and efforts to introduce them are increasing worldwide.

10. **Management of patient**—

   1) Respiratory isolation for 24 hours after start of chemotherapy.
   2) Treatment: ampicillin has been the drug of choice. However, about 30% of strains are now resistant due to beta-lactamase production. Ceftriaxone, cefotaxime, or chloramphenicol is thus recommended concurrently or singly until antimicrobial susceptibility has been ascertained. The patient should be given rifampicin prior to discharge from hospital to ensure elimination of the organism from the nasopharynx.

11. **Management of contacts and the immediate environment—**

   1) Prophylaxis is recommended for Hib but not other serotypes of *H. influenzae*. Rifampicin should be given to all household contacts (including adults) in households with any children younger than 1 year (other than the index case) or with a child aged 1–3 years who is inadequately immunized. When 2 or more cases of invasive disease have occurred within 60 days and unimmunized or incompletely immunized children attend the child care facility, all attenders and supervisory personnel should receive rifampicin. When a single case has occurred, the use of rifampicin prophylaxis is controversial.
   2) Observe contacts younger than 6 years, especially infants, for signs of illness, such as fever.
   3) Educate parents about the risk of secondary cases in siblings younger than 4 years and the need for prompt evaluation and treatment if fever or stiff neck develops.

12. **Special considerations—**

   1) Reporting: case report may be required in some endemic areas.
   2) Monitor for cases occurring in susceptible population settings, such as day care centers and large foster homes.

C. PNEUMOCOCCAL MENINGITIS

   1. Clinical features—Onset is usually sudden with high fever, lethargy or coma, and signs of meningeal irritation. It can be fulminant and occurs with bacteremia but not necessarily with any other focus, although there may be otitis media or mastoiditis. Pneumococcal meningitis has a high case-fatality rate.

   2. Causative agent—*S. pneumoniae,* a Gram-positive diplococcus. Nearly all strains causing meningitis and other severe forms of pneumococcal disease are encapsulated. There are 90 known capsular serotypes. The distribution of serotypes varies regionally and with age. In North America the 13 serotypes in pneumococcal conjugate vaccine are those that cause a substantial proportion of pneumococcal meningitis in children and adults.

   3. Diagnosis—May be by isolation of organisms from blood or cerebrospinal fluid. Pneumococcal capsular polysaccharide may be identified by the Quellung reaction or polymerase chain reaction.

   4. Occurrence—Worldwide. Most prevalent among children aged 2 months to 3 years. In developing countries infants are at highest risk; in North America, risk peaks at 6–18 months old.

5. Reservoir—Humans. Pneumococci are often found in the upper respiratory tract of healthy persons. Carriage is more common in children than in adults.

6. Incubation period—Unknown; probably 1–4 days.

7. Transmission—Through droplet spread and contact with respiratory secretions; direct contact with a person with pneumococcal disease generally results in nasopharyngeal carriage of the organism rather than in disease. The period of communicability lasts as long as organisms are present, which may be for a prolonged period, especially in immunocompromised hosts.

8. Risk groups—A sporadic disease in young infants, the elderly, and other high-risk groups, including asplenic and hypogammaglobulinemic patients. Predisposing factors are cochlear implantation and basilar fracture causing persistent communication with the nasopharynx (see Pneumococcal Pneumonia section in "Pneumonia"). Immunity is associated with the presence of circulating bactericidal and/or anticapsular antibody, acquired transplacentally, from prior infection, or from immunization.

9. Prevention—Vaccination is the mainstay of prevention. In many industrialized countries, pneumococcal conjugate vaccines are recommended for children younger than 2 years and those aged 2–4 years with certain high-risk conditions, such as immunocompromising conditions, sickle cell disease, asplenia, heart or lung disease, or cochlear implantation. The vaccines cover either the 10 or 13 serotypes that often cause pneumococcal meningitis in industrialized countries. Developing countries are introducing pneumococcal conjugate vaccines into their routine infant vaccine schedules. A polysaccharide vaccine containing 23 of the most common serotypes has been available since 1983. This is recommended in several countries for use in persons aged 65 years and older and those aged 2–64 years with immunocompromising conditions or certain chronic illnesses.

10. Management of patient—

1) Concurrent disinfection of nasal and throat secretions.
2) Treatment: penicillin, ceftriaxone, or cefotaxime are the drugs of choice. Because resistance is common in many areas, blood and cerebrospinal fluid culture should be performed for all patients with suspected bacterial meningitis, and susceptibility testing performed on pneumococci. Where resistance is widespread, ceftriaxone or cefotaxime given along with vancomycin are recommended for empirical therapy until susceptibility results are known. Intravenous dexamethasone early in the

course of the illness along with antibiotics has been shown to reduce the long-term complications of pneumococcal meningitis.

11. Management of contacts and the immediate environment— Protection of contacts is not necessary except during an outbreak (see Special Considerations discussed next).

12. Special considerations—

1) Reporting: case report to local health authority may be required in some areas.
2) Epidemic measures: pneumococcal meningitis can occur as part of a cluster of pneumococcal disease in institutional settings. Immunization using either the 23-valent polysaccharide vaccine or a conjugate vaccine, depending on the setting and the serotype, should be used to control outbreaks. Targeted antimicrobial prophylaxis (e.g., penicillin) may be useful in some outbreaks, especially those caused by nonvaccine type strains and when the outbreak strain is not resistant to antimicrobial agents. Widespread antimicrobial prophylaxis is not always effective and can induce resistance.

D. NEONATAL MENINGITIS

Infants with neonatal meningitis develop lethargy, seizures, apneic episodes, poor feeding, hypo- or hyperthermia, and sometimes respiratory distress, usually in their first week of life. The white blood cell count may be elevated or depressed. CSF culture yields group B streptococci, *L. monocytogenes* (see "Listeriosis"), *Escherichia coli* K-1, or other organisms acquired from the birth canal. Infants aged 2 weeks to 2 months may develop similar symptoms, with recovery from the CSF of group B streptococci or organisms of the Klebsiella-Enterobacter-Serratia group, acquired from the nursery environment. Meningitis in both groups is associated with septicemia. Treatment is with ampicillin, plus a third-generation cephalosporin or aminoglycoside until the causal organism has been identified and its antimicrobial susceptibilities determined.

[A. Cohn]

MOLLUSCUM CONTAGIOSUM

DISEASE	ICD-10 CODE
MOLLUSCUM CONTAGIOSUM	ICD-10 B08.1

1. **Clinical features**—A viral infection of the skin resulting in smooth-surfaced, firm, and dome-shaped or hemispherical papules with central umbilication. The lesions may be flesh-colored, white, translucent, or yellow. Most papules are 2-5 mm in diameter; lesions with large size or "giant mollusca" (10-30 mm) are occasionally seen. Lesions in adults are most often on the lower abdominal wall, pubis, genitalia, or inner thighs; on children, they are most often on the face, trunk, and proximal extremities. In immunocompetent hosts the course of infection is usually benign, typically resulting in the development of 15-35 lesions with no other symptoms present. Immunocompromised hosts (e.g., patients with HIV infection) may develop hundreds of disseminated lesions of the body and face. Occasionally the lesions itch and show a linear orientation, which suggests autoinoculation by scratching. In some patients, 50-100 lesions may become confluent and form a single plaque. Without treatment, molluscum contagiosum can persist for 6 months to 2 years. Any one lesion has a life span of 2-3 months. Lesions may resolve spontaneously or as a result of inflammatory response following trauma or secondary bacterial infection. Treatment (including mechanical removal of the lesions) may shorten the course of infection.

2. **Causative agent**—Molluscum contagiosum virus (MCV), a member of *Poxviridae* family, genus *Molluscipoxvirus*; the genus comprises at least 4 distinct genetic types (MCV-1 to -4), differentiated by deoxyribonucleic acid (DNA) endonuclease cleavage maps. The virus has not been grown in cell culture.

3. **Diagnosis**—Can be clinical when multiple lesions are present. Lesions visualized by dermatoscopy, showing orifices and vessels (in crown, radial, or punctiform patterns) are suggestive of molluscum contagiosum. For confirmation, the core can be expressed onto a glass slide and examined by ordinary light microscopy for classic basophilic, Feulgen-positive, intracytoplasmic inclusions, the "molluscum" or "Henderson-Paterson bodies." Histology or molecular analysis (polymerase chain reaction [PCR]) confirms the diagnosis.

4. **Occurrence**—Worldwide. Serological tests are not well standardized and skin inspection is the only screening technique available; epidemiological studies of the disease have therefore been limited. Population surveys have been conducted among specific subpopulations (American Indian and Alaska Natives), and in geographically restricted

areas (Fiji and Papua New Guinea). These surveys have shown that peak disease incidence occurs in childhood.

5. Reservoir—Humans.

6. Incubation period—For experimental inoculation, 19–50 days; clinical reports give 7 days to 6 months.

7. Transmission—Usually through direct skin-to-skin contact, including sexual contact and through handling objects contaminated with virus (towels, swimming pool kick boards). Infections have been observed in individuals who have recently undergone tattooing or cosmetic hair removal. Autoinoculation is also suspected. The period of communicability is unknown but probably exists as long as lesions persist.

8. Risk groups—All ages may be affected; more often seen in children. Disease is more common in HIV-infected patients, in whom lesions may disseminate.

9. Prevention—Avoid contact, or sharing bathtubs, bath towels, or sponges, with affected patients.

10. Management of patient—

1) Infected children with visible lesions should be excluded from close contact sports unless lesions can be fully covered.
2) Treatment: indicated to minimize risk of transmission. No therapy has proven to be uniformly effective for either immunocompetent or immunocompromised patients. Common therapies fall into three general categories: ablative (cryotherapy, curettage, salicylic acid, cantharidin, podophylline, and trichloroacetic acid); immunomodulatory (imiquimod, cimetidine); and virucidal (topical cidofovir).

11. Management of contacts and the immediate environment—Examine sexual partners where applicable. Disinfect surfaces and objects routinely handled by children with lesions.

12. Special considerations—Epidemic measures: suspend direct contact activities. Disinfect surfaces.

[M. Reynolds]

MUCORMYCOSIS
(zygomycosis)

DISEASE	ICD-10 CODE
INFECTIONS DUE TO MUCORALES	ICD-10 B46.0-B46.5
INFECTIONS DUE TO ENTOMOPHTHORALES	ICD-10 B46.8
BASIDIOBOLOMYCOSIS	ICD-10 B46.8
CONIDIOBOLOMYCOSIS	ICD-10 B46.8

I. INFECTIONS DUE TO MUCORALES (mucormycosis)

1. Clinical features—Infections caused by fungi of the order Mucorales result in disease that is typically rapidly progressive, destructive, and associated with high mortality. These fungi have an affinity for blood vessels and cause thrombosis, infarction, and tissue necrosis. The mycosis has an acute or subacute course. In debilitated persons it is the most fulminant fungal infection known.

The 4 main systemic forms of the disease are the rhinocerebral, pulmonary, gastrointestinal, and disseminated types. Cutaneous infection may also occur. The underlying disease influences the portal of entry of the fungus. Rhinocerebral disease represents one-third to one-half of all cases and usually presents as nasal or paranasal sinus infection, most often in patients with poorly controlled diabetes mellitus. Necrosis of the turbinates, perforation of the hard palate, necrosis of the cheek or orbital cellulitis, proptosis, and ophthalmoplegia may occur. Infection may penetrate to the internal carotid artery or extend directly to the brain and cause infarction.

Pulmonary mucormycosis (zygomycosis) appears to occur most commonly among hematological malignancy patients with neutropenia and recipients of hematopoietic stem cell transplants. In this form, the fungus causes thrombosis of pulmonary blood vessels and infarcts of the lung.

Gastrointestinal mucormycosis has been associated with severe malnutrition and has been reported in preterm neonates. In this form, mucosal ulcers or thrombosis and gangrene of stomach or bowel wall may occur.

Disseminated mucormycosis usually occurs in severely immunosuppressed patients, such as those with profound neutropenia and hematological malignancy. Deferoxamine therapy has been associated with disseminated mucormycosis. Nosocomial infections have been reported.

2. Causative agents—Rapidly growing molds of the order Mucorales. *Rhizopus* is the genus most commonly implicated in human disease. One of the most common *Rhizopus* species causing mucormycosis is *Rhizopus* *arrbizus*. Other genera known to cause human disease include *Mucor*, *Rhizomucor*, *Lichtheimia* (formerly *Absidia*), *Cunninghamella*, *Apophysomyces*, *Saksenaea*, and *Syncephalastrum*.

3. **Diagnosis**—Can be challenging. Clinical manifestations in immunosuppressed hosts may be similar to those caused by other invasive mold infections, such as aspergillosis. Definitive diagnosis is usually made through microscopic demonstration of broad, "ribbon-like," nonseptate or pauciseptate hyphae in tissue or body fluids with an accompanying positive culture. Immunohistochemistry reagents and direct deoxyribonucleic acid (DNA)–based detection testing are also available for tissue blocks.

Wet preparations and smears may be examined. Cultures alone are not diagnostic, because mucormycete fungi are found in the environment. However, in an immunosuppressed patient with a compatible clinical syndrome, a positive culture for a mucormycete should be taken very seriously. Similarly, the diagnosis may be difficult to establish based solely upon histopathology, since it may be difficult to appreciate the distinctive characteristics of mucormycete fungal hyphae that differentiate them from those of other molds, such as *Aspergillus* spp., in tissue.

4. **Occurrence**—Worldwide. Incidence may be increasing because of longer survival of patients with immunosuppression, with diabetes mellitus and certain blood dyscrasias (especially acute leukemia and aplastic anemia), and who are treated with deferoxamine for aluminum or iron overload when receiving chronic hemodialysis for renal failure. Some institutions have reported increasing numbers of cases among hematopoietic stem cell transplant recipients in association with the use of voriconazole, a broad-spectrum azole antifungal that has potent activity against *Aspergillus* spp., but not against the mucormycetes.

5. **Reservoir**—Common saprophytes in the environment.

6. **Incubation period**—Unknown. Fungus spreads rapidly in susceptible tissues.

7. **Transmission**—Through inhalation or ingestion of fungal spores by susceptible individuals. Direct inoculation in intravenous (IV) drug users and at sites of IV catheters and cutaneous burns may occur. No direct person-to-person or animal-to-person transmission.

8. **Risk groups**—The rarity of infection in healthy individuals despite the abundance of Mucorales in the environment indicates natural resistance. Corticosteroid use, metabolic acidosis, deferoxamine, and immunosuppressive treatment predispose to infection. Malnutrition predisposes to the gastrointestinal form.

9. **Prevention**—Optimal clinical control of diabetes mellitus to avoid acidosis.

10. **Management of patient**—

1) Treatment: prompt initiation of a lipid formulation of amphotericin B and in some cases surgical resection of infected tissue are essential, given the high mortality rate. Control of the predisposing underlying condition (i.e., glucose control and treatment of acidosis in diabetics, reduction of immunosuppression) is also important. A newer antifungal, posaconazole, has been shown to be effective as salvage treatment in some patients who do not tolerate amphotericin B or whose disease is refractory to amphotericin B. Hyperbaric oxygen has been used as adjunctive therapy but its benefit has not been established.

2) Ordinary cleanliness. Terminal cleaning.

11. **Management contacts and the immediate environment**—Generally a sporadic disease. Investigation of contacts and source of infection is not usually beneficial in sporadic cases, due to the ubiquity of these fungi in the environment. However, outbreaks due to contaminated medical supplies have occurred.

12. **Special considerations**—None.

II. INFECTIONS DUE TO ENTOMOPHTHORALES

Entomophthoromycosis includes 2 histopathologically identical entities: basidiobolomycosis and conidiobolomycosis. Unlike infections due to fungi of the order Mucorales, these infections are typically subcutaneous and slowly progressive. Histopathologically, while infections due to Mucorales are characterized by fungal angioinvasion and tissue infarction, infection due to Entomophthorales usually results in a chronic, eosinophilic inflammatory response without angioinvasion. They are not characterized by thromboses or infarction, do not usually occur in association with serious preexisting disease or cause disseminated disease, and seldom cause death. The Splendore-Höeppli phenomenon may be seen around fungal hyphae in tissue infection due to Entomophthorales. These 2 infections have been recognized principally in tropical and subtropical areas of Asia, Africa, and Latin America.

In terms of Basidiobolomycosis, *Basidiobolus ranarum* causes the subcutaneous form of entomophthoromycosis, presenting as a granulomatous inflammation. The fungus is ubiquitous, occurring in decaying vegetation, soil, and the gastrointestinal tract of amphibians and reptiles. The disease presents as a firm, painless, and sharply circumscribed subcutaneous mass, mainly in children and adolescents, more commonly in males. Common sites of infection are the buttocks, thighs, and chest. The infection may heal spontaneously. Recommended treatment is oral potassium iodide.

In terms of conidiobolomycosis, *Conidiobolus coronatus*, occurring in soil and decaying vegetation, causes the mucocutaneous form of entomophthoromycosis. This usually originates in the paranasal skin or nasal mucosa and presents as nasal obstruction or swelling of the nose or adjacent structures. The lesion may spread to involve contiguous areas, such as lip, cheek, palate, or pharynx. The disease is uncommon and occurs principally in adult males. Recommended treatment is oral potassium iodide or IV amphotericin B.

For both forms of entomophthoromycosis, incubation periods and modes of transmission are unknown. Person-to-person transmission does not occur. A few cases of a rare primary visceral form of conidiobolomycosis due to *Conidiobolus incongruus* have been reported in patients (immunocompromised or not) as lung infections spreading to contiguous organs.

[R. Smith]

MUMPS
(infectious parotitis)

DISEASE	ICD-10 CODE
MUMPS	ICD-10 B26

1. **Clinical features**—An acute viral disease characterized by fever, swelling, and tenderness of one or more salivary glands—usually the parotid, and sometimes the sublingual or submaxillary glands. Parotitis may be unilateral or bilateral, and typically lasts 7-10 days in unvaccinated individuals. Prodromal symptoms are nonspecific, consisting of myalgia, anorexia, malaise, headache, and low-grade fever. Not all cases of parotitis are caused by mumps infection, but other parotitis-causing agents do not produce parotitis on an epidemic scale. Orchitis, most commonly unilateral, occurs in 20%-30% of affected postpubertal males, but sterility is extremely rare. Mumps orchitis has been reported to be a risk factor for testicular cancer. As many as 40%-50% of mumps infections have been associated with respiratory symptoms, particularly in children younger

than 5 years. Mumps can cause sensorineural hearing loss in both children and adults. Pancreatitis, usually mild, occurs in 4% of cases.

Symptomatic aseptic meningitis occurs in up to 10% of mumps cases; patients usually recover without complications, though many require hospitalization. Mumps encephalitis is rare (1–2/100,000 cases) but can result in permanent sequelae, such as paralysis, seizures, and hydrocephalus; the case-fatality rate for mumps encephalitis is about 1%. Mumps infection during the first trimester of pregnancy has been associated with spontaneous abortion, but there is no firm evidence that mumps during pregnancy causes congenital malformations.

2. **Causative agent**—Mumps virus, a member of the family *Paramyxoviridae*, genus *Rubulavirus*.

3. **Diagnosis**—Acute mumps infection can be confirmed through: a positive serological test for mumps-specific immunoglobulin class M (IgM) antibodies; seroconversion—a significant ($\geq$ 4-fold) rise in serum mumps immunoglobulin class G (IgG) titer as determined by a quantitative serological assay; detection of virus by reverse transcription polymerase chain reaction (RT-PCR); or isolation of mumps virus from an appropriate clinical specimen (buccal swab or cerebrospinal fluid [CSF]). Diagnosis may be more challenging in vaccinated populations, in which the IgM response may be absent or short-lived and viral load may be lower. There is some evidence that serum collected at least 5–10 days after parotitis onset may improve the ability to detect IgM among persons who have received 1 or 2 doses of measles, mumps, rubella [MMR]. The ability to confirm cases by ribonucleic acid (RNA) detection using real-time RT-PCR is improved when samples are collected within 2 days after symptom onset, regardless of vaccination status. Absence of a mumps IgM response in a vaccinated or previously infected individual presenting with clinically compatible mumps *does not rule out mumps* as a diagnosis. A positive IgG result is expected among previously vaccinated persons. Older persons with no history of mumps illness or vaccination may have detectable mumps IgG due to a previous subclinical infection.

4. **Occurrence**—In unvaccinated populations, about one-third of patients have inapparent or subclinical infections, especially young children. In temperate climates, winter and spring are peak seasons. In the absence of immunization, mumps is endemic, with an annual incidence usually 100–1,000 per 100,000 population and epidemic peaks every 2–5 years. In many industrialized countries, mumps was a major cause of viral encephalitis. Serosurveys conducted prior to mumps vaccine introduction found that in some countries 90% of persons were immune by age 15 years, while in other countries a large proportion of the adult population remained susceptible. In countries where mumps vaccine has not been introduced, the incidence of mumps remains high, mostly affecting

children 5-9 years of age. By the end of 2012, 120 of 194 WHO Member States included mumps vaccine in their national immunization schedules. In countries where mumps vaccine coverage has been sustained at high levels, the incidence of the disease has dropped markedly.

5. Reservoir—Humans.

6. Incubation period—About 16-18 days (range 12-25).

7. Transmission—By droplet spread; also direct contact with the saliva of an infected person. Virus has been isolated from saliva from 7 days before the onset of parotitis to 9 days afterwards. Maximum infectiousness occurs between 2 days before onset of parotitis and 5 days afterwards. Inapparent infections can be communicable.

8. Risk groups—Immunity is generally long-lasting and develops after either inapparent or clinical infections.

9. Prevention—Public education should encourage mumps immunization for susceptible individuals. Routine mumps vaccination is recommended in countries with an efficient childhood vaccination program and sufficient resources to maintain high levels of vaccine coverage. Mumps vaccination is recommended at age 12-18 months, as part of the MMR vaccine, though most countries have a 2-dose schedule, with the second dose given at least 1 month after the first dose. More than 85% of recipients develop immunity that is long lasting and may be lifelong.

Live attenuated mumps virus vaccines are available as monovalent vaccines or trivalent MMR vaccines. Hydrolyzed gelatin and/or sorbitol are used as stabilizers in mumps vaccine, along with neomycin as a preservative. Mumps vaccines are cold-chain dependent and should be protected from light.

Different strains of live attenuated mumps vaccine have been developed in Japan, Russia, Switzerland, and the USA. All licensed strains are judged acceptable by WHO for public health programs, except the Rubini strain, which is not recommended because of demonstrated low efficacy; persons who received this strain should be revaccinated with another strain. In most industrialized countries, only the Jeryl-Lynn strain, or strains derived from it, are accepted, because they show no confirmed association with aseptic meningitis.

The reported incidence of adverse events depends on the strain of mumps vaccine. The most common adverse reactions are fever and parotitis. Rare adverse reactions include orchitis, sensorineural deafness, and thrombocytopenia. Aseptic meningitis, resolving spontaneously in less than 1 week without sequelae, has been reported at frequencies ranging from 0.1-100 cases per 100,000 vaccine doses. This reflects differences in vaccine strains and their preparation, as well as variations in study design and case ascertainment. Better data are needed to establish more precise estimates of aseptic meningitis incidence in recipients of different strains of mumps vaccine. The rates of aseptic meningitis due to mumps vaccine are at least 100-fold lower than rates of aseptic meningitis due to infection with wild mumps virus.

Accumulated global experience in industrialized countries shows that 2 doses of vaccine afford better protection against mumps than a single dose. The first dose is usually given as MMR vaccine at the age of 12–18 months. The age of administration of the second dose may range from the second year of life to age at school-entry, depending on programmatic considerations aimed at optimizing vaccination coverage. Less commonly, the second vaccination may be delivered through supplementary campaigns in developing countries.

Countries intending to use mumps or MMR vaccine during mass campaigns should give special attention to planning. The mumps vaccine strain should be carefully selected, and health workers should receive training on expected rates of adverse events following immunization and on community advocacy and health education activities.

Mumps vaccine is contraindicated in persons with evidence of severe immunosuppression (e.g., cluster of differentiation 4 glycoprotein [CD4] percentages <15% [all ages] and CD4 <200 cells/mm^3 [age >5 years] for ≥6 months), including those with HIV infection, congenital immunodeficiencies, and immunosuppression due to high doses of steroids or chemotherapeutic agents. Treatment with a low dose of steroids on alternate days, topical steroid use, and aerosolized steroid preparations are not, however, contraindications. Pregnant women, or women planning a pregnancy in the next month, should not receive mumps vaccine, although no evidence exists that mumps vaccine causes fetal damage.

10. **Management of patient—**

1) Respiratory isolation for 5 days after onset of parotitis. Exclude patients from school or workplace for 5 days after onset of parotitis if susceptible contacts (those not immunized) are present.
2) Concurrent disinfection of articles soiled with nose and throat secretions.

11. **Management of contacts and the immediate environment—**

1) Immunize susceptible contacts to reduce likelihood of infection upon future exposures. Immune globulin (IG) is not effective as a preventive measure or as postexposure prophylaxis, and not recommended.
2) Exclude susceptible persons from school or the workplace from the 12th until the 25th day after exposure if other susceptibles are present.

12. **Special considerations—**

1) Reporting: WHO recommends making mumps a notifiable disease in all countries.
2) Epidemic measures: immunize susceptibles, especially those at risk of exposure. Serological screening to identify susceptibles is impractical and unnecessary, since there is no risk in immunizing those who are already immune.

[A. Barskey]

MYCETOMA AND NOCARDIOSIS

DISEASE	ICD-10 CODE
ACTINOMYCETOMA	ICD-10 B47.1
EUMYCETOMA	ICD-10 B47.0
NOCARDIOSIS	ICD-10 A43

Mycetoma has 2 distinct etiologies. Infections caused by fungi are termed eumycotic mycetoma or eumycetoma; those caused by aerobic actinomycetes (filamentous bacteria) are termed actinomycotic mycetoma or actinomycetoma. The latter manifest either as a mycetoma or as a pulmonary infection of varying severity (nocardiosis).

I. EUMYCOTIC MYCETOMA (eumycetoma)

1. Clinical features—A clinical syndrome characterized by formation of small subcutaneous nodules that enlarge and become fixed to the underlying tissue and the skin, eventually forming sinus tracts that drain purulent material with visible granules (or grains) composed of a matrix component and masses of mycelial fungi; this is considered as pathognomonic. Eventually, the lesions result in destruction of structures, deformity, and loss of function. Pain is not a feature; bone invasion is common but pathological fractures are rare. Mycetoma may spread directly or through the lymphatic system with secondary lesions; hematogenous spread occurs but is uncommon.

Lesions are usually on the foot or lower leg; sometimes on the hand, shoulders, and back; and rarely at other sites. Lesions on the head may invade the brain. It is unusual to have lesions on more than one extremity or area of the body.

Eumycetoma may be difficult to distinguish from osteosarcoma, rhabdomyosarcoma, sporotrichosis, chronic osteomyelitis, and botryomycosis (a clinically and pathologically similar entity caused by a variety of bacteria, including *staphylococci* and Gram-negative bacteria).

2. Causative agents—Eumycetoma is mainly caused by *Madurella mycetomatis*; *Trematosphaeria* (formerly *Madurella*) *grisea*; *Pseudallescheria boydii* species complex, *Falciformispora* (formerly *Leptosphaeria*) *senegalensis*.

Some species are more frequent in certain regions depending on the climate (rainfall).

3. Diagnosis—Specific diagnosis depends on visualizing the grains in fresh preparations; the color of the grain may indicate the organism involved. Fine needle aspiration or a biopsy is often required and identification of the causative bacteria or fungus is best made by culture. Molecular methods such as ribosomal deoxyribonucleic acid (rDNA) internal transcribed spacer region sequencing may be used. The extent of the lesion is determined with ultrasound, computerized tomography (CT) scan, or magnetic resonance imaging (MRI); the latter may show the individual grain as the "dot-in-circle" sign.

4. Occurrence—Eumycetoma occurs most commonly in tropical and subtropical regions, in the so-called mycetoma belt between latitudes 15°S and 30°N. Endemic areas typically have a long, hot dry season and a short, heavy rainy season. The highest incidences are in Sudan (70% are eumycetoma); other countries in Africa include Senegal, Mauritania, Niger, Mali, Cameroon, Somalia, Kenya, and Djibouti; in Asia mainly India; Iran; and in Central and South America, Venezuela, Argentina, Colombia, and Chile.

5. Reservoir—Fungi that are etiologic agents of mycetoma are found in soil and decaying vegetation.

6. Incubation period—Can be months to years from exposure.

7. Transmission—Subcutaneous implantation of organisms from a saprophytic source by penetrating wounds (e.g., thorns, splinters). No person-to-person transmission. Causal agents are widespread in nature; there are no data on the occurrence of subclinical infection.

8. Risk groups—Disease is most common in those aged 20–40 years. Men are 5 times more likely to develop disease, which could be related to more occupational exposure to contaminated soil; alternatively there may be a reporting bias. Disease is more common in agricultural and outdoor laborers. It is also more common in warmer climates where less protective clothing, particularly shoes, are worn. Often there are several cases in one family; while genetic factors have been demonstrated, factors related to sharing the same environment may also be important.

9. Prevention—Protect against puncture wounds by wearing shoes and protective clothing. Early diagnosis and treatment can prevent the debilitating effect of chronic disease.

10. Management of patient—Treatment: in eumycetoma smaller lesions may be removed surgically; in larger lesions medical treatment with an azole such as ketoconazole or itraconazole will cause reduction in size thus facilitating conservative surgery, but need to be given up to 12 months; recurrence rates are high as the fungus is not eradicated. Treatment with voriconazole or posaconazole has been helpful in eumycetoma, but experience is limited. Terbinafine has also been successfully used in some cases of eumycetoma. Fluconazole, amphotericin B, 5-flucytosine, and the echinocandins are ineffective.

11. Management of contacts and the immediate environment— None.

12. Special considerations—Medical education on mycetoma: Early detection, correct diagnosis, and proper treatment are important for a good therapeutic outcome.

II. NOCARDIOSIS AND ACTINOMYCETOMA

1. Clinical features—Pulmonary infection is the most common clinical presentation of infection with nocardia and can present as pneumonia, lung abscesses, or cavitary lesions. Contiguous spread within the thoracic cavity and hematogenous dissemination, particularly to the central nervous system (CNS), are common. Superficial abscess or localized cellulitis also occurs following inoculation injuries with contaminated soil. Mycetoma is a specific chronic progressive clinical syndrome involving infection with *Nocardia* spp. (or other aerobic actinomycetes) character-ized by swelling and suppuration of subcutaneous tissues and formation of sinus tracts, predominately located in the distal extremities.

2. Causative agents—*Nocardia asteroides* complex: (including *Nocardia asteriodes, Nocardia farcinica, Nocardia Nova, and Nocardia canea); Nocardia brasiliensis, Nocardia otitidiscaviarum, Nocardia cyriacigeorgica*, and *Nocardia abscessus*.

3. Diagnosis—Diagnosis of nocardiosis is difficult since clinical manifestations are nonspecific, requiring identification from clinical samples. Presumptive diagnosis may be provided from microscopic examination of stained smears of sputum, pus, cerebrospinal fluid, bronchial washings or tissue may reveal beaded Gram-positive, weakly acid-fast, branched filaments; colonies generally appear as snowballs with aerial hyphae. Culture confirmation is desirable but often difficult, and any suspicion of nocardial infection should be passed on to the microbiology laboratory to enhance diagnosis. Biopsy or autopsy usually clearly establishes involvement, although histopathology may be nonspecific. Current serological tests are nonspecific with an exception of a serological test for detecting *N. brasiliensis*. The extent of the lesion is determined with ultrasound, CT scan, or MRI; the latter may show the individual grain as the "dot-in-circle" sign.

4. Occurrence—An occasional sporadic disease in people and animals in all parts of the world. *N. asteroides* complex is the most common cause of nocardial pulmonary and disseminated disease worldwide. *N. brasiliensis* is the most common cause of nocardial cutaneous and lymphocutaneous infections, and mycetomas reported predominantly in tropical and subtropical regions of the southern USA, Central and South America, and Australia.

5. Reservoir—Found worldwide as an environmental saprophyte in soil, water, and organic material.

6. Incubation period—Uncertain; probably a few days to a few weeks.

7. Transmission—Typically acquired through inhalation or skin inoculation. Not directly transmitted from humans or from animals to humans. Organism-specific virulence variation and host exposure are important determinants of susceptibility.

8. Risk groups—Immunocompromised status (e.g., due to alcoholism, diabetes, or steroid use) is a risk factor in more than 60% of infections, but the incidence in those with AIDS is lower than expected, even accounting for sulfamethoxazole prophylaxis. Men have a greater risk than women of becoming infected; the male-to-female ratio is 3 to 1.

9. Prevention—None.

10. Management of patient—

1) Concurrent disinfection of discharges and contaminated dressings.
2) Treatment: most *Nocardia* species maintain a specific antimicrobial susceptibility profile. Therefore, *Nocardia* spp. identification is important as antimicrobial susceptibility profiles can impact patient care. Isolates should be referred to a reference laboratory with expertise in *Norcardia* spp. identification and for susceptibility testing. Treatment guidelines have not been established due to lack of controlled clinical trials. Historically, sulfonamides, specifically trimethoprim-sulfamethoxazole (TMP-SMX), have

been the drugs of choice if in vitro susceptibility testing indicates sulfonamides. However, if the organism is not susceptible to or the patient is intolerant of TMP-SMX, alternative antimicrobial agents with in vitro activity against *Nocardia* include amikacin, imipenem, meropenem, ceftriaxone, cefotaxime, minocycline, moxifloxacin, levofloxacin, linezolid, tigecycline, and amoxicillin-clavulanic acid. In patients with severe disease or immunocompromising conditions, combination therapy might be warranted. The most clinical experience exists for amikacin and imipenem. Depending on the extent of infection, surgical drainage and debridement could be required. Prolonged therapy is required to minimize relapse. A combination of parenteral and oral therapy for 1-3 months for patients with primary cutaneous lesions, 6 months for immunocompetent patients with pulmonary or non-CNS extrapulmonary disease, and 6-12 months for immunocompromised patients or those with CNS disease is recommended. Co-amoxiclavulanic acid has been used as rescue therapy after combinations of dapsone, TMP-SMX, and aminoglycosides, with good result; however acquired resistance may develop and it is not effective against *A. madurae*.

Amikacin combined with a carbapenem such as imipenem or meropenem may also be used in refractory cases. Surgery is rarely required.

11. Management of contacts and the immediate environment—Most disease is sporadic. Occasional outbreaks may occur from environmental sources, and transmission through health care workers is probably rare.

12. Special considerations—None.

[W. Bower, M. Brandt, B. Lasker]

NIPAH AND HENDRA VIRAL DISEASES

DISEASE	ICD-10 CODE
NIPAH VIRUS INFECTION	ICD-10 B33.8
HENDRA VIRUS INFECTION	ICD-10 B33.8

1. **Clinical features**—Nipah virus (NiV) manifests primarily as encephalitis. Hendra virus (HeV) has been identified in seven humans to date and appears to manifest either as a respiratory illness or as a prolonged and initially mild meningoencephalitis.

Symptoms range in severity, from mild to coma and/or respiratory failure and death, and include fever and headaches, sore throat, dizziness, drowsiness and disorientation, or influenza-like symptoms, and atypical pneumonitis. Subclinical infections also occur.

Pneumonitis was prominent in the 2 initial HeV cases—one of which was fatal—whereas NiV cases have been largely encephalitic, and were initially misdiagnosed as Japanese encephalitis. A proportion of NiV patients display pulmonary involvement with atypical pneumonitis, and the majority of patients who survive acute NiV encephalitis make a full recovery, but up to 20% have residual neurologic deficits. Mild late-onset disease and relapse encephalitis have been observed several months after initial infection, and the case-fatality rate varies between 40% and 75%.

2. **Causative agents**—HeV and NiV are members of a new genus, *Henipaviruses*, of the *Paramyxoviridae* family.

3. **Diagnosis**—NiV or HeV infection can be confirmed by direct detection of virus by virus isolation or polymerase chain reaction (PCR) in blood, cerebrospinal fluid (CSF), urine, oropharyngal secretions, nasal or oral swabs, bronchial wash if collected at the early stage of infection. At a later stage, immunoglobulin class M (IgM) and immunoglobulin class G (IgG) antibodies may be detectable in the serum and CSF by enzyme-linked immunosorbent assay (ELISA) or by serum neutralization assays. If death occurs rapidly and only tissues (e.g., brain, spleen) are available, diagnosis should be confirmed by PCR, virus isolation, or by immunohistochemistry in formalin-fixed tissues and paraffin embedded blocks.

4. **Occurrence**—HeV, first recognized in 1994 in Australia, has caused severe respiratory disease in horses in Queensland; in 1994, 3 human cases followed close contact with horses with respiratory or neurological disease, the first 2 during the initial outbreak, the third occurring 13 months after an initially mild meningitis illness, when the virus reactivated to cause a fatal encephalitis. Sporadic cases of disease in horses have continued to occur in coastal Queensland and northern New South Wales, from 1999 to time of

writing, with a spike of outbreaks and cases in 2011. A mild human case occurred in 2004 in a veterinarian, following an autopsy on a euthanized horse in Cairns, North Queensland, and 2 further human cases occurred during an outbreak in horses at a veterinary clinic in Brisbane in 2008, and a fatal case in August 2009 in Cawarral, all presenting with a moderate to severe influenza-like illness requiring hospitalization. All human infections have been associated with contact with infected horses.

NiV was first identified in 1999 in Malaysia, as a cause of severe respiratory disease in domestic swine in the pig-farming provinces of Perak, Negeri Sembilan, and Selangor. Asymptomatic infection in the pigs was common, and the case-fatality rate was generally low (5%). The first human case is believed to have occurred in 1996, although most cases were identified in the first months of 1999 (with 105 confirmed deaths). During 1999, 22 abattoir workers in Singapore developed NiV infection following contact with pigs imported from Malaysia, with 1 fatality. In 2001, NiV emerged for the first time in Bangladesh and West Bengal, India. In all, there have been 11 outbreaks of NiV infection in Bangladesh between 2001 and 2011, with more than 196 cases and a fatality rate of about 77%. In the same period, there have been two confirmed outbreaks in India, with more than 70 cases and a fatality rate of about 70%. The outbreaks in India and Bangladesh differed in a number of significant ways from that in Malaysia: there was no evidence of involvement of the intermediate host, swine; a number of cases presented with an acute respiratory distress syndrome, suggesting that transmission could be by inhalation of large droplets; there was strong suggestive evidence of human-to-human transmission for the first time, including nosocomial infections; and there was evidence to suggest that some of the cases were foodborne, hypothesized due to ingestion of date palm juice contaminated with virus from infected bats.

5. Reservoir—Fruit bats, particularly members of the genus *Pteropus*, are the major reservoir hosts of HeV and NiV viruses, without causing overt disease. HeV has been isolated from all 4 Australian members of the genus *Pteropus*, and NiV has been isolated from *Pteropus hypomelanus* in Malaysia, and from *Pteropus lylei* in Cambodia. Antibodies to Nipah-like or Hendra-like viruses have been found in sera from fruit bats collected in Timor Leste, Indonesia, New Guinea, Thailand, India, and Madagascar. Recently, African fruit bats of the genus Eidolon, family *Pteropodidae*, were found positive for antibodies against Nipah and Hendra viruses, indicating that these, or related viruses, might be present within the geographic distribution of *Pteropodidae* bats in Africa. It is therefore reasonable to assume that related viruses exist throughout the range of Pteropid bats, spanning a geographic area stretching from Oceania to the Middle East, and including Africa.

Testing of other animals has shown variable susceptibility. Cats, pigs, ferrets, guinea pigs, the golden hamster, and inbred mice can all be infected. Recent work has shown that dogs not only succumb to infection, but shed virus, and the risk this shedding poses to humans is unknown.

6. **Incubation period**—From 4-32 days.

7. **Transmission**—There is clear evidence that transmission occurs through direct contact with infected horses (HeV) or swine (NiV), or contaminated tissues. Oral and nasal routes of infection, or infection through contaminated body fluid entering into cuts and abrasions, are suspected in most cases in Australia and Malaysia. In Bangladesh and India, it is hypothesized that transmission can occur as a result of ingestion of contaminated palm sap, and possibly from droplets, but modes of transmission remain to be determined in many instances. In Bangladesh, human-to-human transmission has been reported and is thought to occur through unprotected close contact with infectious human secretions. The period of communicability is unknown. Recurrent infection appears to occur.

8. **Risk groups**—All ages are susceptible. People in contact with swine potentially infected with NiV are at increased risk of infection. All recorded cases of HeV infection in humans have been the result of very close contact with infected horses. People at risk are horse owners, animal technicians, and veterinarians. There is the potential for rural populations in contact with *Pteropus* bats to become infected, though infection in bat carers in Australia has not been recorded; a possible risk group would be people ingesting palm sap contaminated with bat secretions or excreta.

9. **Prevention**—

1) Health education about precautionary measures to be taken, and the need to avoid contact with fruit bats, their guano, and infected animals such as pigs and horses. Ensure that fruit bats are not able to roost close to pig pens or stables.

2) As Nipah virus outbreaks in domestic animals have preceded human cases, establishing an animal health surveillance system to detect new cases is essential for providing early warning for veterinary and human public health authorities.

3) Isolate and cull infected horses or swine using appropriate personal protective equipment, with burial or incineration of carcasses, taking appropriate biosecurity precautions and under official supervision.

4) Restrict movement of horses or pigs from infected farms to other areas.

5) A recombinant subunit vaccine has shown efficacy in animal models and is cross-protective against HeV and NiV. This vaccine has been recently available for horses in Australia, both to protect horses and to negate the risk to humans in contact with them,

though it is unclear how long protection lasts following horse vaccination.

10. **Management of patient—**

1) As evidence for person-to-person transmission continues to be accumulated, contact and droplet precautions appear warranted for humans with infections, as well as when handling body fluids and excreta.
2) There is no specific treatment. Ribavirin may decrease mortality from NiV-infected patients, but seemed to have no activity in 2 HeV-infected patients. A cross-reactive (HeV and NiV) human monoclonal antibody showed excellent results in protecting nonhuman primates and ferrets in postexposure therapy and is in human preclinical development.

11. **Management of contacts and the immediate environment—**

1) Investigation of contacts and source of infection: search for missed cases and veterinary investigation.
2) Disinfection and safe management of clinical waste.

12. **Special considerations—**

1) Reporting: case report to Health Authorities usually mandatory wherever infections occur in livestock.
2) Epidemic measures:

- Precautions for animal handlers: protective clothing, including boots, gloves, gowns, goggles, and face shields; washing of hands and body parts with soap before leaving pig farms.
- Culling of infected horses or swine, with burial or incineration of carcasses, under official supervision and with biosecurity precautions.
- Restrict movement of horses or pigs from infected farms to other areas.
- Isolate infected humans if person-to-person transmission appears to be a possibility.

3) International measures: prohibit exportation of horses or pigs and horse/pig products from infected areas.

[P. E. Rollin, B. Knust, S. Nichol]

❖

NOMA

DISEASE	ICD-10 CODE
NOMA	ICD-10 A69.0

1. **Clinical features**—Noma is a debilitating inflammatory condition that starts as a localized gingival ulceration and spreads rapidly through the orofacial tissues, establishing itself with a fairly well defined perimeter surrounding a blackened necrotic center. The word "noma" derives from the Greek "voun," meaning to devour, emphasizing the rapid progression of the disease. The noma lesion often disrupts anatomic barriers and spreads through muscles and bone. In general, there are 3 stages of noma development, which may overlap with one another: an acute phase, a gangrenous phase, and the final scarring phase. The acute phase is characterized by chronic malnutrition as evidenced by severe stunting and weight loss, as well as hair discoloration and edema of the limbs. Other prominent symptoms include marked depletion of serum level of leptin, a polypeptide involved in the inflammatory response and immune function, halitosis, mouth soreness, excessive salivation, facial swelling, and difficulty eating. A child with noma often presents with a body temperature of 101.3°F (38.5°C) or more, enlarged submandibular lymph nodes, variable degree of loss of interdental papillae with alveolar bone exposure, and a medical history notable for antecedent illnesses such as gastroenteritis, measles, malaria, bronchopneumonia, tuberculosis, or HIV-infection. The gangrenous phase coincides with the spread of the gingival inflammatory lesion to the labiogingival fold, and then to the mucosal surface of the cheek and lip. Subsequently, an area of bluish-black discoloration may appear on the cheek. After this finding appears, rapid progression results in perforation of the cheek—usually a matter of days. This phase is characterized by extensive intraoral tissue destruction. Soft tissue sloughing leaves a fairly well-demarcated deep wound with exposed bones and teeth. The disease is usually unilateral but can occur bilaterally. The scarring phase sets in following the gangrenous stage and results in trismus and facial disfigurement. Sequelae of noma depend on the sites affected and the extent of tissue destruction. The sequelae may include displacement or exfoliation of teeth, facial mutilation, bony fusion between the maxilla and mandible, trismus, poor speech, difficulty feeding, persistent leakage of saliva, and severe emotional problems. Atypical sites of noma lesions may occur (e.g., in the mastoid region, scalp, perineum) concurrently with the orofacial lesions. Noma neonatorum occurs during the first few weeks of life in premature and low birthweight babies, and resembles noma in children. Other infections with similar manifestations include ecthyma gangrenosum (associated

with *Pseudomonas aeruginosa*), Buruli ulcer, leishmaniasis, niocervical necrotizing fasciitis in the elderly (associated with diabetes mellitus or other chronic condition), and necrotizing lesions associated with HIV-infection.

2. Causative agent—Noma is a polymicrobial infection. There is lack of consensus on the specific causative microorganisms. In Nigeria *Fusobacterium necrophorum* has been implicated in early noma cases, along with *Prevotella intermedia, Pseudomonas* spp., *Actinomyces* spp., and *Peptostreptococci micros*. A total of 67 bacterial species have been associated with advanced noma lesions in Nigeria including *Eubacterium, Flavobacterium, Microbacterium, Porphyromonas, Streptococcus, Sphingomonas*, and *Treponema*, possibly from contamination from the extra-oral environment. Culture-independent molecular study in another West African country attributes the cause to an imbalance of oral bacterial flora with a prominently increased proportion of *Prevotella* genus. Noma neonatarum is associated with *P. aeruginosa, Escherichia coli*, klebsiella, and staphylococci.

3. Diagnosis—Diagnosis is frequently predicated on clinical manifestations since no specific causative agent has been identified. Severe growth failure, excessive salivation, facial swelling, prominent fetid breath, and edema of the limbs in an impoverished child are very suggestive signs. The picture becomes more compelling if the child has acute necrotizing gingivitis (ANG), presenting as painful ulceration of the interdental papillae, with exposure of the underlying alveolar bone. Additionally, history of a recent or current debilitating illness (e.g., measles, malaria, diarrhea, bronchopneumonia, HIV-infection) virtually confirms the diagnosis. In the fairly advanced gangrenous stage, diagnosis is straightforward.

4. Occurrence—The current distribution of noma is poorly understood because many patients reside in rural parts of developing countries where health care centers are not readily accessible. Noma was a worldwide disease until the early 20th century when it essentially disappeared from industrialized countries coinciding with improvements in the standard of living and before the discovery of penicillin, except in concentration camps of World War II. Rarely noma is seen in industrialized countries in association with HIV-infection, intense immunosuppressive therapy, familial neutropenia, and in children with severe combined immunodeficiency diseases, particularly among Native Americans. Africa has the greatest disease burden, particularly in the "noma belt" that stretches across western and central Africa towards Sudan; Niger, Nigeria, Senegal, Burkina Faso, and Ethiopia are the most affected. Noma has recently been reported in Lao People's Democratic Republic and Haiti, and

WHO estimates that there are 100,000–140,000 new cases each year, increasing in geographic areas with widespread childhood undernutrition and/or high HIV prevalence.

5. Reservoir—*F. necrophorum* has been primarily associated with diseases of animals including liver abscesses in cattle, foot rot in domestic animals, calf diphtheria, and necrotic lesions of the oral cavity. Necrobacillosis of the body surface of wallabies (*Macropus reforgriseus*) is associated with *Fusobacterium nucleatum* and various *Bacteroides* spp. that are associated with human noma lesions. Outbreaks caused by necrobacillosis have occurred in wild kangaroos in Australia during unusually prolonged droughts when the animals tend to congregate around water holes where there is heavy fecal contamination. Noma-like lesions of the mouth and face have also been observed in stressed nonhuman primates, associated with *Fusobacterium* and the *Bacteroides*.

6. Incubation period—The incubation period is unknown, and incidence of acute noma peaks at 1–4 years of age, although late stages may occur in adolescents and adults. The putative oral precursor lesion for noma is ANG, and the latter has a prevalence rate as high as 18% in some underprivileged African communities. ANG shares many risk factors, including microbiological profile, in common with noma, but for reasons that are still unclear, extremely few cases of ANG evolve into noma.

7. Transmission—Noma has not been shown to be a transmissible disease: cases have not been reported in caregivers of children with the disease.

8. Risk groups—Poverty is the key risk factor for noma in African children, associated with malnutrition, unsatisfactory environmental sanitation, poor oral hygiene practices, limited access to health care services, close residential proximity to unkempt livestock, nomadic lifestyle, and a high prevalence of diseases such as malaria, measles, AIDS, diarrhea, and tuberculosis, among other infections. Intergenerational malnutrition is a common feature of communities at risk for noma, as is intrauterine growth retardation and low birth weight. Other risk factors include acute necrotizing gingivitis as well as the current prevalence of HIV/AIDS.

9. Prevention—Health care workers should be familiar with the key risk factors for and early signs of noma including low birthweight, severe infant stunting, persistent diarrhea, severe malnutrition, presence of oral mucosal ulcers, particularly ANG, and halitosis. Improvement in the living conditions is a key to prevention, particularly good nutrition, clean drinking water, segregation of livestock from human living areas, protective measures against malaria, good oral hygiene and immunization against childhood diseases, particularly measles. Increased awareness of the nutritional and health needs of women during pregnancy and lactation is also important. Adequate community and government attention must be paid to routine health care needs, environmental sanitation, nutrition, and public health awareness.

10. **Management of patient—**

1) Early detection of suspicious oral tissue lesions, including all oral/gingival ulcers in a stunted, deprived child.

2) Treatment with wound care, use of appropriate antibiotics (penicillin in combination with metronidazole; amoxicillin plus metronidazole; or monotherapy with only metronidazole), replacement of needed body fluids and electrolytes.

3) Meticulous wound care to minimize secondary infections: daily dressing with gauze soaked in antiseptic; and daily rinsing of the mouth with a solution of chlorhexidine digluconate (0.12%-0.20%).

4) Nutritional rehabilitation with a high protein diet enriched with essential micronutrients.

5) Immunization against childhood diseases if required.

6) Treatment of associated infections (e.g., malaria, tuberculosis, HIV).

7) Minor surgery in the acute phase for control of secondary hemorrhage, removal of loose teeth, and wound debridement.

8) Later stage surgical repair by excision of fibrous bands restricting jaw opening to correct trismus, followed by simple flap surgery and autoplasty. Occasionally complex procedures involving microsurgery.

9) Because of persisting postsurgical functional and cosmetic defects, the psychosocial needs of the patient constitute an important aspect of the treatment.

11. Management of contacts and the immediate environment— Noma is not considered transmissible from person to person, but there is need for increased surveillance in the community for other potential victims of the disease.

12. **Special consideration—**

1) It is recommended that cases be reported to local health authorities to permit clear identification of the geographic distribution and to stimulate local effective preventive measures.

2) International measures: endemic countries may wish to coordinate their efforts across borders, and if so should inform WHO.

[C. O. Enwonwu]

NOROVIRUS INFECTION
(Norwalk-like virus, winter vomiting disease)

DISEASE	ICD-10 CODE
NOROVIRUS INFECTION	ICD-10 A08.1

1. **Clinical features**—Usually a self-limited, mild to moderate disease that often occurs in outbreaks, with clinical symptoms of nausea, vomiting, diarrhea, abdominal pain, myalgia, headache, malaise, low grade fever, or a combination of these symptoms. Gastrointestinal symptoms typically last 24–72 hours. Dehydration is the most common complication.

2. **Causative agent**—Noroviruses are small (27–32 nm), structured ribonucleic acid (RNA) viruses classified within the family *Caliciviridae*; they are highly contagious and recognized as the most common causal agent of sporadic gastroenteritis across all age groups and of gastroenteritis outbreaks worldwide. Differential diagnoses include other viral agents of gastroenteritis such as sapovirus, rotavirus, astrovirus, and enteric adenovirus.

3. **Diagnosis**—Reverse transcription quantitative real-time polymerase chain reaction (RT-qPCR) assays are the preferred method for norovirus detection on whole stool samples and vomitus. These assays are highly sensitive and are able to differentiate between norovirus genogroups I and II. Conventional polymerase chain reaction (PCR) followed by sequencing of PCR products is used for genotyping. Recently a multiplex nucleic acid-based assay for a panel of gastrointestinal pathogens and an enzyme immunoassay (EIA) for the detection of norovirus antigen have been cleared by the US Food and Drug Administration. However, because the sensitivity of the norovirus EIA is limited, these tests should only be used for testing multiple specimens during outbreaks. EIA negative samples should be confirmed by RT-qPCR.

4. **Occurrence**—Worldwide and common; frequently occur in outbreaks but are also an important cause of sporadic disease. Noroviruses account for 9%–24% of all sporadic gastroenteritis; all age groups are

affected, though rates in children younger than 5 years are elevated, and more severe disease occurs in adults older than 65 years. Outbreaks have their source in restaurants, day care centers, cruise ships, hotels, and nursery homes. In industrialized countries, outbreaks are most often associated with health care settings.

5. Reservoir—Humans are the only known reservoir.

6. Incubation period—In volunteer studies, the range was 10–50 hours.

7. Transmission—Fecal-oral route, including direct person-to-person contact and indirect transmission through contaminated food, water, or environmental surfaces. Vomitus-oral transmission can also occur through aerosolization, followed by direct ingestion or environmental contamination. Food is contaminated most often by infected food handlers but also by using contaminated water during production (e.g., shellfish, produce). Secondary household transmission is common. Most communicable during acute stage of disease, but virus may be shed for 2–3 weeks after symptom resolution.

8. Risk groups—Older adults (>65 years), young children (<5 years), and immunocompromized patients are at elevated risk for severe disease and death.

9. Prevention—Use hygienic measures applicable to diseases transmitted via fecal-oral route (see "Typhoid Fever"). In particular, hand hygiene using soap and water, environmental disinfection, and exclusion of ill individuals (until 24–72 hours after symptom resolution) can help prevent spread. Alcohol-based hand sanitizers can be used in addition to hand washing, but they should not be used as a substitute for washing with soap.

10. Management of patient—

   1) Contact precautions.
   2) Treatment: primarily supportive, including fluid and electrolyte replacement as needed for dehydration (see "Cholera").

11. Management of contacts and the immediate environment— Search for means of spread of infection in outbreak situations. Isolate ill individuals to reduce further exposure, especially in health care settings where those infected can be placed together in isolation.

12. Special considerations—

   1) Reporting: obligatory report to local health authority of epidemics in some countries; no individual case report.

2) Large-scale outbreaks could be a potential problem in any disaster where water supplies, sanitation, or food preparation do not meet accepted hygiene standards.

[A. Hall, B. Lopman]

ONCHOCERCIASIS
(river blindness)

DISEASE	ICD-10 CODE
ONCHOCERCIASIS	ICD-10 B73

1. Clinical features—A chronic, nonfatal filarial disease. Adult worms are found in superficial fibrous nodules in subcutaneous tissues, particularly in the head and shoulders (Americas) or pelvic girdle and lower extremities (Africa). Nodules also occur in deep-seated bundles lying against the periosteum of bones or near joints. Female worms discharge microfilariae that migrate through the skin, often causing an intense pruritic rash as the microfilaria die, with disfiguring skin lesions, including chronic papular and lichenified dermatitis, altered pigmentation, edema, and atrophy of the skin. Pigment changes result in the condition known as "leopard skin," while loss of skin elasticity and lymphadenitis may result in "hanging groin." Microfilariae frequently reach the eye, causing visual impairment and blindness. Symptoms are predominantly due to the inflammatory response to endosymbiotic *Wolbachia* bacteria, which are released upon the death of microfilariae. The greater the body load of microfilariae, the greater the risk of developing skin and eye disease. Microfilariae may be found in organs and tissues other than skin and eye, but the clinical significance is unclear; in heavy infections they may also be found in blood, tears, sputum, and urine. Onchocerciasis has been associated with epilepsy and nodding syndrome.

Disease manifestations vary between geographical zones, with onchocercal blindness most prevalent in the African savanna, while skin manifestations predominate in forest areas. In Yemen and central Sudan, the major disease manifestation is Sowda, a pruritic skin condition usually affecting one limb. In the Americas, the manifestations are most consistent with those in the African savanna.

2. Causative agent—*Onchocerca volvulus*, a filarial worm belonging to the class *Nematoda*.

3. Diagnosis—Laboratory diagnosis is made through microscopic examination of fresh superficial skin biopsies incubated in saline for 24 hours at room temperature with observation of one or more emerging microfilariae or through the finding of adult worms in excised nodules. Different species cannot be distinguished morphologically, but species-specific deoxyribonucleic acid (DNA) probes exist that are routinely used for species differentiation in control programs. Differentiation of the microfilariae from those of other filarial diseases is required where the latter are also endemic. Other diagnostic clues include evidence of ocular manifestations and slit-lamp observations of microfilariae in the cornea, anterior chamber, or vitreous body. Serum antibody testing (using recombinant antigens) may be used for diagnosis.

4. Occurrence—Worldwide. Some 37 million people are thought to be infected with *O. volvulus;* more than 99% of cases occur in sub-Saharan Africa, where the disease is transmitted in an extensive area extending from Senegal to Ethiopia, down to Angola in the west, and Malawi in the east. It also occurs focally in Yemen and remains active in 2 foci in 2 countries in the Americas, Venezuela and Brazil. Regional control programs in both Africa and the Americas have had a major impact on the prevalence of disease, and in some areas it has been eliminated. The most recent maps can be found at: http://www.who.int/apoc/countries/en, http://oepa.net/epidemiologia.html, and http://www.cartercenter.org/health/river_blindness/oepa.html.

5. Reservoir—Humans. The disease can be transmitted experimentally to chimpanzees and has been found, rarely, in nature in gorillas.

6. Incubation period—Microfilariae are found in the skin usually only after 1 year or more from the time of the infective bite, though they have been found in children as young as 6 months. In Africa, vectors could be infective 7 days after a blood meal; in Guatemala the extrinsic incubation period is measurably longer ($\leq$14 days) because of lower temperatures.

7. Transmission—Human onchocerciasis can only be acquired through the bite of infected female blackflies of the genus *Simulium*: the most important vectors in Africa and Yemen are the *Simulium damnosum* complex and the *Simulium neavei* complexes, as well as *Simulium albivirgulatum* in Democratic Republic of Congo; in Central America, mainly *Simulium ochraceum*; and in South America, *Simulium metallicum* complex, *Simulium sanguineum/amazonicum* complex, *Simulium quad-rivittatum*, and other species. Microfilariae, ingested by a blackfly feeding on an infected person, penetrate thoracic muscles of the fly, develop into infective larvae, migrate to the cephalic capsule, are liberated on the skin, and enter the bite wound during a subsequent blood meal. Adult worms live as long as 10–14 years and people can infect flies as long as living microfilariae occur in their skin (i.e., ≤10–14 years after last exposure to *Simulium* bites if untreated). No direct person-to-person transmission occurs. Susceptibility is probably universal. Reinfection of infected people is common.

8. Risk groups.—Those who live or work close to vector-breeding sites are at highest risk. Severity of disease depends on cumulative effects of the repeated infections.

9. Prevention—

1) Individual: avoid bites of *Simulium* flies by wearing protective clothing and headgear as often as possible, or by using an insect repellent such as N,N-Diethyl-meta-toluamide (DEET).

2) Community-level: provide annual or semiannual ivermectin treatment to the eligible population of all endemic communities in an onchocerciasis focus in order to prevent onchocercal morbidity and reduce—and, where possible, interrupt—transmission and prevent new infections.

3) Community-level control and elimination programs: the African Program for Onchocerciasis Control (APOC) was established in 1995 to implement effective and sustainable annual ivermectin community treatment throughout Africa by 2015 to prevent disease from onchocerciasis. APOC now promotes the goal of disease elimination where feasible. APOC ensured treatment of more than 75 million people in 2010. The Onchocerciasis Elimination Program for the Americas uses semiannual mass distribution of ivermectin to prevent disease and eliminate the disease. Transmission of infection has been interrupted in 11 of 13 foci in the Americas as of the end of 2012.

10. Management of patient—

1) Evaluate all patients with suspected onchocerciasis for eye disease with slit lamp and fundoscopic exams.

2) Treatment: ivermectin, given as a single oral dose annually or semiannually, kills microfilariae and blocks release of new microfilariae from the uterus of the adult female worm, effectively reducing the number of microfilariae in the skin and eyes over a period of 6–12 months and reducing symptoms. The duration of the effect of such treatment is not well defined. Repeated treatments every 6 months to one year should be continued for symptom control or for evidence of microfilariae in the eye in patients who do not live in endemic areas.

Some authorities recommend a 6-week course of doxycycline treatment in individuals not at risk for reinfection, as the treatment kills adult worms. However, treatment with doxycycline does not kill microfilariae. Ivermectin should still be used for more immediate symptom relief. Neither diethylcarbamazine citrate (DEC) nor suramin are indicated as treatments because of the risk of severe adverse events.

3) If onchocercal subcutaneous nodules are detected and can be safely removed, they may be excised under local anesthesia.

4) Treatment of individuals coinfected with *Loa loa* with ivermectin can result in life-threatening encephalopathy. Such infection should be excluded when appropriate.

11. Management of contacts and the immediate environment— Not applicable—a community problem.

12. Special considerations—Epidemic measures: in areas of high prevalence, concerted efforts to provide community mass drug administration, as described in Prevention in this chapter.

[P. Cantey]

PARACOCCIDIOIDOMYCOSIS
(South American blastomycosis, paracoccidioidal granuloma)

DISEASE	ICD-10 CODE
PARACOCCIDIOIDOMYCOSIS	ICD-10 B41

1. Clinical features—Paracoccidioidomycosis is a polymorphic disease, often severe and progressive, although some self-limited cases have been reported. In younger patients, the disorder is subacute and carries a severe prognosis; in adults, the course is chronic, and the outcome better if appropriate therapy is given. The lungs are the site of primary infection, but the patient's symptoms may not reflect this. The acute or subacute form (less common) usually affects children, adolescents, and young adults who present clinical manifestations compatible with involvement of the reticuloendothelial system (i.e., lymph node hypertrophy, hepatomegaly, and/or splenomegaly). Cervical and submandibular chains of hypertrophic lymph nodes are the most obvious manifestation. In this clinical form, mucosal and pulmonary involvement is infrequent. In the adult form, most patients present with respiratory problems and seek medical advice as a result of the following symptoms in order of decreasing frequency:

1) Mucosal ulcerations occurring in the upper respiratory and digestive tracts, mostly in the mouth and nose

2) Difficulties in swallowing and changes in voice
3) Cutaneous lesions, often located on the face or limbs
4) Enlarged lymph nodes (mostly patients <30 years), especially in cervical area
5) Respiratory problems such as shortness of breath and persistent cough
6) Purulent or blood-tinged sputum and chest pain
7) Brain lesions

These symptoms are accompanied by weakness, malaise, fever, and weight loss. Haematogenous spread of *Paracoccidioides brasiliensis* can result in widespread dissemination, including lesions of the small or large intestine, adrenal gland destruction, oesteomyelitis, arthritis, and meningoencephalitis or focal cerebral lesions. The disease may require differentiation from tuberculosis, Hodgkin's disease, squamous cell carcinoma, and other cutaneous systemic mycoses.

2. Causative agent—*Paracoccidioides brasiliensis*, a dimorphic fungus geographically restricted to areas of South and Central America. Three phylogenetic species have been recognized to date. *Paracoccidioides lutzii* has been named to designate "Pb01-like" isolates endemic to Central-West Brazil.

3. Diagnosis—Direct examination of histopathology or culture; both may have low sensitivity. Serology may be useful but has low specificity.

4. Occurrence—Endemic in tropical and subtropical regions of Latin America from Mexico to Argentina. Some countries are not affected (e.g., some Caribbean Islands and Chile). Brazil is the area of greatest endemicity with considerably fewer cases reported from Colombia, Venezuela, Belize, Nicaragua, the Guianas, Ecuador, and Argentina. Highest incidence is in adults aged 30–50 years. In adults, paracoccidioidomycosis is more common in males than in females with a mean ratio of 15:1.

5. Reservoir—Presumably soil or fungus-laden dust.

6. Incubation period—Highly variable; from 1 month to many years. There is an indication that the fungus can remain dormant in residual lymph node lesions. Dormancy may be the reason why outbreaks have not been reported.

7. Transmission—The route of infection is still a matter of debate. At present, most investigators accept the inhalation theory. Not transmitted from person to person.

8. Risk groups—Occupational distribution reveals a predilection for agricultural workers.

9. **Prevention**—None.

10. **Management of patient**—

1) Concurrent disinfection of discharges and contaminated articles; terminal cleaning.

2) Treatment: presently, itraconazole is considered the best choice for mild-to-moderate infections as it is effective in 95% of cases with low relapse rates and less toxic. Amphotericin B is usually reserved for severely disseminated or critically ill patients, such as those with juvenile-form presentations or those who are immunosuppressed. Its use is limited by frequency of adverse effects and relapse rate as high as 20%–30%. Oral support therapy with itraconazole is also given to these patients for prolonged periods of time. Sulfonamides are cheaper but less effective than azoles. Central nervous system (CNS) disease requires fluconazole or voriconazole.

11. **Management of contacts and the immediate environment**—None.

12. **Special considerations**—None.

[J. Harris]

PARAGONIMIASIS
(pulmonary distomiasis, lung fluke disease)

DISEASE	ICD-10 CODE
PARAGONIMIASIS	ICD-10 B66.4

1. **Clinical features**—A trematode (flat worm) disease most frequently involving the lungs. Symptoms include cough, hemoptysis, and pleuritic chest pain. Chest X-ray findings may include diffuse and/or segmental infiltrates, nodules, cavities, ring cysts, and/or pleural effusions. Extrapulmonary disease is not uncommon; flukes may be found in organs such as the central nervous system, subcutaneous tissues, intestinal wall, peritoneal cavity, liver, lymph nodes, and genitourinary tract. Patients with cerebral infection can present with headache, mental confusion, behavioral changes, convulsion, visual impairment, and cerebral hemorrhage. Infection usually lasts for years, and the infected person may appear well. The disease may be mistaken for tuberculosis clinically and on chest X-rays.

2. Causative agents—*Paragonimus westermani, Paragonimus skrjabini, Paragonimus heterotremus*, and other species in Asia; *Paragonimus africanus* and *Paragonimus uterobilateralis* in Africa; *Paragonimus mexicanus* (*Paragonimus peruvianus*) and other species in the Americas; *Paragonimus caliensis, Paragonimus kellicotti*, and *Paragonimus Mexicans* in Central and North America. Adults typically reddish-brown in color, 7-16 mm by 4-8 mm.

3. Diagnosis—Sputum generally contains orange-brown flecks, sometimes diffusely distributed, in which masses of eggs are seen microscopically and they establish the diagnosis. However, acid-fast staining for tuberculosis destroys the eggs and precludes diagnosis. Eggs are also swallowed, especially by children, and may be found in feces by some concentration techniques. Serologic tests, including enzyme-linked immunosorbent assay (ELISA) and immunoblot, can aid the diagnosis especially when eggs are not seen in sputum or stool.

4. Occurrence—The disease has been reported in Asia, Africa, and the Americas. China, where an estimated 22.3 million people are infected, is the major endemic area, followed by India (Manipur province), Lao People's Democratic Republic, and Myanmar. The disease has been almost eliminated from Japan, while fewer than 1,000 people are infected in the Republic of Korea. Of the Latin American countries, Ecuador is the most affected with an estimated prevalence of 500,000 infections. Infections have also occurred in Brazil, Colombia, Costa Rica, Mexico, Peru, and Venezuela and rarely occur in Canada and the USA.

5. Reservoir—Humans, dogs, cats, pigs, and wild carnivores are definitive hosts and act as reservoirs.

6. Incubation period—Flukes mature and begin to lay eggs approximately 7-12 weeks after ingestion of the infective larvae. The long, variable, poorly defined interval until symptoms appear depends on the organ invaded and the number of worms involved.

7. Transmission—Through consumption of raw, salted, marinated, or partially cooked flesh of freshwater crabs or crayfish containing infective larvae (metacercariae). Larvae excyst in the duodenum, penetrate the intestinal wall, migrate through the tissues, become encapsulated (usually in the lungs), and develop into egg-producing adults. Eggs, either when expectorated in sputum or if swallowed and passed in the feces, gain access to freshwater and embryonate in 2-4 weeks. Larvae (miracidia) hatch, penetrate suitable freshwater snails, and undergo a cycle of development for several months. Larvae emerge from the snails to encyst in freshwater crabs and crayfish. Pickling of these crustaceans in wine, brine, or vinegar, a common practice in Asia, does not kill encysted larvae. Infections often occur in tourists sampling local foods. Eggs may be discharged by those infected for up to 20 years; duration of infection in mollusk and crustacean hosts is not well defined. Infection can also be acquired by ingestion of raw meat from other infected vertebrate hosts that contain young flukes (e.g., wild boars). In addition, transmission has been implicated from contaminated utensils, such as knives or cutting boards. Not directly transmitted from person to person.

8. Risk groups—Primarily people ingesting raw, salted, marinated, or undercooked freshwater crabs or crayfish.

9. Prevention—

1) Educate the public in endemic areas about the parasite.
2) Stress the importance of thorough cooking of crustaceans.
3) Dispose of sputum and feces in a sanitary manner.

10. Management of patient—

1) Concurrent disinfection of sputum.
2) Treatment: praziquantel, triclabendazole, or bithionol.

11. Management of contacts and the immediate environment— In an endemic area, the occurrence of small clusters of cases, or even sporadic infections, is an important signal for examination of local waters for infected snails, crabs, and crayfish and for determination of reservoir mammalian hosts in order to establish appropriate control.

12. Special considerations—None.

[J. Jones, M. Eberhard]

PEDICULOSIS AND PHTHIRIASIS
(lice)

DISEASE	ICD-10 CODE
PEDICULOSIS AND PHTHIRIASIS	ICD-10 B85

1. **Clinical features**—Infestation by head lice occurs on hair, eyebrows, and eyelashes; infestation by body lice is of the clothing, especially along the seams of inner surfaces. Crab lice usually infest the pubic area, and—more rarely—facial hair (including eyelashes in heavy infestations), axillae, and body surfaces. Infestation may result in severe itching and excoriation of the scalp or body. Secondary infection may lead to regional lymphadenitis (especially cervical).

2. **Causative agents**—The ectoparasites *Pediculus capitis* (head louse), *Pediculus corporis* (body louse), and *Phthirus pubis* (crab louse); adult lice, nymphs, and nits (egg cases) infest people. Lice are host-specific; those that infest nonhuman hosts do not infest humans, although they may be present transiently. Both sexes feed on blood. The body louse is the species involved in outbreaks of epidemic typhus caused by *Rickettsia prowazekii*, trench fever caused by *Bartonella quintana*, and epidemic relapsing fever caused by *Borrelia recurrentis*.

3. **Diagnosis**—A head lice infestation is best diagnosed by finding a live nymph or adult louse in the hair or scalp. However, they are small, move quickly, and can be difficult to see. Use of a fine-toothed louse comb may help in identifying live lice. If they are not found, then finding nits (eggs) on hair shafts (within one-fourth inch of the base of the shaft) suggests but does not confirm a lice infestation. If no nymphs or adults are seen and the only nits seen are more than one-fourth inch from the base of hair shafts, then the infestation is probably old, is no longer active, and does not need to be treated.

An infestation with body lice is usually diagnosed by finding eggs and crawling lice in the seams of clothing. Sometimes a body louse can be seen crawling or feeding on the skin.

Pubic lice infestation is diagnosed by finding "crab" lice (because they are crab-like in appearance) or nits on hair in the pubic region or, less commonly, elsewhere on the body.

4. **Occurrence**—Worldwide. Outbreaks of head lice are common among children in schools and institutions everywhere. Body lice are prevalent among populations with poor personal hygiene, especially in cold climates where heavy clothing is worn and bathing is infrequent, or when people cannot change clothes (e.g., in the case of refugees).

5. Reservoir—Humans.

6. Incubation period—Life cycle of 3 stages: eggs, nymphs, and adults. The most suitable temperature range for egg production and hatching is 29-32°C (84.2-89.6°F). Eggs of human lice do not hatch at temperatures under 22°C (71.6°F). Under optimal conditions, lice eggs hatch in 7-10 days. The nymphal stages last about 9-12 days for head and body lice and 13-17 days for crab lice. The egg-to-egg cycle averages about 3 weeks. The life cycle of the adult louse is about 1 month.

7. Transmission—For head and body lice, by direct contact with infested persons and objects used by them; for body lice, also by contact with the personal belongings of infested persons, especially shared clothing and headgear. Crab lice are most frequently transmitted through sexual contact. Lice leave a febrile host. Fever and overcrowding increase transfer from person to person. The period of communicability lasts as long as lice or eggs remain viable on the infested person or on fomites. The adult's life span on the host is approximately 1 month. Nits remain viable on clothing for 1 month. Body lice can survive for up to a week off the host without feeding, head lice and crab lice only about 2 days. Nymphs can survive 24 hours without feeding. Under suitable environmental conditions, head and crab lice eggs can remain viable away from the host for up to 7-10 days; body lice eggs remain viable for up to a month.

8. Risk groups—Head lice transmission is not related to cleanliness of the person who acquires an infestation. Transmission usually occurs by direct contact with the hair of any infected person, often among children during play or at activities such as slumber parties. Persons at risk for body lice generally have close person-to-person contact in conditions of crowding and poor hygiene. Pubic lice infestation is usually acquired during sexual contact with an infested partner.

9. Prevention—

1) Educate the public about diagnosis, treatment, and prevention, including the value of destroying eggs and lice through early detection, safe and thorough treatment of the hair, laundering clothing and bedding in hot water (55°C or 131°F for 20 minutes), and dry cleaning and/or the use of dryers set on "hot cycle."
2) For head lice, avoid head-to-head contact with an infested person, and avoid contact with items that have been in contact with hair from an infested person (e.g., hats, scarves, combs, brushes, pillowcases, towels). For body and pubic lice, avoid direct physical contact with infested individuals and their belongings, especially clothing and bedding.

3) Perform direct inspection of body and clothing for evidence of body lice when indicated. Evidence does not support the efficacy and cost-effectiveness of regular screening of children in classroom or schoolwide settings for head lice and nits.

10. Management of patient—For head lice, topical application of one of the following medications: permethrin cream rinse (1%), piperonyl butoxide/pyrethrins topical, spinosad topical suspension (0.9%), ivermectin lotion (0.5%), or benzyl alcohol lotion (5%). None of these treatments is 100% effective; re-treatment may be necessary. These treatments differ in regard to minimum age, whether a prescription is required, in the extent to which they are ovicidal, and whether re-treatment is routinely recommended or nit combing is needed. Resistance to permethrin and pyrethrins is widespread. Malathion lotion (5%; an organophosphate) has also been used on persons aged 6 years and older. Resistance to malathion has also been detected. Lindane (an organochlorine) is approved for the treatment of head lice and is available as a shampoo, but because of toxicity, side effects, and low efficacy, its use should be limited to patients who cannot tolerate or have failed treatment with other products that pose less risk.

For pubic lice, use piperonyl butoxide/pyrethrins topical or lindane shampoo.

For body lice, clothing and bedding should be washed using the hot water cycle of an automatic washing machine or dusted with pediculicides using power dusters, hand dusters, or 2-ounce sifter cans. Recommended dusts include 1% malathion and 0.5% permethrin.

11. Management of contacts and the immediate environment—Examine household and close personal contacts; treat those infested at the same time. Some experts believe that prophylactic treatment is indicated for contacts who share the same bed with infested persons.

12. Special considerations—

1) Epidemic measures: mass treatment with the treatments recommended in Prevention in this chapter, using insecticides clearly known to be effective against prevalent strains of lice. In typhus epidemics, individuals may protect themselves by wearing silk or plastic clothing tightly fastened around wrists, ankles, and neck and by impregnating their clothes with repellents or permethrin.

2) Disaster implications: diseases for which body and head lice are vectors are particularly prone to occur at times of social upheaval (see Epidemic Louse-Borne Typhus Fever section in "Typhus Fever").

[M. Deming, M. Eberhard]

PERTUSSIS
(whooping cough)

DISEASE	ICD-10 CODE
PERTUSSIS	ICD-10 A37.0, A37.9
PARAPERTUSSIS	ICD-10 A37.1

1. Clinical features—An acute bacterial infection of the respiratory tract classically characterized by paroxysmal cough and inspiratory whoop. The initial (catarrhal) stage consists of an insidious onset of upper respiratory infection with an irritating cough. Over the course of 1–2 weeks, paroxysms develop (paroxysmal phase) and increase in frequency and intensity before gradually improving after 1–2 months. Paroxysms are characterized by repeated violent coughing; each series of paroxysms has many coughs without intervening inhalation, which may be followed by a characteristic high-pitched inspiratory whoop. Paroxysms frequently end with the expulsion of clear, tenacious mucus often followed by vomiting. Between paroxysms, infected persons may appear well. Infants younger than 6 months may have cough without the typical whoop or may present with apnea.

In many industrialized countries with long-standing infant immunization and high coverage, an increasing number of cases are reported in adolescents and adults. Many such cases occur in previously immunized persons and suggest waning immunity following immunization. In those with partial immunity, symptoms vary from a mild, atypical respiratory illness to the full whooping syndrome.

Complications include pulmonary hypertension, pneumonia, atelectasis, seizures, encephalopathy, weight loss, hernias, and death. Pulmonary complications are the most common cause of death; fatal encephalopathy, probably hypoxic, and inanition from repeated vomiting occasionally occur. The number of fatalities in vaccinated populations is low. Most severe disease and deaths occur in infants younger than 6 months, often in those too young to have completed primary immunization. Case-fatality rates are less than 1 per 1,000 in industrialized countries; in developing countries they are estimated at 3.7% for children younger than 1 year and 1% for children aged 1–4 years. Pertussis remains among the most lethal diseases of unimmunized infants and young children, especially in those with underlying malnutrition and simultaneous enteric or respiratory infections.

Parapertussis is a similar but occasional and milder disease.

2. Causative agents—*Bordetella pertussis*, the bacillus of pertussis *stricto sensu*; *Bordetella parapertussis* causes parapertussis. *Bordetellae* are Gram-negative aerobic bacteria; *B. pertussis* and *B. parapertussis* are similar species, but the latter lacks the expression of the gene coding for pertussis toxin. *Bordetella holmesii* has also been reported to cause a pertussis-like syndrome.

3. Diagnosis—Based on clinical suspicion in the presence of typical signs and symptoms of pertussis. Confirmation requires demonstration of the causal organism from nasopharyngeal specimens obtained during the catarrhal and early paroxysmal stages. Culture is performed on Bordet-Gengou or Regan-Lowe culture media both supplemented with 15% defibrinated sheep or horse blood and is considered the "gold standard" of laboratory confirmation. While it is the most specific diagnosis, culture has limited sensitivity (60%). Polymerase chain reaction (PCR) can be highly sensitive and can be performed on the same biological samples as cultures. Direct fluorescent antibody staining of nasopharyngeal secretions is not recommended because of the occurrence of false positive and negative results. Indirect diagnosis is possible by determining a rise in specific immunoglobulin class G (IgG) antibodies directed against the pertussis toxin (anti–PT IgG) in an acute serum of the infected individual collected at the beginning of cough and in a convalescent serum collected one month later. In many industrialized countries, single-point anti-PT antibody tests are readily available and useful for diagnosis late in the course of illness when culture and PCR may be negative. Single-point serology results should be interpreted with caution as they do not differentiate between antibodies due to vaccination and those due to infection.

Differentiation among *B. parapertussis, B. pertussis,* and *B. holmesii* are based on phenotypic, genetic, biochemical, and immunological differences.

4. Occurrence—An endemic disease common in children everywhere, regardless of ethnicity, climate, or geographic location. Outbreaks occur typically every 3–4 years. In communities with active immunization programs and where good nutrition and medical care are available, pertussis still remains endemic, though at greatly reduced rates. Pertussis resurges when immunization rates fall and drops again when immunization programs are reestablished, as seen in Japan, Sweden, and the UK in the 1970s and 1980s. In 2003, despite an estimated worldwide vaccination coverage of around 75% with 3 doses of pertussis-containing vaccines, there were still an estimated 17.6 million pertussis cases with an estimated 279,000 deaths. The actual rates of disease are unknown because reporting is incomplete, and laboratory confirmation differs from country to country. Since 2004, notable increases in incidence have occurred in Australia, the USA, and some European countries.

5. Reservoir—Humans are believed to be the only host for pertussis. *B. parapertussis* can also be isolated from ovines.

6. Incubation period—Average 9–10 days (range 6–20 days).

7. Transmission—Through direct contact with discharges from respiratory mucous membranes of infected persons by the airborne route, probably via large droplets. Indirect spread through the air or contaminated objects may occur rarely. Pertussis is highly communicable in the early catarrhal stage and at the beginning of the paroxysmal cough stage (first 2 weeks). Thereafter, communicability gradually decreases and becomes negligible by about 3 weeks despite persisting spasmodic cough with whoop. Patients are considered no longer contagious after 5 days of treatment with erythromycin, clarithromycin, or azithromycin. In vaccinated populations, infants are most often exposed to pertussis in the home by a parent, older sibling, or other caregiver.

8. Risk groups—Susceptibility of nonimmunized individuals is universal, and pertussis can be severe in immuno-naïve individuals of any age. The highest incidence of pertussis, as well as the highest risk for severe or fatal pertussis, is in infants, but infection also occurs in adolescents and adults. Incidence, morbidity, and mortality are higher in females than males for unknown reasons. Secondary attack rates of up to 90% have been observed in nonimmune household contacts. Disease confers immunity but not lifelong. Maternal antibodies are actively transported across the placenta, and this observation has formed part of the rationale in certain countries to vaccinate pregnant women to reduce severe and fatal pertussis in young infants.

9. Prevention—

1) Educate the public, particularly parents of infants, about the dangers of whooping cough and the advantages of initiating immunization on time (between 6 weeks and 3 months, depending on the country) and of adhering to the immunization schedule. This is important because of the widespread past and present negative publicity given to adverse immunization reactions associated with pertussis vaccination.

2) Pertussis is generally recalcitrant to routine control measures, and immunization is the best means to control pertussis. Active, primary immunization against *B. pertussis* infection is by administering 3 doses of either killed, whole-cell pertussis (wP) or acellular pertussis (aP) vaccines. The latter contain 1–5 different components of *B. pertussis*. These are usually given in combination with diphtheria and tetanus toxoids adsorbed on aluminum salts (diphtheria/tetanus and whole-cell pertussis vaccine [DTwP] or diphtheria/tetanus and acellular pertussis vaccine [DTaP]). Both aP and wP vaccines are very safe; local and transient systemic reactions are less commonly associated with aP vaccines than with wP vaccines. Similar high efficacy (>80%) is observed with the best aP and wP vaccines, although efficacy

can differ among available vaccine products. Protection is greater against severe disease and wanes over time; many industrialized and middle income countries therefore recommend a fourth dose during the second year of life, a fifth dose before school entry, and a reduced dose booster for adolescents and/or adults. Pertussis vaccination does not protect against parapertussis.

Many industrialized and middle-income countries have completely replaced wP vaccines with aP vaccines. Though wP vaccines have a higher occurrence of local and systemic reactions such as fever, price considerations affect the wider implementation of aP vaccines. In most developing countries, wP vaccines continue to be used and effectively reduce the burden of pertussis. Schedules vary, but in all countries the goal should be to reach at least 90% coverage with a primary series of 3 doses of DTwP/DTaP in infants in all areas. In countries where immunization programs have considerably reduced pertussis incidence, a fourth dose is recommended. The optimal timing of a fourth dose and the need and timing for a fifth dose or adolescent/adult booster doses should be based on the local epidemiology. Vaccines containing wP are not recommended after the seventh birthday, since local reactions may be increased in older children and adults. Formulations of acellular pertussis vaccine for use in adolescents and adults have been licensed and are available in several countries.

DTwP/DTaP can be given simultaneously with oral poliovirus vaccine (OPV) and at different sites from inactivated poliovirus vaccine (IPV); *Haemophilus influenzae* type b (Hib) vaccine; hepatitis B (HB) vaccine; pneumococcal and meningococcal conjugate vaccine; and vaccines for measles, mumps, rubella (MMR). Combination vaccines with Hib, IPV, and HB are available and are widely used in Europe and North America.

Minor adverse reactions such as local redness and swelling, fever, and agitation often occur after immunization with wP vaccine (1 in 2–10). Prolonged crying and febrile seizures are less common (1 in 100); hypotonic-hyporesponsive episodes are rare (1 in 2,000). Although febrile seizures and hypotonic-hyporesponsive episodes may follow DTwP and are disturbing to parents and physicians alike, there is no scientific evidence that these reactions have any permanent consequences. Recent detailed reviews of all available studies conclude that there is no demonstrable causal relationship between DTwP and chronic nervous system dysfunction in children. The only true contraindication to immunization with DTwP/DTaP is an anaphylactic reaction to a previous dose or to any constituent of the vaccine. In young infants with suspected evolving and progressive neurological disease, immunization may be delayed to permit diagnosis and avoid possible confusion about the cause of symptoms.

10. **Management of patient—**

1) Respiratory isolation for known cases. Suspected cases should be removed from the presence of young children and infants, especially nonimmunized infants, until the patients have received at least 5 days of antibiotics. Persons with a suspected case who do not receive antibiotics should be isolated for 3 weeks after onset of paroxysmal cough or until the end of cough, whichever comes first.

2) Disinfection measures are of little impact.

3) Treatment: erythromycin, clarithromycin, and azithromycin can shorten the period of communicability but likely do not reduce symptom severity or duration unless given before the paroxysmal stage develops.

11. **Management of contacts and the immediate environment—**

1) Inadequately immunized household contacts younger than 7 years may be excluded from schools, day care centers, and public gatherings for 21 days after last exposure or until the case patients and contacts have received 5 days of appropriate antibiotics.

2) All contacts should have their immunization status verified and brought up to date. Passive immunization has not been demonstrated to be effective, and there is no such product currently commercially available. The initiation of active immunization following recent exposure is not effective against infection, but it should be undertaken to protect the child against further exposure in case he or she has not been infected. Close contacts younger than 7 years who have not received 4 DTwP/DTaP doses or have not received a DTwP/DTaP dose within 3 years should be given a dose as soon after exposure as possible. A 7-day course of erythromycin or clarithromycin or a 5-day course of azithromycin for household and other close contacts—regardless of immunization status and age—is recommended for households where there is a child younger than 1 year. Prophylactic antibiotic therapy in the early incubation period may prevent disease, but difficulties of early diagnosis, the costs involved, and concerns related to the occurrence of drug resistance all limit the benefits of prophylactic treatment. Prophylactic treatment is specifically recommended for the following:

   • Children younger than 1 year and pregnant women in the last 3 weeks of pregnancy (because of the risk of transmission to the newborn).

- Stopping infection among household members, particularly if the household contains children younger than 1 year and pregnant women in the last 3 weeks of pregnancy.

3) Attempts to identify early, missed, and atypical cases are indicated where a nonimmune infant or young child might be exposed.

12. Special considerations—

1) Reporting: case report to local health authority of suspected and confirmed cases is required in most countries; early reporting may permit better outbreak control. The WHO-recommended clinical case definition is "a case diagnosed as pertussis by a physician or a person with a cough lasting at least 2 weeks and at least one of the following symptoms: paroxysms (fits) of coughing, inspiratory 'whooping,' post-tussive vomiting (vomiting immediately after coughing) without other apparent cause." (see http://www.who.int/immunization_monitoring/diseases/pertussis_surveillance/en)

2) Epidemic measures: a search for unrecognized and unreported cases may be indicated to protect preschool children from exposure and to ensure adequate preventive measures for exposed children younger than 7 years. Accelerated immunization with the first dose as early as 6 weeks of age and the second and third doses at 4-week intervals may be indicated; it is more important to make sure that immunization is completed for those whose schedule is incomplete and that the vaccines are given on time according to the national schedule.

3) Disaster implications: pertussis is a potential problem if introduced into crowded refugee camps containing nonimmunized children.

4) Ensure completion of primary immunization of infants and young children before they travel to other countries if possible; review need for a booster dose.

[T. Clark]

PINTA
(carate)

DISEASE	ICD-10 CODE
PINTA	ICD-10 A67

1. **Clinical features**—Pinta is a chronic, nonvenereal, treponemal skin infection without systemic manifestations. One to eight weeks after exposure, a single or several scaly, pruritic, erythematous papules or small plaques with regional lymphadenopathy appear usually on the extremities or other uncovered area. These primary lesions may resolve entirely without treatment. After 3-12 months, the initial lesions appear smaller, and scaly papules develop over a wider area of the body. These secondary lesions vary in size from less than 0.5 cm to several centimeters and also vary in color and form from macules to small plaques. Over time, these lesions evolve into tertiary patches of altered (dyschromic) skin pigmentation of variable size. These treponema-containing patches sometimes pass through stages of blue to violet to brown pigmentation, finally becoming treponema-free depigmented (achromic) areas. Lesions coexist at different stages of evolution and are most common on the face and extremities. The differential diagnosis includes syphilis, psoriasis, yaws, and fungal infections in early lesions and vitiligo, tinea versicolor, and other pigmentary disorders in late lesions.

2. **Causative agent**—*Treponema carateum*, a spirochete.

3. **Diagnosis**—Spirochetes are demonstrable in primary, secondary, and dyschromic (but not achromic) lesions through dark-field or direct fluorescent antibody microscopic examination. Other diseases in the differential might be ruled out by histological examination of the skin lesions. Serological tests for syphilis usually become reactive before or during the secondary lesions, and thereafter behave as in venereal syphilis.

4. **Occurrence**—Pinta is found only among isolated rural populations living in crowded conditions in the American tropics. It is predominantly a disease of older children and adults. Surveys carried out during the mid-1990s by Pan American Health Organization (PAHO)/WHO in targeted Amazonian populations in Brazil, Peru, and Venezuela found few cases. Isolated foci may still exist in Central America and Cuba.

5. **Reservoir**—Humans.

6. **Incubation period**—Usually 2-3 weeks.

7. **Transmission**—The mechanism of transmission is unknown, but it is presumed to be through direct and prolonged contact with initial and

early dyschromic skin lesions. The disease is mainly transmitted in childhood. Various biting and sucking arthropods, especially blackflies, are suspected, but not proven, biological vectors. Not highly contagious; several years of intimate contact may be necessary for transmission.

8. Risk groups—Persons living in endemic areas, particularly children, are at risk for developing pinta.

9. Prevention—Those applicable to other nonvenereal treponematoses apply to pinta; see "Yaws."

10. Management of patient—See "Yaws."

11. Management of contacts and the immediate environment—See "Yaws."

12. Special considerations—

1) Reporting: report to local health authority may be required in some endemic areas.
2) For disaster implications and international measures, see "Yaws."

[C. E. Introcaso, R. Neblett Fanfair]

PLAGUE
(pestis)

DISEASE	ICD-10 CODE
PLAGUE	ICD-10 A20

1. Clinical features—Plague has 3 possible presentations: bubonic, septicemic, and pneumonic. Initial signs and symptoms for all phases may be nonspecific, with fever, chills, malaise, myalgia, nausea, prostration, sore throat, and headache. With bubonic plague, lymphadenitis often develops in those lymph nodes that drain the site of the flea bite that causes infection and are called buboes. The location of buboes can vary depending on the circumstances of exposure, with flea bites on the legs typically resulting in the appearance of buboes in the inguinal area. Axillary buboes can be associated with flea bites as well and are often seen after the handling of infected animals. Cervical buboes are rare in industrialized countries but are relatively common in many developing countries where people sleep on the dirt floors of flea-infested huts. Regardless of the location, the buboes are inflamed and tender and may suppurate. The septicemic form of plague can occur subsequent to bubonic plague (secondary septicemic plague) or without prior lymphadenopathy (primary septicemic plague) and involves bloodstream dissemination to diverse parts of the body, including in some instances the meninges. Septicemic cases also can experience endotoxic shock and disseminated intravascular coagulation, in some instances without localizing signs of infection. Secondary involvement of the lungs results in pneumonia; mediastinitis or pleural effusion may develop. Secondary pneumonic plague is of special significance since respiratory droplets may serve as the source of person-to-person transfer with resultant primary pneumonic or pharyngeal plague; this can lead to localized outbreaks or more widespread epidemics. Though naturally acquired plague usually presents as bubonic plague, purposeful aerosol dissemination as a result of deliberate use would be manifest primarily as pneumonic plague.

Untreated bubonic plague has a case-fatality rate of about 50%–60%. Untreated primary septicemic plague and pneumonic plague are almost invariably fatal. Modern therapy markedly reduces fatalities from bubonic plague; pneumonic and septicemic plague also responds if recognized and treated early (within ~2 days). Plague is a medical and a public health emergency. Further information on this and other plague-related topics or updates can be found at: http://www.cdc.gov/plague.

2. **Causative agent**—*Yersinia pestis*, the plague bacillus.

3. **Diagnosis**—Visualization of characteristic bipolar staining, "safety pin" ovoid, Gram-negative organisms in direct microscopic examination of material aspirated from a bubo, sputum, or cerebrospinal fluid (CSF) is suggestive, but not conclusive, evidence of plague infection. Examination by fluorescent antibody (FA) test, antigen capture by enzyme-linked immunosorbent assay (ELISA) or dipstick formats, or polymerase chain reaction (PCR) are more specific and particularly useful in some instances. In the USA, cases are considered confirmed following isolation of *Y. pestis* by culture of bubo aspirates, blood, CSF, or sputum samples or by demonstration of a 4-fold or greater rise or fall in antibody titer. Slow growth of the organism at normal incubation temperatures may lead to misidentification by automated systems. The passive hemagglutination test using *Y. pestis* Fraction-1 antigen and ELISA are used for serodiagnosis. Recently, WHO and others proposed the use of dipstick (horizontal flow) assays designed to detect *Y. pestis* antigen in clinical samples as a means for rapid diagnosis of cases, but these tests are not widely available. Medical personnel should be aware of areas where the disease is endemic and should entertain the diagnosis of plague early on; unfortunately, plague is often misdiagnosed, especially in travelers who develop illness after returning from an endemic area, and delays in diagnosis can result in fatalities.

4. Occurrence—Plague continues to be a threat because of vast areas of persistent wild rodent infection; contact of wild rodents with domestic rats occurs frequently in some enzootic areas. While urban rat-associated plague has been controlled in most of the world, wild rodent plague exists in the Americas, with foci in northeastern Brazil, the Andean region near the border of Ecuador and Peru, and the western half of the USA causing sporadic cases and occasional outbreaks; also in scattered locations in east-central and southern Africa, the interior of Algeria, and perhaps other African countries bordering the Mediterranean Sea; central, southwestern, and southeastern Asia; and extreme southeastern Europe near the Caspian Sea. Since 1990 the disease has occurred in several African countries, including Botswana, the Democratic Republic of Congo (DRC), Kenya, Madagascar, Malawi, Mozambique, the United Republic of Tanzania, Uganda, Zambia, Zimbabwe, and Algeria. Plague is endemic in China, India, Lao People's Democratic Republic, Mongolia, Myanmar, Viet Nam, and Indonesia. Outbreaks occasionally appear in areas that have been free of the disease for many decades. Since the beginning of the 1990s, there has been an increase in the annual incidence of human cases of plague; moreover, the disease has reappeared in countries where it had not been reported for decades. Currently, the distribution of plague coincides with the geographical distribution of its natural foci. From 2004–2009 a total of 12,503 cases were reported to WHO; 843 of these were fatal. Among these, 99.7% of cases were reported from 8 African countries. DRC has the most active foci of plague worldwide, averaging more than 1,000 suspected cases a year since 2004; following the eruption of several severe outbreaks of pneumonic plague in DRC, the diagnosis is now systematically evoked when a deadly outbreak with hemorrhagic signs is reported in Central Africa.

Human plague in the western USA is sporadic (typically 5–15 cases/year since 1970), with only single cases or small common source clusters in an area, usually following exposure to wild rodents or their fleas—although cases have also been acquired by persons handling infected rabbits, wild carnivores, or domestic cats. No person-to-person transmission has occurred in the USA since 1924, although secondary plague pneumonia occurred in about 20% of bubonic cases in one reported series. Five instances of primary plague pneumonia through cat-to-human transmission have been recorded.

5. Reservoir—Wild rodents are the natural vertebrate hosts of plague and play a key role in maintaining natural plague cycles by serving as sources of infection (amplifying hosts) for the flea vectors of the disease. Some of these species can survive for weeks to months in the burrows of their hosts and appear to represent a significant reservoir of infection. Certain other mammals, including lagomorphs (rabbits and hares), wild carnivores, and domestic cats may also become infected and act as sources of infection to people. In many developing countries, commensal rats play epidemiologically important roles by moving infected fleas into human dwellings from wild lands or agricultural fields.

6. Incubation period—From 1-7 days; may be a few days longer in immunized persons who develop illness. For primary plague pneumonia, incubation period is short, lasting 1-4 days.

7. Transmission—Two main patterns of transmission for naturally acquired human plague can be distinguished:

1) Human intrusion into the zoonotic (sylvatic) cycle during or following an epizootic. Cases typically result from being bitten by infectious wild rodent fleas. Some of these flea species may remain infective for months under suitable conditions of temperature and humidity. Human cases also have been linked to handling infected animals and domestic pets, particularly house cats and dogs, which can carry *Y. pestis*-infected wild rodent fleas into homes. Cats may occasionally transmit infection through bites, scratches, or respiratory droplets; cats develop plague abscesses that have been a source of infection to veterinary personnel.

2) Infection in commensal rodents and their fleas, themselves infected by contact with peridomestic mammals, leads to an entry of the bacteria into human habitat. In that case, the disease is the manifestation of poverty and insufficient conditions of hygiene. Person-to-person transmission by *Pulex irritans* fleas is believed to be important in the South American Andes and a few other places around the world where plague occurs, and this flea is abundant in homes or on domestic animals. Risk of exposure concerns the community as a whole in Africa, India, and South America. On a worldwide basis, the most frequent source of exposure for human cases are the bites of infectious infected rat fleas, especially the oriental rat flea (*Xenopsylla cheopis*). In some countries, wild rodent hosts of plague live in close proximity to humans, as is the case for certain ground squirrels infested with *Oropsylla montana*, the primary vector of plague to humans in North America.

Other important sources of human infection include the handling of infected animals, especially rodents and rabbits but also wild carnivores and domestic cats; rarely, airborne droplets from human patients or household cats with plague pharyngitis or pneumonia; and careless manipulation of laboratory cultures. Human cases acquired by inhalation (primary pneumonic plague) have been reported in the past couple of decades in developing countries. Bubonic plague is not usually transmitted directly unless there is contact with pus from suppurating buboes. Pneumonic plague may be highly communicable under appropriate climatic conditions; overcrowding and cool temperatures facilitate transmission.

In the case of deliberate use, plague bacilli would possibly be transmitted as an aerosol. For more information on the deliberate use of infectious agents to cause harm, see "Outbreak Response in Case of Deliberate Use of Biological Agents to Cause Harm."

8. Risk groups—Susceptibility among humans is general. Immunity after recovery is relative; it may not protect against a future large inoculum. Those who live in areas with poor rodent sanitation practices and hunters, trappers, trekkers, veterinary staff, and farmers operating during or following an epizootic are at increased risk.

9. Prevention—The basic objective is to reduce the likelihood of people being bitten by infectious fleas, having direct contact with infective tissues and exudates, or being exposed to patients with pneumonic plague.

1) Educate the public in enzootic areas on the modes of human and domestic animal exposure; on rat-proofing buildings and preventing access to food and shelter by peridomestic or wild rodents through appropriate storage and disposal of food, garbage, and refuse; and on the importance of avoiding flea bites by use of insecticides and repellents. In sylvatic or rural plague areas, the public should be advised to use insect repellents when walking or working in suspect areas and be warned not to camp near rodent burrows and not to handle rodents. Dead or sick animals should be reported to health authorities or other appropriate persons. Dogs and cats in such areas should be protected periodically with appropriate insecticides to reduce the risk that infectious fleas will be transported into human environs and should not be allowed to roam freely in plague-affected areas. Any animal carcasses brought home by these animals should be disposed of safely.

2) Survey rodent populations periodically to determine whether epizootics are in progress or conditions indicate that one is likely. The effectiveness of rodent sanitation measures in homes and public areas also should be evaluated. Although flea control is the primary means for controlling plague, rat suppression by poisoning (see next paragraph on control of rats) may be used to augment basic environmental sanitation measures; rat control should always be preceded by measures to control fleas. Areas of plague activity can be identified by surveillance of natural foci by testing of fleas collected from rodents and their burrows or nests, by bacteriologic testing of sick or dead wild rodents, and by serological analyses of samples from wild carnivores and outdoor ranging dogs and cats. Regular testing should take place to ensure the effectiveness of insecticides on target flea populations.

3) Control rats on ships, on docks, and in warehouses by rat-proofing or periodic fumigation, combined when necessary with destruction of rats and their fleas in vessels and in cargoes, especially containerized cargoes, before shipment and on arrival from locations endemic for plague.

4) Wear gloves when hunting and handling wildlife. Veterinarians and their staff should wear gloves and masks when examining sick cats.

5) Plague vaccine is unavailable in most countries and should not be relied upon as the sole preventive measure, and immunized persons should take other appropriate prevention precautions as indicated in this chapter. Live attenuated vaccines are used in some countries but can produce adverse reactions, and their efficacy has not been proven. Different vaccination strategies have been used in the past involving both a killed and a live attenuated vaccine, but these strategies have only conferred protection against bubonic plague and not against primary pneumonic plague. Currently, the next generation of plague vaccines is being researched, and, in some cases, vaccines are in clinical trials.

10. **Management of patient—**

1) Rid patients living in rat- and flea-infested dwellings of fleas and treat their clothing and baggage with an appropriate insecticide; hospitalize if practical. Strict isolation is only required for patients with pneumonic plague for whom precautions against airborne spread are required until 48 hours of appropriate antibiotic therapy have been completed and there has been a favorable clinical response. For patients with bubonic plague (if there is no cough and the chest X-ray is negative), drainage and secretion precautions are indicated for 48 hours after start of effective treatment.

2) Disinfect articles and surfaces contaminated with potentially infectious sputum and purulent discharges. Human cadavers and animal carcasses should be handled with strict aseptic precautions.

3) Treatment: rapid diagnosis and treatment are essential to reduce complications and fatality. The laboratory confirmation is of first importance but must not delay treatment. Although streptomycin (adults—2 g/day in 2 equal doses; children—30 mg/kg/day in 2 equal doses) is the drug of choice, gentamicin (adults—3 mg/kg/day in 3 equal doses; children—6.0-7.5 mg/kg/day in 3 equal doses) can be used when the former is not readily available; tetracyclines (adults—2 g/day in 4 equal doses; children >8 years—25-50 mg/day in 4 equal doses) and chloramphenicol (children and adults—50 mg/kg/day in 4 equal doses) are alternative choices. Chloramphenicol is required for

treatment of plague meningitis. All are highly effective if used early. After a satisfactory response to drug treatment, reappearance of fever may result from a secondary infection or a suppurative bubo that may require incision and drainage.

11. **Management of contacts and the immediate environment—**

1) Quarantine measures have been shown to be ineffective in controlling plague outbreaks and can trigger panic in the population. Those who have been in household or face-to-face contact with patients with pneumonic plague should be provided chemoprophylaxis (see next paragraph on protection of contacts) and placed under surveillance for 7 days; those who refuse chemoprophylaxis should be maintained in strict isolation with careful surveillance for 7 days.

2) Protection of contacts: in epidemic situations where human dwellings are invaded by flea-infested rats or harbor human fleas (*Pulex irritans*) that also might act as vectors, consideration should be given to treating family members and other close contacts with an appropriate insecticide. All close contacts should be evaluated for chemoprophylaxis. Close contacts of confirmed or suspected plague pneumonia cases (including medical personnel) should be provided with chemoprophylaxis for a period of 7 days using tetracycline (2 g/day in 2 or 4 equal doses for adults; 25–50 mg/kg/day in 2 or 4 equal doses for children >8 years), doxycyline (100 mg twice daily for persons >45 kg; 2.2 mg/kg for those >8 years <45 kg), or chloramphenicol (30 mg/kg daily in 4 divided doses). Contacts also should be advised about appropriate measures they can take to protect themselves and their families from plague and should be placed under surveillance.

3) Search for sick or dead rodents and their fleas and, if possible, submit these for laboratory analysis. Identify household members and others likely to have had potential similar plague exposures to the cases under investigation. If pneumonic plague is involved, identify household members and others who are likely to have had face-to-face contact with pneumonic plague patients. Determine whether case contacts show evidence of plague and provide medical care, treatment, and chemoprophylaxis as needed.

12. **Special considerations—**

1) Reporting: report any suspected case to the local health authority. In many developed countries, because of the rarity of naturally acquired primary plague pneumonia, even a single case should initiate prompt investigation, and in the unlikely circumstance that a natural source of infection cannot be

identified, public health and law enforcement authorities might be reasonably suspicious of deliberate use. For more information, see Measures in the Case of Deliberate Use later in this section and "Outbreak Response in Case of Deliberate Use of Biological Agents to Cause Harm."

Any event of potential international concern is subject to a notification to WHO under the International Health Regulations. Plague cases are to be reported to WHO only if the assessment done by the country shows that the public health impact can be considered as serious with at least one of the following characteristics: unusual or unexpected event, risk of international spread, significant risk of international travel, or trade restriction. Thus, the occurrence of a pneumonic plague case in a well-known focus should not be systematically notified. Conversely, the appearance of a bubonic case in a nonendemic region is typically an event to be notified.

2) Epidemic measures:

- Investigate all suspected plague deaths with autopsy and laboratory examinations when indicated. Develop and carry out case finding. Establish the best possible facilities for diagnosis and treatment. Alert existing medical facilities to report cases immediately and to use full diagnostic and therapeutic services.

- Attempt to prevent or mitigate public hysteria by appropriate informational and educational releases through the news media, information leaflets, websites, and social media channels.

- Institute intensive flea control in affected areas and during epidemics. Apply flea control measures in expanding circles from known outbreak sites. Flea control should precede antirodent measures, and the latter should not be executed until the efficacy of the flea control measures has been demonstrated. To control fleas, apply insecticidal dusts to rodent runs, harborages, nests, and burrows in and around known or suspected plague areas. All insecticides used for such control should be safe for human residents, labeled for flea control, and known to be effective against local fleas. If nonburrowing rodents are involved, insecticide bait stations can be used. If urban rats are involved, disinsect houses and other structures with insecticidal dusts; dust the bodies and clothing of all residents in the immediate vicinity. After appropriate flea control measures have been taken, rat populations can be suppressed by environmental modifications intended to reduce rodent food and harborage, and applications of appropriate rodent poisons can be considered.

- Implement tracing of contacts and medical surveillance/ chemoprophylaxis.
- Protect field workers against fleas; dust clothing with insecticide powder and use insect repellents daily. Antibiotic prophylaxis should be provided for those with documented close exposure.

3) Disaster implications: plague could become a significant problem in or near endemic areas when there are social upheavals, crowding, and unhygienic conditions.

4) International measures:

- Notify WHO if necessary (see Reporting in Special Considerations in this chapter).
- Measures applicable to ships, aircraft, and land transport arriving from plague areas are specified in the IHR.
- All ships should be free of rodents or periodically deratted.
- Rat-proof buildings at seaports and airports; apply appropriate insecticides; eliminate rats with effective rodenticides.

WHO Collaborating Centres provide support as required. Further information can be found at: http://www.who.int/ collaboratingcentres/database/en.

5) Measures in the case of deliberate use: *Y. pestis* is distributed worldwide; techniques for mass production and aerosol dissemination are thought to exist. The fatality rate of primary pneumonic plague is high, and there is a real potential for secondary spread, particularly in those circumstances where cases are treated in home environments without modern medical care. For these reasons, the risk of a biological attack with plague is considered to be a serious public health concern. In some countries, a few sporadic cases may be missed or not attributed to a deliberate act, particularly in those with natural foci. Any suspect case of pneumonic plague should be reported immediately to the local health department. The sudden appearance of many patients presenting with fever, cough, a fulminant course, and high case-fatality rate should provide a suspect alert for plague; if cough is primarily accompanied by hemoptysis, this presentation favors the tentative diagnosis of pneumonic plague. For a suspected or confirmed outbreak of pneumonic plague, follow the treatment and containment measures outlined in this chapter. Depending on the extent of dissemination, mass prophylaxis of potentially exposed populations may be considered. For more information on the deliberate use of infectious agents to cause harm, see

"Outbreak Response in Case of Deliberate Use of Biological Agents to Cause Harm."

[E. Bertherat, K. Gage]

PNEUMONIA

DISEASE	ICD-10 CODE
PNEUMOCOCCAL PNEUMONIA	ICD-10 J13
MYCOPLASMA PNEUMONIA	ICD-10 J15.7
PNEUMOCYSTIS PNEUMONIA	ICD-10 B59
PNEUMONIA DUE TO *CHLAMYDIA TRACHOMATIS*	ICD-10 P23.1
PNEUMONIA DUE TO *CHLAMYDIA PNEUMONIAE*	ICD-10 J16.0
OTHER PNEUMONIAS	ICD-10 J12, J15, J16.8, J18

I. PNEUMOCOCCAL PNEUMONIA

1. **Clinical features**—Clinical manifestations include sudden onset, high fever, rigors, pleuritic chest pain, dyspnea, tachypnea, and cough productive of "rusty" sputum. Onset may be less abrupt, especially among the elderly; fever, shortness of breath, or altered mental status may provide the first evidence of pneumonia. In infants and young children, fever, vomiting, and convulsions may be the initial manifestations. Laboratory findings include leukocytosis (neutrophilia) and elevated C-reactive protein. Typical chest radiograph findings show lobar or segmental consolidation; consolidation may be bronchopneumonic, especially in children and the elderly. Pneumococcal pneumonia is an important cause of death in infants and the elderly.

Infection can be complicated by empyema, acute respiratory distress syndrome, septic shock, and purpura fulminans. The case-fatality rate varies widely from 5%-35%, depending on the setting (e.g., outpatients vs. inpatients) and the population (e.g., healthy adults vs. persons with alcoholism). In developing countries, case-fatality rates among children are often greater than 10%, and as great as 60% among infants younger than 6 months. Pneumococcal pneumonia among previously healthy individuals with other respiratory infections (e.g., influenza) is well described.

2. Causative agent—*Streptococcus pneumoniae* (pneumococcus), a Gram-positive, lancet-shaped, encapsulated diplococcus that often asymptomatically colonizes the human nasopharynx. Children are colonized with *S. pneumoniae* more often than adults. Current data suggest that 6 serotypes (1, 5, 6B, 14, 19F, 23F) account for the majority of invasive disease worldwide.

3. Diagnosis—A microbiologic diagnosis of pneumococcal pneumonia can guide antibiotic therapy. The presence in sputum of many Gram-positive diplococci together with polymorphonuclear leukocytes suggests pneumococcal pneumonia; however, Gram stain and culture of respiratory secretions are often not performed, largely due to technical aspects of obtaining good quality specimens and the difficulty of distinguishing infection from respiratory tract colonization. Definitive diagnosis of pneumococcal pneumonia is established by isolation of pneumococci from blood or, less commonly, pleural fluid. Among adults, the diagnosis can also be established by identification of pneumococcal polysaccharide in urine. For children, urine antigen testing is not useful because nasopharyngeal colonization can cause excretion of pneumococcal antigen in urine. Most pediatric cases are diagnosed by isolation of pneumococci from blood. Patients suspected of having pneumococcal pneumonia should be treated promptly, preferably after collection of appropriate diagnostic specimens according to established guidelines. If pneumococcus is isolated, susceptibility testing should be performed, and antimicrobial therapy tailored to susceptibility results.

4. Occurrence—*Streptococcus pneumoniae* (pneumococcus) is the most common bacterial etiology of community-acquired pneumonia among all ages. Pneumococcal pneumonia is an endemic disease among the elderly and those with underlying medical conditions. Infection is more frequent among malnourished populations and lower socioeconomic groups, especially in developing countries. It occurs in all climates and seasons, peaking in winter in temperate zones. Certain serotypes may cause epidemics, especially among institutionalized populations, the homeless, and those in developing countries. Incidence is high in certain geographic areas (e.g., Papua New Guinea) and in certain ethnic groups, such as Alaska Natives and Australian Aboriginals. In Europe and North America, estimates of the rate of pneumococcal pneumonia vary widely from approximately 30 cases per 100,000 to nearly 100 per 100,000 adults each year, depending on the population studied and the diagnostic tests used. An increased incidence often accompanies epidemics of influenza.

5. Reservoir—Humans. Pneumococci are commonly found in the upper respiratory tract of healthy people worldwide.

6. Incubation period—Not well determined; may be as short as 1–3 days. Infection is thought to be preceded by asymptomatic colonization.

7. **Transmission**—By droplet spread. Person-to-person transmission is common, but illness among casual contacts and attendants is infrequent. The disease remains communicable presumably until discharges of mouth and nose no longer contain infectious numbers of pneumococci, which usually occurs within 24 hours of initiation of effective antibiotic therapy.

8. **Risk groups**—Susceptibility is increased among certain populations, including infants, the elderly, and persons with underlying illnesses such as anatomical or functional asplenia, sickle cell disease, cardiovascular disease, diabetes mellitus, cirrhosis, Hodgkin's disease, lymphoma, multiple myeloma, chronic renal failure, nephrotic syndrome, HIV infection, and recent organ transplantation. Malnutrition and low birth weight are important risk factors for infection among infants and young children in developing countries. Susceptibility to infection is also increased by processes affecting the integrity of the lower respiratory tract, including influenza, pulmonary edema, aspiration following alcoholic intoxication or other causes, chronic lung disease, or exposure to irritants (e.g., cigarettes, cooking fire smoke). Previously healthy persons can develop pneumococcal pneumonia.

9. **Prevention**—

1) Avoid crowding in living quarters whenever practical, particularly in institutions. Prevent malnutrition and encourage physical activity. Bedridden patients should lie in an upright position at a 30- to 45-degree incline.

2) Protein-polysaccharide conjugate vaccines including 10 or 13 of the commonest serotypes are included in routine infant immunization schedules in many countries. Pneumococcal conjugate vaccines have been shown to be highly effective at preventing invasive pneumococcal disease and pneumococcal pneumonia, with important reductions in disease incidence demonstrated in the target age population (direct effects) and those too old or too young to receive the vaccine (indirect, or herd, effects). It should be noted that the evidence for this is mostly from developed countries, and, at the time of writing, encouraging information about the effectiveness of these vaccines in developing countries is just becoming available.

   WHO considers it a priority to include pneumococcal conjugate vaccines in all national immunization programs and recommends that decisions about which conjugate vaccine to introduce should be left to individual country-level policy makers.

3) A 23-valent pneumococcal polysaccharide vaccine (PPV23) is available for persons older than 2 years. In some countries it is recommended for high-risk persons (individuals aged ≥65 years and those with anatomic or functional asplenia, sickle cell

disease, HIV infection, and a variety of chronic systemic illnesses, including heart and lung disease, cirrhosis of the liver, renal insufficiency, and diabetes mellitus). In resource-poor settings, WHO recommends placing greater emphasis on the introduction of conjugate vaccine for children, given their proven efficacy and their demonstrated indirect benefits for adults.

PPV23 is not effective in children younger than 2 years and has no impact on pneumococcal carriage. For most eligible patients, vaccine needs to be given only once; however, reimmunization is generally safe, and vaccine should be offered to eligible patients whose immunization status cannot be determined. Reimmunization is recommended once for persons older than 2 years who are at highest risk for serious pneumococcal infection and those likely to have a rapid decline in pneumococcal antibody levels, provided that 5 years or more have elapsed since receipt of the first dose of vaccine. In addition, persons aged 65 years and older should be given another dose of vaccine if they received the vaccine more than 5 years previously and were younger than 65 years at the time of primary immunization.

10. **Management of patient—**

1) Respiratory isolation may be warranted for hospitalized patients with a highly antibiotic-resistant infection who may transmit it to patients at high risk of pneumococcal disease.

2) Hand hygiene and cough etiquette.

3) Treatment: antibiotic treatment of infants and young children with pneumonia should start presumptively based on a clinical diagnosis. If tachypnea and chest in-drawing are present, infants younger than 2 months should be transferred to hospital care without delay; if pneumococcal pneumonia is identified, parenteral penicillin G or ampicillin are preferred treatments (or erythromycin for those hypersensitive to penicillin). Based on a clinical trial in Pakistan, immediate treatment of children aged 3–59 months with severe pneumonia with oral amoxicillin may result in equivalent outcome compared to hospitalization and intravenous ampicillin. Because pneumococcal resistance to penicillin and other antimicrobials is increasingly recognized, sensitivities of strains isolated from normally sterile sites, including blood or cerebrospinal fluid (CSF), should be determined. Caution should be exercised in interpreting susceptibility results, as the same isolate may be considered susceptible or resistant to antibiotics (e.g., penicillin, third-generation cephalosporins) depending on potential antibiotic penetration at the site of infection (e.g., blood vs. meninges). WHO guidelines recommend ampicillin or

amoxicillin for home treatment of nonsevere pneumonia for children younger than 5 years (recommended duration of treatment in nonsevere pneumonia is 3 days instead of the standard 5 days); they are not intended for industrialized countries where professional societies have published recommendations for the treatment of community-acquired pneumonia and pneumonia in children.

11. Management of contacts and the immediate environment—
None.

12. Special considerations—

1) Reporting: obligatory report of epidemics in some countries.
2) Epidemic measures: in outbreaks in institutions or in other closed groups, immunization with pneumococcal conjugate or 23-valent polysaccharide vaccine may be carried out unless it is known that the type causing disease is not included in the vaccines. Due to theoretical concerns that immunization with PPV23 may be followed by a period of a few days of increased susceptibility to infection if PPV23 is used, or if the outbreak is particularly explosive, antibiotic prophylaxis may also need to be considered.
3) Disaster implications: crowding of populations in temporary shelters bears a risk of disease, especially for the very young and the elderly.

II. MYCOPLASMA PNEUMONIA

1. Clinical features—Predominantly a febrile lower respiratory infection causing about 20% of pneumonias; less often, a pharyngitis that sometimes progresses to tracheobronchitis or pneumonia. Clinical pneumonia occurs in about 3%–30% of infections with *Mycoplasma pneumoniae*. Disease varies from mild afebrile pharyngitis to febrile illness of the upper or lower respiratory tract. Onset is gradual with headache, malaise, cough (often paroxysmal), sore throat, and sometimes chest discomfort that may be pleuritic. Sputum, scant at first, may increase later. Early patchy infiltration of the lungs is often more extensive on X-ray than clinical findings suggest. In severe cases, the pneumonia may progress from one lobe to another and become bilateral. Leukocytosis occurs after the first week in approximately one-third of cases. Duration varies from a few days to a month or more. Complications such as central nervous system (CNS) involvement (e.g., encephalitis, acute disseminated encephalomyelitis) and Stevens-Johnson syndrome are infrequent; fatalities are rare.

Differentiation is required from atypical pneumonia due to many other agents: other bacteria; adenoviruses; influenza; respiratory syncytial virus; parainfluenza; measles; Q fever; psittacosis; certain mycoses; severe acute respiratory syndrome (SARS or other coronavirus infections); and tuberculosis.

2. Causative agent—*Mycoplasma pneumoniae* belongs to the mycoplasmas (Molicutes) placed between bacteria and viruses. Because mycoplasmas lack cell walls, cell wall synthesis inhibitors such as the penicillins and cephalosporins are not effective in treatment. Along with *Streptococcus pneumoniae* and *Haemophilus influenzae*, *M. pneumoniae* is one of the most common agents of community-acquired pneumonia.

3. Diagnosis—Although serology-based tests are commercially available and widely used, many have proven to be unreliable due to inherent difficulties in interpretation. A 4-fold rise in antibody titers between acute and convalescent sera collected 3-6 weeks apart may provide some diagnostic utility, and serological assays may add value when used as supportive evidence of infection in concert with other testing modalities. Molecular diagnostics, most notably quantitative real-time polymerase chain reaction (qPCR) assays, have become a more common and reliable method for rapid diagnosis of *M. pneumoniae*. Respiratory specimens such as nasopharyngeal and oropharyngeal sputum are acceptable specimen types for qPCR testing. These tests are commercially available in some specialty public health laboratories, but their main drawback is the lack of standardization between laboratories. Some specialized laboratories can also perform culture using special media. However, due to the low recovery rate and lengthy incubation time required, culturing is not routinely attempted for rapid diagnosis.

4. Occurrence—Worldwide; sporadic, endemic, and occasionally epidemic, especially in institutions and military populations. Outbreaks often occur in schools and households. Attack rates vary from 5 to more than 50 per 1,000 persons per year in military populations and 1-3 per 1,000 persons per year in civilians. Epidemics occur more often in late summer and autumn; endemic disease is not seasonal, but there can be variation from year to year and among different geographic areas. Men and women of all ages are equally affected. Infection is most frequent among school-age children and young adults.

5. Reservoir—Humans.

6. Incubation period—6-32 days.

7. Transmission—Probably by droplet inhalation and direct contact with an infected person (including those with subclinical infections). Secondary cases of pneumonia among contacts, family members, and attendants are frequent. The period of communicability is probably less than 20 days. Treatment reduces carriage but does not reliably eradicate the organism from the respiratory tract where it may persist for weeks. Duration of immunity is uncertain. Second attacks of pneumonia may occur. Protection against repeat infection has been correlated with humoral antibodies that persist up to 1 year.

8. Risk groups—Primarily school-age children and young adults, although the disease can occur at any age.

9. Prevention—Avoid crowded living and sleeping quarters whenever possible, especially in institutions, barracks, and ships.

10. Management of patient—

1) Respiratory secretions may be infectious.
2) Hand hygiene and cough etiquette.
3) Treatment: azolides (e.g., azithromycin, clarithromycin), erythromycin, or a tetracycline. Azolides or macrolides are preferred for children younger than 8 years.

11. Management of contacts and the immediate environment— Investigation of contacts and source of infection allows for treatment of clinical infection among family members.

12. Special considerations—

1) Reporting: obligatory report of epidemics in some countries.
2) Epidemic measures: no reliably effective measures for control are available, although antimicrobial prophylaxis has been used in some institutional outbreak settings.

More information can be found at: http://www.who.int/collaboratingcentres/database/en.

III. PNEUMOCYSTIS PNEUMONIA
(interstitial plasma cell pneumonia, PCP)

1. Clinical features—An acute to subacute, often fatal, pulmonary disease, especially in persons with immunosuppression and in malnourished, premature infants. Clinically, patients present with dyspnea on exertion, dry, nonproductive cough, and fever. Auscultatory signs are usually minimal or absent. Chest radiographs typically show bilateral diffuse interstitial infiltrates.

2. Causative agent—*Pneumocystis jiroveci* (previously known as *Pneumocystis carinii* and classified as a protozoa). Currently, it is considered a fungus, based on nucleic acid and biochemical analysis.

3. Diagnosis—Established through demonstration of the causative agent in material from induced sputum, bronchoalveolar lavage, or transbronchial or open lung biopsy. Staining with methenamine silver or

Giemsa can identify the organism. There is no commercially available routine culture method or serological test at present, though several exist in research laboratories.

4. Occurrence—Worldwide; may be endemic and epidemic in debilitated, malnourished, or immunosuppressed infants. It affected approximately 60% of patients with HIV infection in the USA, Europe, and Australia before the routine use of prophylactic medication and antiretroviral therapy. It is a common cause of pneumonia in HIV-infected young infants in developing countries with high HIV prevalence, particularly in sub-Saharan Africa.

5. Reservoir—Humans. Organisms have been demonstrated in rodents, cattle, dogs, and other animals, but the ubiquitous presence of the organism and its subclinical persistence in humans render these potential animal sources of little public health significance.

6. Incubation period—Unknown. Analysis of data from institutional outbreaks and animal studies indicates that the onset of disease often occurs 1–2 months after establishment of the immunosuppressed state.

7. Transmission—The mode of transmission in people is not known. Airborne animal-to-animal transmission has occurred in rats. In one study in the USA, approximately 75% of healthy individuals were reported to have humoral antibody to *P. jiroveci* by 4 years old, suggesting that subclinical infection is common. Pneumonitis in the compromised host is thought to result either from a reactivation of latent infection or a newly acquired infection.

8. Risk groups—Susceptibility is enhanced by prematurity, chronic debilitating illness, and disease or treatments that impair immune mechanisms. Infection with HIV is a predominant risk factor.

9. Prevention—Among immunosuppressed patients—especially those with HIV infection, those treated for lymphatic leukemia, and those with organ transplants—prophylaxis with either oral trimethoprim-sulfamethoxazole, atovaquone, dapsone, or the combination of dapsone, pyrimethamine, and leucovorin is effective in preventing endogenous reactivation for the period during which the patient receives treatment.

10. Management of patient—Treatment: trimethoprim-sulfamethoxazole is the drug of choice. Alternate drugs are pentamidine (intramuscular [IM] or intravenous [IV]), dapsone with trimethoprim, atovaquone, and clindamycin-primaquine.

11. Management of contacts and the immediate environment—No specific measures required unless close or intimate contacts are immunosuppressed, at which time chemoprophylaxis may be considered.

12. **Special considerations—**

1) Reporting: when cases occur in people with evidence of HIV infection, case report may be required in some countries.

2) Epidemic measures: knowledge of the source and mode of transmission is so incomplete that there are no generally accepted measures.

IV. CHLAMYDIAL PNEUMONIAS

A. PNEUMONIA DUE TO *CHLAMYDIA TRACHOMATIS* (neonatal eosinophilic pneumonia, congenital pneumonia due to *Chlamydia*)

1. **Clinical features—**A subacute chlamydial pulmonary disease typically occurring between 4–11 weeks of age among infants whose mothers have chlamydial infection of the cervix. Clinically, the disease is characterized by insidious onset, cough (characteristically staccato), lack of fever, patchy infiltrates on chest radiograph with hyperinflation, eosinophilia, and elevated immunoglobulin class M (IgM) and immunoglobulin class G (IgG). About half of cases show prodromal rhinitis and conjunctivitis. Duration of illness is commonly 1–3 weeks but may extend as long as 2 months. The illness is usually moderate but can progress to severe pneumonia. One study suggests that infants with chlamydial pneumonia are at increased risk of chronic cough and abnormal lung function.

2. **Causative agent—***Chlamydia trachomatis* of immunotypes D to K.

3. **Diagnosis—**A wide variety of diagnostic tests are available, including direct fluorescent antibody tests, enzyme immunoassays, deoxyribonucleic acid (DNA) probes, and nucleic acid amplification systems. Although elevated serum IgM suggests recent infection, microimmunofluorescent assays, considered optimal for detection of antibody, are not widely available.

4. **Occurrence—**Probably coincides with the worldwide distribution of genital chlamydial infection. The disease has been recognized in many countries, and epidemics do not appear to occur.

5. **Reservoir—**Humans. Experimental infection with *C. trachomatis* has been induced in nonhuman primates and mice; animal infections are not known to occur in nature.

6. **Incubation period—**Pneumonia may occur in infants from 1–18 weeks of age (more commonly between 4–11 weeks). Nasopharyngeal infection is usually not recognized before 2 weeks of age.

7. Transmission—From the infected cervix to an infant during birth, with resultant nasopharyngeal infection (and occasionally chlamydial conjunctivitis). Respiratory transmission does not appear to occur.

8. Risk groups—Infants of mothers with chlamydial infection. Maternal antibody does not protect the infant from infection.

9. Prevention—See Chlamydial Conjunctivitis section in the "Conjunctivitis/Keratitis."

10. Management of patient—

1) Universal precautions in hospitals and nurseries.
2) Concurrent disinfection of discharges from nose and throat of infants.
3) Treatment: oral erythromycin is the drug of choice for infants. Sulfisoxazole is a possible alternative.

11. Management of contacts and the immediate environment—Examine parents for infection and treat if positive.

12. Special considerations—None.

B. PNEUMONIA DUE TO *CHLAMYDIA PNEUMONIAE*

1. Clinical features—An acute respiratory disease with cough, frequently a sore throat and hoarseness, and fever at the onset; sputum is scanty and chest pain is rare. Inflammatory signs are sometimes subtle. Pulmonary rales are usually present. The clinical picture is similar to pneumonia caused by *Mycoplasma*. Radiographic abnormalities include bilateral infiltrates, sometimes with pleural effusions. Illness is usually mild, but recovery is slow with cough persisting for 2-6 weeks. Death is rare in uncomplicated cases.

2. Causative agent—*Chlamydophila pneumoniae* is the species name for the human-specific organism with distinct morphological and serological differences from *C. psittaci* and *C. trachomatis*.

3. Diagnosis—Historically, laboratory diagnosis has been primarily serological. Microimmunofluorescence testing of paired sera collected 4-8 weeks apart is commercially available but requires a fluorescent microscope, and there are specificity problems due to cross-reaction with chlamydial antigens of other species. More recently, real-time polymerase chain reaction (PCR) assays have been employed to provide rapid, specific, and sensitive antigen detection of nasopharyngeal/oropharyngeal sputum or other respiratory tract specimens. The organism can be isolated from throat swab specimens in special cell lines, but this is not routinely performed due to cost, length of time to result, and low recovery rates.

4. Occurrence—Presumably worldwide. Age distribution has 2 peaks: one among children between 5 and 15 years of age and one in persons aged 60 years and older. Antibodies are rare in children younger than 5 years; seroprevalence increases among teenagers and young adults to a plateau of about 50% by age 20-30 years, which persists into old age. No seasonality has been noted. Outbreaks in communities, households, day care centers, and schools are often reported.

5. Reservoir—Presumably humans.

6. Incubation period—Unknown; may be 3-4 weeks.

7. Transmission—The mode of transmission has not been defined, although droplet transmission is most likely. The period of communicability also has not been defined but is presumably long; some military outbreaks have lasted as long as 8 months.

8. Risk groups—Susceptibility is thought to be universal with increased likelihood of clinical disease in the presence of preexisting chronic disease. Serological evidence of recall type immune response suggests immunity after infection; second episodes of pneumonia have been observed in military recruits with a secondary type of serological response to the second attack.

9. Prevention—

1) Avoid crowding in living and sleeping quarters.
2) Apply personal hygiene measures: cover mouth when coughing and sneezing and wash hands frequently.

10. Management of patient—

1) Universal precautions should be practiced.
2) Concurrent disinfection of discharges from nose and throat.
3) Treatment: a definite diagnosis is difficult at the early stages of illness. Current recommendations for empiric treatment of community-acquired pneumonia in adults include regimens effective against *C. pneumoniae*, including macrolides, azolides, and tetracyclines. In children, macrolides are the drug of choice. Fluoroquinolones are alternative agents. Treatment may have to be as long as 6 weeks for *C. pneumoniae*.

11. Management of contacts and the immediate environment—Examine all members of the family for infection and treat if positive.

12. Special considerations—

1) Reporting: report epidemics to local health authority.
2) Epidemic measures: case finding and appropriate treatment.

V. OTHER PNEUMONIAS

Among the known viruses, pneumonitis can be caused by adenoviruses, respiratory syncytial virus, parainfluenza viruses, human bocavirus, and probably others as yet unidentified. Because these agents cause upper respiratory disease more often than pneumonia, they are presented in "Common Cold and Other Acute Viral Respiratory Diseases." Measles, influenza, and chickenpox cause pneumonitis and pneumonia. Pulmonary infection with *Chlamydia psittaci* is presented in "Psittacosis." Pneumonia is also caused by infection with rickettsiae (see "Q Fever") and *Legionella* (see "Legionellosis"). Pneumonia can be associated with the invasive phase of nematode infections, such as ascariasis, and with mycoses, such as aspergillosis, histoplasmosis, and coccidioidomycosis.

Various pathogenic bacteria commonly found in the mouth, nose, and throat, such as *Haemophilus influenzae* (see "Meningitis"), *Staphylococcus aureus, Klebsiella pneumoniae, Streptococcus pyogenes* (group A hemolytic streptococci), *Neisseria meningitidis, Bacteroides* species, *Moraxella catarrhalis,* and anaerobic cocci, can cause pneumonia, either as a primary pathogen or as a complication of chronic pulmonary disease or after aspiration of gastric contents or tracheostomy. With increased use of antimicrobial and immunosuppressive treatment, pneumonias caused by enteric Gram-negative bacilli have become more common, especially those caused by *Escherichia coli, Pseudomonas aeruginosa,* and *Proteus* species. Management depends on the organism involved.

[M. Moore]

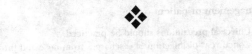

POLIOMYELITIS
(polioviral fever, infantile paralysis)

DISEASE	ICD-10 CODE
POLIOMYELITIS	ICD-10 A80

1. **Clinical features**—A viral infection recognized by acute onset of flaccid paralysis. Infection occurs in the gastrointestinal tract with spread to regional lymph nodes and, in a minority of cases, to the central nervous system. Flaccid paralysis occurs in less than 1% of infections; the rate of paralysis among infected nonimmune adults is higher than that among nonimmunized infants and young children. Approximately 90% of infections are unapparent or result in nonspecific fever. Aseptic meningitis occurs in about 1% of infections. Fever, malaise, headache, nausea, and vomiting are recognized in 10% of infections. If disease progresses to major illness, severe muscle pain and stiffness of the neck and back with flaccid paralysis may occur. Paralysis is usually asymmetric with fever present at onset; maximum extent is usually reached within 3–4 days. The site of paralysis depends on the location of nerve cell destruction in the spinal cord or brain stem; legs are affected more often than arms. Paralysis of the respiration and/or swallowing muscles can be life-threatening. Some improvement in paralysis may occur during convalescence, but paralysis still present after 60 days is likely to be permanent. Infrequently, recurrence of muscle weakness following recovery may occur many years after the original infection has resolved ("postpolio syndrome"); this is not believed to be related to persistence of the virus itself.

With progress made towards global eradication, poliomyelitis must now be distinguished from other paralytic conditions by isolation of virus from stool. Other enteroviruses (notably types 70 and 71), echoviruses, and coxsackieviruses have been reported to cause an illness simulating paralytic poliomyelitis. The most frequent cause of acute flaccid paralysis (AFP) that must be distinguished from poliomyelitis is Guillain-Barré syndrome. Paralysis in Guillain-Barré syndrome is typically symmetrical and may progress for periods as long as 10 days. Fever, headache, nausea, vomiting, and pleocytosis characteristic of poliomyelitis are usually absent in GBS; high protein and low cell counts in cerebrospinal fluid (CSF) and sensory changes are seen in the majority of Guillain-Barré syndrome cases. Acute motor axonal neuropathy ("China paralytic syndrome") is an important cause of AFP in northern China and is probably present elsewhere; it is seasonally epidemic and closely resembles poliomyelitis. Fever and CSF pleocytosis are usually absent, but paralysis may persist for several months. Other causes of AFP include transverse myelitis, traumatic neuritis, infectious and toxic neuropathies, tick paralysis, myasthenia gravis, porphyria, botulism, insecticide poisoning, polymyositis, trichinosis, and periodic paralysis. Differential diagnosis of acute nonparalytic poliomyelitis includes other forms of acute nonbacterial meningitis, purulent meningitis, brain abscess, tuberculous meningitis, leptospirosis, lymphocytic choriomeningitis, infectious mononucleosis, the encephalitides, neurosyphilis, and toxic encephalopathies.

2. Causative agent—Poliovirus (genus *Enterovirus*) types 1, 2, and 3; all types cause paralysis. Wild poliovirus type 1 is isolated from paralytic cases most often, and type 3 less so. Circulating wild type 2 poliovirus has not been detected since October 1999. Type 1 most frequently causes epidemics. Paralytic polio cases have also been reported due to outbreaks caused by circulating vaccine–derived polioviruses (cVDPVs) types 1, 2, and 3. Presently most cVDPVs are caused by type 2 viruses. Paralytic polio also occurs in association with vaccination (vaccine-associated paralytic poliomyelitis) in vaccine recipients or their healthy contacts at a rate of approximately 1 in every 2.5 million doses administered, or 1 in 800,000 first vaccinations.

3. Diagnosis—Definitive laboratory diagnosis requires isolation of the poliovirus from stool samples, cerebrospinal fluid, or oropharyngeal secretions. Specialized laboratories can differentiate "wild" from "vaccine-derived" and vaccine virus strains. Rises in antibody levels (>4-fold) are less helpful in the diagnosis of wild poliomyelitis infection; type-specific neutralizing antibodies may already be present when paralysis develops, and significant titer rises may therefore not be demonstrable in paired sera. Antibody response following immunization mimics the response after infection with wild type viruses, and the widespread use of live polio vaccines makes interpretation of antibody levels difficult, except to rule out polio in cases where no antibody has developed in immunocompetent children. Poliovirus is demonstrable in throat secretions as early as 36 hours and in feces 72 hours after exposure to infection in both clinical and inapparent cases.

4. Occurrence—Historically, poliomyelitis occurred worldwide sporadically and as epidemics with an increase during the late summer and autumn in temperate countries. In tropical countries, a less pronounced seasonal peak occurred in the hot and rainy season. With improved immunization and the global initiative to eradicate poliomyelitis, wild polioviruses at the time of writing were endemic in only 3 countries that had not succeeded in interrupting transmission (Afghanistan, Nigeria, Pakistan). However, type 2 cVDPVs were circulating in 5 countries (Afghanistan, Chad, Nigeria, Pakistan, Somalia), and sporadic polio importations continued to occur in areas of West/Central Africa and the Horn of Africa. Poliomyelitis remains primarily a disease of infants and young children. In the 3 countries that have not yet succeeded in interrupting transmission, 80%–90% of cases are in children younger than 3 years, and virtually all cases are in those younger than 5 years.

Although wild poliovirus transmission has ceased in most countries, importation remains a threat. A large outbreak of poliomyelitis occurred in 1992–1993 in the Netherlands among members of a religious group that refuse immunization, and virus was also found among members of a related religious group in Canada, although no cases occurred. Since 2000, imported wild poliovirus has caused outbreaks and paralytic cases in more than 30 countries, primarily in Africa, Asia, and the Middle East. In recent years, outbreaks following wild poliovirus importations into polio-free countries have often affected adults due to the increasing susceptibility of older populations in areas with gaps in routine immunization coverage. Until recent changes in immunization policy with the exception of rare imported cases, the few cases of poliomyelitis recognized in industrialized countries were caused by vaccine virus strains. About half of vaccine-associated paralytic poliomyelitis cases occurred among adult contacts of vaccinees. Between 2000 and 2012, polio outbreaks due to cVDPVs were reported from 20 countries, all of which continue to use oral poliovirus vaccine (OPV) for routine immunization. These outbreaks have been associated with areas of low OPV coverage, and the cases were clinically indistinguishable from polio caused by wild poliovirus.

5. Reservoir—Humans, most frequently people with inapparent infections, especially children. No long-term carriers of wild type poliovirus have been detected. Chronic carriage of vaccine-derived poliovirus has been reported, all from industrialized countries or emerging economies and all associated with primary immunodeficiency syndromes; at end of 2012 one such carrier was known to be continuing to excrete virus.

6. Incubation period—Commonly 7–14 days for paralytic cases; reported range of 3 to possibly 35 days.

7. Transmission—Primarily person-to-person spread, principally through the fecal-oral route; virus is detectable more easily and for a longer period in feces than in throat secretions. Where sanitation levels are high, pharyngeal spread may be relatively more important. In rare instances, milk, foodstuffs, and other materials contaminated with feces have been implicated as vehicles. No reliable evidence of spread by insects. Transmission is possible as long as the virus is excreted. Virus typically persists in the throat for approximately 1 week and in feces for 3–6 weeks. Cases are most infectious during the days before and after onset of symptoms. Type-specific immunity, apparently of lifelong duration, follows both clinically recognizable and inapparent infections. Second attacks of polio are rare and result from infection with a poliovirus of a different type.

8. Risk groups—Groups that refuse immunization; minority populations, migrants, and other unregistered children, nomads, refugees, and the urban poor are at high risk, as well as those in areas in geographic proximity to endemic countries and those that are inaccessible due to insecurity. Intramuscular injections, trauma, or surgery during the incubation period or prodromal illness may provoke paralysis in the affected extremity. Tonsillectomy increases the risk of bulbar involvement. Excessive muscular activity in the prodromal period may predispose to paralysis. Infants born of immune mothers have transient passive immunity.

9. **Prevention—**

1) Educate the public on the advantages of immunization in early childhood.

2) Both a trivalent live, attenuated OPV and an injectable inactivated poliovirus vaccine (IPV) are commercially available for routine immunization. Since 2005 monovalent OPV types 1 and 3 have been developed and licensed for use in mass campaigns and, since 2009 bivalent OPV, for provision of higher, type-specific seroconversion rates in areas where one or both of these serotypes are circulating.

OPV simulates natural infection by inducing both circulating antibody and resistance to infection of the pharynx and intestine (mucosal immunity) and also immunizes some susceptible contacts through secondary spread. In developing countries, lower rates of seroconversion and reduced vaccine efficacy for OPV have been reported; this can be overcome by administration of numerous extra doses in immunization programs and/or supplemental campaigns. Breastfeeding does not cause a significant reduction in the protection provided by OPV. WHO recommends the use of OPV for immunization programs in developing countries because of the capacity to induce mucosal immunity, low cost, ease of administration, and superior capacity to provide population immunity through secondary spread.

IPV, like OPV, provides excellent individual protection by inducing circulating antibody that blocks the spread of virus to the central nervous system and also protects against pharyngeal infection, but it does not induce intestinal immunity comparable to OPV (though IPV may substantially boost intestinal immunity in children who have previously been vaccinated with OPV). Many middle-income countries and most industrialized countries have switched to IPV alone for routine immunization because wild type polioviruses have been eliminated in those settings, ongoing global eradication efforts have reduced the risk of importations, and the risk of paralysis from OPV in these countries is considered greater than that from wild poliovirus.

A few individuals with underlying primary immune deficiency disorders who chronically excreted an OPV-derived poliovirus have been identified in industrialized countries and emerging market economies; the significance of these chronic excreters for polio eradication is under review. More troublesome are outbreaks of poliomyelitis caused by circulating vaccine-derived polioviruses (cVDPVs). These are capable of spreading through populations and infecting nonvaccinated or incompletely vaccinated individuals. The extent of this problem has become clearer in recent years, with at least 4 such outbreaks being detected each year since 2008, arising primarily in areas of low OPV coverage.

3) Recommendations for routine and supplementary childhood immunization: in developing countries, WHO recommends 4 doses of OPV at 6, 10, and 14 weeks of age, with an additional dose at birth and/or at the measles contact (usually 9 months of age), depending on the endemicity and/or risk of polio in the country. In endemic countries and countries at high risk of importations or cVDPV emergence, WHO recommends annual national supplemental immunization campaigns to administer 2 or more doses of OPV at least 1 month apart to all children younger than 5 years regardless of prior immunization status. These campaigns should be conducted during the cool, dry season to achieve maximum effect. On the attainment of a high level of control in an endemic country, targeted house-to-house mop-up immunization campaigns in infected and high-risk areas are recommended to interrupt the final chains of transmission. Where polio is still endemic or at high risk of importation and spread, WHO recommends the use of OPV for all infants, including those who may be infected with HIV in whom study has shown OPV to be safe. Diarrhea is not a contraindication to OPV. In industrialized countries, contraindications to OPV frequently include congenital immunodeficiency (B lymphocyte deficiency, thymic dysplasia), current immunosuppressive treatment, disease states associated with immunosuppression (e.g., lymphoma, leukemia, and generalized malignancy), and the presence of immunodeficient individuals in the households of potential vaccine recipients. IPV should be used in such people, but this is no longer an issue in most industrialized countries as they have now shifted to IPV.

With progress towards eradication, the risk profile of paralytic poliomyelitis is changing, particularly in industrialized and high/middle income countries, and many have either replaced OPV with IPV for routine immunization or introduced mixed OPV/IPV use, for instance using IPV for routine immunization and OPV for mass campaigns to control possible outbreaks.

Recognizing the long-term risks posed by vaccine-derived polioviruses and the fact that the type 2 wild poliovirus had been eradicated globally by 1999, the World Health Assembly in 2012 recommended that all countries should begin planning for the phased removal of the OPV strains from their routine immunization programs in a globally coordinated manner, beginning with the type 2 Sabin strain. It is recommended that all countries introduce at least 1 dose of IPV into their national vaccination schedule and routine immunization program in advance of OPV2 withdrawal.

4) Immunization of adults: routine immunization for adults is not considered necessary. Primary immunization is advised for previously nonimmunized adults traveling to endemic countries and countries at high risk of importations, members of communities or population groups in which poliovirus disease is present, laboratory workers handling specimens containing poliovirus, and health care workers who may be exposed to patients excreting wild type polioviruses. In most industrialized countries, IPV is recommended for adult primary immunization. Those having previously completed a course of immunization and currently at increased risk of exposure are often given an additional dose of IPV. A single, lifetime booster is recommended for previously immunized adults traveling to polio-infected areas.

Travelers from polio-infected areas are recommended to have an additional dose of OPV at least 6 weeks before each international journey to reduce the risk of transient virus carriage and international spread. In case of urgent travel, a minimum of 1 dose of OPV should be given ideally 4 weeks before departure. Some polio-free countries have established special immunization requirements for travelers from polio-endemic and reinfected countries (e.g., receipt of an additional dose on arrival), and travelers should check immunization requirements prior to departure. All travelers are advised to carry their written vaccination record in the event that evidence of polio vaccination is requested for entry into countries being visited, preferably using the IHR International Certificate of Vaccination or Prophylaxis. The certificate is available at: http://www.who.int/ihr/IVC200_06_26.pdf.

10. **Management of patient—**

1) Enteric precautions in the hospital for wild virus disease; of little value under home conditions because many household contacts are infected before poliomyelitis has been diagnosed.

2) Concurrent disinfection of throat discharges, feces, and articles soiled therewith. In communities with modern and adequate

sewage disposal systems, preliminary disinfection is not necessary. Terminal cleaning.

3) Treatment: none; attention during acute illness to complications of paralysis requires expert knowledge and equipment, especially for patients in need of respiratory assistance. Physical therapy is used to attain maximum function after paralytic poliomyelitis and can prevent many deformities that are late manifestations of the illness.

11. Management of contacts and the immediate environment—

1) Immunization of familial and other close contacts is recommended but may not contribute to immediate control; the virus has often infected susceptible close contacts by the time the initial case is recognized.

2) Occurrence of a single case of poliomyelitis due to wild poliovirus or a cVDPV in a country that has interrupted transmission is a public health emergency prompting immediate investigation and planning for a large-scale response. A thorough search for additional cases of AFP in the area around the case assures early detection, facilitates control, and permits appropriate treatment of unrecognized and unreported cases.

12. Special considerations—

1) Reporting: poliomyelitis is a disease under surveillance by WHO and targeted for eradication. Since 2007, countries party to the IHR are required to inform WHO immediately of individual cases of paralytic polio due to wild poliovirus and to report details and extent of virus transmission. Countries should also report wild poliovirus isolated from other sources (e.g., environmental sampling) and polio cases due to cVDPV. In countries undertaking poliomyelitis eradication and/or certification, each case of AFP, including Guillain-Barré syndrome, in children younger than 15 years must be reported and fully investigated, as well as each case of suspected polio in people of any age. Nonparalytic infections should also be reported to the local health authority.

2) Epidemic measures: in any country that has previously interrupted transmission of wild poliovirus, a single case of poliomyelitis must now be considered a public health emergency, requiring an extensive supplementary immunization response over a large geographic area. Responses should be initiated within 4 weeks of confirmation of the index case and should consist of a minimum of 5 mass immunization rounds spaced 4–6 weeks apart (with ≥2 rounds after the last detected case) using bivalent OPV or the appropriate type-specific monovalent OPV, covering a minimum of 2–5 million children, and achieving at least 95% coverage in

each administrative area. cVDPVs require a similar intensity of response but use trivalent OPV where the causative agent is a type 2 vaccine-derived poliovirus.

3) Disaster implications: overcrowding of nonimmune groups and collapse of the sanitary infrastructure pose an epidemic threat.

4) International measures: cases must be reported to WHO under the IHR (see Reporting in Special Considerations in this chapter). Planning of a large-scale immunization response must begin immediately, be completed within 72 hours, and, if appropriate, be coordinated with bordering countries. Primary isolation of the virus is best accomplished in a designated Global Polio Eradication Laboratory. Once a wild poliovirus is isolated, molecular epidemiology can help trace the source. At-risk countries should submit weekly reports on cases of poliomyelitis, AFP cases and AFP surveillance performance to their respective WHO offices until the world has been certified polio-free.

International travelers visiting polio-infected areas should be adequately immunized. For further information, see the WHO publication *International Travel and Health*.

WHO Collaborating Centres provide support as required. More information can be found at: http://www.who.int/collaboratingcentres/database/en. Further information can be found at: http://www.who.int/gpv.

[R. B. Aylward]

PRION DISEASES
(transmissible spongiform encephalopathies)

DISEASE	ICD-10 CODE
CREUTZFELDT-JAKOB DISEASE	ICD-10 A81.0
GERSTMANN-STRÄUSSLER-SCHEINKER SYNDROME	ICD-10-CM A81.09
VARIANT CREUTZFELDT-JAKOB DISEASE	ICD-10-CM A81.01
FATAL FAMILIAL INSOMNIA	ICD-10-CM A81.09

A group of brain diseases characterized by a clinical and neuropathologic picture of progressive neurodegeneration resulting from tissue deposition of prions, which are believed to be an abnormally folded form of a host-encoded cellular protein (the prion protein). Prions are believed to be the causative agents, and their deposition in neurons is the hallmark of prion disease pathology and pathogenesis. Human prion diseases comprise:

- Creutzfeldt-Jakob disease (CJD), occurring in 3 different forms: sporadic CJD (~85% of cases), familial CJD (10–15% of cases), and iatrogenic CJD (<1% of cases).
- Variant CJD (vCJD), which has been causally linked with bovine spongiform encephalopathy (BSE), a prion disease of cattle.
- Gerstmann-Sträussler-Scheinker syndrome (GSS).
- Fatal familial insomnia (FFI).

The most common prion disease in humans, sporadic CJD, is not thought to be exogenously acquired, and it occurs sporadically. Other prion diseases not thought to be exogenously acquired include familial CJD, GSS, and FFI, and they are associated with mutations of the prion protein gene and inherited within families. Still, other prion diseases in humans (Kuru, vCJD, iatrogenic CJD) are thought to be acquired exogenously, incubation periods are generally long (many years), and there is no demonstrable inflammatory or immune response. Even those diseases thought not to be acquired exogenously, and some that are genetically associated, may be transmissible to others in certain settings (e.g., iatrogenic CJD, vCJD).

1. Clinical features—Signs and symptoms of CJD are limited to central nervous system (CNS) dysfunction. It typically presents as a subacute illness in the middle-aged and elderly (median age at death, 68 years) as a rapidly progressive encephalopathy with confusion, dementia, and other neurologic signs such as cerebellar dysfunction and myoclonus. However, clinical heterogeneity and atypical presentations have been reported. Patients have no fever, and routine blood tests and cerebrospinal fluid (CSF) cell count are normal. Typical periodic high-voltage complexes are present in the electroencephalogram (EEG) in about 70% of cases, and the CSF 14-3-3 and tau proteins are elevated in the majority of patients. Brain magnetic resonance imaging (MRI) shows signal hyperintensity in the caudate/putamen in many cases, especially on fluid attenuation inversion recovery sequences. High signal may be seen in some cerebral cortical regions.

Variant CJD (vCJD), first identified in 1996, has a longer clinical course (median 14 months vs. 4 months for sporadic CJD) and usually presents with psychiatric or behavioral disturbances, followed by signs of neurologic dysfunction, usually delayed by several months after the onset of illness. The typical EEG changes of sporadic CJD are seen only rarely in vCJD. MRI scan in vCJD shows high signal in the pulvinar area of the posterior thalamus in more than 90% of cases, especially on fluid attenuation inversion recovery sequences. The CSF 14-3-3 may be elevated, but in only about 45% of cases. All tested confirmed cases of vCJD to date have been homozygous for methionine (MM) at the polymorphic codon 129 of the prion protein gene. It remains unclear whether or not vCJD will occur in non-MM individuals who may be infected at present.

The clinical picture for genetic prion diseases is highly variable, and traditionally they have been classified as familial CJD, GSS, and FFI. GSS is used to describe a heterogeneous group of inherited prion diseases that are characterized by long illness duration and the presence of amyloid plaques, primarily in the cerebellum. FFI predominantly involves the thalamus, resulting in an illness characterized by intractable insomnia and autonomic nervous system dysfunction.

CJD must be differentiated from other forms of dementia (especially Alzheimer's disease), other infections (including encephalitis and vasculitis), and toxic, endocrine, autoimmune, and metabolic encephalopathies.

2. Causative agent—CJD and other related diseases are believed to be caused by prions, which are abnormally folded versions of the self-replicating, host-encoded prion protein. The normal cellular prion protein is a structural component of cell membranes of neurons and other mammalian cells. Genetic prion diseases are associated with one of several mutations in the prion protein gene located on chromosome 20 that encodes for the normal prion protein. The pattern of inheritance is variable, but up to 40% of cases may have no family history of a prion disease. Many prion diseases are transmissible in the laboratory to other species, including wild and transgenic mice and nonhuman primates.

3. Diagnosis—All forms of CJD are diagnosed based on clinical features, and EEG, CSF 14-3-3, and MRI findings. In vCJD, immunohistochemical or Western blot testing of tonsil biopsy can be very helpful but is probably best reserved for those cases with atypical features and/or without the MRI pulvinar sign. A definite diagnosis of all prion diseases depends on brain tissue testing and is usually undertaken at postmortem examination. Genetic testing on a simple blood sample is of importance in the diagnosis of suspect genetic prion disease. Brain biopsy can provide antemortem diagnosis, but this is an invasive procedure and is arguably best reserved for those cases in which an alternative diagnosis is otherwise not possible.

4. Occurrence—Sporadic CJD has been reported worldwide with annual mortality rate of 1-2 per million population. The highest age-specific average mortality rate (>5 cases/million) occurs in the 65-79 year age group. Genetic prion disease foci have been reported in familial clusters in Chile, Israel, and Slovakia. Variant CJD typically affects a younger age group than sporadic CJD (median age at death: 28 vs. 68 years). As of mid-2012, 226 vCJD cases had been identified worldwide, including 176 patients in the UK and 26 in France. Although the incidence of vCJD cases is falling because of human dietary protection measures and changes in animal feeding and slaughtering practices, concerns about iatrogenic transmission by blood, surgery, and dentistry still remain. Five instances of bloodborne vCJD transmission have been reported in the UK.

5. Reservoir—Humans are the only species affected by the CJD prions in nature, with the exception of vCJD, which represents zoonotic spread of BSE from its reservoir, thought to be in cattle. Subclinical infection with the BSE prion appears to be present in human populations (especially in the UK where the estimated prevalence ranges between 1 in 1,250 and 1 in 3,500). The magnitude of the risk from such infections is unknown, but they may represent a potential reservoir of infection for secondary, human-to-human spread by blood transfusion, organ transplantation, or surgery.

6. Incubation period—The concept of incubation period from the time of an external source exposure may not be applicable to sporadic and genetic prion diseases. For acquired forms of human prion diseases (e.g., iatrogenic CJD and variant CJD), incubation periods could range from 15 months to more than 30 years. The route of exposure influences the incubation period: a mean of 12 years (range, 1.3–30 years) with direct CNS exposure (dura mater grafts) and a mean of 17 years (range, 5–42 years) with peripheral exposure (human pituitary hormones given by injection). The incubation period for 3 patients with vCJD infected by blood transfusion ranged from 6.6–8.5 years. The estimated mean incubation period for vCJD from consuming BSE-contaminated cattle products is between 10 and 20 years.

7. Transmission—There is no firm evidence that sporadic CJD is an exogenously acquired disease. De novo spontaneous generation of the self-replicating, abnormally folded protein has been hypothesized as a source of the disease. Some case-control studies have suggested that surgery may be a risk factor for some sporadic CJD patients. Iatrogenic transmission of CJD has occurred following the use of contaminated cadaver-derived human pituitary hormone, dura mater and corneal grafts, EEG depth electrodes, and neurosurgical instruments. In all these cases, it is presumed that infection from a case, or cases, of sporadic CJD was inadvertently transmitted to another person in the course of medical/surgical treatment.

The mechanism of transmission of BSE from cattle to humans has not been established, but the favored hypothesis is that humans are infected through dietary consumption of the BSE agent. Three cases of vCJD have resulted from red cell transfusion, and a fourth patient heterozygous at codon 129 was positive for the vCJD agent but died of another condition. This agent was also found in a spleen sample of a fifth patient, who received fractionated plasma products partly sourced from a donor who went on to develop vCJD. To date, blood products have not been shown to be a risk factor for other forms of prion diseases in humans.

The highest levels of prion infectivity are associated with CNS tissues. In sporadic CJD, infectivity may be present in non-CNS tissues, but at much lower levels and probably essentially during the period of clinical illness. In vCJD, infection is present in lymphoid tissues and blood during the incubation period and during clinical illness. The level of infectivity in the CNS rises late in the incubation period, and high levels of infectivity occur in the CNS throughout symptomatic illness.

8. Risk groups—The following persons have been regarded as "at risk" for developing a prion disease: recipients of human dura mater graft, human cadaver-derived pituitary hormones (especially human cadaver-derived growth hormone), and cornea transplants; persons undergoing neurosurgery; and members of families with heritable CJD.

Mutations of the prion protein gene are associated with genetic or familial forms of human prion diseases. In human prion diseases, the polymorphic codon 129 of the prion protein gene, which codes for either methionine or valine, influences susceptibility and phenotypical expression of the disease.

9. Prevention—

1) Avoid organ or tissue transplants from infected patients and reuse of potentially contaminated surgical instruments. WHO guidelines to minimize the risk of transmission of CJD and sterilization protocols for CJD-contaminated surgical instruments are available at: http://www.who.int/csr/resources/publications/bse/WHO_CDS_CSR_APH_2000_3/en.

2) Avoid iatrogenic exposures:

   - Specific precautions should be taken in the management of persons with confirmed or suspected prion disease.
   - When determining the risk of iatrogenic transmission, infectivity of a given tissue should be considered together with the route of exposure. Infectivity is found most often, and in the highest concentration, in the CNS. Precautions have been proposed when performing certain interventions on prion disease patients (dental, diagnostic, surgical procedures) and when handling instruments or cleaning and decontaminating instruments, work surfaces, and waste.
   - Blood transfusion has resulted in the transmission of vCJD. This has not been demonstrated for other forms of prion disease.

3) Avoid exposures to BSE-causing agent in food of bovine origin because BSE is a risk to animal and public health; it is transmissible to humans, and food is considered the most likely source of exposure. Bovines, bovine products, and byproducts potentially carrying the BSE agent have been traded worldwide,

giving this risk a global dimension with possible repercussions for public health, animal health, and trade. At this time, the 2 key methods used to protect public health are minimizing or eliminating BSE in livestock populations and excluding from human food bovine tissues with the likely potential to contain the BSE agent if an animal were infected. For further information, see the report of the Joint WHO/FAO/OIE (World Health Organization/Food and Agriculture Organization/World Organisation for Animal Health) technical consultation on *BSE: Public Health, Animal Health and Trade* available at: http://whqlibdoc.who.int/publications/2001/9290445556.pdf

10. **Management of patient—**

1) No specific treatment is available; only supportive care is provided.
2) Prions are remarkably resistant to standard disinfection and sterilization methods, but a combination of sodium hydroxide (2M for 1 hour) or sodium hypochlorite (20,000 ppm for 1 hour) with porous load autoclaving can be used to inactivate prions. If they cannot be discarded, one of the three most stringent chemical and autoclave sterilization methods recommended by WHO should be used to reprocess heat-resistant instruments that come in contact with high infectivity tissues (brain, spinal cord, and eyes) or low infectivity tissues (cerebrospinal fluid, kidneys, liver, lungs, lymph nodes, spleen, olfactory epithelium, and placenta) of patients with suspected or confirmed CJD. These and the necessary precautions that need to be followed are available at: http://www.cdc.gov/ncidod/dvrd/cjd/qa_cjd_infection_control.htm.

11. **Management of contacts and the immediate environment—**
In investigation of contacts and source of infection, it is important to obtain a detailed history of past surgical procedures, exposure to human pituitary hormones or human dura mater grafts, family history, and blood transfusion or donation history.

12. **Special considerations—**

1) Reporting: many countries have made CJD (including vCJD) a notifiable disease. The OIE lists BSE as a reportable disease for international trade in livestock and livestock products.
2) International measures for the prevention of vCJD: to avoid human exposures to the BSE agent in food of bovine origin, no part or product of any animal that has shown signs of a prion disease should enter the human food chain. Countries should

not permit tissues that are likely to contain the BSE agent to enter any (human or animal) food chain.

- Managing BSE in cattle:

  o All countries should determine the BSE risk status of their cattle population through the outcome of an annual risk assessment, identifying all potential factors for BSE introduction, recycling, and amplification. A BSE surveillance system fitting the estimated level of risk should be put into place.

  o Whenever a risk of BSE is identified, countries can consider taking immediate steps to define the specified risk materials; tissues that have been shown to contain infectivity should be removed and destroyed. If the BSE risk is considered higher, other tissues that under certain conditions may carry infectivity can be added to the specified risk materials list for removal and destruction. Additional precautions may be taken, such as prohibiting cattle over a certain age from entering food or feed chains. WHO, FAO, and OIE continuously review this approach specifically in relation to public health issues.

  o Countries should monitor the effective application of the regulatory measures that have been decided upon, in particular the effectiveness of their ban (if in place) on feeding ruminant tissues to ruminants.

  o International trade in food products may disseminate tissues containing BSE; control transborder passage of cattle and bovine meat from areas where cattle are infected with BSE. WHO, FAO, and OIE continue to work together to mitigate the risk of dissemination of BSE agents.

- Prevention of bloodborne transmission: as a precautionary measure to reduce the risk of transmission of vCJD through blood or blood products, some countries—including Canada, the USA, and some continental European countries—have requested that blood centers exclude potential blood donors who have resided for a specified period in the UK.

[E. Belay]

❖

PSITTACOSIS

(*Chlamydia* [or *Chlamydophila*] *psittaci* infection, ornithosis, parrot fever, avian chlamydiosis)

DISEASE	ICD-10 CODE
PSITTACOSIS	ICD-10 A70

1. Clinical features—An acute disease with systemic presentations and respiratory symptoms. Acute onset of fever, headache, myalgia, and dry cough are typical clinical features. Respiratory symptoms are often mild when compared with pneumonia demonstrable by chest X-ray. Cough is initially absent or nonproductive; when present, sputum is mucopurulent and scant. Pleuritic chest pain and splenomegaly occur infrequently; pulse may be slow in relation to temperature. Respiratory failure, hepatitis, endocarditis, and encephalitis are occasional complications; relapses may occur. Although usually mild or moderate, human disease can be severe, especially in untreated elderly persons.

2. Causative agent—the bacterium *Chlamydophila* (formerly *Chlamydia*) *psittaci*.

3. Diagnosis—May be suspected in patients presenting with symptoms, a history of exposure to birds, and appropriate laboratory tests (serology). Due to a lack of specific laboratory testing, there is a possibility that reported cases of psittacosis may have been caused by the recently described *Chlamydophila pneumoniae* rather than *C. psittaci*. Isolation of the infectious agent from sputum, blood, or postmortem tissues, cultured in mice, eggs, or cell culture and under safe laboratory conditions only, confirms the diagnosis. Recovery of the infectious agent from human specimens may be difficult, especially if the patient has received broad-spectrum antibiotics.

4. Occurrence—Worldwide. It is primarily an infection of birds. Outbreaks occasionally occur in households, pet shops, aviaries, avian exhibits, and pigeon lofts. Most human cases are sporadic; many infections are probably not diagnosed.

5. Reservoir—Birds are the primary reservoir—mainly birds of the parrot family (psittacine birds—including parakeets and parrots); less often poultry, pigeons, and canaries. Apparently healthy birds can be carriers and shed the infectious agent, particularly when subjected to stress through crowding and shipping. Birds may shed the bacteria intermittently, and sometimes continuously, for weeks or months.

6. Incubation period—From 1–4 weeks.

7. **Transmission**—By inhaling the agent from desiccated droppings, secretions, and dust from feathers of infected birds. Imported psittacine birds are the most frequent source of exposure, followed by turkey and duck farms; processing and rendering plants have also been sources of occupational disease. Geese and pigeons are occasionally responsible for human disease. Rarely, person-to-person transmission may occur during acute illness with paroxysmal coughing.

8. **Risk groups**—Susceptibility is general, and postinfection immunity is incomplete and transitory. Older adults may be more severely affected.

9. **Prevention**—

1) Educate the public to the danger of exposure to infected pet birds. Medical personnel responsible for occupational health in animal processing plants should be aware that febrile respiratory illness with headache or myalgia among employees exposed to birds may be psittacosis.
2) Regulate the importation, raising, and trafficking of birds of the parrot family.
3) Prevent or eliminate avian infections through quarantine of infected farms (or premises with infected birds) until the buildings have been disinfected and diseased birds destroyed or adequately treated with tetracycline.
4) Psittacine birds offered for sale should be raised under psittacosis-free conditions and handled in such a manner as to prevent infection. Tetracyclines can be effective in controlling disease in psittacines and other companion birds if properly administered to ensure adequate intake for at least 30 and preferably 45 days.
5) Conduct surveillance at pet shops and aviaries where psittacosis has occurred or where birds epidemiologically linked to cases were obtained and at farms or animal processing plants to which human psittacosis was traced. Infected birds must be treated or destroyed, and the area where they were housed must be thoroughly cleaned and disinfected with a phenolic compound.

10. **Management of patient**—

1) Coughing patients should be instructed to cough into paper tissue (which must be discarded properly) or upper arm.
2) Treatment: antibiotics of the tetracycline group until 10–14 days after temperature returns to normal. Macrolides (e.g., erythromycin) are an alternative when tetracycline is contraindicated.

11. **Management of contacts and the immediate environment**—
Trace origin of suspected birds. If they cannot be killed, ship swab-cultures

of their cloacae or droppings to the laboratory in appropriate transport media and shipping containers in compliance with postal regulations; after the cultures are taken, the birds should be treated with a tetracycline drug. If they are to be killed, place bodies in plastic bags, close securely, and ship frozen (on dry ice) to nearest laboratory capable of isolating *Chlamydia*.

12. **Special considerations—**

1) Reporting: obligatory case report to health authorities in many countries.
2) Epidemic measures: cases are usually sporadic or confined to families, but outbreaks related to infected aviaries or bird suppliers may be extensive. Report outbreaks of avian psittacosis to agricultural and public health authorities. In poultry flocks, large doses of tetracycline can suppress, but not eliminate, infection and thus may complicate investigations.
3) International measures: compliance with national regulations to control importation of psittacine birds.

[H. Badaruddin]

Q FEVER
(query fever)

DISEASE	ICD-10 CODE
Q FEVER	ICD-10 A78

1. **Clinical features**—Q fever is an acute febrile disease characterized by chills, headache, malaise, myalgia, and sweats. There is considerable variation in severity and duration; infections may be unapparent or present as a fever of unknown origin. A pneumonitis may be found on X-ray examination, although radiographic patterns are nonspecific and do not allow for differentiation from other etiologies. Abnormal liver function tests are common. Acute and chronic granulomatous hepatitis, which can be confused with tuberculous hepatitis, has been reported. Chronic Q fever manifests primarily as culture negative endocarditis or vascular infection and occurs primarily in patients with preexisting risk factors such as valvular or vascular defects. Other rare clinical syndromes, including neurological syndromes, have been described. The case-fatality rate in untreated acute cases is usually less than 1%. Q fever endocarditis is fatal if untreated, whereas with treatment the 10-year mortality rate is 19%. A post-Q fever fatigue syndrome has been described.

2. Causative agent—*Coxiella burnetii*. The organism can be found in biological excreta of infected animals such as urine, feces, and milk, with the highest numbers of bacteria shed in birth products (e.g., placenta, amniotic fluid). The bacterium is highly resistant to many disinfectants and environmental conditions.

3. Diagnosis—Facilitated by use of 2 antigenic preparations: phase I, which represents the infectious agent, and phase II, which is a laboratory-generated attenuated form of the infectious agent with truncated lipopolysaccharide. For acute Q fever, a demonstration of a 4-fold rise in phase II immunoglobulin class G (IgG) antibody between acute and convalescent serum taken 3–6 weeks apart is the standard for confirmed diagnosis. A single high serum phase II IgG titer may be considered evidence of probable acute infection in a clinically compatible patient. Laboratory diagnosis by polymerase chain reaction (PCR) of blood or serum can also be used in the first 2 weeks after symptom onset and prior to antibiotic administration. Diagnosis of chronic Q fever requires an antiphase I IgG antibody titer greater than or equal to 1:1024 and a compatible clinical presentation. Anti-*C. burnetii* antibodies may be detectable for 10–15 years as long as sensitive methods such as immunofluorescence (IF) are used for detection. Bacteria may be identified in tissues (liver biopsy or heart valve) by immunohistochemistry and electronic microscope.

4. Occurrence—Reported from all continents. It is endemic in areas where reservoir animals are present. Outbreaks have occurred among workers in stockyards, in meatpacking and rendering plants, in laboratories, and in medical and veterinary centers that use sheep (especially pregnant ewes) in research. An epidemic occurred in the Netherlands from 2007–2010 that was linked to infected goat farms. Individual cases may occur where no animal contact can be demonstrated. The lack of animal contact should not preclude a clinical suspicion of diagnosis as infections that are caused by airborne transmission of *C. burnetii* often present with no direct animal exposure history.

5. Reservoir—Sheep, cattle, and goats are the primary reservoirs for *C. burnetii*. However, infection has been confirmed in multiple vertebrate species including cats, dogs, wild mammals, birds, and ticks. Transovarial and transstadial transmission are common in ticks that participate in wildlife cycles in rodents, larger animals, and birds. Infected animals are often asymptomatic but shed massive numbers of organisms in placental tissues and birth fluids at parturition. Abortions may occur in sheep and goats, particularly in naive populations where the agent has recently been introduced.

6. Incubation period—Dose-dependent; typically 2–3 weeks; range: 3–30 days.

7. Transmission—Transmission occurs most commonly through airborne dissemination of *Coxiella* in dust or aerosols from premises contaminated by placental tissues, birth fluids, and excreta of infected animals. Airborne particles containing organisms may be carried downwind for a distance of 1 kilometer or more. Contamination also occurs through direct contact with contaminated materials, such as wool, straw, and laundry. Raw milk from infected cattle or goats contains viable organisms and may be responsible for human transmission. Direct transmission by blood or marrow transfusion has been rarely reported. Sporadic cases of nosocomial transmission have been reported during autopsies and obstetrical procedures of infected women.

8. Risk groups—Veterinarians; sheep, goat, and dairy farmers; veterinary researchers; and abattoir workers are at risk for *C. burnetii* infection. Persons with valvular heart disease or vascular defects, pregnant women, and persons who are immunosuppressed are at risk for chronic Q fever after an acute infection.

9. Prevention—

1) Educate persons in high-risk occupations on sources of infection and the necessity for adequate disinfection and disposal of animal birth products; restrict access to sheds, barns, and laboratories with potentially infected animals; and stress the value of pasteurization of milk.
2) Immunization with vaccines prepared from formalin inactivated *C. burnetii* is useful in protecting laboratory workers and is strongly recommended for those working with live *C. burnetii*. It should also be considered for abattoir workers and others in hazardous occupations, including those carrying out medical research with pregnant sheep. To avoid severe local reactions, vaccine administration should be preceded by a skin sensitivity test with a small dose of diluted vaccine. Vaccine should not be given to individuals with a positive skin or antibody test or a documented history of Q fever. A Q fever vaccine was previously available through the US Army's Special Immunizations Program, but currently the only commercially available vaccine for humans is in Australia.
3) Research workers using pregnant sheep or goats should be identified and enrolled in a health education and surveillance program. This should include a baseline serum evaluation, followed by yearly evaluations. Persons at risk for chronic infection should be advised of the risk of serious illness that may result from Q fever. Laboratory clothes must be appropriately bagged and washed to prevent infection of laundry personnel. Animal-holding facilities should be away from populated areas, and measures should be

implemented in order to prevent airflow to other occupied areas. No casual visitors should be permitted.

10. **Management of patient—**

   1) Treatment: acute disease: doxycycline administered orally for 14 days. For acute Q fever in pregnancy, cotrimoxazole should be given throughout the pregnancy. For children, cotrimoxazole can be given for 14 days, but in severe cases doxycycline should be used. Q fever patients at risk for chronic disease should be monitored serologically and clinically at 3, 6, 12, 18, and 24 months after the acute infection. Chronic disease: doxycycline in combination with hydroxychloroquine for 18–24 months. Surgical replacement of the infected valve may be necessary in some patients with endocarditis.

11. **Management of contacts and the immediate environment—**

   1) Search for history of contact with sheep, cattle, or goats on farms or in research facilities or with parturient cats; consumption of raw milk; or direct or indirect association with a laboratory that handles *C. burnetii*.
   2) Disinfection: autoclaving is recommended to sterilize research materials, veterinary byproducts, and contaminated clothing. Gamma irradiation is effective for inactivation of live bacteria but is typically limited to small volumes such as antigen preparations. Quaternary ammonium compounds combined with detergents (MicroChem, Enviro-Chem) or 70% ethanol may be used for surface disinfection.
   3) Universal precautions should be used during postmortem examination or when performing any aerosol-generating procedure (e.g., bone sawing) on suspected cases in humans or animals.

12. **Special considerations—**

   1) Reporting: Q fever is a notifiable disease in many countries.
   2) Epidemic measures: control measures involve elimination of sources of infection, observation of exposed people, and administration of doxycycline to symptomatic persons. The 2007–2010 Netherlands epidemic resolved after widespread culling of infected goats and repopulation with vaccinated goats nationwide. Detection is particularly important in pregnant women, the immunosuppressed, and patients with cardiac valve and vascular lesions.
   3) International measures: measures to ensure the safe importation of goats, sheep, cattle, and their products (e.g., wool, hides). WHO Collaborating Centres provide support as required.

Further information can be found at: http://www.who.int/collaboratingcentres/database/en.

4) Deliberate use: *C. burnetii* is easy to produce in animals, can be desiccated and transmitted through aerosol. The agent is listed as a category B bioterrorism agent by the US Centers for Disease Control.

[G. J. Kersh, A. D. Anderson]

RABIES
(hydrophobia)

DISEASE	ICD-10 CODE
RABIES	ICD-10 A82

1. Clinical features—An acute viral zoonotic disease that causes a progressive viral encephalomyelitis that is nearly always fatal. Onset is generally heralded by a sense of apprehension, headache, fever, malaise, and sensory changes (paresthesia) at the site of an animal bite. Excitability and aero- and/or hydrophobia, often with spasms of swallowing muscles, are frequent symptoms. Delirium with occasional convulsions follows. Such classic symptoms of furious rabies are noted in two-thirds of cases, whereas the remaining present as paralysis of limbs and respiratory muscles with sparing of consciousness. Phobic spasms may be absent in the paralytic form. Coma and death ensue within 1–2 weeks, mainly due to cardiac failure.

2. Causative agents—Lyssaviruses, such as the classical rabies virus, are in the family *Rhabdoviridae* in the genus *Lyssavirus*. Genus *Lyssavirus* currently contains 14 species and is divided into 3 phylogroups. Only one of the species, classical rabies virus, is currently present in the Americas. Classical rabies virus is the most important for public health as it causes 99.9% of all human rabies cases worldwide. Lyssaviruses in Africa (Mokola and Duvenhage) and Eurasia (European bat lyssaviruses 1 and 2) and the Australian bat lyssavirus, which was first identified in 1996 in several species of flying foxes in Australia, have been associated with human deaths from rabies. All members of the genus are antigenically related, but use of monoclonal antibodies and nucleotide sequencing demonstrates differences according to animal species and/or geographical origin. Rabies caused by other lyssaviruses may be diagnosed by the standard direct fluorescent antibody test on brain tissue or by suggested antemortem tests. Several other lyssaviruses (e.g., Aravan virus, Irkut virus, Khujand virus,

Lagos bat virus, West Caucasian bat virus, Shimoni bat virus, Bokeloh bat lyssavirus, Ikoma lyssavirus, Lleida bat lyssavirus) have been characterized as etiological agents of rabies in mammals but have not so far been identified in human infections.

3. Diagnosis—Rabies can present in atypical forms, and medical personnel unfamiliar with the disease may misdiagnose it. Confirmatory diagnosis is made through specific postmortem fluorescent antibody (FA) staining of brain tissue or virus isolation in mouse or cell cultures. Antemortem diagnosis can be made by specific FA staining of viral antigens in frozen skin sections taken from the back of the neck at the hairline, detection of viral antibodies in serum and cerebrospinal fluid (CSF), and specific amplification of viral nucleic acids in saliva or skin biopsies by reverse transcription polymerase chain reaction (RT-PCR). Serological diagnosis is based on neutralization tests in cell culture or in mice. Viral shedding in body secretions is intermittent, and therefore the absence of virus or nucleic acids in those secretions does not exclude rabies as a diagnosis. A combination of tests for detection of rabies specific antibodies, antigens, and nucleic acids is needed for conclusive antemortem diagnosis.

4. Occurrence—Worldwide; more than 10 million human exposures and approximately 55,000 rabies deaths are estimated to occur each year, almost all in developing countries, particularly in Asia (31,000 deaths) and Africa (24,000 deaths). The disease is underreported worldwide, in part due to misdiagnosis. Most human deaths follow dog bites for which adequate postexposure prophylaxis was not or could not be provided. In Latin America, a regional dog rabies control program coordinated by Pan American Health Organization (PAHO) since 1983 has led to a reduction of almost 95% in the number of human deaths with only 9 cases reported in 2012, 46% of which followed contact with hematophagous bats. During the past 12 years, although reduction of the numbers of human cases have been reported in several Asian countries (particularly Thailand), increases have occurred in China—where since 1996 the number of notified human rabies deaths has continuously increased, reaching on average 3,000–4,000 in recent years. Western, Central, and Eastern Europe, including Russia, report fewer than 50 human rabies deaths annually. In the USA between 2000–2012, 30 of 40 human rabies cases were acquired domestically, and almost all were bat-associated infections.

Given the global distribution of bat rabies, few areas are truly free of autochthonous rabies in the animal population. Some sites include insular locations in the western Pacific and parts of the Caribbean. By 2000, many Western European countries had successfully eliminated fox rabies by oral immunization via the distribution of vaccine-laden baits. In Canada and the USA, oral immunization of free-ranging wild terrestrial carnivores has likewise helped to control rabies over large areas.

5. Reservoirs—All mammals are susceptible. Reservoirs and important vectors include wild and domestic Canidae, such as dogs, foxes, coyotes, wolves, and jackals and also skunks, raccoons, raccoon dogs, mongooses, and other common carnivores, such as cats in North America. In developing countries, dogs remain the principal reservoir. Infected populations of vampire, frugivorous, and insectivorous bats occur in Mexico and Central and South America, and infected insectivorous bats are present throughout Canada, the USA, and Eurasia. In Africa, Asia, and Australia, infected frugivorous and insectivorous bat species are involved in transmission. Many other mammals, such as rabbits, squirrels, chipmunks, rats, mice, and opossums are very rarely infected.

6. Incubation period—Highly variable but usually 3-8 weeks, and very rarely as short as a few days or as long as several years. The length of the incubation period depends in part on wound severity, wound location in relation to nerve supply, and relative distance from the brain; the amount, species, and variant of virus; the degree of protection provided by clothing; and other factors.

7. Transmission—Dogs are the main transmitter of rabies to humans in most developing countries, whereas in many developed countries, rabies is a disease of wild carnivores with sporadic spillover infection to domestic animals. The most common form of exposure is virus-laden saliva from a rabid animal introduced though a bite or scratch (and very rarely into a preexisting fresh break in the skin or through intact mucous membranes). Person-to-person transmission is theoretically possible but is rare and not well documented. Several cases of rabies transmission by transplant of cornea, solid organs, and blood vessels from persons dying of undiagnosed central nervous system (CNS) disease have been reported from Asia, Europe, and North America. Airborne spread has been suggested in a cave where heavy infestations of bats were roosting and demonstrated in laboratory settings, but this is thought to occur very rarely. Transmission from infected vampire bats feeding on domestic animals is common in Latin America. Rabid insectivorous or frugivorous bats can transmit rabies to terrestrial animals, wild or domestic.

Defined periods of communicability before onset of clinical signs of animal hosts are only known with reliability in domestic dogs, cats, and ferrets and are usually for 3-10 days before onset of clinical signs (rarely >4 days) and throughout the course of the disease. Longer periods of excretion before onset of clinical signs (14 days) have been observed with certain canine rabies virus variants in experimental infections, but these are the exception. Excretion in other animals is highly variable. For example, in one study bats shed virus for 12-16 days before evidence of illness, whereas in another, skunks shed virus for at least 8 days before onset of clinical signs. In general, 10 days communicability period with intermittent shedding preceding clinical onset for dogs, cats, and ferrets and 14 days for other mammals (including humans) has been assumed in risk assessments in the majority of countries.

8. Risk groups—Persons exposed to rabid animals, particularly veterinarians and veterinary technicians, animal control staff, wildlife researchers, cavers, staff of quarantine kennels, rehabilitators, laboratory and field personnel working with rabies virus or other lyssaviruses, and long-term travelers to rabies-endemic areas. All mammals are susceptible to varying degrees; the degree of susceptibility may be influenced by the virus species and variant, as well as by certain host parameters (e.g., age, health, nutrition).

9. Prevention—Many preventive measures are possible at the level of the primary animal host(s) and transmitter(s) of rabies to humans. Such measures are part of a comprehensive rabies control program.

1) Register, license, and vaccinate all owned dogs, cats, ferrets, and other pets, when feasible, in enzootic countries; manage population of ownerless animals and strays. Educate pet owners and the public on the importance of local community responsibilities. Pets should be leashed in congested areas when not confined on the owner's premises; strange-acting or sick animals of any species—domestic or wild—should be avoided and not handled; animals that have bitten a person or another animal should be reported to relevant authorities, such as the police or local health departments; if possible, such animals should be confined and observed as a preventive measure or euthanized and tested in a laboratory. Wildlife should be appreciated in nature and not be kept as pets. Where animal population reduction is impractical, animal contraception and repetitive vaccination campaigns may prove effective.

2) Maintain active surveillance for animal rabies. Laboratory capacity should be developed to perform FA diagnosis on all wild mammals involved in human or domestic animal exposures, and all domestic animals clinically suspected of having rabies.

3) Detain and observe for 10 days any healthy-appearing dog, cat, or ferret known to have bitten a person (stray or ownerless dogs, cats, or ferrets may be euthanized and examined for rabies by fluorescent microscopy); animals showing suspicious clinical signs of rabies should be euthanized and tested for rabies. If the biting animal was infective at the time of the bite, it usually develops signs of rabies within 4–10 days, such as change in behavior, excitability, or paralysis, followed by acute death. All wild mammals that have bitten a person should be euthanized and the brain examined for evidence of rabies.

4) In a timely manner, submit to a qualified laboratory the intact head of suspect animals, packed in ice (not frozen), for rabies diagnosis.

5) Euthanize unvaccinated domestic animals bitten by known rabid animals; if detention is elected, hold the animal in a secure facility for at least 6 months under veterinary supervision, and vaccinate against rabies at least 30 days before release. If previously vaccinated, booster immediately with rabies vaccine, and detain for at least 45 days.

6) Immunize wild carnivore reservoirs and free-ranging domestic dogs, using vaccine-laden baits containing attenuated or recombinant rabies viral vectors, as utilized in Europe and North America.

7) Cooperate with wildlife conservation authorities in programs to reduce the carrying capacity of wildlife hosts of sylvatic rabies with vaccine-laden baits and to reduce exposures to domestic animals and human populations—such as in circumscribed enzootic areas near campsites and in areas of dense human habitation.

8) Vaccinate individuals at high risk of exposure (see Risk Groups in this chapter). Such persons should receive preexposure immunization, using potent and safe cell-culture vaccines. Vaccine can be administered in doses of 1.0 ml or 0.5 ml intramuscularly (IM) on days 0, 7, and 21 or 28. Results with intradermal (ID) immunization (using WHO recommended schedules) for human diploid cell rabies vaccine (HDCV), purified chick embryo (PCECV), and purified Vero cell vaccines have been equivalent to what is expected from the intramuscular schedule. Antibody response to ID immunization has, however, been less than ideal in some groups receiving chloroquine for antimalarial chemoprophylaxis and may be the same in persons receiving antimalarials structurally related to chloroquine (e.g., mefloquine, hydroxychloroquine). The HDCV was the original gold standard for modern human rabies prophylaxis, but other less expensive cell-culture vaccines fulfilling basic WHO requirements for the ID route, such as purified vero cell and chick embryo cell vaccines, are widely and successfully used in many canine rabies-endemic countries.

If a risk of exposure continues, single booster doses are given, preferably after serological testing every 6 months to 2 years, depending upon the defined level of exposure, as long as the risk remains.

Cell-culture vaccines are considered to be safe and well tolerated, although reported reaction rates to primary immunization have varied with the monitoring system. Following IM immunization with the human diploid cell vaccine, mild and self-limited local reactions, such as pain at the site of injection, redness, and swelling, occur in 21%–74% of cases. Mild systemic reactions, such as fever, headache, dizziness, and gastrointestinal symptoms, occur in 5%–40% of cases, and systemic hypersensitivity following booster injections occurs in 6% of vaccines but is less common following primary immunization. When further purification steps are added, systemic hypersensitivity reactions become very rare. With chick embryo and vero cell-based vaccines, the rates of local and mild systemic reactions are similar to those of the human diploid cell vaccine, but no systemic hypersensitivity reactions have been reported. Compared with IM vaccination, the ID application is at least as safe and well tolerated.

9) Prevention of rabies after animal bites (postexposure prophylaxis [PEP]) consists of first aid, passive immunization, and vaccination as follows:

- First aid: clean and flush the wound immediately with soap or detergent and water, then apply either 70% ethanol, tincture of aqueous solution of iodine or povidone iodine, or Dakins solution (household bleach: 3 tablespoons of bleach plus one-half teaspoon baking soda in 1 liter of boiled water). The wound should not be sutured unless unavoidable. Sutures, if required, should be placed after local infiltration of immune globulin (see Passive Immunization in next paragraph); they should be loose and should not interfere with free bleeding and drainage.

- Passive immunization: infiltrate the wound with human (HRIG) or equine (ERIG) rabies immune globulin as soon as possible after exposure to neutralize the virus. HRIG should be used in a single dose of 20 IU/kg and ERIG in a single dose of 40 IU/kg. All, or as much as possible, of the rabies immune globulin (RIG) should be infiltrated into and around the bite wound; the remainder, if any, should be given IM. Where serum of animal origin (ERIG) is used, an intradermal or subcutaneous test dose preceding administration may detect potential allergic sensitivity, but the utility of this testing for predictive risk has been questionable.

  In previously vaccinated persons, RIG and ERIG are not required or recommended as part of PEP.

  No significant adverse reactions have been attributed to HRIG; however, immune globulin from a nonhuman source produces serum sickness in 5%–40% of recipients. Newer, commercially produced purified animal globulins, in particular purified equine globulin, have only a 1%–6% risk of serum sickness reactions. The commonly used skin test for ERIG will not predict serum sickness. Serious anaphylaxis is extremely rare with purified ERIG products (2 in >150,000 cases in 1 series). The risk of contracting fatal rabies outweighs the risks for allergic reactions.

Animal studies suggest that passive immunization with HRIG and ERIG, combined with vaccination, is effective after exposure to majority of known lyssavirus species (phylogroup I). However, currently available rabies biologics do not provide adequate protection against phylogroup II (Mokola, Lagos bat, and Shimoni bat viruses) and putative group III lyssaviruses (West Caucasian bat virus and Ikoma). Regardless, although postexposure prophylaxis may not always be effective for the management of some bat lyssavirus infections, it should always be used no matter what the geographic location.

- Vaccination: WHO-approved cell-culture vaccines should be applied according to the WHO and USA-CDC (Advisory Committee on Immunization Practices [ACIP]) approved "Modified Essen Regimen" in 4 IM doses of 0.5 or 1.0 ml on days 0, 3, 7, and 14 in the deltoid region or for small children in lateral thigh muscles. This is to start as soon as possible after exposure. In Europe, Asia, Africa, South and Central America, 2 additional WHO-approved regimens are widely used and found to be safe and effective; these are referred to as the "Essen Regimen" with 5 IM doses of vaccine on days 0, 3, 7, 14, and 28 as well as "2-1-1" or "Zagreb Regimen," which consists of 2 full intramuscular doses at 2 sites on day 0 and 1 injection each on days 7 and 21, thus saving 1 vaccine dose and 1 clinic visit.

Reduced-dose vaccination, WHO-approved, multisite intradermal postexposure schedules have been approved by local authorities in several rabies-endemic countries of Asia and Africa where the cost of vaccine is a significant deterrent to proper postexposure prophylaxis. WHO recommends 2 ID multisite regimens with cell-culture vaccines known to be safe and immunogenic: (1) the 2-site Thai Red Cross regimen (2-2-2-2) and (2) the 8-site Oxford regimen (8-0-4-0-1-1). If properly applied using potent modern vaccines, these schedules result in an antibody response equivalent to that seen with the 3 WHO-approved intramuscular regimens.

As for passive prophylaxis, animal studies suggest that vaccination should be provided as a part of PEP after exposure to any lyssaviruses no matter what the geographic location.

It has been well documented that subjects with severe immunodeficiency will not respond well to rabies vaccination, and some may not develop neutralizing antibody. Careful wound cleansing and the use of immunoglobulin is thus of great importance in such patients, with the vaccination mandatory and administered in the usual full 5-doses regimen.

A serum specimen should be collected at the time of the last dose of vaccine and tested for rabies antibodies. If sensitization reactions appear in the course of immunization, consult the health department or infectious disease consultants for guidance. If the immunodeficient person has had a previous full course of preexposure or postexposure rabies immunization with an approved vaccine, only 2 doses of vaccine need to be given—one immediately and one 3 days later.

- The combination of local wound treatment, passive immunization with RIG, and active vaccination is recommended for all severe exposures (category III, see end of this paragraph), the combination providing reliable, adequate protection. Pregnancy and infancy are never contraindications to PEP. Persons presenting even months after the bite must be dealt with in the same way as recent exposures. Factors to be considered in the initiation of PEP are the nature of the contact; rabies endemicity at the site of encounter or origin of the animal; the animal species involved; vaccination/clinical status of the animal and of the exposed person; availability of animal for observation; and laboratory results of animal for rabies, if available.

10. **Management of patient with clinical rabies—**

   1) Contact with salivary secretions or tears of a rabid patient should be avoided during the illness.
   2) Concurrent disinfection of saliva and articles soiled therewith. Although transmission from a patient to attending personnel has not been documented, immediate attendants should be warned of the potential hazard of infection from saliva and should wear gloves, protective gowns, face shield, and other appropriate personal protection equipment to avoid exposure from a coughing patient.
   3) Treatment: for clinical rabies, intensive supportive medical care.

11. **Management of contacts and the immediate environment—**

   1) Following appropriate risk assessment, contacts who are bitten by the patient or who have an open wound or mucous membrane exposure to the patient's saliva or tears should receive specific PEP.
   2) Search for rabid animal(s) and for people and other animals bitten.

12. **Special considerations—**

   1) Reporting: obligatory case report to local health authority is required in most countries.

2) Epidemic (epizootic) measures: applicable only to animals; a sporadic disease in humans.

- Establish control area under authority of laws, regulations, and ordinances in cooperation with appropriate human, agricultural, and wildlife conservation authorities.
- Immunize dogs and cats through officially sponsored, intensified mass programs that provide immunizations at temporary and emergency stations. For protection of other domestic animals, use approved vaccines appropriate for each animal species.
- In urban areas of industrialized countries, strict enforcement of regulations requiring collection, detention, and euthanasia of ownerless and stray dogs and of nonimmunized dogs found off owners' premises; control of the dog population by castration, spaying, or drugs, as well as through policies for proper waste management, have been effective in breaking transmission cycles.
- Mass immunization of wildlife with baits containing vaccine has contained red fox rabies in Western Europe and southern Canada and coyote, gray fox, and raccoon rabies in the USA.

3) Disaster implications: a potential problem exists if the disease is freshly introduced or enzootic in an area where there are many stray dogs or wild reservoir animals. Similarly, in disaster areas—for example after earthquakes, hurricanes, or tsunamis—stray animals may be present after human evacuations with subsequent bites to animal control or humane society personnel taking part in future rescue attempts.

4) International measures:

- Strict compliance by common carriers and travelers with national laws and regulations (http://www.who.int/ith/en). Immunization of animals, certificates of health and origin, and microchip identification of animals may be required.
- WHO Collaborating Centers and other international organizations and institutions are prepared to collaborate with national services on request. See WHO Expert Consultation on Rabies, Second Report, TRS 982, and WHO, Geneva, 2013, annex 8. Further information on Collaborating Centers can be found at: http://www.who.int/collaboratingcentres/database/en.

POSTEXPOSURE PROPHYLAXIS GUIDE

WHO recommendations for PEP rabies management follow—

Category of exposure	Type of exposure/contact to a domestic or wild animal[a] suspected or confirmed to be rabid or to an animal unavailable for testing	Who recommended postexposure prophylaxis
Category I (no exposure)	Touching or feeding of animal; licks on intact skin. Contact of intact skin with secretions or excretions of a rabid animal or human case.	None, if reliable case history is available.
Category II	Nibbling of uncovered skin. Minor scratches or abrasions without bleeding.	Administer vaccine immediately.[b] Stop prophylaxis if animal remains healthy throughout an observation period of 10 days[c] or is proven to be negative for rabies by a reliable laboratory, using appropriate diagnostic techniques.
Category III	Single or multiple transder-mal bites[d] or scratches; contamination of mucous membranes with saliva (licks); licks on broken skin. Exposure to bats.[e]	Administer rabies vaccine immedi-ately and rabies immunoglobulin, preferably as soon as possible after initiation of postexposure prophylaxis. Rabies immunoglobulin can be injected up to 7 days after first vaccine dose administration. Stop prophylaxis if animal remains healthy throughout an observation of 10 days, or is proven to be negative for rabies by a reliable laboratory using appropriate diagnostic techniques.

[a]Exposure to most small mammals, such as insectivores (e.g., shrews), rodents (e.g., mice, rats, squirrels), and lagomorphs (e.g., rabbits and hares) seldom, if ever, requires specific rabies prophylaxis.

[b]The placing of an apparently healthy dog or cat in or from a low-risk area under careful supervision may warrant delaying prophylaxis.

[c]This observation period applies only to dogs, cats, and ferrets. Except for threatened or endangered species, other domestic and wild animals suspected of being rabid should be euthanized and their tissues examined for the presence of rabies antigen by appropriate laboratory techniques.

[d]Bites especially on the head, neck, face, hands, and genitals are category III exposures because of the rich innervation of these areas.

[e]Postexposure prophylaxis should be considered when contact between a human and a bat has occurred, unless the exposed person can rule out a bite or scratch or exposure of a mucous membrane.

US recommendations for postexposure management follow—

ACIP: human rabies prevention—United States, 2008: recommendations of the Advisory Committee on Immunization Practices. *MMWR Recomm Rep.* 2008;57(RR-3):1–28.

ACIP: use of a reduced (4-dose) vaccine schedule for postexposure prophylaxis to prevent human rabies: recommendations of the advisory committee on immunization practices. *MMWR Recomm Rep.* 2010;59(RR-2): 1–9.

Vaccination Status	Regimen[a]
Not previously vaccinated	**Wound cleansing** All PEP to begin with immediate and thorough cleansing of all wounds with soap and water. If available, a virucidal agent such as a povidone-iodine solution should be used to irrigate the wounds. **HRIG** Administer 20 IU/kg body weight. If anatomically feasible, the full dose should be infiltrated around the wound(s); any remaining volume should be administered IM at an anatomic site distant from that of vaccine administration (such as deltoid or the anterior-lateral aspect of the thigh). RIG should not be administered in the same syringe or location as the vaccine. Because HRIG may partially suppress active production of antibody, no more than the recommended dose should be given. **Vaccine** HDCV or PCECV, 1.0 ml, IM (deltoid area[b]); one each on days 0, 3, 7, and 14 in immunocompetent individuals and on days 0, 3, 7, 14, and 28 in immunosuppressed individuals
Previously vaccinated[d]	**Wound cleansing** All postexposure prophylaxis to begin with immediate and thorough cleansing of all wounds with soap and water. If available, a virucidal agent such as a povidone-iodine solution should be used to irrigate wounds. **RIG** RIG should not be administered. **Vaccine** HDCV or PCEV, 1.0 mL, IM (deltoid area[b]); one each on days 0 and 3.

[a]Regimens are applicable for all age groups, including children.

[b]The deltoid area is the only acceptable site of vaccination for adults and older children. For younger children, the outer aspect of the thigh may be used. Never administer vaccine in the gluteal area.

[c]Day 0 is the day the first dose of vaccine is administered.

[d]History of preexposure vaccination with HDCV, RVA (rabies vaccine, adsorbed), or PCECV; prior postexposure prophylaxis with HDCV, RVA, or PCECV; or previous vaccination with any other type of rabies vaccine and a documented history of antibody response to the prior vaccination.

In addition to PEP as described, consult regional, provincial, local, state, or national health officials if questions arise about the need for rabies prophylaxis.

[R. Franka]

RAT-BITE FEVER
(Streptobacillary fever, Haverhill fever, epidemic arthritic erythema, spirillary fever, sodoku)

DISEASE	ICD-10 CODE
STREPTOBACILLOSIS	ICD-10 A25.1
SPIRILLOSIS	ICD-10 A25.0

1. Clinical features—The general term "rat-bite fever" refers to 2 rare bacterial zoonoses—Streptobacillosis and spirillosis—that have similar clinical features. In Streptobacillosis, an abrupt onset of fever, headache, vomiting, and muscle pain is followed within 2–4 days by a maculopapular rash most marked on the extremities. The rash can also be petechial, purpuric, or pustular. A nonsuppurative polyarthritis can develop in over half of cases. There is usually a history of a rodent bite, which healed normally within the previous 10 days. Bacterial endocarditis, pericarditis, parotitis, tenosynovitis, and focal abscesses of soft tissues or the brain can occur late in untreated cases. Symptoms usually resolve within 2 weeks without treatment, but relapses often occur, with an approximate case-fatality rate of 7%–10%. Spirillosis disease differs from streptobacillosis in the presence of an indurated or ulcerated lesion at the site of the bite when fever develops, in the rarity of arthritic symptoms, and in the presence of a distinctive rash of reddish or purplish plaques. Complications may resemble those of streptobacillosis. Untreated, the case-fatality rate is approximately 10%.

2. Causative agents—*Streptobacillus moniliformis* for streptobacillosis, *Spirillum minus* for spirillosis.

3. Diagnosis—Laboratory methods are essential for differentiation, and serological testing is not reliable. Laboratory confirmation of Streptobacillosis is through isolation of the organism by inoculating material from the primary lesion, lymph node, blood, joint fluid, or pus into the appropriate bacteriological medium enriched with 20% serum or ascitic fluid or into laboratory animals (guinea pigs or mice that are not naturally infected). Growth has been most successful on heart infusion agar plates with 5% rabbit blood with addition of sterile rabbit or horse serum spread on the agar and dried. The organism is a fastidious, slow-growing organism; therefore, cultures should be maintained for 10 days following inoculation. Animal inoculation alone is used for isolation of *S. minus*, since it has not been successfully cultured on artificial media.

4. Occurrence—Rat-bite fever is a rare disease that can occur worldwide. Streptobacillosis is more common in North and South America and Europe, while spirillosis occurs in Asia and Africa.

5. Reservoir—Infected rats, rarely other rodents (squirrels, mice, gerbils), and cats, dogs, ferrets, and weasels, which may become infected when hunting rodents.

6. Incubation period—For streptobacillosis, usually from 3–10 days; can range from 2 days to 3 weeks. For spirillosis, usually between 7 and 21 days with a range of 1 day to 6 weeks.

7. Transmission—*S. moniliformis* and *S. minus* are commensal organisms of rats and can be found in the oral, nasal, and conjunctival secretions and urine of an infected animal. Transmission most frequently occurs through biting, but sporadic cases may occur without history of a bite. Direct contact with rats is not necessary; infection has occurred in people working or living in rat-infested buildings. In outbreaks of Haverhill fever, milk, or water contaminated by rat urine or feces has usually been suspected as the vehicle of infection. No direct person-to-person transmission has been reported.

8. Risk groups—Persons having direct or indirect contact with rats and other animal reservoirs.

9. Prevention—Rat-proof dwellings and reduce rat and other reservoir populations. Prevent contamination of food and water sources by rodents. For pet owners and laboratory animal technicians, use appropriate restraining techniques and protective equipment when handling rodents. Penicillin may be used as prophylaxis following a rodent bite, since up to 10% of rodent bites may result in rat-bite fever.

10. Management of patient—Treatment: penicillin, tetracyclines, or erythromycin for 7–10 days. Prompt treatment may shorten clinical course and reduce occurrence of complications.

11. Management of contacts and the immediate environment—
Investigate contacts and source of infection to establish whether there are
additional unrecognized cases.

12. Special considerations—

1) Reporting: report of an epidemic to the local health authority is
   obligatory in most countries; no case report required although
   encouraged.
2) Epidemic measures: a cluster of cases requires search for a
   common source, possibly contaminated food and water.

[M. Guerra, J. McQuiston]

RELAPSING FEVER
(borrelia recurrentis, louse-borne relapsing fever)

DISEASE	ICD-10 CODE
RELAPSING FEVER	ICD-10 A68

1. Clinical features—A systemic louse-borne epidemic or tickborne
sporadic spirochetal disease in which periods of fever lasting 2–7 days
alternate with afebrile periods of 4–14 days; the number of relapses varies
from 1–10 or more. Total duration of louse-borne relapsing fever (LBRF)
averages 13–16 days; usually longer for tickborne relapsing fever (TBRF).
Other nonspecific signs and symptoms include headache, myalgia, arthralgia,
shaking chills, and gastrointestinal pain or illness. Patients with LBRF are
more likely to have jaundice, central nervous system (CNS) involvement,
petechial rashes, blood-tinged sputum, and epistaxsis. In contrast, acute
respiratory distress syndrome has been reported more frequently in TBRF.
Predisposing factors (poor nutrition and thiamine or vitamin B deficiency)
may lead to more severe disease and neurological involvement. The overall
case-fatality rate in untreated cases is between 2% and 10%.

2. Causative agents—Helical and motile spirochetes of the genus
Borrelia. Borrelia recurrentis is the sole agent of human-specific LBRF and
is spread from person to person by the human body louse. *Borrelia
duttoni* also appears to be a human-specific pathogen but is one of more
than 10 species that cause TBRF; all TBRF species are transmitted by soft-
bodied (argasid) ticks. Both LBRF and TBRF spirochetes demonstrate
antigenic variation in parallel with successive relapses. In North America,

most human cases are caused by *Borrelia hermsii* transmitted by the soft-bodied tick *Ornithodoros hermsi*. The classical agent of relapsing fever in Europe is *Borrelia hispanica*, also tickborne.

3. Diagnosis—The spiral shaped bacteria range in length from 7-30 um and in width from 0.2-0.5 um and stain poorly with Gram stain reagents. They are best detected in peripheral blood (febrile periods most sensitive) and visualized in wet mounts by dark-field microscopy (where corkscrew motility assists detection) or in Giemsa- or Wright-based stained smears with bright-field microscopy. Detection of spirochetes during afebrile and late-stage febrile periods is generally insensitive. Weanling mice and specialized liquid culture media (Barbour-Stoenner, Kelly, or BSK) may serve as amplifying environments to increase the sensitivity of subsequent microscopic detection.

4. Occurrence—Relapsing fever has been reported from all parts of the world except Australia and New Zealand. Louse-borne relapsing fever occurs in limited areas in Asia, eastern Africa (Burundi, Ethiopia, and Sudan), highlands of central Africa, and South America. Tickborne disease is endemic throughout tropical Africa with other foci in India, the Islamic Republic of Iran, Portugal, Saudi Arabia, Spain, northern Africa, central Asia, and North and South America. Sporadic human cases and occasional outbreaks of tickborne disease occur in portions of Europe, western Canada, and the USA. In parts of the world, such as Senegal and Tanzania for TBRF and Ethiopia for LBRF, these diseases are among the top 10 bacterial causes of mortality and hospital admissions.

5. Reservoir—For the singular agent of LBRF (*B. recurrentis*) and one species (*B. duttoni*) of TBRF, humans are the reservoir. For other species of TBRF, wild rodents are the primary reservoir. The long life span (years) of argasid (soft) tick vectors of TBRF and transovarial transmission of spirochetes from adult females to eggs may enable ticks themselves to serve as reservoirs during periods of mammalian blood-host absence. With the exception of *B. recurrentis* and *B. duttoni*, humans are incidental and dead-end hosts.

6. Incubation period—Louse-borne relapsing fever, usually 8 days (range 5-15 days). Tickborne relapsing fever, about 7 days (range 2-18 days).

7. Transmission—The epidemic form (LBRF) is spread by lice, whereas the endemic or sporadic forms are spread by argasid ticks. Repeated infections may occur. There is no direct person-to-person transmission (exception—transplacental transmission in infected pregnant women). LBRF is acquired by crushing an infected louse, *Pediculus humanus*; this results in contamination of the bite wound or an abrasion of the skin. Lice become infective 4-5 days after ingestion of blood from an infected person and remain so for life (20-30 days). In tickborne disease, people are infected by the bite of an argasid tick, principally *Ornithodoros moubata* and *Ornithodoros hispanica* in Africa, *Ornithodoros rudis* and *Ornithodoros talaje* in Central and South America, *Ornithodoros tholozani* in the Near and Middle East, and *Ornithodoros hermsi* and *Ornithodoros turicata* in the USA. Most argasid ticks are rapid (<30 minutes) and nocturnal feeding ticks and bites are often not recognized. Infected ticks can live and remain infective for several years without feeding, and they may pass the infection transovarially to their progeny.

8. Risk groups—Various risk groups in endemic regions. For LBRF, those living in crowded conditions with poor sanitary resources and practice, particularly those sharing clothing and bedding with infected individuals. For TBRF, persons disturbing or habitating environments (caves and abandoned human dwellings) where infected ticks and reservoirs are present. Most argasid ticks are indiscriminate feeders and will prey upon humans when their usual blood-meal host is purposely displaced by human intervention or unwittingly displaced by human activity. The developing human fetus is particularly vulnerable to often fatal infection as spirochetes are able to cross the placental barrier and establish a persistent fetal infection while the mother may clear the infection.

9. Prevention—

1) Control lice using measures prescribed for louse-borne typhus (see Epidemic Louse-Borne Typhus Fever section in "Typhus").
2) Control ticks by measures prescribed for spotted fever (see "Rickettsioses"). Soft tick-infested human habitations may present a major problem, and eradication of the ticks may be difficult. Closing crevasses in wall structures and installing rodent proofing to prevent future colonization by rodents and their soft ticks are the mainstay of prevention and control. Spraying with approved acaricides, such as diazinon, chlorpyrifos, propoxur, pyrethrum, or permethrin, may be tried.
3) Use personal protective measures, including repellents and permethrin on clothing and bedding, for people with exposure in endemic foci. Dimethyl phthalate (5%) and 10% carbolic soap are effective.
4) Antibiotic chemoprophylaxis with tetracyclines may be taken after exposure (arthropod bites) when the risk of acquiring the infection is high.

10. Management of patient—

1) Blood/body fluid precautions. Patients, clothing, household contacts, and immediate environment must be deloused or freed of ticks.

2) Treatment: erythromycin, tetracycline, chloramphenicol, or doxycycline for 7 days.

11. Management of contacts and the immediate environment— For individual tickborne cases, search for additional associated cases and sources of infection; for louse-borne disease, application of appropriate lousicidal preparation to infested contacts (see "Pediculosis and Phthiriasis").

12. Special considerations—

1) Reporting: report to local health authority of louse-borne relapsing fever required as a Disease Under Surveillance by WHO; tickborne disease, reporting required in some areas.

2) Epidemic measures: for louse-borne relapsing fever, when case reporting has been properly done and cases are localized, dust or spray contacts and their clothing with 1% permethrin and apply permethrin spray at 0.03-0.3 kg/hectare (2.47 acres) to the immediate environment of all reported cases. Provide facilities for washing clothes and for bathing to affected populations; establish active surveillance, especially in refugee camps. Where infection is known to be widespread, apply permethrin systematically to all people in the community. For tickborne relapsing fever, apply permethrin or other acaricides to target areas where vector ticks are thought to be present; for sustained control, an application cycle of 1 month is recommended during the transmission season. Since animals (horses, camels, cows, sheep, pigs, and dogs) can also play a role in tickborne relapsing fever, persons entering tick-infested areas (hunters, soldiers, vacationers, and others) should be educated regarding tickborne relapsing fever.

3) Disaster implications: a serious potential hazard among louse-infested populations. Epidemics are common in wars, famines, and other situations with increased prevalence of pediculosis (e.g., overcrowded, malnourished populations with poor personal hygiene), especially with important population movements and in refugee camps.

4) International measures: prompt notification by governments to WHO and adjacent countries of an outbreak of louse-borne relapsing fever in any areas of their territories with further information on the source and type of the disease and the number of cases and deaths.

[M. Schriefer]

RICKETTSIOSES
(spotted fever group)

DISEASE	CAUSATIVE AGENT	ICD-10 CODE
ROCKY MOUNTAIN SPOTTED FEVER	*Rickettsia rickettsii*	ICD-10 A77.0
MEDITERRANEAN SPOTTED FEVER (BOUTONNEUSE FEVER)	*Rickettsia conorii* and closely related organisms	ICD-10 A77.1
AFRICAN TICK-BITE FEVER	*Rickettsia africae*	ICD-10 A77.8
QUEENSLAND TICK TYPHUS	*Rickettsia australis*	ICD-10 A77.3
NORTH ASIAN TICK TYPHUS	*Rickettsia sibirica*	ICD-10 A77.2
TICKBORNE LYMPHADENOPATHY (TIBOLA)	*Rickettsia slovaca*	ICD-10 A77.x
FLINDERS ISLAND SPOTTED FEVER	*Rickettsia honei*	ICD-10 A77.x
AUSTRALIAN SPOTTED FEVER	*Rickettsia marmionii*	ICD-10 A77.x
FAR-EASTERN SPOTTED FEVER	*Rickettsia heilong-jiangensis*	ICD-10 A77.x
JAPANESE SPOTTED FEVER	*Rickettsia japonica*	ICD-10 A77.x
MACULATUM INFECTION	*Rickettsia parkeri*	ICD-10 A77.x
RICKETTSIALPOX	*Rickettsia akari*	ICD-10 A79.1

I. TICKBORNE SPOTTED FEVERS
ROCKY MOUNTAIN SPOTTED FEVER (RMSF, febre maculosa)
MEDITERRANEAN SPOTTED FEVER (Mediterranean tick fever,
boutonneuse fever, Marseilles fever, Kenya tick typhus, India tick
typhus, Israeli tick typhus, Astrakhan fever)
AFRICAN TICK-BITE FEVER
NORTH ASIAN TICK FEVER (Siberian tick typhus)
TICKBORNE LYMPHADENOPATHY (TIBOLA; Dermacentor-borne
necrosis and lymphadenopathy [DEBONEL])
FLINDERS ISLAND SPOTTED FEVER (Thai tick typhus)
AUSTRALIAN SPOTTED FEVER
FAR-EASTERN TICKBORNE RICKETTSIOSIS
JAPANESE SPOTTED FEVER
MACULATUM INFECTION

1. Clinical features—Spotted fever group rickettsial infections are a closely related group of primarily tickborne bacterial infections causing clinically similar diseases characterized by fever, rash, and vasculitis. Although clinical presentations and severity vary by species, some spotted fever infections can be associated with multiorgan involvement such as respiratory failure, hepatosplenomegaly, heart failure, renal failure, bleeding, and neurological complications.

1) Rocky Mountain spotted fever (RMSF) ranges greatly in severity and can be mild if treated early, or rapidly fatal in some patients if appropriate treatment is not initiated before day 5 of symptoms. It is characterized by the sudden onset of moderate to high fever, significant malaise, deep muscle pain, severe headache, chills, and conjunctival injection. A maculopapular rash appears on the extremities on the third to fifth day in many patients; the rash includes the palms and soles in about 30% and spreads rapidly to the body trunk. A petechial exanthem generally occurs on or after the sixth day and is often associated with vascular and end organ damage. Every effort should be made to treat the disease before this time and prevent petechia from developing. The case-fatality rate ranges between 20% and 80% in different regions in the absence of treatment; with prompt recognition and treatment, death is uncommon. Median duration between symptom onset and death is 8 days in fatal cases, even in previously healthy people. The primary risk factor associated with more severe disease and death is delayed antibiotic therapy. Factors that make the disease more difficult to diagnose increase the risk of delayed treatment and therefore death. These factors include absence or delayed appearance of the typical rash, or failure to recognize it, especially in dark-skinned individuals; occurrence of the disease outside the typical seasonality; or occurrence of disease outside the established geographic distribution. Tick exposure reports are often misleading as tick bites are typically painless and go unrecognized by patients. Low platelets, low sodium, and elevated liver enzymes are frequently observed in RMSF patients. The early stages of RMSF may be confused with ehrlichiosis, meningococcemia (see "Meningitis"), enteroviral infection, dengue, and many other febrile illnesses.

2) Mediterranean spotted fever (MSF) is a mild to severe febrile illness with abrupt onset; there may be a primary lesion or eschar at the site of a tick bite. This eschar (tache noire), often evident at the onset of fever, is a small ulcer 2–5 mm in diameter with a black center and red areola; regional lymph nodes are often enlarged. A generalized maculopapular erythematous rash occurs about the fourth to fifth day. With

appropriate antibiotic therapy, fever typically resolves within 48 hours. The case-fatality rate varies by region.

3) African tick-bite fever is similar to MSF but typically has a milder course. Fatalities are rarely reported. Abrupt onset of fever, nausea, headache, and myalgia are common and may be accompanied by one or multiple inoculation eschars. Regional draining lymphangitis and aphthous stomatitis may occur. Rash is noticed in only half the cases and may be maculopapular or vesicular. Complications are rare and symptoms typically resolve after 10 days but resolve more quickly with appropriate antibiotics.

4) Queensland tick typhus is clinically similar to MSF; the rash may be vesicular.

5) North Asian tick typhus is clinically similar to MSF; rash and lymphadenitis are common.

6) Tickborne lymphadenopathy is a mild rickettsiosis; main symptoms include an eschar, often found on the head; regional lymphadenopathy; low-grade fever; and, in some cases, alopecia at eschar site.

7) Flinders Island spotted fever is a mild disease with maculo-papular rash; eschar and adenopathy are rare.

8) Australian spotted fever manifests with eschar, maculopapular or vesicular rash, and adenopathy; fatalities have been reported.

9) Far-Eastern tickborne rickettsiosis is characterized by eschar, faint macular or maculopapular rash, lymphadenopathy, and lymphangitis, and conjunctival papulae may be present.

10) Japanese spotted fever similarly involves eschar, macular, or maculopapular rash (which may become petechial) lymphadeno-pathy, and enlarged lymph nodes; fatalities have been described.

11) Maculatum infection is a mild febrile illness with eschar and maculopapular-to-vesicular rash.

2. Causative agents—See earlier table.

3. Diagnosis—The indirect immunofluorescence assay (IFA) is the gold standard for serological diagnosis confirmation. Serological diagnosis is confirmed by a 4-fold or greater rise in specific antibody (immunoglo-bulin class G [IgG]) titer when comparing a patient's acute and convalescent sera. The acute sample should be taken in the first week of illness and the convalescent should be taken 3–4 weeks after the acute sample. IFA tests become positive generally in the second to third week of illness. Therefore, an acute titer taken in the first week of illness should be used as a baseline for comparison to the convalescent sample, and a negative acute result does not rule out active infection, nor does a positive acute result confirm the diagnosis. Older Weil-Felix tests using Proteus OX-19 and Proteus OX-2 antigens are less sensitive and less specific and are not recommended. During acute stages of infection and prior to doxycycline treatment, rickettsiae may sometimes be detected by polymerase chain reaction (PCR) in blood and serum. More frequently detection can be achieved in skin biopsies using immunostains or PCR. Culturing blood or buffy coats on cell culture monolayers permits isolation of the organisms and facilitates precise confirmatory diagnosis.

4. **Occurrence—**

   1) RMSF: throughout the USA and in Argentina, Brazil, Canada, Colombia, Mexico, and Central America. In most of the USA, infections occur primarily from April through September, mainly in the southeast and south central regions; highest incidence rates are seen in North Carolina and Oklahoma. A focus of RMSF in the US southwest has cases occurring year-round with most cases reported March–November.

   2) MSF: widely distributed throughout the African continent, in India, and in those parts of Europe and the Middle East adjacent to the Mediterranean and the Black and Caspian seas. In more temperate areas, the highest incidence is during warmer months when ticks are numerous; in tropical areas, disease occurs throughout the year. In some areas such as the Negev in Israel and Astrakhan, Russia, tache noir lesions are less frequently seen with MSF infections than occurs in other areas.

   3) African tick-bite fever: sub-Saharan Africa, including Botswana, South Africa, Swaziland, and Zimbabwe; the Lesser Antilles and the West Indies. Outbreaks of disease may occur when groups of travelers (such as people on safari in Africa) are bitten by ticks. Cases are occasionally imported into the USA and Europe.

   4) Queensland tick typhus: Queensland, New South Wales, Tasmania, and coastal areas of eastern Victoria, Australia.

   5) North Asian tick fever: North China, Mongolia, and Asiatic areas of Russia.

   6) Tickborne lymphadenopathy: Europe and Asia.

   7) Flinders Island spotted fever: Australia, Thailand, Flinders Island, and Tasmania.

   8) Australian spotted fever: Australia.

   9) Far-Eastern tickborne rickettsiosis: Far East of Russia, northern China.

   10) Japanese spotted fever: Japan.

   11) Maculatum infection: coastal regions of southeastern USA; southern South America, including Argentina, Uruguay, and parts of Brazil.

5. Reservoir—Maintained in nature among a variety of tick species by transovarial and transstadial passage. Organisms from both RMSF and MSF can be transmitted to dogs, rodents, and other animals; animal infections may be subclinical, but persistent infections in rodents and disease in dogs have been observed. Dogs are useful sentinels for spotted fever group rickettsiae. Clustered cases of RMSF in humans and dogs may occur at the same time. Rodents and reptiles are the reservoir for Australian spotted fever and Japanese spotted fever; rodents and lagomorphs for Far-Eastern tick-borne rickettsiosis. The reservoir for Flinders Island spotted fever is not well determined; however, reptiles, migratory birds, and rodents are suspected.

6. Incubation periods—Incubation periods for all spotted fever group rickettsial infections range from 2–21 days.

7. Transmission—Most spotted fever infections are transmitted by ixodid (hard) ticks, which are widely distributed throughout the world; tick species differ markedly according to geographical area. Primary route of transmission is via tick exposure; however, diagnosis should not depend on the recollection of a tick bite as they are often painless and not recognized. Contamination of breaks in the skin or mucous membranes with crushed tissues, feces of the tick, or aerosolized particles (RMSF) may also lead to infection. The disease is not directly transmitted from person to person; however, household clusters may occur because of the possible proximity to the infected tick population.

Common vectors are as follows:

1) RMSF: *Dermacentor variabilis* (American dog tick), *Dermacentor andersoni* (Rocky Mountain wood tick), *Rhipicephalus sanguineus* (brown dog tick), and *Amblyomma cajennense* (cayenne tick).
2) Mediterranean spotted fever: *R. sanguineus* (brown dog tick).
3) African tickbite fever: *Amblyomma hebraeum* (African bont tick) and *Amblyomma variegatum* (tropical bont tick).
4) Queensland tick typhus: *Ixodes holocyclus* (paralysis tick).
5) North Asian tick fever: *Dermacentor* and *Haemaphysalis* ticks.
6) Tickborne lymphadenopathy: *Dermacentor marginatus* (ornate sheep tick).
7) Flinders Island spotted fever: *Aponomma hydrosauri* (southern reptile tick), *Ixodes tasmanii* (common marsupial tick), and *Ixodes granulatus*.
8) Australian spotted fever: *Ixodes holocyclus* (Australian paralysis tick) and *Haemaphysalis novaeguineae*.
9) Far-Eastern tickborne rickettsiosis: *Dermacentor silvarum*, *Haemaphysalis concinna* (relict tick) and *Haemaphysalis japonica douglasii*.

10) Japanese spotted fever: *Haemaphysalis flava*, *Haemaphysalis longicornis* (bush tick), *Dermacentor taiwanensis*, and *Ixodes ovatus*.

11) Maculatum infection: *Amblyomma maculatum* and *Amblyomma triste*.

8. Risk groups—Susceptibility is general. Risk factors for severe or fatal outcome include young age, advanced age, alcoholism, glucose-6-phosphate dehydrogenase (G6PD) deficiency, or immunocompromise; however, fatal outcome can occur in previously healthy people of all ages in severe diseases such as RMSF. Patients with a history of alcoholism may be at increased risk for delayed diagnosis and treatment, because abnormal laboratory values may be seen as symptomatic of alcohol abuse and not alert the physician to an acute rickettsial infection.

9. Prevention—

1) See also Prevention in "Lyme Disease." Search for and remove attached or crawling ticks immediately after exposure to tick-infested habitats.

2) Minimize tick populations near residences by removing ticks from dogs and using acaridal collars or other treatment.

3) Vaccine is not available. Antibiotic prophylaxis following a tick bite is not recommended.

10. Management of patient—

1) Carefully remove all ticks from patients.

2) Treatment: doxycycline is the drug of choice for adults and children of all ages and should be initiated as soon as a rickettsial infection is suspected to avoid treatment delay and risk of severe illness and death. Doxycycline has not been shown to cause dental staining at the dose and duration used to treat rickettsial infections. The adult dose is 100 mg twice a day, while the pediatric dose is 2.2 mg/kg twice a day, for 3 days after resolution of fever (usually a 5- to 10-day course). In cases of documented life-threatening allergies to tetracyclines, or pregnancy, chloramphenicol may be considered as an alternative. However, it may be less effective at preventing death than doxycycline. If patient symptoms worsen, expert opinion should be consulted regarding the need for possible doxycycline use during pregnancy or in patients with life-threatening tetracycline allergies (which are rare). Most broad-spectrum antibiotics have no efficacy against rickettsial infections and limited evidence suggests that sulfa-containing antibiotics and fluoroquinolones may worsen the outcome of these diseases. Therefore, extreme caution should be

used when treating rickettsial infections with antibiotics other than doxycycline.

11. Management of contacts and the immediate environment— Spotted fever group rickettsiae infections can occur in clusters due to similar environmental exposures. People with similar exposures should be notified to be alert for symptoms and be treated if they become febrile. Tick checks should be performed by people at risk. Patients should be advised to treat homes, yards, and pets with acaracide containing products if ticks are present.

12. Special considerations—Reporting: case reporting is obligatory for many of the spotted fever group rickettsial diseases in some countries.

WHO Collaborating Centres provide support as required. More information can be found at http://www.who.int/collaboratingcentres/database/en.

II. RICKETTSIALPOX (vesicular rickettsiosis)

1. Clinical features—An acute febrile illness in which an initial skin lesion at the site of a mite bite, often associated with lymphadenopathy, is followed by fever; a disseminated vesicular skin rash appears, which generally does not involve the palms and soles, and lasts only a few days. It may be confused with chickenpox. Death is uncommon. Acute hepatitis may be one of the leading symptoms after infection and before development of specific vesicular rash.

2. Causative agent—*Rickettsia akari*.

3. Diagnosis—Serology, PCR, or immunostains of biopsied tissues as described in Diagnosis in "Rickettsioses."

4. Occurrence—Urban areas of the eastern USA; most cases have been described from New York City. *R. akari* has also been reported in Russia and neighboring countries, in Africa, and in the Republic of Korea.

5. Reservoir—Mice (*Mus musculus*) in urban sites in the USA. Commensal rats are reported to be the reservoir in Russia, and *Apodemus* in the Republic of Korea.

6. Incubation period—6–15 days.

7. Transmission—Rickettsialpox is acquired from *Liponyssoides sanguineus*, the house mouse mite, either through a bite or similar contamination of broken skin with the feces of infected mites. The disease is not directly transmitted from person to person; however, household clusters may occur because of the possible proximity to the infected mite population.

9. **Prevention**—Includes rodent elimination and mite control.

10. **Management of patient**—The infection is responsive to tetra-cyclines, and doxycycline is the treatment of choice in adults and children of all ages. Clinical improvement typically occurs with a 3-day course.

11. **Management of contacts and the immediate environment**—Household contacts of cases should be educated about symptoms and treatment. Simultaneous control of household rodent population and rodent mites has been effective at controlling epidemics.

12. **Special considerations**—None.

[J. Regan, C. Kato]

RIFT VALLEY FEVER

DISEASE	ICD-10 CODE
RIFT VALLEY FEVER	ICD-10 A92.4

1. **Clinical features**—Rift Valley fever (RVF) is a viral zoonosis that primarily affects animals but also has the capacity to infect humans. RVF virus infection can be unapparent or characterized by a brief, self-limiting febrile illness with a sudden onset of fever, myalgia, chills, dizziness, and headache, lasting for 3–4 days. Recovery is usually without sequelae. In a small proportion of cases (1%), the clinical syndrome progresses to a severe disease of 3 forms: ocular, meningoencephalitis, or hemorrhagic with liver failure. The appearance of shock, multiorgan failure, and disseminated intravascular coagulation are of poor prognosis. Laboratory findings may include elevated liver enzyme levels, thrombocytopenia, leukopenia, anemia, and elevated blood urea nitrogen and creatinine. Variable neurological sequelae are observed in survivors of RVF encephalitis. In about 1–5% of all RVF patients, unilateral or bilateral retinal hemorrhages occur, resulting in transitory or permanent scotoma visual field defects. The overall case-fatality rate is low (1–5%) but can reach 50% in hospitalized patients.

2. **Causative agent**—RVF virus is a member of the genus *Phlebovirus* family *Bunyaviridae*.

3. **Diagnosis**—During the acute phase of disease, virus can be detected from blood or serum by conventional or real-time polymerase chain reaction (PCR), virus isolation, or antigen detection enzyme-linked immunosorbent

assay (ELISA). Serological diagnosis (immunoglobulin class M [IgM], immunoglobulin class G [IgG]) is made by ELISA. RVF virus-specific neutralizing antibodies persist for years. Antibodies appear a few days after onset of symptoms and virus is very rapidly cleared. In fatal cases, the virus can be detected in tissues (liver) by molecular techniques, virus isolation, or by immunohistochemistry.

4. Occurrence—A RVF compatible disease in lambs and humans was first reported in East Africa in the 1910s, and RVF virus was first isolated in 1930 in Kenya. Since then, it has been reported in most sub-Saharan African countries, Egypt, Madagascar, and in the past 10 years in the Arabian Peninsula (Yemen and Saudi Arabia), marking the first reported occurrence of the disease outside the African continent and raising concerns that it could extend to other parts of Asia and Europe. Large livestock and human outbreaks have recurred in East Africa, Egypt, Sudan, Mauritania, South Africa, and Madagascar.

5. Reservoirs—RVF is a predominantly epizootic virus, is maintained in nature in *Aedes* sp. mosquitoes. Virus has been isolated from male and female mosquitoes suggesting transovarial transmission. Hatching of infected *Aedes* eggs follows abnormally high rainfall and flooding, infected mosquitoes feeding on susceptible wildlife species or livestock, resulting in abortion storms and virus amplification. Horizontal transmission to other mosquito species (i.e., *Culex* sp.) is facilitated by the high viremia observed in domestic ruminants.

6. Incubation period—Usually 2-7 days.

7. Transmission—Through bites of infected mosquitoes or by direct contact with the blood, body fluids, or abortion products of infected domestic ruminants (e.g., sheep, goat, cattle, camels). The virus infects humans through inoculation, for example via a wound from an infected knife, through contact with broken skin, or through inhalation of aerosols produced during the slaughter of infected animals. The aerosol mode of transmission has also led to infection in laboratory workers. Human-to-human transmission has not been reported, but accidental laboratory infections with RVF viruses have been frequently described.

8. Risk groups—Humans become infected from contact with blood of infected animals (and their tissues) or from a mosquito bite. Farmers, herders, owners of livestock, abattoir workers, and veterinary personnel are at risk of RVF infection. Numerous laboratory infections were described before the systematic use of personnel protective equipment.

9. Prevention—

1) Human RVF vaccines are not available. Contact and droplet precautions are recommended for management of RVF patients

(discussed later). Personal protective equipment and high containment laboratories are recommended for RVF virus manipulations.

2) Application of insect repellents on clothes in endemic areas; see "Arboviral Encephalitides" for preventive measures against mosquitoes.

3) Handling potentially infected animals or their tissues should be done with protective equipment, using contact and droplet precautions.

4) RVF infections of humans are most effectively prevented by preventing animal infections through vaccination of livestock.

10. Management of patient—Although no human-to-human transmission has been described, patients with acute RVF can have high levels of viremia, and so precautions are advised. Patient isolated in a single room. Strict contact, droplet, blood, and body fluid precautions needed. Persons handling biological specimens or materials contaminated with blood or body fluid from suspect or confirmed RVF patients should also take proper safety precautions. No specific treatment available. General measures including early hospitalization and symptomatic management of the patients.

11. Management of contacts and the immediate environment—There is no human-to-human transmission. Use proper management (isolation, destruction) of potentially infectious animals and animal products. Use of insecticide-treated bed nets and insect repellent is recommended to prevent mosquito transmission of RVF virus.

12. Special considerations—

1) Reporting: individual cases should be reported to the local health authority, and confirmed cases could be notifiable to national authorities in some countries. Security authorities in some countries require notification of RVF virus isolation. RVF is listed as agent that must be assessed in terms of potential to cause Public Health Emergencies of International Concern under the IHR. Suspicion or confirmation of RVF in animal should be reported to the Office International des Epizooties.

2) Epidemic measures: limit contact with potentially infected animals. Use of insecticide-treated bed nets and insect repellent is recommended to prevent mosquito transmission of RVF virus. See "Arboviral Encephalitides."

[B. Knust, P. E. Rollin]

ROTAVIRUS INFECTION

(sporadic viral gastroenteritis, severe viral gastroenteritis of infants and children)

DISEASE	ICD-10 CODE
ROTAVIRUS INFECTION	ICD-10 A08.0

1. Clinical features—A sporadic, seasonal, often severe gastroenteritis of infants and young children, characterized by vomiting, fever, and watery diarrhea. Rotavirus infection is occasionally associated with severe dehydration and death in young children. Secondary symptomatic cases among adult family contacts can occur, although subclinical infections are more common. Infection has occasionally been found in pediatric patients with a variety of other clinical manifestations, but the virus is probably coincidental rather than causative in these conditions. Rotavirus is a major cause of nosocomial diarrhea of newborns and infants. Although rotavirus diarrhea is generally more severe than acute diarrhea due to other agents, illness caused by rotavirus is not distinguishable from that caused by other enteric viruses for any individual patient.

2. Causative agent—The 70-nm rotavirus belongs to the *Reoviridae* family. Group A is common in humans, group B is uncommon in infants but has caused large epidemics in adults in China, and group C appears to be uncommon in humans. Groups A, B, C, D, E, and F occur in animals. There are 6 major serotypes of group A human rotavirus, based on antigenic differences. The major neturalization antigen is the VP7 outer capsid surface protein, and another outer capsid protein, VP4, is associated with virulence and also plays a role in virus neutralization.

3. Diagnosis—Commercially available enzyme-linked immunosorbent assay (ELISA) kits are the standard method for diagnosis and the most commonly used worldwide. Electron microscopy, latex agglutination, and other immunological techniques, some of which are commercially available, can also identify rotavirus in stool specimens or rectal swabs but are not commonly used. Evidence of rotavirus infection can be demonstrated by serological techniques, but diagnosis is usually based on the demonstration of rotavirus antigen in stools. False-positive ELISA reactions are common in newborns, and thus positive reactions in newborns require confirmation by an alternative test.

4. Occurrence—In both industrialized and developing countries, rotavirus is associated with about one-third to one-half of hospitalized cases of diarrheal illness in infants and children younger than 5 years. Neonatal rotaviral infections are frequent in certain settings but are usually asymptomatic. Essentially all children are infected by rotavirus in their first 2-3 years of life with peak incidence of clinical disease in the 6-24-month age group. Outbreaks occur among children in day care settings. Rotavirus is more frequently associated with severe diarrhea than other enteric pathogens; in developing countries, it is responsible for an estimated 200,000–250,000 diarrheal deaths each year. Although not consistent in all settings, in temperate climates, rotavirus diarrhea often occurs in seasonal peaks during cooler months; in tropical climates, diarrhea usually occurs throughout the year with a moderate peak in the cooler dry months. Rotavirus infection of adults is usually asymptomatic but occasionally manifests as travelers' diarrhea; diarrhea in the immunocompromised (including those with HIV infection); diarrhea in parents of children with rotavirus infection; and diarrhea in the elderly, sometimes in outbreaks in geriatric units.

5. Reservoir—Probably humans. The animal viruses do not typically produce disease in humans.

6. Incubation period—Approximately 24–72 hours.

7. Transmission—Probably fecal-oral with possible contact or respiratory spread. Although rotaviruses do not effectively multiply in the respiratory tract, they may be encountered in respiratory secretions. There is some evidence that rotavirus may be present in contaminated water. The virus is communicable during the acute stage and later while virus shedding continues. Rotavirus is not usually detectable after about the eighth day of infection, although excretion of virus for 30 days or more has been reported in immunocompromised patients. Symptoms last for an average of 4–6 days.

8. Risk groups—Susceptibility is greatest between 6 and 24 months of age. By 3 years, most children have acquired rotavirus antibodies. Diarrhea is uncommon in infected infants younger than 3 months. Immunocompromised individuals are at particular risk for prolonged rotavirus antigen excretion and intermittent rotavirus diarrhea.

9. Prevention—

1) WHO has prequalified 2 new vaccines against rotavirus in 2006: Rotarix and Rota Teq and recommends these vaccines for all children worldwide. Clinical trials in both developed and developing countries have demonstrated their safety and efficacy in preventing rotavirus-associated severe gastroenteritis. Data from many countries in the developed world that have implemented routine rotavirus vaccination show marked declines in the incidence of severe diarrhea, including declines in diarrhea mortality.

2) The effectiveness of other preventive measures is undetermined. Hygienic measures applicable to diseases transmitted via the fecal-oral route may not be effective in preventing transmission. The virus survives for long periods on hard surfaces, in water, and on hands. It is relatively resistant to some commonly used disinfectants but is inactivated by chlorine.

3) Prevent exposure of infants and young children to individuals with acute gastroenteritis in family and institutional (day care or hospital) settings by maintaining a high level of sanitary practices.

4) Exclusively breastfed infants are protected against rotavirus infection during the period of breastfeeding; however, some data indicate that breastfeeding may not reduce the overall population rate of severe rotavirus gastroenteritis during the first 2 years of life.

10. Management of patient—

1) Enteric precautions, with frequent hand washing by caretakers of infants.

2) Sanitary disposal of diapers; place overalls over diapers to prevent leakage.

3) Treatment: oral rehydration therapy with oral glucose-electrolyte solution is adequate in most cases. Parenteral fluids are needed in cases with vascular collapse or uncontrolled vomiting (see "Cholera and Other Vibrioses"). In children younger than 5 years, give elemental zinc for 10–14 days. Antibiotics and antimotility drugs are contraindicated.

11. Management of contacts and the immediate environment—
Source and vehicle(s) of infection should be sought in high-risk populations and those with the risk of prolonged rotavirus shedding through epidemiological investigation.

12. Special considerations—

1) Reporting: obligatory report of epidemics in some countries; no individual case report required.

2) A potential problem with dislocated populations.

[M. Patel]

RUBELLA
(German measles)

DISEASE	ICD-10 CODE
RUBELLA	ICD-10 B06

1. **Clinical features**—Rubella is most often a mild febrile viral disease with a diffuse punctate and maculopapular rash. Clinically, rubella is indistinguishable from febrile rash illness due to measles, dengue, parvovirus B19, human herpesvirus 6, coxsackievirus, echovirus, adenovirus, or scarlet fever. Children usually present few or no constitutional symptoms, but adults may experience a 1-5 day prodrome of low-grade fever, headache, malaise, mild coryza, and conjunctivitis. Postauricular, occipital, and posterior cervical lymphadenopathy is the most characteristic clinical feature and precedes the rash by 5-10 days. Thrombocytopenia can occur, but hemorrhagic manifestations are rare. Arthralgia and, less commonly, arthritis complicate a substantial proportion of infections, particularly among adult females. Encephalitis is seen in 1 out of 6,000 cases and occurs with a higher frequency in adults. Up to 50% of rubella infections are either without rash or subclinical.

Rubella is important because it can produce a constellation of anomalies in the developing fetus, called congenital rubella syndrome (CRS). CRS may occur in up to 90% of infants born to women who are infected with rubella during the first 10 weeks of pregnancy. Fetuses infected early are at greatest risk of intrauterine death, spontaneous abortion, and CRS. Clinical manifestations of CRS include single or combined defects or symptoms such as hearing impairment, cataracts, microphthalmia, congenital glaucoma, microcephaly, meningoencephalitis, developmental delay, congenital heart defects (e.g., patent ductus arteriosus, atrial or ventricular septal defects), purpura, hepatosplenomegaly, jaundice, and radiolucent bone disease. Moderate and severe CRS is usually recognizable at birth; mild CRS with only slight cardiac involvement or hearing impairment may not be detected for months or even years after birth. Insulin-dependent diabetes mellitus is recognized as a frequent late manifestation of CRS. Congenital malformations and fetal death can also occur following inapparent maternal rubella. Defects are rare when maternal infection occurs after the 20th week of gestation.

2. **Causative agent**—Rubella virus (family *Togaviridae*, genus *Rubivirus*).

3. **Diagnosis**—Laboratory diagnosis of rubella is required since clinical diagnosis is often inaccurate. Laboratory confirmation is usually based on a positive rubella-specific immunoglobulin class M enzyme-linked immunosorbent assay (IgM ELISA) test on a blood specimen obtained within 28 days after the rash onset. An epidemiologically confirmed rubella case is a patient with suspected rubella with an epidemiological link to a laboratory-confirmed case.

Other methods for rubella diagnosis include paired serum specimens that show seroconversion, or at least a 4-fold rise in rubella-specific immunoglobulin class G (IgG) antibody titer, positive rubella reverse transcription polymerase chain reaction (RT-PCR) test, and virus isolation; RT-PCR and virus isolation may be only available in higher-level reference laboratories.

Laboratory confirmation of CRS in an infant is based on a positive rubella-specific IgM ELISA test on a blood specimen, the persistence of a rubella-specific IgG antibody titer in a blood specimen beyond the time expected from passive transfer of maternal IgG antibody, isolation of the virus from a throat swab or urine specimen, or detection of rubella virus by PCR. Almost all infants with CRS have a positive rubella IgM test from 0–3 months old, and more than 30% of infants remain positive from 4–9 months old. Rubella virus has been isolated from throat and urine specimens of infants with CRS and from cataract surgery aspirates in children up to 3 years of age.

4. Occurrence—In the absence of generalized immunization, rubella occurred worldwide at endemic levels with epidemics every 5–9 years. Large rubella epidemics resulted in very high levels of morbidity. For example, the US epidemic in 1964–1965 led to an estimated 12.5 million cases of rubella, more than 20,000 cases of CRS, and 11,000 fetal deaths; the incidence of CRS during endemic periods was 0.1–0.2 per 1,000 live births and 1–4 per 1,000 live births during epidemics. In countries where the rubella vaccine has not been introduced, rubella remains endemic. In 2010, an estimated 103,000 CRS cases occurred worldwide. Since 2009, surveillance data has provided evidence that the interruption of rubella virus transmission among countries has occurred in the WHO Region of the Americas, and rubella is now only endemic in the rest of the world.

As of the end of 2013, 135 countries/territories (70% of the world total) have introduced rubella vaccine in their national immunization programs, with the highest percentage in the WHO Region of the Americas (100% of countries) and Europe (100%), followed by the Western Pacific Region (81%), the Eastern Mediterranean Region (64%), the Southeast Asia Region (45%), and the African Region (13%). In many countries, sustained high levels of rubella immunization have drastically reduced or eliminated rubella and CRS.

5. Reservoir—Humans.

6. Incubation period—From 14–17 days with a range of 14–21 days.

7. Transmission—Through contact with nasopharyngeal secretions of infected people. Infection is by droplet spread or direct contact with patients. Infants with CRS shed large quantities of virus in their pharyngeal secretions and urine and serve as a source of infection to their contacts. The disease is highly communicable. The period of communicability is about 1 week before and at least 4 days after onset of rash. Infants with CRS may shed virus for up to 1 year after birth.

8. Risk groups—Immunity is usually permanent after natural infection and thought to be long term, probably lifelong, after immunization; infants born to immune mothers are ordinarily protected for 6-9 months, depending on the amount of maternal antibodies acquired transplacentally.

9. Prevention—Rubella control is needed primarily to prevent fetal death and/or CRS in the offspring of women who acquire the disease during pregnancy.

1) Educate the general public on modes of transmission, and stress the need for rubella immunization. Health care providers must be aware of the risks caused by rubella in pregnancy.

2) A single dose of live, attenuated rubella virus vaccine elicits a significant and long-lasting antibody response in about 95%-100% of susceptible individuals aged 9 months or older. Rubella vaccines are cold-chain dependent and should be protected from light. Several rubella vaccines are available as single antigen, that is, measles and rubella (MR), measles, mumps, rubella (MMR), or measles, mumps, rubella, and varicella vaccines. Most of the currently licensed vaccines are based on the live attenuated RA27/3 strain of rubella virus; other live attenuated rubella virus strains are used in China and Japan.

3) WHO recommends use of the vaccine in all countries where control or elimination of rubella and CRS are considered a public health priority. The primary purpose of rubella vaccination is to prevent the occurrence of congenital rubella infection, including CRS. This can be done using combined vaccines (measles, rubella or measles, mumps, rubella), and current efforts in global measles control should be used as an opportunity to pursue control of rubella. Two general approaches are recommended to prevent the occurrence of CRS:

   - Prevention of CRS only through immunization of adolescent girls or women of childbearing age.
   - Elimination of rubella as well as CRS. For countries undertaking the elimination of rubella and CRS, the preferred approach is to begin with MR vaccine or MMR vaccine in a campaign targeting a wide range of ages that is followed immediately by the introduction of MR or MMR vaccine into the routine childhood vaccination program. The first dose of a rubella containing vaccine should be delivered with MCV1 (first dose of measles vaccine either at 9 months or 12 months), depending on the level of measles virus transmission. All subsequent follow-up campaigns should use MR vaccine or MMR vaccine. In addition, countries should make efforts to reach women of childbearing age by immunizing adolescent girls or women of

childbearing age, or both, through routine services. If countries conduct any supplementary immunization activities targeting immunity gaps in adults, the supplementary immunization activity should include both males and females.

Depending on the burden of disease and the available resources, countries may choose to accelerate their progress towards elimination by conducting campaigns targeting a wide range of ages of both adult males and females. The precise target population depends on the country's susceptibility profile, cultural acceptability, and operational feasibility. Following well-designed and well-implemented programs, rubella and CRS have disappeared from many countries. Two regions—the Americas and Europe— have adopted a goal of rubella elimination.

Inadequately implemented childhood vaccination programs may run the risk of increasing the number of susceptibles among women—and the possibility of increased numbers of cases of CRS—but the risk decreases as immunized child cohorts become adults. To avoid the potential of an increased risk of CRS, countries should achieve and maintain immunization coverage of 80% or greater with at least 1 dose of a rubella containing vaccine delivered through routine services with MCV1 or regular SIAs, or both.

Following the introduction of large-scale rubella vaccination, coverage should be measured periodically by age and locality. In addition, surveillance is needed for rubella and CRS. If resources permit, longitudinal serological surveillance can be used to monitor the impact of the immunization program, especially through assessing rubella IgG antibody in serum samples from women attending antenatal clinics.

Rubella vaccine should be avoided in pregnancy because of the theoretical—but never demonstrated—teratogenic risk. To date, CRS has not occurred in almost 3,000 susceptible pregnant women who were unknowingly pregnant and received RA27/3 rubella vaccine in early pregnancy. If pregnancy is being planned, however, an interval of 1 month should be observed after rubella immunization. Receipt of rubella vaccine during pregnancy is not an indication for abortion. Rubella vaccine should not be given to anyone with an immunodeficiency or who receives immunosuppressive therapy. Asymptomatic HIV-infected persons can, however, be safely immunized.

4) In case of infection with wild rubella virus early in pregnancy, culturally appropriate counseling should be provided. Abortion may be considered in those countries where this is an option.

5) Intramuscular immune globulin (IG) given within 72 hours of rubella exposure may decrease clinical disease, viral shedding, and the rate of viremia in exposed susceptible persons. IG may be considered for a susceptible pregnant woman exposed to the disease who would not be in a position to consider abortion. The absence of clinical signs in a pregnant woman who has received IG does not guarantee that fetal infection has been prevented. Infants with congenital rubella have been born to mothers who were given IG shortly after exposure.

10. Management of patient—

1) In hospitals, patients suspected of having rubella should be managed under droplet isolation precautions; attempts should be made to prevent exposure of nonimmune pregnant women. Exclude children from school and adults from work for 7 days after onset of rash. Infants with CRS may shed virus for 12 months. All persons having contact with infants with CRS should be immune to rubella either naturally or through immunization; contact between these infants and pregnant women should be avoided. In hospitals, contact isolation precautions should be applied to infants younger than 12 months with CRS unless urine and pharyngeal virus cultures are negative for rubella virus.
2) Treatment: none.

11. Management of contacts and the immediate environment—

1) Immunization of contacts will not necessarily prevent infection or illness. Passive immunization with IG is not indicated (except possibly as indicated earlier).
2) Identify pregnant female contacts, especially those in the first trimester. Such contacts should be tested serologically for susceptibility (IgG antibody) or early infection (IgM antibody) and advised accordingly.

12. Special considerations—

1) Reporting: in countries where rubella elimination is a goal, all cases of rubella and of CRS should be reported. In many countries, reporting is obligatory. Early reporting of suspected cases permits early establishment of control measures.
2) For surveillance purposes, the WHO-recommended case definition of a suspected rubella case is any person with fever, nonvesicular (maculopapular) rash, and adenopathy (cervical, suboccipital, or postauricular).
3) Epidemic measures: prompt reporting of all confirmed and suspected cases; the country's established goal for rubella

control/elimination will dictate the level of investigation required. During an outbreak, a limited number (5-10) of suspect cases (definition discussed earlier) should be investigated with laboratory tests to confirm that disease is due to rubella. However, during an outbreak, all rash illnesses in pregnancy should be investigated. The medical community and general public should be informed about rubella epidemics in order to identify and protect susceptible pregnant women. Active surveillance for infants with CRS should be carried out until 9 months after the last reported rubella case.

[S. Reef]

SALMONELLOSIS

DISEASE	ICD-10 CODE
SALMONELLOSIS	ICD-10 A02

"Salmonellosis" is about illness caused by nontyphoidal *Salmonella* organisms. Illness caused by *Salmonella* serotypes Typhi and Paratyphi is described in "Typhoid Fever and Paratyphoid Fever."

1. Clinical features—A bacterial disease commonly manifested by sudden onset of diarrhea, abdominal pain, fever, nausea, and often vomiting. Diarrhea, which may be bloody, usually persists for several days. Dehydration, especially among infants and the elderly, may be severe. Deaths are uncommon, except in the very young, the frail elderly, the debilitated, and the immunosuppressed. Morbidity and costs from medical care and absenteeism may be high. More illness occurs than is confirmed by culture.

Infection may begin as acute enterocolitis and develop into septicemia or focal infection. In enterocolitis, fecal excretion of infectious organisms usually persists for days or weeks after illness has resolved; administration of antimicrobial agents may increase the duration of shedding. Occasionally, the agent localizes in a normally sterile site, producing abscess, septic arthritis, osteomyelitis, cholecystitis, endocarditis, meningitis, pericarditis, pneumonia, cystitis, or pyelonephritis. In the USA, 9% of laboratory-confirmed cases are extra-intestinal infections. Severity of the disease is related to serotype, number of organisms ingested, and host factors; severity can be increased when the organism is resistant to antimicrobial agents used to treat the patient.

2. Causative agent—Nontyphoidal *Salmonella* bacteria. Approximately 2,500 serotypes have been identified. Most are spread from animal reservoirs, which are usually asymptomatic. In most areas, a small number of serotypes account for the majority of infections; nearly all *Salmonella* isolated from ill persons are serotypes of *Salmonella enterica* subsp. *enterica*. In most countries with surveillance for *Salmonella* infections, *S. enterica* subsp. *enterica* serotypes Typhimurium and Enteritidis are the most commonly reported. There is much variation in the relative prevalence of other serotypes from country to country.

3. Diagnosis—In cases with diarrhea or septicemia, *Salmonella* may be isolated from feces or blood, respectively, on enteric media during acute stages of illness. *Salmonella* may also be isolated from other sites, such as cerebrospinal fluid and urine. Serological tests are not useful in diagnosis.

4. Occurrence—Worldwide; more extensively reported in North America and Europe, no doubt because of more frequent use of cultures and better reporting. The incidence rate is highest in infants and children younger than 5 years. The proportion of laboratory-confirmed infections that are part of outbreaks depends partly on each country's surveillance for sporadic cases and outbreaks; in the USA, it is about 6%. *Salmonella* causes many outbreaks in restaurants, nursing homes, schools, and hospitals, usually from food contaminated at its source, that was inadequately cooked or that cross-contaminated other foods, and, much less often, through handling by an ill person who is infected or a carrier. Infections can also result from direct or indirect contact with infected animals or their environments. *Salmonella* can also cause outbreaks due to widely distributed commercial products that are contaminated; these cases may appear to be sporadic, appearing in many jurisdictions or geographical locations. For example, a large USA outbreak due to improperly pasteurized milk affected 285,000 persons. *Salmonella* also causes widespread outbreaks through contact with animals that carry *Salmonella* including turtles and other reptiles, chicks and ducklings, backyard poultry, and frogs.

5. Reservoir—Domestic and wild animals, including poultry (e.g., chickens [especially chicks], ducks, geese, turkeys), reptiles (e.g., turtles, iguanas, snakes), amphibians (e.g., frogs, toads), swine, cattle, rodents (e.g., hamsters, mice, rats), and pets (e.g., dogs, cats, guinea pigs, hedgehogs); also humans (i.e., persons with diarrhea and convalescent carriers). Chronic human carriers are rare (except for serotype Typhi) but are prevalent in animals, particularly in birds and reptiles.

6. Incubation period—From 6–72 hours, usually about 12–36 hours. Longer incubation periods of up to 16 days have been documented and may not be uncommon following low-dose ingestion.

7. Transmission—Salmonellosis is a zoonotic disease. Direct or indirect contact with infected animals or their environments may lead to infection and has resulted in many outbreaks. Infected animals typically appear healthy and clean, but their bodies (hide, fur, feathers, and scales) and their environments (e.g., water in a turtle tank) can be contaminated with *Salmonella*.

Salmonellosis is classified as a foodborne disease because ingestion of contaminated food, most times of animal origin, is the predominant mode of transmission. Food sources include raw and undercooked foods of animal origin (e.g., eggs, raw milk and milk products, meat, poultry), as well as other foods such as produce and processed foods. In 2005, investigators in the USA who cultured 40,000 random samples of meat, including chicken, pork, and beef, found that 5.7% of all samples and 33% of poultry yielded *Salmonella*. Highest prevalence is often found in poultry products—isolation rates from poultry of 40–50%. Widespread outbreaks have been linked to ingestion of eggs, poultry, ground beef, tomatoes, leafy greens, and melons from single suppliers and from commercially processed foods including frozen pot pies, peanut butter, dry snack foods, and cereals. Inadequate cooking and cross-contamination of other foods are important risk factors.

In the USA, numerous large outbreaks have also been linked to contact with high-risk animals, including live poultry in backyard flocks, reptiles, especially small turtles and amphibians. Dry dog food and pet treats, such as pig ears, have been sources of recent human outbreaks, suggesting that contaminated pet products may be an underrecognized source of human infections. One way *Salmonella* can be transmitted to farm animals is by feeds and fertilizers prepared from contaminated meat scraps, fish meal, and bones; crowding and inadequate hygiene can facilitate the spread from one animal to another.

Contaminated water is also an important mode of transmission, especially in areas where drinking water supplies are not disinfected. Fecal contamination of nonchlorinated public water supplies has caused large outbreaks. Recreational water has also been a source of infection.

Person-to-person fecal-oral transmission is possible, especially when diarrhea is present; persons with diarrhea and those in diapers (e.g., infants and incontinent adults) likely pose a greater risk of transmission than do asymptomatic continent carriers. Hospital epidemics were common decades ago and tended to be protracted, with organisms persisting in the environment through transmission via the hands of personnel or contaminated instruments. Maternity units with infected (at times asymptomatic) infants can also be sources. The probability of infection is related to the dose ingested, and it is estimated that from 100–1,000 organisms are usually required for infection. Models suggest a 10–20% probability for infection with a dose of 100 organisms and a 60–80% probability for infection at 1,000,000 organisms. Fewer organisms may cause infection if ingested in vehicles that buffer gastric acid.

The period of communicability extends throughout the course of infection and carriage. A temporary carrier state may continue for months, especially in infants. Depending on the serotype, approximately 1% of infected adults and 5% of children younger than 5 years, may excrete the organism for up to 1 year.

8. Risk groups—Susceptibility is universal and is increased by achlorhydria, antacid treatment, gastrointestinal surgery, prior or current antimicrobial therapy, neoplastic disease, immunosuppressive treatment, and debilitating conditions, including malnutrition. Whereas most cases are a self-limited gastroenteritis, immunosuppressed patients, including HIV-infected persons, and persons at the extremes of age, especially infants, are at increased risk for invasive infection. In such cases, antimicrobial treatment is advised. Septicemia in people with sickle-cell disease increases the risk of focal systemic infection (e.g., osteomyelitis).

9. Prevention—A multifaceted approach to prevention is needed that should include consumers, health care providers, veterinarians, regulatory agencies, public health officials, and industry. Key elements are:

1) Food safety education

- Educate consumers, patients, and food handlers about the importance of

  o thoroughly cooking all foods of animal origin, particularly poultry, meat, and egg products;
  o handwashing before, during, and after food preparation;
  o refrigerating prepared foods in small containers at a safe temperature (between 32° and 40°F [0–4°C]); refrigerating cooked foods within 2 hours;
  o using a food thermometer to ensure that poultry and meat reach a safe minimum internal temperature;
  o avoiding recontamination in the kitchen after cooking is completed;
  o keeping uncooked meats separate from produce, cooked foods, and ready-to-eat foods;
  o washing hands, cutting boards (one for raw meat, one for other foods when possible), counters, knives, and other utensils thoroughly after they contact uncooked foods; and
  o maintaining a sanitary kitchen and protecting prepared foods against rodent and insect contamination.

- Educate consumers to avoid consuming certain high-risk foods:

  o Raw or incompletely cooked eggs (e.g., eggs "over easy" or "sunny side up") and dirty or cracked eggs. Use pasteurized eggs or egg products in recipes that would result in consumption of raw or lightly cooked eggs (e.g., Hollandaise sauce, Caesar salad dressing, eggnog, home-made ice cream).

○ Raw milk, raw milk yogurt, and unpasteurized soft cheese.
○ Ciders and juices that are not pasteurized.
○ Raw or undercooked meat and poultry.
○ Children, older adults, pregnant women, and persons with weakened immune systems should avoid eating raw sprouts of any kind (including alfalfa, clover, radish, and mung beans).

- Educate known carriers about the need for careful hand washing after defecation and before handling food, and discourage them from handling food for others as long as they shed organisms.

2) Education about zoonotic salmonellosis from pets and other animals: recognize that healthy pets and other animals may carry and transmit *Salmonella* and that young children are at particular risk.

- Wash hands thoroughly after handling animals and pet foods, and after cleaning animal enclosures, especially before handling food, drinks, or other items that will be touched by babies (e.g., bottles).
- Keep high-risk animals (live poultry, reptiles, and amphibians) out of child care facilities that have children younger than 5 years and out of nursing homes and other facilities with high-risk individuals. Because small turtles are particularly hazardous to young children, their distribution has been banned in the USA since 1975.
- Avoid giving pets raw foods of animal origin because they may transmit pathogens to pets and to people.

3) Food industry measures:

- Restaurants and stores should buy meat, poultry, produce, and other foods only from suppliers that meet or exceed performance standards for contamination of food with pathogens at all stages of production from farm to fork.
- In fields, orchards, and produce packing plants, decrease contamination of foods eaten with no or minimal cooking by using *Salmonella*-free fertilizers and uncontaminated water,

limiting wild animal incursions, and providing toilets and handwashing facilities for workers.

- In food animal production, establish *Salmonella* control programs (feed control, cleaning and disinfection, vector control, and other sanitary and hygienic measures).
- Pet food and fodder manufacturers should adequately treat animal-derived foods prepared for animal consumption (e.g., meat, bone, fish meal) to eliminate pathogens and then prevent recontamination.
- Evaluate measures to decrease prevalence in flocks and herds, including combined sanitation and vaccination strategies. (In some countries a radical policy of eradication of *Salmonella*-positive chicken flocks has resulted in significantly lower salmonellosis incidence in humans.)
- Establish facilities for and encourage the use of food irradiation for meats, spices, and eggs.

4) Public health and regulatory policies:

- Conduct public health surveillance with molecular subtyping and interviews of reported ill persons to track trends and detect outbreaks.
- Investigate outbreaks of *Salmonella* infections using both human and animal surveillance data, and collaborate with agriculture and animal health colleagues to identify sources and devise prevention measures.
- Inspect for sanitation and adequately supervise abattoirs, food-processing plants, feed-blending mills, egg grading stations, restaurants, and butcher shops.

10. Management of patient—

1) Health care providers should collect patient stool specimens for culture testing when appropriate.
2) Proper handwashing should be stressed. For hospitalized patients, enteric precautions in handling feces and contaminated clothing and bed linen. Exclude symptomatic individuals from food handling and from direct care of infants and young children, older adults, and immunocompromised and institutionalized patients. Exclusion of asymptomatic infected individuals is indicated for those with questionable hygienic habits and may be required by local or national regulations. When exclusion is mandated, release to return to work handling food or in patient care generally requires 2 consecutive negative stool cultures for *Salmonella*, collected not less than 24 hours apart; if

antimicrobial agents have been given, the initial culture should be taken at least 48 hours after the last dose.

3) Concurrent disinfection of feces and soiled articles. In communities with adequate sewage disposal systems, feces can be discharged directly into sewers without preliminary disinfection.

4) Treatment: for uncomplicated gastroenteritis, none generally indicated, except rehydration and electrolyte replacement with oral rehydration solution (see "Cholera"). Infants, the elderly, persons whose immune systems are compromised (e.g., by sickle-cell disease, HIV, certain drugs such as immunosuppressives, antineoplastics), and patients with continued fever or manifestations of extra-intestinal infection should receive antimicrobial agents. In adults, treatment with ciprofloxacin is highly effective, but its use is not approved for children; ampicillin or amoxicillin may be used for children. Antimicrobial resistance is variable. The use of antimicrobial agents for the acute infection may increase the duration of carriage.

Awareness of the resistance patterns of strains in the patient's location can help in choosing initial therapy. In the 1990s, multiresistant serotype Typhimurium definitive phage-type 104 emerged throughout the world. These strains are usually resistant to ampicillin, chloramphenicol, streptomycin, sulfonamide, and tetracycline, and the associated genes are chromosomally encoded. Similarly, serotype Newport strains resistant to 7 antimicrobial classes, including third-generation cephalosporins, emerged in the 2000s. The emergence of these strains is thought to be linked to the use of antimicrobial agents in agriculture.

5) Patient Education: provide educational materials on prevention of foodborne illness and zoonotic salmonellosis in patient waiting rooms. Many organizations have developed free educational materials available in multiple formats and languages.

11. Management of contacts and immediate environment—Culture stools of household contacts who are involved in food handling, direct patient care, or care of young children or elderly people in institutional settings.

12. Special considerations—

1) Reporting: case report obligatory.
2) A risk in a situation in which large numbers of people must be fed in an area with poor sanitation.

WHO Collaborating Centres provide support as required. More information can be found at:

- http://www.who.int/collaboratingcentres/database/en
- http://www.who.int/foodsafety/publications/consumer/manual_keys.pdf
- http://www.who.int/gfn/en
- http://www.cdc.gov/salmonella

[C. Barton Behravesh, P. M. Griffin]

SARS, MERS, AND OTHER CORONAVIRUS INFECTIONS

DISEASE	ICD-10 CODE
SEVERE ACUTE RESPIRATORY SYNDROME	ICD-10 U04.9 (provisional)
MIDDLE EAST RESPIRATORY SYNDROME	
OTHER NOVEL CORONAVIRUSES	

I. SEVERE ACUTE RESPIRATORY SYNDROME (SARS)

1. Clinical features—Early signs and symptoms of SARS are nonspecific and consistent with influenza-like illness, with a spectrum of disease ranging from milder or atypical presentations to severe respiratory illness. SARS should be considered in the differential diagnosis in an individual presenting with fever above 38°C (100.4°F) and with symptoms of lower respiratory tract illness (e.g., cough, dyspnea, shortness of breath), with radiological evidence of lung infiltrates consistent with pneumonia or adult respiratory distress syndrome (ARDS), or with autopsy findings consistent with pneumonia or ARDS without an identifiable cause and with no alternative diagnosis that can fully explain the illness. Cases can become severe quickly, progressing to respiratory distress coinciding with peak viremia that occurs during the second week of illness (e.g., 10 days), with about 20%–30% requiring intensive care.

2. Causative agent—SARS is caused by the SARS-coronavirus (CoV). CoVs are enveloped, single-stranded positive strand ribonucleic acid (RNA) viruses that infect mammals and birds. In humans, CoVs are mainly associated with upper respiratory tract infections but can cause severe disease. Bats are most likely the natural reservoirs for SARS-CoV. Other animals, such as the masked palm civet, probably serve as intermediate hosts between bats and humans.

3. Diagnosis—SARS is diagnosed by exclusion of more usual causes of severe respiratory disease. It is unlikely that sporadic cases of SARS will be detected unless a patient with pneumonia gives a history of one or more of the following:

1) Exposure to an animal host.
2) SARS-CoV-related laboratory work.
3) Travel to southern China or another area with increased likelihood of animal-to-human transmission of SARS-CoV-like viruses from wildlife or other animal reservoirs.

Diagnosis requires both a compatible clinical illness and definitive laboratory tests for SARS-CoV infection. As there has been no documented human-to-human transmission of SARS-CoV worldwide since 2004, the number of qualified laboratories that test for SARS-CoV is limited. WHO recommends that testing for SARS-CoV only be undertaken when there is compelling clinical and/or epidemiological evidence that SARS may be the cause of an individual case or cluster of acute respiratory illness.

A variety of diagnostic tests are available. Their reliability depends on the type of clinical specimens collected and the timing of collection relative to symptom onset. Respiratory samples and stool samples should be routinely collected for nucleic acid detection by reverse transcription polymerase chain reaction (RT-PCR) or virus isolation during the first and second weeks of illness, as these specimens are most likely to yield virus. Sensitivity of newer RT-PCR assays has improved with approximately 80% SARS-CoV RNA detected in stored respiratory specimens that had been collected within the first few days of symptom onset. When upper respiratory tract specimens are negative, lower respiratory specimens may be useful. Persons infected with CoVs often shed virus in stool for days to weeks. In stool, RT-PCR assays can detect SARS-CoV RNA for more than 4 weeks after illness onset. A confirmed positive PCR test for the global surveillance of SARS requires at least 2 different clinical specimens (e.g., nasopharyngeal and stool), the same type of specimen collected on 2 or more days during illness (e.g., 2 or more nasopharyngeal aspirates), 2 different assays, or repeat PCR using a new extract from the original clinical sample on each occasion of testing. Serologic testing is also available, and acute and convalescent phase sera should also be collected if possible.

All positive test results should be independently verified by a WHO International SARS Reference and Verification Network laboratory.

WHO has published guidance on the clinical and laboratory diagnosis of SARS:

- http://www.who.int/csr/resources/publications/WHO_CDS_CSR_ARO_2004_1/en/index.html
- http://www.who.int/csr/sars/guidelines/en/SARSLab meeting.pdf

- http://www.who.int/csr/resources/publications/en/ SARSReferenceLab. pdf

4. Occurrence—SARS is thought to have first appeared in human populations in November 2002. The 2002–2003 epidemic was characterized by outbreaks worldwide including in Canada, Singapore, Viet Nam, and China (originating in Guangdong Province and spreading to major cities in other areas, including Beijing, Taipei, and the Special Administrative Region of Hong Kong). The disease spread internationally along major airline routes and resulted in 8,096 reported SARS cases in 29 countries with 774 deaths (9.6%). The last reported cases of SARS were in a cluster linked to a laboratory worker in China who was thought to have been infected in April 2004 at a laboratory where the virus was being studied.

It remains very difficult to predict when or whether SARS will reemerge in epidemic form. China has implemented strict market and food safety and other measures to prevent the transmission of SARS-like coronaviruses from animal hosts to humans. However, clustering of SARS-like illness in persons exposed to potential animal hosts—among health care workers or others exposed to a health care facility—remains an important sentinel event that may indicate the reemergence of SARS.

5. Reservoir—The Himalayan masked palm civet (*Paguma larvata*) is considered the main source of animal-to-human transmission of SARS-CoV. Cave-dwelling Chinese horseshoe bats (of the genus *Rhinolophus*) are a reservoir of SARS-like coronaviruses that are closely related to those responsible for the SARS epidemic but display greater genetic variation than SARS-CoV isolated from humans or civets. Initial studies in Guangdong Province, China, showed similar coronaviruses in civets and in a small number of other wildlife species sold in wet markets.

6. Incubation period—From 2–10 days (mean of 5–6 days), with isolated reports of longer incubation periods.

7. Transmission—SARS-CoV-like viruses are thought to have been introduced into the human population from wildlife hosts in 2002. SARS is usually transmitted from person to person by direct contact and respiratory droplets and in some situations by fomites. Caring for or living with an infected person or having direct contact with respiratory secretions, body fluids, and excretions from someone infected with SARS-CoV are high-risk exposures in the absence of appropriate levels of infection control. In one recorded instance, it is thought the virus was transmitted by an environmental vehicle, possibly aerosolized sewerage or transport of sewerage by mechanical vectors. Nosocomial transmission of SARS-CoV was common early in the 2002–2003 outbreak but subsequently declined as a result of early diagnosis and strengthening infection control practices. Transmission studies have suggested that each SARS patient infected an average of 3 additional persons. During the 2002–2003 outbreak several SARS patients were recognized as superspreaders because of the high number of persons secondarily infected (average ~36 patients). The superspreading phenomenon was associated with several factors, including a large number of close contacts, delayed diagnosis, more severe illness, and poor infection control practices.

The period of communicability is not yet completely understood. Epidemiological and virological studies and clinical follow-up during the epidemic indicated that transmission does not occur before onset of clinical signs and symptoms, and that maximum period of communicability is usually less than 21 days.

8. Risk groups—The primary risk factor is contact with a person infected with SARS-CoV or the SARS-CoV itself secondary to a laboratory breach in infection control. Health workers are at great risk of infection, especially before the diagnosis of SARS is suspected and when involved in aerosol-generating procedures such as intubation or nebulization.

9. Prevention—Health services should develop clinical algorithms to assist clinicians in assessing patients with acute febrile respiratory infection for their risk of SARS, based on the national and global risk assessment of SARS reemergence. *WHO Guidelines for the Global surveillance of SARS* and *WHO SARS Risk Assessment and Preparedness Framework* provide detailed guidance on SARS alert and triage of acute respiratory illness in the current epidemiological situation (http://www.who.int/csr/resources/publications/WHO_CDS_CSR_ARO_2004_2/en).

1) Identify all suspect and probable cases using the WHO case definitions for SARS.
2) Health care workers (HCWs) involved in the triage process should wear a face mask (N/R/P 95/99/100 or filtering face piece 2/3 or equivalent national manufacturing standard) with eye protection, wear gloves, and wash hands before and after contact with any patient, especially after activities likely to cause contamination and after removing gloves. Triage and waiting areas need to be adequately ventilated.
3) Soiled gloves, stethoscopes, and other equipment must be treated with care as they have the potential to spread infection. Broad-spectrum disinfectants of proven antiviral activity, such as fresh bleach solutions, must be widely available at appropriate concentrations and must be used according to manufacturers' instructions.

10. Management of patient—Measures should include preparedness planning for the detection, investigation, containment, and control of unexplained clusters of acute respiratory disease.

1) Anyone arriving at health care facilities and requiring SARS assessment must be rapidly diverted by triage nurses to a separate area to minimize transmission to health care workers, patients, and visitors. If tolerated, the patient must be given a face mask to wear, preferably one that filters expired air.

2) Isolate anyone under investigation for SARS and implement infection control procedures.

3) Obtain samples (e.g., respiratory, blood, serum, stool) to exclude standard causes of pneumonia, including atypical causes. Consider the possibility of coinfection with SARS-CoV and carry out appropriate chest radiography. Preliminary testing of blood/serum should include white blood cell count, platelet count, creatinine phosphokinase, liver function tests, urea, and electrolytes.

4) At the time of admission, prescription of antibiotics for the treatment of community-acquired pneumonia is recommended until diagnoses of treatable causes of ARDS have been excluded. Ribavirin and corticosteroids have been used with little success. The effectiveness of other therapeutic options, such as interferon and antiviral drugs, are not known. No vaccine is available.

5) Strict standard droplet and airborne precautions for infection control must be applied to avoid direct contact with body fluids, respiratory droplets, and aerosols. All staff, including ancillary staff, must be fully trained in infection control and must use appropriate personal protective equipment.

6) Disposable equipment should be used wherever possible in the treatment and care of patients with SARS, and it should be disposed of appropriately. If medical devices are to be reused, they must be sterilized according to manufacturers' instructions. Surfaces should be cleaned with broad-spectrum disinfectants of proven antiviral activity, since SARS-CoV loses infectivity after exposure to commonly used disinfectants and fixatives.

7) Movement of patients outside the isolation unit should be avoided. If moved, patients should wear a face mask if tolerated. Visitors should be kept to a minimum and personal protective equipment used under supervision.

8) Proper handwashing is crucial before and after contact with any patient, after activities likely to cause contamination, and after removing gloves. Alcohol-based skin disinfectants can be used if there is no obvious contamination with organic material.

9) Particular attention should be paid to interventions such as use of nebulizers, chest physiotherapy, bronchoscopy, gastroscopy, and other procedures that may disrupt the respiratory tract or place the health care worker close to the patient and potentially infected secretions. All sharp and cutting instruments must be

handled safely and patients' linen must be prepared on site for the laundry staff and placed into biohazard bags.

11. **Management of contacts and the immediate environment—**

1) Trace contacts. A contact is defined as a person who cared for or lived with a confirmed case of SARS or a person under investigation or who had direct contact with their respiratory secretions, body fluids, and/or excretions (e.g., feces). Contact tracing must be systematic for contacts during an agreed period prior to the onset of symptoms in the index case.

2) Information about the signs, symptoms, and means of transmission of SARS should be provided to each contact. Place contacts under active surveillance for 10 days and educate them about self-monitoring for fever by recording temperature daily. Stress to the contact that fever is the most consistent first symptom to appear in SARS. Ensure the contact is visited or telephoned daily by a member of the public health care team to determine whether fever or other signs and symptoms of SARS are developing. If such signs and symptoms do develop, a follow-up examination should be conducted at a suitable health care facility under appropriate levels of infection control.

3) If a suspect or probable SARS case is removed from surveillance because an alternative diagnosis can fully explain the illness, contacts can also be removed from surveillance and discharged from follow-up. Voluntary home quarantine of asymptomatic contacts was used routinely as a control measure in some of the affected cities during the 2002–2003 outbreak, and characteristics of viral excretion were well described; however, its efficacy in reducing transmission was not formally evaluated.

12. **Special considerations—**

1) Reporting: SARS is a notifiable disease under the International Health Regulations (IHR).

2) Should SARS reemerge, WHO will provide regular information updates and evidence-based travel recommendations to limit the international spread of infection in accordance with the IHR. A global response, facilitating exchange of information among scientists, clinicians, and public health experts, has been shown to be effective in providing information and real-time evidence-based policies and strategies.

3) The laboratory-associated outbreaks of SARS highlight the importance of strict adherence to biosafety procedures and practices for laboratory work with SARS-CoV. WHO strongly

recommends Biosafety Level 3 (BSL3) for working with live SARS-CoV material.

4) During an epidemic, establish a multisectoral national SARS advisory group to oversee control measures. Traditional public health measures, including active case finding, case isolation, strict adherence to infection control in health care settings, contact tracing, fever monitoring, and enhanced surveillance, have been successful in controlling the spread of SARS. Ensure adequate triage facilities and clearly indicate to the general public where they are located and how they can be accessed.

5) Risk communication and community education should be an integral part of epidemic control measures. Establish telephone hotlines or other means of dealing with enquiries from the general public, health professionals, and the media. Ensure that all stakeholders have access to these resources.

II. MIDDLE EAST RESPIRATORY SYNDROME (MERS) CORONAVIRUS (CoV)

1. Clinical features—Since its emergence in 2012, signs and symptoms of MERS coronavirus infections in the majority of primary human cases have been reported as severe respiratory disease as judged by admission to intensive care, mechanical ventilation, use of extra corporeal membrane oxygenation and vasopressors, and death; however, recently milder clinical presentations and even some asymptomatic cases have been reported. Secondary human cases have had a spectrum of disease ranging from milder influenza-like illness to severe respiratory illness. There have also been cases with atypical presentation, such as immunosuppressed individuals presenting with gastric involvement. Coinfections with other respiratory viruses (in particular influenza A [H1N1], herpes simplex virus, rhinovirus, parainfluenza virus, influenza B) have been reported.

2. Causative agent—MERS-CoV. CoVs are enveloped, single-stranded positive strand RNA viruses that infect a wide range of mammals and birds. In humans, CoVs are mainly associated with seasonal upper respiratory tract infections similar to the common cold but can cause severe disease.

3. Diagnosis—All cases to date have had a direct or indirect link to the Middle East, and so relevant travel history should be obtained in any individual presenting with a febrile acute respiratory illness.

Both upper and lower respiratory and serum samples should be collected for nucleic acid detection. If available, serologic testing should be considered. Rapid real-time PCR diagnostic assays have been developed for the specific detection and confirmation of MERS-CoV. WHO has published guidance on the clinical and laboratory diagnosis of MERS-CoV and defines laboratory confirmation of a case as a person testing positive in at least 2 different PCR targets on the viral genome or positive for a single PCR target with sequence confirmation from a different genomic site. A number of laboratories have successfully established a PCR screening assay and accept samples from probable cases for confirmation. Within the Middle East, MERS-CoV screening of severe acute respiratory illness cases with no known etiology is encouraged.

Only laboratories with adequate biosafety containment should attempt virus culture. Further information can be found at:

- http://www.who.int/csr/disease/coronavirus_infections/ MERS_Lab_recos_16_Sept_2013.pdf
- http://www.who.int/csr/disease/coronavirus_infections/ InterimRevisedSurveillanceRecommendations_nCoVinfection_ 27Jun13.pdf

4. Occurrence—MERS-CoV was first identified in a fatal case of acute pneumonia with renal failure in a 60-year-old man from the Kingdom of Saudi Arabia in June 2012, but phylogenetic analyses of the MERS-CoV full genome sequences currently available indicate that it likely was introduced into the human population in mid-2011. By June 11, 2014, 699 laboratory-confirmed cases, including at least 209 deaths, had been officially reported to WHO. Sporadic cases have been identified in a number of countries in the Middle East, Europe, North Africa, and North America, all with a direct/indirect link to the Middle East. Retrospective testing of a cluster of fatal pneumonia cases (with no known etiology), which occurred in Jordan April 2012, identified this cluster to have been the earliest known human infections with MERS-CoV. Full genome analyses of viruses to date suggest there have been multiple introductions into the human population rather than a single common source with undetected transmission. The level of undetected circulation in the human population remains unknown. Sporadic human cases of MERS-CoV infections are likely to continue until the source of infection and risk factors for transmission have been definitely established and prevention is possible, or the presumed epizootic ends.

5. Reservoir—Although the reservoir remains unknown, the search for the source of MERS-CoV infection has uncovered many closely related beta-coronaviruses in numerous bat species including insectivorous bats common in the Middle East (e.g., the Egyptian tomb bat, *Taphozous perforates*). None of the full genomes detected thus far have been similar enough to MERS-CoV to suggest it as the parental strain. Other animals common to the area have also been implicated. Serological cross-sectional studies in dromedary camels across the Middle Eastern region have demonstrated a high seropositivity rate to MERS-CoV or a virus very antigenically similar to MERS-CoV. Sequence comparisons between the viruses detected in the human and camel samples cannot firmly conclude the direction of transmission or rule out a potential common infection source for both and studies are ongoing.

6. Incubation period—The incubation period for primary cases with environmental exposure is unknown, as the source of infection has not yet been identified. However, from case-contact studies following person-to-person transmission events, the incubation period is estimated to be between 2 and 14 days (median 5–6 days).

7. Transmission—The source of infection for index cases with environmental exposure is still unknown; however, person-to-person transmission is thought to be by direct contact, by fomites, and by respiratory droplets. Transmission has occurred in household, hospital, and work settings. Nosocomial transmission of MERS-CoV has been seen across the Middle East with nonsustained human-to-human transmission, including secondary cases in health care workers who sometimes remain asymptomatic. The period of communicability is not yet understood, and studies are ongoing. Further information can be found at: http://www.who.int/csr/disease/coronavirus_infections/Healthcare_MERS_Seroepi_Investigation_27Jan2014.pdf.

8. Risk groups—A variety of comorbidities have been associated with either MERS-CoV severe disease or death in sporadic cases, with diabetes, immunosuppression and heart disease being the most commonly reported comorbidity conditions. The main risk factor for infection is contact with a person infected with MERS-CoV. Health care workers involved in aerosol-generating procedures, such as intubation or nebulization, are at greatest risk of infection, especially before the diagnosis of MERS-CoV is suspected and when infection control may not have been adequately instigated.

9. Prevention—

1) Identify all possible and probable cases using the WHO case definitions for MERS.
2) Apply standard infection control measures, including hand hygiene, and use of personal protective equipment, including eye protection, to avoid direct contact with patients' blood, body fluids, secretions (including respiratory secretions), and nonintact skin.
3) When working within 1 m (3 ft) of the patient, droplet precautions should be taken by placing patients in single rooms when possible, limit patient movement, and ensure that patients wear appropriate personal protective equipment when outside their rooms.

4) Health care workers performing aerosol-generating procedures should use personal protective equipment, including gloves, long-sleeved gowns, eye protection, and particulate respirators (N95 or equivalent). Whenever possible, use adequately ventilated single rooms when performing aerosol-generating procedures.

10. Management of suspect and confirmed patients—Same as for SARS (see SARS section in this chapter).

In addition, prescription of antibiotics for the treatment of community-acquired pneumonia is recommended at the time of admission until diagnoses of treatable causes of respiratory infection or ARDS have been excluded. Empiric therapy can be adjusted when laboratory results are available. There are currently no specific antiviral therapies or vaccines for MERS-CoV, but several therapeutic options, including convalescent plasma, are being studied.

The WHO guidelines *Clinical Management of Severe Acute Respiratory Infections When Novel Coronavirus Is Suspected* provide detailed guidance on MERS alert and triage of acute respiratory illness in the current epidemiological situation (http://www.who.int/csr/disease/coronavirus_infections/InterimGuidance_ClinicalManagement_NovelCoronavirus_11Feb13u.pdf).

11. Management of contacts and the immediate environment—

1) All close contacts of a confirmed case should be identified. A contact is a person who cared for or lived with a confirmed case or had direct unprotected contact with that person's respiratory secretions, body fluids, and/or excretions while that person was symptomatic.

2) Contacts should be placed under active surveillance for 10–14 days with self-monitoring for respiratory symptoms. Ensure the contact is visited or telephoned daily by a member of the public health care team to determine whether signs and symptoms of MERS are developing. If such signs and symptoms do develop, follow-up examination should be conducted under appropriate levels of infection control with upper and if possible lower respiratory tract samples taken for MERS-CoV PCR testing. As part of case-contact studies, paired serum samples (as soon after exposure as possible and 4–6 weeks later in lieu of acute and convalescent sampling) should be taken from each identified contact to identify all MERS-CoV infection, including asymptomatic infection.

3) A suspect or probable MERS diagnosis can be discarded if an alternative diagnosis can fully explain the illness.

4) The need for coordinated seroepidemiology studies has been well recognized and in response WHO has provided a detailed study protocol for the serological investigation of contacts. This study can be found at: http://www.who.int/csr/disease/coronavirus_infections/WHO_Contact_Protocol_MERSCoV_19_November_2013.pdf.

12. Special considerations—

1) Reporting: MERS is a notifiable disease under the IHR.
2) WHO provides regular information updates and evidence-based travel recommendations during an outbreak to limit the international spread of infection in accordance with the IHR. A global response, facilitating exchange of information among scientists, clinicians, and public health experts, has been an effective means to support the development of evidence-based policies and intervention strategies.
3) WHO strongly recommends Biosafety Level 3 (BSL3) for working with live MERS-CoV material.
4) Implementation of infection control in health care settings appears to prevent onward transmission of MERS-CoV to health care workers and patients without spread to the wider community.
5) Establishing good communication routes with regular updates to clinicians and other health care workers to keep awareness of MERS-CoV high both inside and outside the affected countries. Establish easily accessible web tools or other means of dealing with enquiries from health professionals, the general public, and the media.

[E. Schneider, A. Bermingham, R. Pebody, J. M. Watson]

SCABIES
(sarcoptic itch, sarcoptic acariasis)

DISEASE	ICD-10 CODE
SCABIES	ICD-10 B86

1. **Clinical features**—A parasitic infestation of the skin caused by a mite whose presence is evident as papules, vesicles, or tiny linear burrows containing the mites and their eggs. Itching is intense, especially at night, but complications are limited to lesions secondarily infected by scratching.

Lesions are prominent around finger webs, anterior surfaces of wrists and elbows, anterior axillary folds, and belt line and thighs. Nipples, abdomen, and the lower portion of the buttocks are frequently affected in women as are external genitalia in men. In infants, the head, neck, palms, and soles may be involved; these areas are usually spared in older individuals.

In immunodeficient individuals and in senile patients, infestation often appears as a generalized dermatitis more widely distributed than the burrows with extensive scaling and sometimes vesiculation and crusting (Norwegian or crusted scabies); the usual severe itching may be reduced or absent. When scabies is complicated by beta-hemolytic streptococcal infection, there is a risk of acute glomerulonephritis.

2. **Causative agent**—*Sarcoptes scabiei* var *hominis*, a mite. Other *Sarcoptes* species and other animal mites, including other variants of *S. scabiei,* can live but not reproduce on humans; such infestations are self-limiting.

3. **Diagnosis**—Typically done by clinical examination of papules. Diagnosis can be confirmed by recovery from a burrow and microscopic identification of the mite, eggs, or mite feces (scybala). Care should be taken to choose lesions for scraping or biopsy that have not been excoriated by repeated scratching. Prior application of mineral oil facilitates collecting the scrapings and examining them under a cover slip. Applying ink to the skin and then washing it off will disclose the burrows.

4. **Occurrence**—Widespread and endemic in many countries. Causes of epidemics are not clear, but past epidemics were attributed to poverty, poor sanitation, and crowding associated with war, mass movement of people, and economic crises. Recent epidemics have affected people of all socioeconomic levels and standards of personal hygiene.

5. **Reservoir**—Humans.

6. **Incubation period**—In persons without previous exposure, 2-6 weeks. Persons who have been previously infested develop symptoms 1-4 days after reexposure.

7. Transmission—Transfer of parasites commonly occurs through prolonged direct contact with infested skin and also during sexual contact. Transfer from undergarments and bedding occurs only if these have been contaminated by an infested person immediately beforehand. Mites can burrow beneath the skin surface in about 1 hour. Persons with the crusted scabies are highly contagious because of the large number of mites present in the exfoliating scales.

Transmission can occur until mites and eggs are destroyed by treatment, ordinarily after 1 or occasionally 2 courses of treatment 1 week apart. Crusted scabies can require multiple treatments with one or more agents to eliminate an infestation.

8. Risk groups—Household members and sexual partners of persons infested with scabies and other persons living in conditions in which close body and skin contact is common. When scabies outbreaks occur, they tend to be in nursing homes, child care centers, extended-care facilities, and prisons. The risk groups for crusted (Norwegian) scabies are immunocompromised, elderly, disabled, or debilitated persons

9. Prevention—Educate the public and medical community on mode of transmission, early diagnosis, and treatment of infested patients and contacts.

10. Management of patient—

1) Isolation: exclude infested individuals from school or work until the day after treatment. For hospitalized patients, contact isolation for 24 hours after start of effective treatment. Twenty-four hours may be insufficient in crusted scabies because viable mites can remain after a single treatment. In an institutional outbreak of crusted scabies, 10-day isolation of the index patient is suggested.

2) Concurrent disinfestation: laundering clothing and bedding worn or used by the patient in the 48–72 hours prior to treatment may not be needed for most infestations. However, it is important for patients with crusted scabies because potential for fomite transmission is high. Using hot cycles of both washer and dryer will kill mites and eggs.

3) Treatment: the treatment of choice, particularly for children and pregnant or nursing women, is topical permethrin (5%). Other topical therapies are crotamiton (10%) and lindane (1%; an organochloride). The safety of crotamiton in children and during pregnancy has not been confirmed. Because of concerns about neurologic toxicity, lindane should only be used in patients who cannot tolerate or have failed treatment with safer medication. Benzyl benzoate is an inexpensive scabicide widely used in developing countries. Oral ivermectin has been shown to be effective against scabies but is not licensed for this use. A repeat treatment with oral ivermectin may be necessary after 7–10 days

if eggs survive the initial treatment. A combination of benzyl benzoate and oral ivermectin may prove useful in HIV-infected persons with severe scabies. Resistance has been reported for all scabicides.

Topical agents are applied to the whole body except the head, left on for the prescribed time, and then washed off as directed. On the following day, the patient should have a cleansing bath and change to fresh clothing and bedding. Itching may persist for 1–2 weeks; this should not be regarded as a sign of drug failure or reinfestation. Overtreatment is common and should be avoided because of toxicity of some of these agents, especially lindane.

Multiple courses of treatment with one or more scabicides may be necessary for patients with crusted scabies. Close supervision of all treatment, including bathing, is necessary.

11. **Management of contacts and the immediate environment—**

1) Search for unreported or unrecognized cases among companions and household members. Single infestations in a family are uncommon. All affected members of a household or close community should be treated at the same time to avoid reinfestation. Those who have had skin-to-skin contact with infested persons (including family members and sexual contacts) should be treated prophylactically.

2) Epidemic measures:

- Provide treatment and educate infested individuals and others at risk.
- Cooperation of nonhealth authorities is often needed.
- Coordinated mass treatment.
- Extend screening to whole families, military units, or institutions. Segregate infested individuals if possible.
- Soap and facilities for mass bathing and laundering are essential. Tetmosol soap may help prevent infestation.

12. **Special considerations—**A potential nuisance in situations of overcrowding.

[M. Deming, M. Eberhard, D. Martin]

SCHISTOSOMIASIS
(bilharzia, snail fever)

DISEASE	ICD-10 CODE
SCHISTOSOMIASIS	ICD-10 B65

1. **Clinical features**—A blood fluke (trematode) infection with adult worms living within mesenteric veins or the venous plexus of the bladder of the host over a life span of many years. Mated female worms release eggs into the circulation; depending on the species, eggs make their way through the bowel or bladder wall and are shed in feces (*Schistosoma mansoni, Schistosoma japonicum*) or urine (*Schistosoma haematobium*). Eggs that fail to pass out of the body may produce granulomata and fibrosis in organs where they lodge.

Symptoms are related to host immune responses to schistosome eggs in the human host and vary by the number and location of the eggs. *S. mansoni* and *S. japonicum* give rise primarily to hepatic and intestinal pathology. Signs and symptoms include diarrhea, abdominal pain, and hepatosplenomegaly. Long duration and high intensity of infection can lead to liver fibrosis and portal hypertension. *S. haematobium* gives rise to urinary manifestations. Signs and symptoms include dysuria, urinary frequency, and hematuria at the end of urination; chronic infection can also cause hydronephrosis or changes to the female genital tract and has been associated with increased risk of bladder cancer in both sexes. Rarely, neuroschistosomiasis may develop when aberrant eggs lodge in the spinal cord (more common with *S. mansoni* or *S. haematobium*) or brain (more often *S. japonicum*).

Acute infection can cause systemic manifestations (Katayama fever), which have been reported in travelers to endemic countries. Signs and symptoms of acute schistosomiasis include fever, headache, myalgia, rash, diarrhea, and respiratory symptoms.

The larvae of certain schistosomes of birds and mammals may penetrate the human skin and cause dermatitis, sometimes known as "swimmer's itch"; these schistosomes do not mature in humans.

2. **Causative agents**—*S. mansoni*, *S. haematobium*, and *S. japonicum* are the major species causing human disease. *Schistosoma mekongi* and *Schistosoma intercalatum* are only important in limited areas.

3. **Diagnosis**—Through demonstration of eggs in the stool by direct smear or using the Kato-Katz technique (*S. mansoni* or *S. japonicum*). *S. haematobium* infection is diagnosed by the examination of a urine sediment or Nuclepore filtration. Serologic testing is useful for diagnosis of traveler infections, but current available methods do not distinguish

between past and current infection. Useful immunological tests include immunoblot analysis, the circumoval precipitin test, immunofluorescence assay (IFA), and enzyme-linked immunosorbent assay (ELISA) with egg or adult worm antigen; positive results on serological antibody detection tests could be indicative of prior infection and are not proof of current infection.

4. Occurrence—*S. mansoni* is found in Africa; the Arabian Peninsula; Brazil, Suriname, and Venezuela in South America; and in some Caribbean islands. *S. haematobium* is found in Africa and the Middle East. *S. japonicum* is found in China, the Philippines, and Sulawesi in Indonesia.

S. mekongi is found in the Mekong River area of Cambodia and the Lao People's Democratic Republic. *S. intercalatum* occurs in parts of central and western Africa.

5. Reservoir—Humans are the principal reservoir of *S. haematobium*, *S. intercalatum*, and *S. mansoni*. Humans, dogs, cats, pigs, cattle, water buffalo, and wild rodents are potential hosts of *S. japonicum*; their relative epidemiological importance varies in different regions. Epidemiological persistence of the parasite depends on the presence of an appropriate snail as intermediate host (i.e., species of the genera *Biomphalaria* for *S. mansoni*; *Bulinus* for *S. haematobium* and *S. intercalatum*; *Oncomelania* for *S. japonicum*; and *Tricula* for *S. mekongi*).

6. Incubation period—Acute systemic manifestations (Katayama fever) may occur in primary infections 2-6 weeks after exposure, immediately preceding and during initial egg deposition.

7. Transmission—Infection occurs when cercariae (free-swimming larval forms) penetrate the skin. In the human host, cercariae become schistosomula and migrate through various tissues before developing into adult worms. Adult forms of *S. mansoni, S. japonicum, S. mekongi,* and *S. intercalatum* usually remain in mesenteric veins; those of *S. haematobium* usually migrate to the venous plexus of the urinary bladder. Eggs are deposited in venules and escape into the lumen of the bowel or urinary bladder, or end up lodging in other organs including the liver and the lungs. The eggs of *S. haematobium* leave the body mainly in the urine, those of the other species in the feces. The eggs hatch in water and the liberated larvae (miracidia) penetrate into suitable freshwater snail intermediate hosts. After several weeks of amplification through asexual reproduction, the cercariae emerge from the snail; infected snails continue to release cercariae for as long as they live.

Schistosomiasis is not communicable directly from person to person. Infected persons who are shedding eggs maintain transmission in areas with appropriate snail hosts and poor sanitation. *S. mansoni* and *S.*

haematobium worms can survive for more than 10 years in infected humans.

8. Risk groups—Susceptibility is universal. Risk is higher in groups with greatest exposure to water containing infectious cercariae. Any immunity developing as a result of infection is variable and not yet fully understood.

9. Prevention—

1) In endemic areas, regular mass drug treatments with praziquantel for populations at risk, including school-age children, women of childbearing age, and certain groups with occupational water exposure, are recommended.

2) Dispose of feces and urine so that viable eggs will not reach bodies of fresh water containing intermediate snail hosts. Control of animals infected with *S. japonicum* is desirable but difficult.

3) Improve irrigation and agriculture practices. Reduce snail habitats by removing vegetation, draining and filling marshy areas, or lining canals with concrete.

4) Where appropriate, treat snail-breeding sites with molluscicides. Cost and environmental impact may limit the utility of these agents.

5) Minimize exposure to contaminated water (e.g., by wearing rubber boots). Application of topical water-resistant preparations containing N,N-diethyl-meta-toluamide (DEET) may prevent cercarial penetration, but total coverage is difficult. Immediate vigorous towel drying of exposed skin has been suggested to reduce cercarial penetration after accidental water contact but is ineffective for all but the briefest of exposures.

6) Provide water for drinking, bathing, and washing clothes from sources free of cercariae or treated to kill them. Effective measures for inactivating cercariae include water treatment with iodine or chlorine, although these treatments may not inactivate other pathogens in contaminated water. Allowing water to stand for 48–72 hours before use is also effective.

7) Travelers visiting endemic areas should be advised of the risks and informed about preventive measures. Local tourist information suggesting fresh water bodies are free of schistosomiasis is not always reliable.

10. Management of patient—

1) Treatment: praziquantel is the drug of choice against all species.
2) Sanitary disposal of feces and urine.

11. Management of contacts and the immediate environment— Investigate contacts for infection from a common source.

12. **Special considerations**—

1) Reporting: reporting requirements vary by country and region.
2) Surveillance case definition: for endemic areas, screening for urinary schistosomiasis is based on detection of visible hematuria, positive reagent strip for hematuria, or *S. haematobium* eggs in urine. Screening for intestinal schistosomiasis is based on detection of eggs in stools.
3) Epidemic measures: examine for schistosomiasis and treat all who are infected, but especially those with disease and/or moderate to heavy intensity of infection; pay particular attention to children. Provide clean water, warn people against contact with water potentially containing cercariae, and prohibit contamination of water with urine and feces. Treat areas that have high snail densities with molluscicides as appropriate.

Further information may be found at:

- http://www.who.int/topics/schistosomiasis/en
- http://www.cdc.gov/parasites/schistosomiasis/index.html

[S. Montgomery]

SHIGELLOSIS
(bacillary dysentery)

DISEASE	ICD-10 CODE
SHIGELLOSIS	ICD-10 A03

1. **Clinical features**—An acute bacterial disease involving the distal small intestine and colon, characterized by loose stools accompanied by fever, nausea, and sometimes toxemia, vomiting, cramps, and tenesmus. Stools may contain blood and mucus (dysentery) resulting from mucosal ulcerations and confluent colonic crypt microabscesses caused by the invasive organisms; however, many cases present with nonbloody diarrhea. Convulsions may be an important complication in young children. Bacteremia is uncommon. Severity and case-fatality rate vary with the host (age and preexisting nutritional state) and serotype. *Shigella dysenteriae* type 1 (Shiga bacillus) spreads in epidemics and is often associated with serious disease and complications including toxic megacolon, intestinal

perforation, and the hemolytic uremic syndrome; case-fatality rates have been as high as 20% among hospitalized cases even in recent years.

Mild and asymptomatic infections occur. These are usually self-limited, lasting on average 4-7 days. Many infections with *Shigella sonnei* result in a short clinical course and an almost negligible case-fatality rate except in immuno-compromised hosts. Certain strains of *Shigella flexneri* can cause a reactive postinfectious arthropathy (formerly known as Reiter syndrome), especially in persons who are genetically predisposed by having HLA-B27 antigen.

2. Causative agents—*Shigella* strains are Gram-negative, facultatively anaerobic, nonmotile rods classified in the family *Enterobacteriaceae*. *Shigella* strains cause dysentery symptoms by invading and destroying the cells that line the large intestine. These symptoms are mediated by several invasion-related factors including *ipaC* and *ipaH*, which are encoded on a characteristic large 120- to 140-MDa plasmid. The *ipaH* factor is also chromosomally encoded. The severity of symptoms associated with infection by *Shigella dysenteriae* type 1 is thought to be related to its production of Shiga toxin type 1. Rarely, nontype 1 strains of *S. dysenteriae* and certain strains of *S. flexneri* also produce Shiga toxin type 1. With the exception of *Shigella boydii* serotype 13, *Shigella* and *Escherichia coli* represent a single genomospecies. *S. boydii* 13 has been determined to be a separate species, *Escherichia albertii*. There are 4 subgroups of *Shigella*, which have traditionally been regarded as separate species:

1) Group A: *S. dysenteriae*;
2) Group B: *S. flexneri*;
3) Group C: *S. boydii*;
4) Group D: *S. sonnei*.

Groups A, B, and C are further divided into 15, 8, and 19 serotypes, respectively, and *S. flexneri* serotypes 1 through 5 further subdivided into 11 subserotypes designated by numbers and lowercase letters (e.g., *S. flexneri* 2a). *S. sonnei* (Group D) consists of a single serotype.

3. Diagnosis—Isolation of *Shigella* from feces or rectal swabs provides bacteriological diagnosis. Outside the human body, *Shigella* remains viable only for a short period, which is why stool specimens for culture must be processed rapidly after collection. *Shigella* isolates should be tested for antimicrobial susceptibility. Commercial rapid diagnostic tests or antigen detection assays are not available.

4. Occurrence—Shigellosis causes an estimated 125 million illnesses and 14,000 deaths per year. Shigellosis is endemic in both tropical and temperate climates. Reported cases represent only a small proportion of cases, even in developed areas. Mixed infections with other intestinal pathogens also occur.

The geographical distribution of the 4 *Shigella* serogroups is different, as is their pathogenicity. More than one serotype is commonly present in a community. In general, *S. flexneri*, *S. boydii*, and *S. dysenteriae* account for most isolates from developing countries. *S. dysenteriae* type 1 is of particular concern in developing countries and complex emergency situations where huge outbreaks can occur. *S. sonnei* is most common in industrialized countries where the disease is generally less severe. Multidrug-resistant *Shigella* (including *S. dysenteriae* type 1) with considerable geographical variations have appeared worldwide in association with the widespread use of antimicrobial agents.

5. Reservoir—The only significant reservoir is humans, although prolonged outbreaks have occurred in primate colonies.

6. Incubation period—Usually 1–3 days, but may range from 12–96 hours and up to 1 week for *S. dysenteriae* type 1.

7. Transmission—Mainly by direct or indirect fecal-oral transmission from a symptomatic patient or asymptomatic carrier. The infective dose can be as low as 10–100 organisms. Individuals primarily responsible for transmission include those who fail to clean hands and under fingernails thoroughly after defecation. They may spread infection to others directly by physical contact or indirectly by contaminating food, water, or fomites. Transmission via drinking or recreational water may also occur as the result of direct fecal contamination. Flies can transfer organisms from latrines to uncovered food items. Certain sexual practices, particularly among men who have sex with men, also increase risk of transmission.

The period of communicability continues during the acute infection and until the infectious agent is no longer present in feces, usually for less than 4 weeks after illness. Very rarely, the asymptomatic carrier state may persist for months or longer; appropriate antimicrobial treatment usually reduces duration of carriage to a few days.

8. Risk groups—Two-thirds of the cases and most of the deaths are in children younger than 10 years. Illness in infants younger than 6 months is unusual, and breastfeeding is protective for infants and young children. The elderly, the debilitated, and the malnourished of all ages and those infected with HIV are particularly susceptible to severe disease and death. Secondary attack rates in households can be as high as 40%. Outbreaks occur in crowded conditions and where contact with fecal material is possible such as in prisons, institutions for children, child care centers, mental health facilities, and crowded refugee camps, as well as among men who have sex with men.

9. Prevention—

    1) General measures to improve hygiene are important. An organized effort to promote careful hand washing with soap

and water is the single most important control measure to decrease transmission rates in most settings. Provide soap and hand dryers or individual paper towels in public settings if otherwise not available. Prophylactic administration of antibiotics is not recommended.

2) Use of barriers during oral-, digital-, and genital-anal contact, accompanied by washing hands and genitals with soap before and after sexual contact, may help prevent transmission.

3) Studies with experimental serotype-specific live oral vaccines and parenteral polysaccharide conjugate vaccines show protection of short duration (1 year) against infection with the homologous serotype.

4) Closure of or prolonged exclusion of ill children from affected child care centers may lead to placement of infected children in other centers with subsequent transmission in the latter, and few data exist to assess whether these are effective control measures.

10. **Management of patient—**

1) Early recognition and report of outbreaks in child care centers and institutions are especially important.

2) Fluid and electrolyte replacement is important when there are signs of dehydration (see "Cholera and Other Vibrioses"). Antibiotics, selected according to the current, local prevailing antimicrobial sensitivity pattern, appear to slightly shorten the duration and severity of illness. They should be used in individual cases if warranted by the severity of illness or to protect vulnerable contacts.

3) *Shigellae* have shown a propensity to acquire resistance against new antimicrobials that were initially highly effective. Multidrug resistance to most of the low-cost antibiotics (ampicillin, trimethoprim-sulfamethoxazole) is common, and the choice of specific agents will depend on the antibiogram of the isolated strain or during outbreaks on local antimicrobial susceptibility patterns. In many areas, high prevalence of *Shigella* resistant to trimethoprim-sulfamethoxazole, ampicillin, and tetracycline has resulted in a reliance on fluoroquinolones (such as ciprofloxacin) as first-line treatment, but resistance to these has also emerged, particularly in Asia and Africa. Ceftriaxone and azithromycin may also be considered for the treatment of shigellosis, especially in children, although standards for assessing susceptibility of *Shigellae* to azithromycin do not exist. The use of antimotility agents (such as loperamide) is contraindicated in children and generally discouraged in adults since these drugs may prolong illness.

4) During acute illness, use enteric precautions. Because of the small infective dose, patients with known *Shigella* infection

should not be employed to handle food or to provide child or patient care until one or more successive fecal samples or rectal swabs (collected ≥24 hours apart but not sooner than 48 hours after discontinuance of antimicrobials) are found to be *Shigella*-free. Patients must be told of the importance and effectiveness of hand washing with soap and water after defecation or changing diapers to reduce transmission. Patients should also be advised to avoid recreational water exposures while symptomatic.

5) Ensure concurrent disinfection of feces and contaminated articles. In communities with an adequate sewage disposal system, feces can be discharged directly into sewers without preliminary disinfection. Terminal cleaning is also important in health care settings.

11. **Management of contacts and the immediate environment—**

1) Whenever feasible, ill contacts should be excluded from handling food and from caring for children or patients until diarrhea ceases and one or more successive negative stool cultures are obtained at least 24 hours apart and at least 48 hours after discontinuation of antibiotics. Thorough hand washing after defecation and before handling food or caring for children or patients is essential if such contacts are unavoidable.

2) The search for unrecognized mild cases and convalescent carriers among contacts may be unproductive and seldom contributes to the control of an outbreak. Cultures of contacts should generally be confined to food handlers, attendants and children in hospitals, and other situations where the spread of infection is particularly likely.

3) Investigate water and food supplies and recreational water exposures, and use general sanitation measures. The potentially high case-fatality rate in infections with S. *dysenteriae* type 1, coupled with antibiotic resistance, calls for measures comparable to those for typhoid fever, including the need to identify the source(s) of all infections. In contrast, this is not necessary in an isolated infection with S. *sonnei* in a private home.

12. **Special considerations—**

1) Reporting: case report to local health authority obligatory in many countries. Any group of cases of acute diarrheal disorder should be reported at once to the local health authority, even without specific identification of the causal agent.

2) Common-source foodborne or waterborne outbreaks require prompt investigation and intervention whatever the infecting species. Institutional outbreaks may require special measures, including separate housing for cases and new admissions, a

vigorous program of supervised hand washing, and repeated cultures of patients and attendants. The most difficult outbreaks to control are those that involve groups of young children (not yet or recently toilet-trained) or the mentally disabled, and those where there is an inadequate supply of water.

3) Shigella infection, particularly that caused by *S. dysenteriae* type 1, is a potential problem in a disaster situation where personal hygiene and environmental sanitation are deficient (see "Typhoid Fever and Paratyphoid Fever").

[A. Bowen]

SMALLPOX AND OTHER POXVIRUS DISEASES

DISEASE	ICD-10 CODE
SMALLPOX	ICD-10 B03
VACCINIA	ICD-10 B08.0
MONKEYPOX	ICD-10 B04
ORF VIRUS DISEASE	ICD-10 B08.0

I. SMALLPOX

The last naturally acquired case of smallpox in the world occurred in October 1977 in Somalia; global eradication was certified 2 years later (1979) by WHO and by the World Health Assembly in May 1980. Except for a limited outbreak after a laboratory accident at the University of Birmingham, UK, in 1978, no further cases have been identified. All known smallpox (variola) virus stocks are held under security in 2 places: at CDC, Atlanta, Georgia, USA; and at the State Research Centre of Virology and Biotechnology, Koltsovo, Novosibirsk Region, Russia. In response to concerns that the world would not be equipped to respond to and contain the disease in the event that smallpox should reemerge as result of accidental or intentional release, the World Health Assembly has authorized the retention of virus at the laboratories in Russia and the USA for the purposes of essential research, has set up a biosafety inspection program for the 2 laboratories, and has appointed a group of experts to determine and oversee the research. Because few health care workers today have ever encountered smallpox or have ever managed cases of the illness, it is important that they become familiar with the clinical and epidemiological features of smallpox and how it can be distinguished from chickenpox and other rash illnesses. Laboratory confirmation of variola virus from suspect smallpox patients is performed at the 2 WHO Collaborating Centre laboratories where the virus stocks are held, using appropriate biosafety containment practices.

1. Clinical features—Smallpox was a systemic viral disease generally presenting with a characteristic skin eruption. Preceding the appearance of the rash was a prodrome of sudden onset with high fever (40°C/104°F), malaise, headache, prostration, severe backache, and occasional abdominal pain and vomiting—a clinical picture that resembled influenza. After 2–4 days, the fever began to fall, and a deep-seated rash developed in which individual lesions containing infectious virus progressed through successive stages of macules, papules, vesicles, pustules, then crusted scabs that fell off 3–4 weeks after the appearance of the rash. The lesions first appeared on the face and extremities, including the palms and soles, and subsequently on the trunk—the so-called centrifugal rash distribution. They were well circumscribed and at the same stage of development in a given area.

Two types of smallpox were recognized during the 20th century: variola minor (including a genetically and biologically distinct subgroup described as alastrim), which had a case-fatality rate of less than 1%; and variola major, which had a case-fatality rate among unvaccinated populations of 20%–50% or more (30% on average). Fatalities normally occurred between the fifth and seventh day after onset of illness, occasionally as late as the second week. Fewer than 3% of variola major cases experienced a fulminant hemorrhagic course, characterized by a severe prodrome, prostration, and bleeding into the skin and mucous membranes; such hemorrhagic cases were rapidly fatal. In hemorrhagic smallpox the usual vesicular rash did not appear, and the disease might have been confused with severe leukemia, meningococcemia, or idiopathic thrombocytopenic purpura. The rash of smallpox could also be significantly modified in previously vaccinated persons to the extent that only a few highly atypical lesions might be seen. In such cases, prodromal illness was not modified, but the maturation of lesions was accelerated with crusting by the 10th day.

Smallpox was most frequently confused with chickenpox (varicella), in which skin lesions commonly occur in successive crops with several stages of maturity visible at the same time. The chickenpox rash is more abundant on covered than on exposed parts of the body, is centripetal rather than centrifugal, and is usually intensely itchy. However, the appearance of the rash in the early florid stage of a very severe chickenpox case may generate diagnostic confusion for those unfamiliar with smallpox or monkeypox. The smallpox vesicles are firm ("bullet-like") and deep-seated, whereas the chickenpox vesicles are more superficial and easily deroofed.

2. Causative agent—Variola virus, a species of *Orthopoxvirus*.

3. Diagnosis—Smallpox was indicated by a clear-cut prodromal illness; the more or less simultaneous appearance of all lesions when the fever broke; the similarity of appearance of all lesions in a given area rather than successive crops; and deep-seated lesions with no surrounding inflammatory flare, often involving sebaceous glands and scarring of the pitted lesions. In contrast, chickenpox lesions are superficial, not well circumscribed, and manifested with irregular borders; the vesicle or pustule is surrounded by an inflammatory flare, and chickenpox rash is usually pruritic. Smallpox lesions were virtually never seen at the apex of the axilla, and chickenpox lesions are rarely, if ever, seen on the palms and soles of the feet—a distribution characteristic of smallpox in many cases. Outbreaks of variola minor were recognized by low case-fatality rates in the late 19th century. Although the rash was like that in ordinary smallpox, patients generally experienced less severe systemic reactions, and hemorrhagic cases were virtually unknown.

Prior to eradication, laboratory confirmation of smallpox used isolation of the virus on chorioallantoic membranes or tissue culture from the scrapings of lesions, from vesicular or pustular fluid, from crusts, and sometimes from blood during the febrile prodrome. Electron microscopy or immunodiffusion technique often permitted a rapid provisional diagnosis—though eradication was made possible on the basis of clinical, not laboratory, diagnosis. It should be remembered that all orthopoxviruses look alike on electron microscopy, so it cannot distinguish smallpox from other orthopoxviruses that infect humans, such as vaccinia or monkeypox. Molecular methods, such as polymerase chain reaction (PCR), are now available for rapid diagnosis of smallpox and other orthopoxvirus infections. Should smallpox infection be suspected, immediate communication by national authorities to WHO is obligatory under the International Health Regulations (IHR). Advice will be provided on appropriate laboratories to confirm the diagnosis and for guidance on management of the suspected case and follow-up of contacts.

4. Occurrence—Formerly a worldwide disease; no known human cases since 1978.

5. Reservoir—As epidemiologically described in the 19th and 20th centuries, smallpox was exclusively a human disease with no known animal or environmental reservoir. Currently, the virus is maintained only in 2 WHO-designated laboratories.

6. Incubation period—From 7-19 days; commonly 10-14 days to onset of illness and 2-4 days more to onset of rash.

7. Transmission—Infection usually occurred via the respiratory tract (droplet spread) or skin inoculation. The conjunctivae or the placenta were occasional portals of entry. The period of communicability extended from the time of development of the earliest rash lesions to disappearance of all scabs, about 3 weeks. Risk of transmission appears to have been highest in the first week after appearance of the earliest lesions through droplet spread from the oropharyngeal enanthem and subsequent oropharyngeal excretion of virus.

8. Risk groups—Smallpox research scientists. Susceptibility among the unvaccinated is universal.

9. Prevention—Prevention and eradication of smallpox was based on vaccination (vaccinia virus). Because of the relatively long period of incubation for smallpox, vaccination within a 4-day period after exposure prevented or attenuated clinical illness. Two newer, more attenuated, vaccines have been developed and have been approved for specified uses by several national regulatory authorities.

10. Management of patient—Antiviral therapy was not effective and, apart from vaccination, control of smallpox in the preeradication era was based on identification and isolation of cases and supportive treatment. New antivirals are in advanced stages of regulatory assessment but have not yet been approved.

11. Management of contacts and the immediate environment—The historical control strategy included vaccination of contacts and those living in the immediate vicinity (ring vaccination), surveillance of contacts (including daily monitoring of temperature), and isolation of those contacts in whom fever developed. This approach would be implemented if an outbreak of the disease were to recur in the present-day setting.

12. Special considerations—Reporting: should a nonvaricella, smallpox-like case be suspected, immediate telephone communication with local and national health authorities is obligatory. National health authorities should inform WHO immediately. Notification of smallpox is mandatory under the IHR.

Further information can be found at: http://www.who.int/csr/disease/smallpox.

II. VACCINIA

Vaccinia virus is the live, fully replicative orthopoxvirus immunizing agent that was used to eradicate smallpox. Discovery of vaccinia variants causing human infection in the Indian subcontinent and in South America (Brazil) has led to the consideration that vaccine may have "escaped" into animal populations; alternatively, these occurrences may be indicative of the origins of vaccinia virus. Vaccinia virus has been genetically engineered and biologically derived into candidate and approved vaccines (some are in clinical trials) with low potential for spread to nonimmune contacts.

Vaccination with licensed (fully replicative) smallpox vaccine is recommended for all laboratory workers at high risk of contracting infection, such as those who directly handle cultures or animals contaminated or infected with vaccinia or other orthopoxviruses that infect humans. It may also be considered for other health care personnel who are at lower risk of infection, such as doctors and nurses whose contact with these viruses would be limited to contaminated dressings. WHO does not recommend vaccination in the general public, because the risk of death (1/1,000,000 doses) or serious side effects are greater than the known risk of infection with smallpox. Vaccination is contraindicated in persons with deficient immune systems, persons with eczema or certain other dermatitis disorders, and pregnant women. Vaccine immune globulin can be obtained for laboratory workers in the USA through the CDC Drug Service (1-404-639-3670) and in other industrialized countries from public health agencies. Vaccination should be repeated unless a major reaction (one that is indurated and erythematous 7 days after vaccination) or "take" has developed. Booster vaccinations are recommended within 10 years in categories for which vaccine is recommended. WHO maintains a supply of the vaccine seed lot (vaccinia virus strain Lister Elstree) at the WHO Collaborating Centre for Smallpox Vaccine at the National Institute of Public Health and Environmental Protection in Bilthoven, The Netherlands. WHO also maintains a stockpile of vaccine to be used if needed to control a proven outbreak of smallpox.

III. MONKEYPOX

1. Clinical features—Human monkeypox is a sporadic zoonotic infection first identified in 1970 from remote rural villages in Central and West African rainforest countries, as smallpox disappeared. Clinically, the disease closely resembles ordinary or modified smallpox, but lymphadenopathy is a more prominent feature in many cases and occurs in the early stage of the disease. Pleomorphism and "cropping" similar to that seen in chickenpox are observed in 20% of patients, depending on strain. The case-fatality rate among children not vaccinated against smallpox ranges from 1%–14%.

2. Causative agent—Monkeypox virus is a species of the genus *Orthopoxvirus* with biological properties and a genome distinct from variola virus. At least 2 genetically distinct clades of monkeypox exist with different human clinical and epidemiologic manifestations. To date, West African clade monkeypox manifests without apparent human-to-human transmission and without human mortality, whereas the Congo Basin clade is associated with human-to-human transmission and case-fatality rates historically reported at an average of approximately 10% in unvaccinated persons.

3. Diagnosis—Identification of the characteristic lesion; ascertainment of a history of direct or indirect contact with animals of West and

Central African origin; through electron microscopy demonstration of poxvirions in the lesion; by growth of the virus primate cell cultures; or through positive molecular (e.g., PCR) or serological tests.

4. Occurrence—Between 1970 and 1994, more than 400 cases of human monkeypox were reported from West and Central Africa; the Democratic Republic of the Congo (DRC, formerly Zaire) accounted for about 95% of reported cases during a 5-year surveillance period from 1981–1986. Poor public health infrastructure and other factors complicate accurate case reporting. A 2003 introduction of monkeypox in the USA related to importation and sale of exotic animals from West Africa as pets resulted in infection of North American prairie dogs for sale in pet shops and at least 50 probable and confirmed human cases, mainly among prairie dog owners and animal handlers. In the late 1990s, a prolonged outbreak of human monkeypox was recognized in DRC; it has been postulated that lack of vaccination and an epizootic allowed multiple virus transmission events to humans across the species barrier. In 2003, a prolonged and efficient chain of human-to-human transmission was described, also in DRC. Outbreaks of monkepox continue to be reported in DRC; outbreaks have also been identified in the Republic of Congo, and sporadic cases have been identified elsewhere. The disease affects all age groups; children younger than 16 years have historically constituted the greatest proportion of cases.

5. Reservoir—The natural history of the disease is unclear; humans, primates, and squirrels appear to be involved in the enzootic cycle. Ecological studies in the 1980s point to squirrels (*Funisciurus* and *Heliosciurus*), abundant among the oil palms surrounding the villages at the study sites, as a significant local reservoir host. Monkeypox virus has also been demonstrated in terrestrial giant pouched Gambian rats (*Cricetomys* sp.) and dormice (*Graphiurus* spp.) Maintenance of an animal reservoir and animal contact appear to be required to sustain the disease among humans.

6. Incubation period—7–17 days; usually around 12 days.

7. Transmission—In the 1980s about 75% of reported cases of human monkeypox were attributable to contact with affected animals; in one recent 1996–1997 DRC outbreak, it appeared that a larger number of cases were attributable to person-to-person contact. Unaccustomed conditions of crowding at the start of that event due to civil disruption may have contributed to this unusual pattern. The longest chain of person-to-person transmission was 7 reported serial cases, but serial transmission usually does not extend beyond secondary cases. Epidemiological data suggest a secondary attack rate of about 8%. Most cases have occurred either singly or in clusters in small remote villages, usually in tropical rainforest where the population has multiple contacts with several types of wild animals.

8. Risk groups—Hunters in tropical rainforests of West and Central Africa and their families, laboratory workers, and others exposed either directly or indirectly to rodent populations from West and Central Africa.

9. Prevention—

1) Smallpox vaccination is believed to be protective. However, the protection provided by childhood smallpox vaccination is waning in the general populations at risk since the cessation of smallpox vaccination in the 1980s.

2) Human infection may be controllable to some extent by education to limit contact with infected cases and potentially infected animals. However, in areas where the disease is endemic in the zoonotic reservoirs and the population relies on hunting as an important food source, sporadic infections continue to occur.

3) The 2003 outbreak in the USA clearly demonstrates potential for monkeypox to be a public health threat outside enzootic areas, and there is evidence that infection has also emerged in nature outside of historic "known" enzootic areas. It is not fully understood whether this represents a real extension of enzootic areas or is the result of ascertainment of human infection.

    Full evaluation of the ecology, epidemiology, and virology associated with monkeypox outbreaks in endemic areas will enable understanding of prevention and control measures.

4) Currently, due to adverse event profiles and anticipated clinical and epidemiologic risk-benefit ratios, cross-protective prophylactic vaccination with "smallpox vaccine" (fully replicative vaccinia) is not routinely recommended by WHO.

10. Management of patient—Patients should be managed symptomatically and, if hospitalized, placed under strict infection control measures with sterilization of any implements used in patient management and safe disposal of bandages by boiling, autoclaving, or incineration; physical contact with others should be avoided until lesions have completely resolved.

11. Management of contacts and the immediate environment—No special management is required for persons who have had contact with a case of human monkeypox except for self-monitoring, and, if signs and symptoms occur, patients should then be examined by a medical worker.

12. Special considerations—Smallpox (vaccinia) vaccination was used as an outbreak response intervention in the USA outbreak in 2003. A WHO Technical Advisory Committee on monkeypox has recently recommended continued studies of human monkeypox—in particular, intensified prospective surveillance and ecological studies in order to

568 / SMALLPOX AND OTHER POXVIRUS DISEASES

determine the risk/benefit of the potential use of vaccine to prevent monkeypox in humans in relevant areas.

IV. ORF VIRUS DISEASE (contagious pustular dermatitis, human orf, ecthyma contagiosum)

1. Clinical features—A proliferative cutaneous viral disease in which the lesion, usually solitary and located on hands, arms, or face, is a red to violet vesiculonodule, maculopapule, or pustule, progressing to a weeping nodule with central umbilication. There may be several lesions, each up to 3 cm in diameter and lasting 3-6 weeks. With secondary bacterial infection, lesions may become pustular. Regional adenitis occurs in a few cases. A maculopapular rash may occur on the trunk. Erythema multiforme and erythema multiforme bullosum are rare complications. Disseminated disease and serious ocular damage have been reported but are uncommon. The disease has been confused with cutaneous anthrax and malignancy.

2. Causative agent—Orf virus, a deoxyribonucleic acid (DNA) virus belonging to the genus *Parapoxvirus* of poxviruses (family *Poxviridae*). The agent is closely related to other parapoxviruses that can be transmitted to humans as occupational diseases, such as milkers' nodule virus of dairy cattle and bovine papular stomatitis virus of beef cattle. Contagious ecthyma parapoxvirus of domesticated camels may infect people on rare occasions.

3. Diagnosis—Identification of the characteristic lesion, ascertainment of a history of contact with sheep, goats, or wild ungulates, in particular their young; through electron microscopy demonstration of ovoid parapoxvirions in the lesion or by growth of the virus in ovine, bovine, or primate cell cultures; or through positive molecular (e.g., PCR) or serological tests.

4. Occurrence—Probably worldwide among farm workers.

5. Reservoir—Probably in various ungulates (sheep, goats, reindeer, musk oxen). The virus is very resistant to physical factors, except ultraviolet (UV) light, and may persist for months in soil and on animal skin and hair.

6. Incubation period—Generally 3-6 days.

7. Transmission—Through contact with infected sheep and goats and, occasionally, wild ungulates (deer, reindeer). Direct contact with the mucous membranes of infected animals, with lesions on udders of nursing dams, or through intermediate passive transfer from apparently normal animals contaminated by contact, knives, shears, stalls mangers and sides, trucks, and clothing. Human infection may follow production and administration of vaccines to animals. Person-to-person transmission is rare. Human lesions show a decrease in the number of virus particles as the disease progresses.

Susceptibility is probably universal; recovery produces variable levels of immunity.

8. Risk groups—A common infection among shepherds, veterinarians, and abattoir workers in areas producing sheep and goats and an important occupational disease in New Zealand.

9. Prevention—

1) Good personal hygiene and use of gloves.
2) Washing of hands and exposed areas with soap and water.
3) Domestic and wild ungulates should be considered a potential source of infection. Ensure general cleanliness of animal housing areas. The efficacy and safety of parapoxvirus vaccines in animals has not been fully determined.

10. Management of patient—Boil, autoclave, or incinerate dressings. There is no specific treatment.

11. Management of contacts and the immediate environment— Determine history of contact.

12. Special considerations—Reporting: check local reporting requirements. Case report to local health authority is not usually required but may be desirable when a human case occurs in areas not previously known to have the infection.

[C. Roth]

SPOROTRICHOSIS

DISEASE	ICD-10 CODE
SPOROTRICHOSIS	ICD-10 B42

1. Clinical features—A fungal disease, usually of the skin, often of an extremity. It begins as a nodule. As this grows, lymphatics draining the area become firm and cord-like and form a series of nodules, which in turn may soften and ulcerate. Osteoarticular, pulmonary, and multifocal infections occur but are relatively rare, except multifocal disseminated infections in HIV patients. Fatalities are uncommon.

2. Causative agent—*Sporothrix schenckii* species complex, consisting of *S. schenckii*, *Sporothrix mexicana*, *Sporothrix globosa*, and *Sporothrix* *brasiliensis. Sporothrix luriei, Sporothrix albicans*, and *Sporothrix inflata* are genetically different species.

3. Diagnosis—Culture of a biopsy, pus, or exudate confirms the diagnosis in skin lesions. Organisms are rarely visualized by direct smear. Biopsied tissue should be examined with fungal stains. Serologic testing is available for detection of antibodies.

4. Occurrence—Reported worldwide but characteristically sporadic and relatively uncommon. An epidemic of respiratory infection among approximately 3,000 gold miners in South Africa was caused by the fungus growing on mine timbers. Contact with infected cats was an exposure risk in a Brazilian outbreak of lymphocutaneous infection in 2003. Outbreaks of cutaneous infection have occurred among children playing in baled hay and adults working with it. A cluster of cutaneous infections was also reported in gardeners who had stuffed topiaries with contaminated sphagnum moss.

5. Reservoir—Soil, decaying vegetation, wood, moss, and hay.

6. Incubation period—The lymphatic form develops 1 week to 3 months after injury.

7. Transmission—Fungus is introduced through skin pricks from thorns or barbs, handling of sphagnum moss, or slivers from wood or lumber. Pulmonary sporotrichosis presumably arises through inhalation of conidia. Person-to-person transmission has only rarely been documented.

8. Risk groups—Farmers, gardeners, and horticulturists are occupational groups at risk of infection from environmental reservoirs. As cats are often infected and have exudative lesions, persons handling sick cats are also at risk.

9. Prevention—Treat lumber with fungicides in industries where pulmonary disease is a risk. Wear gloves and long sleeves when working with sphagnum moss and when gardening. Use personal protection when handling sick cats.

10. Management of patient—

1) In lymphocutaneous infection, itraconazole, terbinafine, or saturated solution of potassium iodide given orally 3 times daily, increased drop by drop, is effective. In extracutaneous forms, amphotericin B is the drug of choice, but itraconazole is also useful.
2) Concurrent disinfection of discharges and dressings. Terminal cleaning.

11. Management of contacts and the immediate environment—

   1) Search for undiagnosed and untreated cases.
   2) Determine source to limit future exposures. In the South African epidemic, mine timbers were sprayed with a mixture of zinc sulfate and triolith in order to control the epidemic.

12. Special considerations—None.

[A. E. Purfield]

STAPHYLOCOCCAL DISEASES

DISEASE	ICD-10 CODE
BOILS, CARBUNCLES, FURUNCLES, ABSCESSES	ICD-10 L02; B95.6-B95.8
IMPETIGO	ICD-10 L01
CELLULITIS	ICD-10 L03
STAPHYLOCOCCAL SEPSIS	ICD-10 A41.0-A41.2
STAPHYLOCOCCAL PNEUMONIA	ICD-10 J15.2
ARTHRITIS	ICD-10 M00.0
OSTEOMYELITIS	ICD-10 M86
ENDOCARDITIS	ICD-10 133.0
IMPETIGO NEONATORUM	ICD-10 L00
ABSCESS OF THE BREAST	ICD-10 P39.0
STAPHYLOCOCCAL DISEASE ON HOSPITAL MEDICAL AND SURGICAL WARDS	ICD-10 T81.4
TOXIC SHOCK SYNDROME	ICD-10 A48.3
Staphylococcal food poisoning (see "Foodborne Intoxications")	

Staphylococci produce a variety of syndromes. Clinical manifestations range from a single pustule to sepsis and death. A pus-containing lesion (or lesions) is the primary clinical finding in skin infection. An abscess is the typical pathological manifestation. Production of toxins may also lead to staphylococcal diseases such as toxic shock syndrome.

Virulence of bacterial strains varies greatly. The most important human pathogen is *Staphylococcus aureus*. Most strains ferment mannitol and are coagulase-positive. However, coagulase-negative strains are increasingly important, especially in bloodstream infections among patients with intravascular catheters, in infections of prosthetic materials, and in other health care–associated infections. Antibiotic resistance of staphylococci has risen over the last 60 years and continues to cause adverse health-economic outcomes.

Staphylococcal disease has different clinical and epidemiological patterns in the general community, in newborns, in menstruating women, and among hospitalized patients; each will be presented separately in this chapter. Staphylococcal toxic shock syndrome represents a rare but potentially lethal complication of staphylococcal carriage and is presented at the end of this chapter.

I. STAPHYLOCOCCAL DISEASE IN THE COMMUNITY

1. Clinical features—The common bacterial skin lesions are impetigo, folliculitis, furuncles (boils), carbuncles, abscesses, and infected lacerations. The basic lesion of impetigo is described in this chapter (see Clinical Features under Staphylococcal Disease in Hospital Nurseries section). A distinctive "scalded skin" syndrome is associated with certain strains of *Staphylococcus aureus*, which produce an epidermolytic toxin. Other skin lesions are localized and discrete. Constitutional symptoms are unusual. If lesions extend or are widespread, fever, malaise, headache, and anorexia may develop. Usually, lesions are uncomplicated, but seeding into the bloodstream may lead to lung abscess, osteomyelitis, arthritis, endocarditis, or meningitis. In addition to primary skin lesions, staphylococcal conjunctivitis occurs in newborns and the elderly. Staphylococcal pneumonia is a well-recognized complication of influenza. Staphylococcal endocarditis and other complications of staphylococcal bacteremia may result from parenteral use of illicit drugs or nosocomially from intravenous catheters and other devices. Embolic skin lesions are frequent complications of endocarditis due to *S. aureus*. Coagulase-negative staphylococci may cause sepsis, meningitis, endocarditis, or female urinary tract infections. These are increasing in frequency, usually in connection with prosthetic devices or indwelling catheters.

2. Causative agent—Various coagulase-positive strains of *S. aureus*. Epidemics are caused by relatively few strains. The majority of clinical isolates of *S. aureus*, whether community- or hospital-acquired, are resistant to penicillin G, and multiresistant (including methicillin-resistant) strains have become widespread. Community-associated methicillin-resistant *S. aureus* (CA-MRSA) is spreading quickly in many parts of the world;

however, its prevalence and molecular epidemiology varies considerably from continent to continent.

Evidence suggests that slime-producing strains of coagulase-negative staphylococci may be more pathogenic, but the data are inconclusive. *S. saprophyticus* is a common cause of urinary tract infection in young women.

3. Diagnosis—Confirmed by isolation of the organism on culture. Most strains of staphylococci can be characterized through molecular methods such as antibiotic resistance profile, spa-typing, multilocus sequence typing, and whole genome sequencing.

4. Occurrence—Worldwide. Highest incidence is in areas where hygiene conditions are suboptimal and people are crowded together; common among children, especially in warm weather. The disease occurs sporadically and as small epidemics in families, sport teams, and summer camps, with various members developing recurrent illness due to the same staphylococcal strain. Asymptomatic carriers may serve as unrecognized reservoir. Also a problem in nursing homes and other health care institutions.

5. Reservoir—Humans; rarely animals. The animal reservoir of CA-MRSA (mostly farm pigs but also horses and companion animals) appears to be increasing with new implications for MRSA control in human medicine.

6. Incubation period—Variable and indefinite.

7. Transmission—The major site of colonization is the anterior nasal passages; 20%-30% of the general population are nasal carriers of coagulase-positive staphylococci. Autoinfection is responsible for at least two-thirds of infections. Persons with a draining lesion or purulent discharge are the most common sources of epidemic spread. Transmission is through contact with a person who has a purulent lesion or is an asymptomatic carrier of a pathogenic strain. Some carriers are more effective disseminators of infection than others. Hands are the most important instruments for staphylococcal transmission. The role of contaminated objects has been overstressed. Airborne spread is rare but has been demonstrated in patients with associated viral respiratory disease. The period of communicability continues as long as purulent lesions continue to drain or the carrier state persists. Autoinfection may continue for the period of nasal colonization or duration of active lesions.

8. Risk groups—Immune mechanisms depend mainly on an intact opsonization/phagocytosis axis involving neutrophils. Susceptibility to infection is therefore greatest among the newborn and the chronically ill. Elderly and debilitated people, drug abusers, and those with diabetes mellitus, cystic fibrosis, chronic renal failure, agammaglobulinemia, disorders of neutrophil function (e.g., chronic granulomatous disease), neoplastic disease, and burns are particularly susceptible. Use of steroids also increases susceptibility.

9. **Prevention**—Educate the public and health personnel in personal hygiene, especially handwashing and the importance of not sharing bath towels. Treat initial cases in children and families promptly. Staphylococcal decolonization with topical antiseptics may be a reasonable preventive option in patients with multiple documented recurrences of staphylococcal infection or ongoing transmission in a close cohort of individuals (i.e., household spread).

10. **Management of patient**—

1) Isolation is not practical in most communities. Infected people should avoid contact with infants and debilitated people.
2) Search for draining lesions.
3) Treatment: in localized skin infections, systemic antimicrobials are not indicated unless infection spreads significantly or complications ensue. Local skin cleaning followed by an appropriate topical antimicrobial (such as mupirocin, 3 times/day) is adequate. Hot dry compresses may help to cure localized infections. Avoid wet compresses, which may spread infection. Incise abscesses to drain pus and possibly remove foreign bodies. For severe staphylococcal infections, use penicillinase-resistant penicillin; if there is hypersensitivity to penicillin, use a cephalosporin active against staphylococci (unless there is a history of immediate hypersensitivity to penicillin) or clindamycin. CA-MRSA skin infections can be treated with cotrimoxazole, tetracycline, or clindamycin. In severe systemic infections, choice of antibiotics should be governed by local epidemiologic data and results of susceptibility tests on isolates. Vancomycin is the treatment of choice for severe infections caused by coagulase-negative staphylococci and MRSA; prompt parenteral treatment is important.
4) Place dressings from open lesions and discharges in disposable bags; dispose of these in a practical and safe manner.

11. **Management of contacts and the immediate environment**—Occasionally, determination of nasal carrier status of the pathogenic strain among family members or health care workers (as appropriate) is useful.

12. **Special considerations**—

1) Reporting: outbreaks in schools, summer camps and other population groups should be reported to the local health authority. In many industrialized countries, any recognized clusters of cases in the community should also be reported.

2) Epidemic measures:

- Search for and treat those with clinical illness, especially those with draining lesions.
- Strict personal hygiene with emphasis on handwashing should be encouraged. Culture for nasal carriers of the epidemic strain and treat locally with mupirocin or, if unsuccessful, oral antimicrobials.
- Investigate unusual or abrupt prevalence increases in community staphylococcal infections for a possible common source (e.g., an unrecognized hospital epidemic).

II. STAPHYLOCOCCAL DISEASE IN HOSPITAL NURSERIES

1. Clinical features—Impetigo or pustulosis of the newborn and other purulent skin manifestations are the staphylococcal diseases most frequently acquired in nurseries. Characteristic skin lesions develop secondary to colonization of the nose, umbilicus, circumcision site, rectum, or conjunctivae. Colonization of these sites with staphylococcal strains is a normal occurrence and does not imply disease. Lesions most commonly occur in diaper and intertriginous areas. They are initially vesicular, rapidly turning seropurulent, surrounded by an erythematous base. Rupture of pustules favors their spread. Complications are unusual, although lymphadenitis, furunculosis, breast abscess, pneumonia, arthritis, osteomyelitis, and others have been reported.

Though uncommon, staphylococcal scalded skin syndrome (Ritter disease, pemphigus neonatorum) may occur. Clinical manifestations range from diffuse scarlatiniform erythema to generalized bullous desquamation. Like bullous impetigo, it is caused by strains of *S. aureus*, which produce an epidermolytic toxin.

2. Causative agent; 3. Diagnosis—Same as for Staphylococcal Disease in the Community section in this chapter.

4. Occurrence—Worldwide. Problems occur mainly in hospitals, are promoted by lax aseptic techniques, and are amplified by emergence and transmission of antibiotic-resistant strains, in particular CA-MRSA.

5. Reservoir—Same as for Staphylococcal Disease in the Community section in this chapter.

6. Incubation period—Commonly 4-10 days; disease may not occur until several months after colonization.

7. Transmission—Primarily spread by hands of hospital personnel; rarely airborne. The period of communicability is the same as for Staphylococcal Disease in the Community section in this chapter.

8. Risk groups—Susceptibility of newborns appears to be general. For the duration of colonization with pathogenic strains, infants remain at risk of disease.

9. Prevention—

1) Use aseptic techniques when necessary and clean hands with alcohol-based hand rubs before contact with each infant in nurseries.
2) Personnel with minor lesions (pustules, boils, abscesses, paronychia, conjunctivitis, severe acne, otitis externa, or infected lacerations) must not be permitted to work in nurseries.
3) Surveillance and supervision through an active hospital infection control committee, including a regular system for investigating, reporting, and reviewing hospital-acquired infections.
4) Some experts advocate routine application of antibacterial substances such as gentian violet, acriflavine, chlorhexidine, or bacitracin ointment to the umbilical cord stump while in the hospital.

10. Management of patient—

1) Without delay, place all known or suspected cases in the nursery on contact isolation precautions.
2) Treatment for localized impetigo: cleanse skin and apply a topical antibiotic such as mupirocin ointment (3 times/day); widespread lesions may be treated orally with an antistaphylococcal antimicrobial such as cephalexin or cloxacillin. Serious infections require parenteral treatment (see Treatment under Staphylococcal Disease in the Community section in this chapter). Nasal decontamination with mupirocin is indicated to prevent recurrence.
3) Place dressings from open lesions and discharges in disposable bags; dispose of these in a practical and safe manner.

11. Management of contacts and the immediate environment—See Control Measures in Case of Outbreaks under Staphylococcal Disease in Hospital Nurseries section in this chapter.

12. Special considerations—

1) Reporting: obligatory reporting of epidemics to local health authority.
2) Control measures in case of outbreaks:

- Two or more concurrent cases of staphylococcal disease related to a nursery or maternity ward is presumptive evidence of an outbreak and warrants investigation. Culture all lesions to determine antibiotic resistance pattern and type of epidemic strain. Laboratories should keep clinically important isolates for genotyping to support epidemiological investigations.

- In nursery outbreaks, start isolation precautions for cases and contacts until all have been discharged. Colonized or infected infants should be grouped ("cohorting"). Assignments of personnel should be restricted to specific cohorts.

- Before admitting new patients, wash cribs, beds, and other furniture with an approved disinfectant.

- Examine all personnel for draining lesions anywhere on the body. Perform an epidemiological investigation, and, if one or more personnel are associated with the disease, culture nasal specimens from them and all others in contact with infants. It may become necessary to exclude and treat all carriers of the epidemic strain until cultures are negative. Treatment of asymptomatic carriers aims to suppress the nasal carrier state, usually through local application of appropriate antibiotic ointments to the nasal vestibule, sometimes with concurrent systemic antibiotics for 5–7 days.

- Investigate adequacy of nursing procedures, especially availability of alcohol-based hand rubs. Emphasize strict hand hygiene. Personnel assigned to infected or colonized infants should not work with noncolonized newborns.

III. STAPHYLOCOCCAL DISEASE ON HOSPITAL MEDICAL AND SURGICAL WARDS

1. Clinical features—Lesions vary from simple furuncles or stitch abscesses to extensively infected bedsores or surgical wounds, septic phlebitis, acute or chronic osteomyelitis, pneumonia, meningitis, endocarditis, or sepsis. A toxic state can complicate infection if the strain produces toxins. This is an ever-present risk.

2. Causative agent—*S. aureus*; see Causative Agent under Staphylococcal Disease on Hospital Medical and Surgical Wards section in this chapter. Resistance to penicillin occurs in up to 95% of strains and increasing proportions are resistant to semisynthetic penicillins (e.g., oxacillin), aminoglycosides (e.g., gentamicin), macrolides, and quinolones.

3. Diagnosis—Verification depends on isolation of *S. aureus*, associated with a clinical illness compatible with the bacteriological findings.

4. Occurrence—Worldwide. Staphylococcal infection is a major cause of hospital-acquired infection in the general wards of hospitals. Attack rates may assume epidemic proportions, and community spread may occur when hospital-infected patients are discharged. Misuse of antimicrobials has increased the prevalence of antibiotic-resistant staphylococci.

5. Reservoir; 6. Incubation period; 7. Transmission—See Reservoir, Incubation Period, and Transmission under Staphylococcal Disease in the Community section in this chapter.

8. Risk groups—Postoperative staphylococcal infection is a constant threat to the convalescence of the hospitalized surgical patient. Increased use of prosthetic devices and indwelling catheters accounts for increased incidence of nosocomial staphylococcal infections.

9. Prevention—

1) Educate hospital medical staff to use narrow-spectrum antimicrobials for simple staphylococcal infections for short treatment durations and to reserve certain antibiotics for specific situations (e.g., reserve cephalosporins for penicillin-resistant staphylococcal infections and vancomycin for beta-lactam resistant staphylococcal infections).
2) A hospital infection control committee must enforce strict aseptic technique and provide programs to monitor nosocomial infections.
3) Promote hand hygiene compliance with alcohol-based hand rubs throughout the hospital.

10. Management of patient—

1) Isolation: whenever staphylococci are known or suspected to be abundant in draining pus or the sputum of a patient with pneumonia, the patient should be placed in a private room. This is not required when wound drainage is scanty, provided an occlusive dressing is used and care is taken in changing dressings to prevent environmental contamination. Health care workers must practice appropriate hand hygiene, gloving, and gowning techniques.
2) Place dressings from open lesions and discharges in disposable bags; dispose of these in a practical and safe manner.

3) Treatment: appropriate antimicrobials as determined through antibiotic sensitivity tests. Life-threatening staphylococcal infections should be treated with vancomycin pending test results.

11. Management of contacts and the immediate environment— See Control Measures in Case of Outbreaks under Staphylococcal Disease on Hospital Medical and Surgical Wards section in this chapter.

12. Special considerations—

1) Reporting: obligatory report of epidemics; no individual case report.
2) Control measures in case of outbreaks:

   • The occurrence of 2 or more cases with epidemiological association is sufficient to suspect epidemic spread and to initiate investigation.
   • See Control Measures in Case of Outbreaks under Staphylococcal Disease in Hospital Nurseries section in this chapter.
   • Review and enforce strict aseptic techniques.

IV. TOXIC SHOCK SYNDROME

Toxic shock syndrome (TSS) is a severe illness characterized by sudden onset of high fever, vomiting, profuse watery diarrhea, and myalgia, followed by hypotension and—in severe cases—shock. More than three-quarters of cases occur in females. An erythematous "sunburn-like" rash is present during the acute phase, about 1–2 weeks after onset, with desquamation of the skin, especially of palms and soles. Fever is usually high (39°C/102°F), with hypotension, and 3 or more of the following organ systems are involved:

• Gastrointestinal (GI)
• Muscular (severe myalgia and/or creatine phosphokinase level >twice the normal upper limit)
• Mucous membranes (vaginal, pharyngeal, and/or conjunctival hyperemia)
• Renal (blood urea nitrogen or creatinine >twice normal and/or sterile pyuria)
• Hepatic (aspartate aminotransferase or alanine transferase [AST or ALT] >twice normal)
• Hematological (platelets <100,000/mm^3)

- Central nervous system (CNS; disorientation or alterations in consciousness without focal neurological signs)

Blood, throat, and cerebrospinal fluid (CSF) cultures are negative for pathogens; the recovery of *S. aureus* from any of these sites does not, however, invalidate a case. Serological tests for Rocky Mountain spotted fever, leptospirosis, and measles are negative.

Most cases of TSS have been associated with strains of *S. aureus* producing toxic shock syndrome toxin 1. These strains, rarely present in vaginal cultures from healthy women, are regularly recovered from women with menstrually associated TSS or in those with TSS after gynecological surgery.

Although almost all early cases of TSS occurred in women during menstruation, and most with vaginal tampon use; only 55% of cases now reported are associated with menses. Other risk factors include use of contraceptive diaphragms and vaginal contraceptive sponges and infection following childbirth or abortion. Instructions for sponge use, advising that these should not be left in place for more than 30 hours, must be heeded.

Menstrual TSS can be prevented by avoiding use of highly absorbent vaginal tampons; risk may be reduced by using tampons intermittently (i.e., not all day and all night throughout the period) and using less absorbent tampons. Women who develop a high fever and vomiting or diarrhea during menstruation must discontinue tampon use immediately and consult a physician.

A TSS virtually identical to that occurring with *S. aureus* infection occurs with infection caused by group A beta-hemolytic streptococci.

Treatment of TSS is largely supportive. Efforts should be made to eradicate potential foci of *S. aureus* infection through drainage of wounds, removal of vaginal or other foreign bodies (e.g., wound packing) and use of beta-lactam resistant antistaphylococcal drugs. Clindamycin or linezolid may help reduce toxin production.

[S. Harbarth]

STREPTOCOCCAL DISEASES

DISEASE	ICD-10 CODE
STREPTOCOCCAL SORE THROAT	ICD-10 J02.0
IMPETIGO	ICD-10 L01.0
ERYSIPELAS	ICD-10 A46
SCARLET FEVER	ICD-10 A38
PUERPERAL FEVER	ICD-10 O85
OTHER GROUP A STREPTOCOCCAL INFECTIONS	ICD-10 A49.1
GROUP B STREPTOCOCCAL SEPSIS OF THE NEWBORN	ICD-10 P36.0
STREPTOCOCCAL DENTAL CARIES IN EARLY CHILDHOOD	ICD-10 K02
STREPTOCOCCAL TOXIC SHOCK SYNDROME	ICD-10: B95.0
Streptococcus pneumoniae infections (see ''Pneumonia'')	

Group A streptococci cause a variety of diseases (see Group A Streptococcal Infections section in this chapter). Streptococci of other groups can also produce infections in humans. Group B beta-hemolytic streptococci, found in the human vagina and gastrointestinal tract, may cause neonatal sepsis and suppurative meningitis (see Group B Streptococcal Disease of the Newborn section in this chapter), as well as urinary tract infections, postpartum endometritis, and other systemic disease in adults, especially those with diabetes mellitus. Group D organisms (including enterococci), both hemolytic and nonhemolytic, are involved in bacterial endocarditis and urinary tract infections. Groups C and G organisms have produced outbreaks of streptococcal tonsillitis, usually foodborne; their role in sporadic cases is less well defined, but they can both cause invasive diseases similar to group A infections. Glomerulonephritis has followed group C infections but has very rarely been reported after group G infection; neither group is known to cause rheumatic fever. Group C and G pharyngeal infections are more common in adolescents and young adults.

I. GROUP A STREPTOCOCCAL INFECTIONS
(streptococcal sore throat, group A strep infection, scarlet fever, impetigo, erysipelas, puerperal fever, rheumatic fever)

1. Clinical features—The most frequently encountered group A streptococcal (GAS) conditions are pharyngitis/tonsillitis and superficial skin infections such as impetigo or pyoderma. Other acute infections include scarlet fever, puerperal fever, septicemia, erysipelas, cellulitis, mastoiditis, otitis media, pneumonia, peritonsillitis, wound infections, and, rarely, necrotizing fasciitis and a toxic shock-like syndrome. One or other form of clinical disease often predominates during outbreaks. Acute glomerulonephritis may develop after pharyngeal or skin infection with a limited number of ("nephritogenic") strains of GAS associated with specific types of M protein (M-types).

1) Streptococcal sore throat: patients with streptococcal sore throat typically exhibit sudden onset of fever, exudative tonsillitis or pharyngitis (sore throat), and tender, enlarged anterior cervical lymph nodes. The pharynx, the tonsillar pillars, and soft palate may be injected and edematous; petechiae may be present against a background of diffuse redness. Coincident or subsequent otitis media or peritonsillar abscess may occur. Possible nonsuppurative complications include acute rheumatic fever (an average of 19 days following pharyngitis) and acute glomerulonephritis (an average of 10 days following pharyngitis or ≥3 weeks after skin infection). Rheumatic heart (valvular) disease occurs days to weeks after acute streptococcal infection, and Sydenham chorea (in the past often referred to as Saint Vitus' Dance) several months following infection.

2) GAS skin infection (pyoderma, impetigo): usually superficial and may proceed through vesicular, pustular, and encrusted stages. Glomerulonephritis may occur later, usually 3 weeks after the skin infection.

3) Scarlet fever: a form of GAS infection characterized by a skin rash, occurring when the infecting strain produces a pyrogenic exotoxin (erythrogenic toxin) and the patient is sensitized, but not immune, to the toxin. Clinical characteristics may include all symptoms associated with a streptococcal sore throat (or with a streptococcal wound, skin, or puerperal infection) as well as enanthem, strawberry tongue, and exanthem. The rash is usually a fine erythema, commonly punctate, blanching on pressure, often felt (like sandpaper) better than seen, and appearing most often on the neck, chest, folds of the axilla, elbow, groin, and inner surfaces of the thighs. Typically, the scarlet fever rash does not involve the face, but there is flushing of the cheeks and circumoral pallor. High fever, nausea, and vomiting often accompany severe infections. During convalescence, skin peeling occurs at the tips of fingers and toes and less often over wide areas of trunk and limbs, including palms and soles; it is more pronounced where the exanthem was severe. The case-fatality rate in some parts of the world has occasionally been as high as 3%. Scarlet fever may be followed by the same sequelae as streptococcal sore throat.

4) Erysipelas: an acute skin infection characterized by fever, constitutional symptoms, leukocytosis, and a red, tender, edematous spreading lesion of the skin, typically with a definite raised border. The central point of origin tends to clear as the periphery extends. Face and legs are common sites. Recurrences are frequent and disease is more common among persons with underlying skin conditions. The disease has a good prognosis with early diagnosis and treatment but may be especially severe in patients suffering from debilitating disease. Erysipelas due to GAS is to be distinguished from erysipeloid caused by *Erysipelothrix rhusiopathiae*, a localized cutaneous infection (typically without fever or systemic symptoms) seen primarily as an occupational disease of people handling fresh-water fish or shellfish, infected swine or turkeys or their tissues, or—rarely—sheep, cattle, chickens, or pheasants.

5) Perianal cellulitis (due to GAS): recognized more frequently in the past decade and, though it occurs among all ages, is primarily a disease of early childhood. It can also result in disease outbreaks.

6) GAS puerperal fever: an acute disease, usually febrile, with local and general symptoms and signs of bacterial invasion of the genital tract and sometimes the bloodstream in the postpartum or postabortion patient. Case-fatality rate is low when strepto-coccal puerperal fever is adequately treated. Puerperal infec-tions may be caused by organisms other than hemolytic streptococci; they are clinically similar but differ bacteriologi-cally and epidemiologically (see "Staphylococcal Disease").

7) Streptococcal toxic shock syndrome (STSS) and necrotizing fasciitis: the most severe forms of invasive GAS infection. Although the incidence of these manifestations of GAS likely increased in the late 1980s and early 1990s, active surveillance in the USA indicates that rates of STSS and necrotizing fasciitis due to GAS have been fairly stable during the last 15 years. Necrotizing fasciitis (sometimes called "flesh-eating bacteria") can be caused by multiple pathogens, but the most common etiology is GAS. It is a rapidly progressive disease that destroys muscles, fat, and skin tissue. Patients often present with skin that is erythematous, edematous, and hot to the touch. The pain is often described as out of proportion to what is expected by physical exam. Patients often have fever and chills, fatigue, vomiting, and diarrhea. In the USA the mortality rate is approximately 25%. STSS clinical features include hypotension and one or more of the following: renal impairment; thrombo-cytopenia; disseminated intravascular coagulation; serum glu-tamic oxaloacetic transaminase or bilirubin elevation; adult respiratory distress syndrome; a generalized erythematous macular rash; or soft-tissue necrosis (necrotizing fasciitis).

STSS may occur with either systemic or focal (throat, skin, lung sites) group A streptococcal infections, and mortality rates are as high as 35%–40%. For both necrotizing fasciitis and STSS, rapid diagnosis, aggressive management, and early use of appropriate antibiotics are critical.

2. **Causative agent**—*Streptococcus pyogenes*—or GAS—are Gram-positive, β-hemolytic bacteria. While the critical virulence factor, the M protein, generates type-specific immunity, distinct GAS serotypes are increasingly being identified through *emm* typing—a system that determines the *emm* gene encoding the M-protein. Over 240 distinct *emm* types that vary by geographic and time distributions have been recognized. Skin infections caused by GAS usually differ serologically from GAS-associated with throat infections. In scarlet fever, 3 immunologically different types of erythrogenic toxin (pyrogenic exotoxins A, B, and C) have been demonstrated. In STSS, 80% of isolates produce pyrogenic exotoxin A. Phenotypically mucoid strains have been involved in recent outbreaks of rheumatic fever.

3. **Diagnosis**—Provisional laboratory findings are based on the isolation of the organisms from affected tissues (e.g., blood, wounds) using blood agar or other appropriate media, or on identification of GAS antigen in pharyngeal secretions (the rapid antigen detection test). Colony morphology and the production of clear beta-hemolysis on blood agar made with sheep's blood identify streptococci on cultures; inhibition by special antibiotic discs containing bacitracin (0.02–0.04 units) constitutes tentative identification. Specific serogrouping procedures provide definitive identification. Antigen detection tests also allow rapid identification, demonstrating a rise in serum antibody titer (antistreptolysin O, antihyaluronidase [not commercially available], anti-DNA-ase B) between acute and convalescent stages of illness; high titers may persist for several months.

In many industrialized countries, current recommended practice for diagnosis of strep pharyngitis is to first do a rapid antigen detection test (high specificity but low sensitivity) or a throat culture and, if this is positive, assume the patient has a GAS infection. If the result of a rapid test used in a child or adolescent is negative or equivocal, a throat culture should be done to guide management and prevent superfluous use of antibiotics.

4. **Occurrence**—Streptococcal (GAS) pharyngitis/tonsillitis and scarlet fever are common in temperate zones, well recognized in semitropical areas, and less frequently recognized in tropical climates. Unapparent infections are at least as common in tropical as in temperate zones, and in temperate zones streptococcal diseases may be endemic, epidemic, or sporadic. In these zones, streptococcal pharyngitis is unusual before the age of 3 years, peaks among 6–12 year olds, and declines thereafter. Both

pharyngitis and invasive infections occur year round but peak in late winter and spring.

Acute rheumatic fever (ARF) is a nonsuppurative complication of streptococcal pharyngitis/tonsillitis. In developing countries ARF tends to occur sporadically. Rheumatic fever remains a major cause of cardiovascular disease in the developing world. It is estimated that 15.6 million people worldwide have rheumatic heart disease with 470,000 new cases of rheumatic fever occurring each year. People aged between 5 and 15 years and military and school populations have been most often affected. Many reported cases have followed infections by specific GAS serotypes, such as M-types 3, 5, 6, and 18, particularly among highly mucoid strains of M18. The highest incidence, during late winter and spring, corresponds to that of pharyngitis. ARF has virtually disappeared from industrialized countries; however, it can reappear as demonstrated in North America in the mid-1980s when ARF occurred in scattered communities.

In the USA, of the estimated 11,000–13,300 annual severe (invasive) GAS infections, 1,250–1,600 patients die. Approximately 6% and 7% of persons with invasive infection develop STSS and necrotizing fasciitis, respectively. Globally, the incidence of invasive GAS infections ranges from 2.5–46 cases per 100,000 population, with the highest reported rates in indigenous populations of the USA and Australia.

The highest incidence of streptococcal impetigo occurs in young children (aged 2–5 years) in the latter part of the hot season in tropical climates. Poststreptococcal glomerulonephritis following skin infections is associated with a limited number of streptococcal M-types that generally differ from those associated with nephritis following infections of the upper respiratory tract. Among indigenous populations in Australia and the Pacific, high rates of impetigo accompanied by a great diversity of skin-associated strains and low rates of GAS pharyngitis suggest that ARF can also occur as a complication of impetigo, although this has not been confirmed.

Geographical and seasonal distribution of erysipelas is similar to those for scarlet fever and streptococcal sore throat; erysipelas is most common in infants and those older than 20 years. Occurrence is sporadic, even during epidemics of streptococcal infection.

Reliable morbidity data do not exist for puerperal fever. In industrialized countries, morbidity and mortality have declined, although outbreaks may still occur in institutions where aseptic technique is faulty.

5. Reservoir—Humans.

6. Incubation period—Short, usually 1–3 days, for pharyngitis; estimated 7–10 days for impetigo.

7. Transmission—Through large respiratory droplets or direct contact with patients or carriers; extremely rarely through indirect contact with contaminated objects. Individuals with acute upper respiratory tract (especially nasal) infections are particularly likely to transmit infection. Casual contact rarely leads to infection. In populations where impetigo is prevalent, GAS may be recovered from normal skin for 1-2 weeks before skin lesions develop; the same strain may appear in the throat (without clinical evidence of throat infection), usually late in the course of the skin infection.

Anal, vaginal, skin, and pharyngeal carriers have been responsible for nosocomial outbreaks of serious streptococcal infection, particularly following surgical procedures. Many such outbreaks have been traced to operating room personnel or other health care workers. Identification of the carrier often involves intensive epidemiological and microbiological investigation; eradication of the carrier state typically requires a different antibiotic regimen than that used for treatment of disease and may require multiple courses of specific antibiotic regimens (see Patient Management in this chapter). Dried streptococci reaching the air via contaminated items (floor dust, lint from bedclothes, handkerchiefs) may be viable but apparently do not infect mucous membranes and intact skin.

Explosive outbreaks of streptococcal sore throat may follow ingestion of contaminated food. Milk and milk products have been associated most frequently with foodborne outbreaks; egg salad and similar preparations have recently been implicated. Direct contamination of milk or egg products by humans appears to be the important source of foodborne episodes; infected food preparers are often implicated as the original source of infection. GAS may also be indirectly transmitted to cattle from human carriers, then spread through raw milk from these cattle (although cows do not contract the disease). Milkborne group C outbreaks have been traced to infected cows. Foodborne outbreaks of group G streptococcal pharyngitis have also been reported.

Transmissibility of GAS pharyngitis generally ends within 24 hours of beginning appropriate antibiotic treatment. Patients with untreated streptococcal pharyngitis may carry the organism for weeks or months, usually in decreasing numbers; contagiousness of these patients decreases sharply in 2-3 weeks after onset of infection. In untreated, uncomplicated impetigo, the period of communicability extends 10-21 days; in untreated conditions with purulent discharges, it lasts weeks or months.

8. Risk groups—Patients with skin breakdown (e.g., burns, wounds) are highly susceptible to streptococcal infections of the affected area. Persons with chronic underlying medical conditions (e.g., diabetes) and the elderly are at increased risk for invasive GAS infections.

Susceptibility to streptococcal pharyngitis/tonsillitis and scarlet fever is general, although many people develop either antitoxin or type-specific antibacterial immunity, or both, through unapparent infection. Antibacterial immunity develops against the specific M-type of GAS that induced infection and may last for years. Antibiotic therapy may interfere with the development of type-specific immunity. Repeated attacks of pharyngitis/tonsillitis or other disease due to different types of streptococci are not uncommon. However, when a child or adolescent experiences multiple episodes of culture-positive or rapid test-positive acute pharyngitis within a period of months to years, this person is most likely a pharyngeal carrier of GAS who is actually experiencing viral pharyngitis. Immunity against erythrogenic toxin, and hence against rash, develops within a week after onset of scarlet fever and is usually permanent; second attacks of scarlet fever are rare but may occur because of the 3 immunological forms of toxin. Some degree of passive immunity to group A streptococcal disease occurs in newborns with transplacental maternal type specific antibodies. Patients who have had one attack of rheumatic fever have a significant risk of recurrence of rheumatic fever following GAS infections, often with further cardiac damage. Individuals who have had erysipelas appear predisposed to subsequent attacks. Recurrence of glomerulonephritis is unusual, possibly because very few M-types are "nephritogenic."

9. **Prevention—**

   1) Educate the public, parents, and health workers about modes of transmission; importance of hand hygiene; relationship of streptococcal infection to acute rheumatic fever, Sydenham chorea, rheumatic heart disease, and glomerulonephritis; and need for prompt diagnosis and completion of the full course of antibiotics prescribed.
   2) Provide easily accessible laboratory facilities for recognition of GAS.
   3) Pasteurize milk and exclude infected people from handling milk or dairy products.
   4) Prepare potentially dangerous foods just prior to serving, or adequately refrigerate in small quantities at 4°C (39°F) or less.
   5) Exclude people with skin lesions from food handling.
   6) Infection control: critical assessment of adherence to infection control practices should be undertaken in GAS outbreaks in facilities housing highly vulnerable populations (e.g., nursing homes, acute and long-term rehabilitation facilities). Outbreaks in such facilities are often due to, or perpetuated by, poor routine infection control practices.

10. **Management of patient—**

1) Drainage and secretion precautions may be terminated after 24 hours of effective antibiotic therapy; antibiotics should be continued for 10 days to avoid development of rheumatic heart disease.

2) Concurrent disinfection of purulent discharges and all articles soiled therewith. Terminal cleaning.

3) Treatment of streptococcal pharyngitis: penicillin (oral penicillin V or intramuscular [IM] benzathine penicillin G) or oral amoxicillin for individuals without a penicillin allergy. To date there has never been a documented penicillin-resistant strain of GAS. Treatment must provide adequate levels for 10 days. While antibiotics may shorten clinical illness somewhat, it is also recognized that patients with streptococcal pharyngitis improve in 3–4 days without antibiotics. Appropriate antibiotic use reduces the frequency of suppurative complications, prevents the development of most cases of acute rheumatic fever, prevents further spread of the organism in the community, and may reduce the risk of acute glomerulonephritis after pharyngeal infection (not confirmed for acute nephritis after skin infections). For penicillin-sensitive patients the following antibiotics are recommended: an oral first-generation cephalosporin, clindamycin, or clarithromycin for 10 days; or azithromycin for 5 days. Resistance to macrolides has been noted to be common in some countries; local data on prevalence of resistance should be used to guide therapy.

   Treatment of necrotizing fasciitis and STSS: in addition to prompt use of broad spectrum intravenous antibiotics, treatment for necrotizing fasciitis almost always requires immediate surgical exploration and debridement of infected tissue; amputation of the affected limb may be necessary. Treatment of STSS includes hemodynamic support with fluids and intravenous antibiotics. For both necrotizing fasciitis and STSS, once GAS is identified, penicillin and clindamycin are the recommended antibiotics. Clindamycin suppresses the synthesis of bacterial toxins, causes suppression of tumor necrosis factor, and is effective regardless of the inoculum size or stage of growth of GAS.

4) Secondary prevention of complications: to prevent streptococcal reinfection and possible recurrence of rheumatic fever or chorea among patients with acute rheumatic fever, monthly injections of long-acting benzathine penicillin G (or daily oral penicillin in compliant patients) should be given for at least 5 years (for those with mild mitral regurgitation, at least 10 years; for those with severe valve disease or after valve surgery, life-

long prophylaxis is recommended). Those who do not tolerate penicillin may be given sulfadiazine orally or erythromycin if necessary. Prophylactic IM or oral penicillin may be used in some patients with recurrent erysipelas.

11. Management of contacts and the immediate environment— Investigation of contacts and source of infection: culture symptomatic contacts. Search for and treat carriers in situations where contacts may be at high risk for developing sequelae of GAS infections (e.g., evidence of streptococcal infection in families with multiple cases of rheumatic fever or streptococcal toxic shock syndrome; occurrence of cases of rheumatic fever or acute nephritis in a population group such as a school; outbreaks of postoperative wound or postpartum infections). Identification and treatment of carriers may also be undertaken in well-documented epidemics of severe streptococcal infection, such as outbreaks of invasive GAS infections among nursing home residents, in order to halt ongoing transmission among a highly vulnerable population.

12. Special considerations—

1) Reporting: obligatory report of epidemics in some countries. Acute rheumatic fever and/or STSS or other invasive GAS infections are also reportable in some localities.
2) Epidemic measures:

- Determine source and manner of spread (person-to-person or single-source outbreaks due to contaminated milk or food). Single-source foodborne or nosocomial outbreaks can often be traced to an individual with an acute or persistent streptococcal infection, or who is carrying streptococci (nose, throat, skin, vagina, or perianal area), through identification of the M-type or *emm* type of the streptococcus.
- Investigate promptly any unusual grouping of cases to identify possible common sources.
- For extensive or protracted outbreaks in special close contact groups (e.g., military recruits, day-care centers, nursing homes), it may be necessary to administer antibiotic prophylaxis to the entire group to terminate spread. In these settings, the benefits of such widespread use of antibiotics should be carefully weighed against the potential side effects.

WHO Collaborating Centres provide support as required. Further information can be found at: http://www.who.int/collaboratingcentres/database/en.

II. GROUP B STREPTOCOCCAL SEPSIS OF THE NEWBORN

1. Clinical features—Human subtypes of group B streptococci (*Streptococcus agalactiae*) produce invasive disease in the newborn of 2 distinct forms. Early onset disease (from 1-7 days) with sepsis, pneumonia, and less frequently meningitis, osteomyelitis, or septic arthritis is acquired in utero or during delivery. Late onset disease (7 days to several months) is acquired in about half the cases through person-to-person contact and presents mostly as meningitis or sepsis. Advances in neonatal care have led to a fall in the case-fatality rate from 50%-4%. Survivors may have speech, hearing, visual problems, psychomotor retardation, or seizure disorders if there has been meningeal involvement.

2. Causative agents—*S. agalactiae*, group B, is the cause of sepsis in the newborn. About 10%-30% of pregnant women harbor group B streptococci (GBS) in the genital tract, and about 1% of their offspring may develop symptomatic infection. GBS found in bovine mastitis are not a cause of this disease.

3. Diagnosis—Culture and isolation of GBS from blood, cerebrospinal fluid, or other normally sterile body fluid.

4. Occurrence—Thought to occur worldwide, but most studies at time of writing are from North America and Europe.

5. Reservoir—Humans; commonly found in the gastrointestinal, reproductive, and urinary tracts.

6. Incubation period—From 1-6 days after birth (early onset disease).

7. Transmission—Early onset disease: transmitted to infants during the intrapartum period, especially to infants delivered at under 37 weeks, and/or when rupture of membranes occurs 18 hours or more before delivery.

8. Risk groups—Babies born prematurely, when there is rupture of membranes more than 18 hours prior to delivery, or when their mothers have fever during labor are at particularly high risk. However, most babies who develop disease (75%) are full term.

9. Prevention—Two preventive approaches have been used successfully:

  1) Risk-based method: identify candidates for intrapartum chemoprophylaxis according to the presence of any of the following intrapartum risk factors for early-onset disease:

- Delivery at under 37 weeks.
- Intrapartum temperature greater than or equal to 38°C (≥100.4°F).
- Rupture of membranes for 18 hours or more.

2) Screening-based method: screen all pregnant women for vaginal and rectal GBS colonization at 35–37 weeks' gestation, and offer women with colonization intrapartum antibiotics during labor. In both cases, women with GBS bacteriuria during the current pregnancy or who previously gave birth to an infant with early-onset GBS disease are candidates for intrapartum antibiotic prophylaxis.

3) Compelling evidence for a strong protective effect of the screening-based method relative to the risk-based strategy has led to the current recommendation in many countries of prenatal screening by vaginal-rectal culture for group B streptococcus colonization at 35–37 weeks' gestation and chemoprophylaxis for all pregnant women identified as GBS carriers at the time of labor or rupture of membranes. Women whose culture results are unknown at the time of delivery should be managed according to the risk-based method.

10. **Management of patient—**

1) In hospitals and institutions, patients should be isolated, especially in maternity wards and nurseries.

2) Infection control measures (see "Infection Prevention and Control").

3) Treatment: routine use of antimicrobial prophylaxis for newborns whose mothers received intrapartum chemoprophylaxis for GBS infection is not recommended, although therapeutic use of these agents is appropriate for infants with clinically suspected sepsis.

11. **Management contacts and the immediate environment—**The administration of intravenous penicillin or ampicillin to women colonized with group B streptococci at the onset of and throughout labor interrupts transmission to newborn infants, decreasing infection and mortality. Penicillin is the preferred agent in women without penicillin allergy. No GBS isolates with confirmed resistance to penicillin or ampicillin have been observed to date. Alternative regimens for allergic women include clindamycin and cefazolin.

12. **Special considerations—**A vaccine for pregnant women to stimulate antibody production against invasive disease in newborns is under development.

III. STREPTOCOCCAL DENTAL CARIES IN EARLY CHILDHOOD (nursing bottle caries, baby bottle tooth decay)

While the cause of dental caries in young children is multifactorial, the subject is included in this section because of the involvement of a streptococcal species. In early childhood a characteristic pattern of dental caries occurs in which maxillary primary incisors are routinely affected with carious lesions, but mandibular primary incisors are rarely involved; involvement of other primary teeth varies. Because of the association of this pattern with a specific feeding habit, the process was called nursing bottle caries or baby bottle tooth decay, but it also occurs in children using feeding cups.

Streptococcus mutans is present in these carious lesions. These Gram-positive facultative anerobes produce caries in young experimental animals in the presence of dietary sugar. They are members of the viridans group of streptococci; hemolysis of blood agar is usually alpha or gamma. They require a nonshedding oral surface for colonization and are common residents of dental plaque.

Early childhood caries occur worldwide with highest prevalence in developing countries. Disadvantaged children, regardless of ethnicity or culture, and those with low birth weight are most frequently affected; enamel hypoplasia, which may occur because of compromised nutritional status during formative stages of primary dentition, is often associated.

The main reservoir from which infants acquire mutans streptococci is the mother; strains isolated from mothers and their babies show similar or identical bacteriocin profiles and identical plasmid or chromosomal deoxyribonucleic acid (DNA) patterns.

Mother-to-child transmission occurs through transfer of infected saliva by kissing the baby on the mouth or, more likely, by moistening the nipple or pacifier, or by tasting food on the baby's spoon before serving it. Colonization by maternal organisms largely depends on inoculum size; mothers with extensive dental caries usually have high levels of mutans streptococci in their saliva.

To prevent dental caries of early childhood, promote good oral hygiene in mothers and encourage early weaning from the bottle. Counsel parents and caretakers about the dangers of dental caries from milk and beverages containing sugar and of transferring saliva to a baby's mouth when mothers and other caretakers have untreated carious teeth.

[C. Van Beneden]

STRONGYLOIDIASIS

DISEASE	ICD-10 CODE
STRONGYLOIDIASIS	ICD-10 B78

1. **Clinical features**—An often asymptomatic helminthic infection with clinical manifestations that include transient dermatitis when larvae of the parasite penetrate the skin on initial infection; cough, rales, and sometimes demonstrable pneumonitis when larvae pass through the lungs; or abdominal symptoms caused by adult worms in the intestinal mucosa. Symptoms of chronic infection may be mild or severe, depending on the intensity of infection. Classic symptoms of chronic infection include abdominal pain (usually epigastric, often suggesting peptic ulcer), diarrhea, and urticaria; and sometimes also nausea, weight loss, vomiting, weakness, and constipation. Intensely pruritic dermatitis (larva currens) radiating from the anus may occur, as can stationary wheals lasting 1–2 days, as well as a migrating serpiginous rash moving several centimeters per hour across the trunk. Rarely, intestinal autoinfection with increasing worm burden (hyperinfection) may lead to disseminated strongyloidiasis with wasting, pulmonary involvement, and death, particularly, but not exclusively, in the immunocompromised host. In these cases, secondary Gram-negative sepsis is common. Eosinophilia is usually moderate (10%–25%) in the chronic stage but may be normal or low with dissemination. Immunosuppressed persons, including those with human T-cell lymphotrophic virus (HTLV-1), those on oral or intravenous steroids, those receiving chemotherapy for malignancies, or transplant patients, are at increased risk for disseminated or hyperinfection strongyloidiasis.

2. **Causative agents**—*Strongyloides stercoralis* and *Strongyloides fulleborni*, nematodes.

3. **Diagnosis**—Entails identifying motile larvae in concentrated stool specimens of freshly passed feces, on nutrient agar plate cultures, in duodenal aspirates, or occasionally in sputum. Ruling out the diagnosis may require repeat examinations. Held at room temperature for 24 hours or more, feces may show developing stages of the parasite, including rhabditiform (noninfective) and filariform (infective) larvae (these must be distinguished from larvae of hookworm species) and free-living adults. Serological tests based on larval stage antigens are positive in 80%–85% of infected patients.

4. **Occurrence**—Throughout tropical and temperate areas; more common in warm, wet regions. Prevalence in endemic areas is not

594 / STRONGYLOIDIASIS

accurately known. May be prevalent in residents of institutions where personal hygiene is poor. Human infection with *S. fulleborni* has been reported only in Africa and in Papua New Guinea.

5. Reservoir—Humans are the principal reservoir of *S. stercoralis*, with occasional transmission of dog and cat strains to humans. Nonhuman primates are the reservoir of *S. fulleborni* in Africa.

6. Incubation period—2-4 weeks from penetration of the skin by filariform larvae until rhabditiform larvae appear in the feces; the period until symptoms appear is indefinite and variable.

7. Transmission—Infective (filariform) larvae develop in feces or moist soil contaminated with feces, penetrate the skin, enter the venous circulation, and are carried to the lungs. They penetrate capillary walls, enter the alveoli, ascend the trachea to the epiglottis, and descend into the digestive tract to reach the upper part of the small intestine where development of the adult female is completed. The adult worm, a parthenogenetic female, lives embedded in the mucosal epithelium of the intestine, especially the duodenum, where eggs are deposited. These hatch and liberate rhabditiform (noninfective) larvae that migrate into the intestinal lumen, exit in feces, and develop after reaching the soil into either filariform (infective) larvae or free-living adults. The free-living fertilized females produce eggs that hatch and liberate rhabditiform larvae, which may become filariform larvae within 24-36 hours. In some individuals, rhabditiform larvae may develop to the infective stage before leaving the body and penetrate through the intestinal mucosa or perianal skin, resulting in autoinfection that can cause persistent infection for many years. Person-to-person transmission may also occur; the period of communicability lasts as long as living worms remain in the intestine, up to 75 years in cases of continuous autoinfection.

8. Risk groups—Immunosuppressed patients including those on corticosteroid therapy, with HTLV-1, with hematologic malignancies, or with organ transplants are at risk of dissemination.

9. Prevention—

1) Dispose of human feces in a safe manner.
2) Pay strict attention to hygienic habits, including use of footwear in endemic areas.
3) Rule out suspected strongyloidiasis through serologic or stool testing before initiating immunosuppressive treatment for any reason.
4) Examine and treat infected dogs, cats, and monkeys in contact with humans.

10. Management of patient—Treatment: because of the potential for autoinfection and dissemination, all infections, regardless of worm burden, should be treated. Ivermectin for 2 days is the regimen of choice; albendazole for 7 days is a less efficient alternative. Repeated courses of treatment (or longer courses in the case of disseminated disease) may be required.

11. Management of contacts and the immediate environment— Members of the same household or institution should be examined for evidence of infection. Patients hospitalized with strongyloidiasis should be placed on contact precautions.

12: Special considerations—None.

[L. Fox]

SYPHILIS
(lues)

DISEASE	ICD-10 CODE
SYPHILIS	ICD-10 A50-A52

1. Clinical features—Syphilis is a systemic treponemal infection characterized by 3 possible clinical stages and variable periods of latency. The primary stage is characterized by an indurated, painless ulcer known as a chancre. About 3 weeks after contact with another person's infectious lesions, the primary chancre develops at the site of exposure. Chancres can appear anywhere on the skin or mucous membranes, and although they commonly occur on the penis, vulva, mouth, or perianal skin, they might occur internally on the cervix or anus and go unnoticed. Firm, nonfluctuant, painless, regional lymphadenopathy frequently develops with the primary lesion. Without treatment, the chancre involutes in 4-6 weeks.

Within several weeks to months of the primary lesion, and occasionally at the same time as the primary lesion, a secondary skin eruption appears. Symmetric macular-to-papulosquamous skin lesions develop, classically occurring on the trunk, palms, and soles. Mucous patches (glistening, white-to-red patches) are seen in the mouth or on other mucous membranes, and condyloma lata (white, smooth papules or plaques) are seen in the genital area. The secondary stage is often accompanied by fever, sore throat, malaise, and generalized lymphadenopathy. Secondary manifestations resolve without treatment in weeks to 12 months; all untreated cases will go on to latent infection. In the early years of latency, there might be recurrences of lesions of the skin and mucous membranes. Up to one-third of untreated patients will eventually exhibit signs and symptoms of tertiary syphilis.

In the primary and secondary stages, treponemal invasion of the central nervous system (CNS) and abnormalities in the cerebrospinal fluid (CSF) are common. Patients are most often asymptomatic, but some might develop acute syphilitic meningitis with cranial nerve palsies and deafness. CNS disease in the form of meningovascular syphilis might develop 5-12 years after initial infection, and paresis or tabes dorsalis might develop 15-20 years after initial infection.

Most untreated patients do not go on to develop tertiary syphilis but remain in the latent period for the rest of their lives. Five to twenty years after initial infection some untreated patients develop gummas of the skin, musculoskeletal system, or internal organs; syphilitic endarteritis with aortic and coronary artery disease; or CNS disease described earlier. The widespread use of antimicrobials has decreased the frequency of these tertiary manifestations.

Concurrent HIV infection might change the appearance and behavior of the primary and secondary mucocutaneous lesions and increase the risk of CNS disease in patients with syphilis. Neurosyphilis must be considered in the differential diagnosis of HIV-infected individuals with CNS symptoms and ocular and otologic complaints.

A woman with untreated early (primary, secondary, or early latent) syphilis during pregnancy has a very high risk of transmitting the infection to her fetus. Congenital syphilis can cause stillbirth, prematurity, neonatal death, or a live-born infant with a spectrum of clinical manifestations of congenital syphilis. Although these infants often appear normal at birth, early manifestations of congenital syphilis appear by 2 months of age and include failure to thrive, mucocutaneous abnormalities similar to those seen in secondary syphilis, organomegaly, anemia, bony lesions, and CNS abnormalities. Congenital infection might also result in late manifestations that appear by 2 years of age. These late manifestations include CNS abnormalities, such as interstitial keratitis, deafness, and bony or dental abnormalities such as notched incisors, saddle-nose deformities, or saber shins.

2. Causative agent—*Treponema pallidum*, subsp. *pallidum*, a spirochete.

3. Diagnosis—Testing usually begins with a nontreponemal serologic test such as the rapid plasma reagin. If that test is positive, the patient should have a confirmatory treponemal serologic test, such as the *T. pallidum* particle agglutination. When both tests are positive and the patient has never been treated for syphilis, the diagnosis is confirmed. For patients with a history of treatment for syphilis, reinfection is determined by a 4-fold increase in nontreponemal test titer compared to previous titers.

If testing begins with a treponemal test, such as an enzyme immunoassay (EIA) or a chemiluminesence immunoassay, patients who test positive should be tested with a nontreponemal test. When both are positive, results are interpreted as earlier. If only the treponemal test is positive, and the patient has never been treated for syphilis, the patient might have old untreated syphilis or early primary syphilis. In that case, a second treponemal test could be done, and if positive (or no second test is available), the patient should be treated. Patients do not require additional treatment if they have a positive treponemal test, a negative nontreponemal test, and a history of treatment for syphilis.

Patients in the early stage of disease with primary lesions may have negative serologic tests. Smears of lesion exudate can be examined for spirochetes using dark-field microscopy or polymerase chain reaction (PCR), or biopsy of the lesion can be performed for histology with immunofluorescent or other specific staining for spirochetes; however, these techniques may not be available in many laboratories. In cases where confirmatory tissue diagnosis is not available, patients should be treated based on clinical findings. Other causes of genital ulcers should also be considered and treated.

Infants should be screened by testing the mother's serum. This is because the infant's serum may be nonreactive if the mother's serologic test result is of low titer or if the mother was infected late in pregnancy. If maternal serum is not available, infant serum is preferred to cord blood. Syphilis patients with neurologic abnormalities or evidence of treatment failure may have neurosyphilis and should have CSF testing performed.

4. Occurrence—Syphilis occurs worldwide and is usually more prevalent in urban areas. After a period of decline from the late 1970s to the late 1990s, incidence in developed countries has increased again in recent years, notably in Western Europe and the USA, among men who have sex with men.

5. Reservoir—Humans.

6. Incubation period—10 days to 3 months, usually 3 weeks.

7. Transmission—Transmission of syphilis occurs when a person comes into direct contact with the primary or secondary lesions of an infected person. These lesions contain infectious spirochetes. Exposure is almost always through sexual contact during oral, vaginal, or anal sex. Because primary lesions might occur internally and secondary lesions may go unnoticed or undiagnosed, transmission might occur without either partner being aware of the disease. Transmission can also occur through blood transfusion if the donor is in the early stages of disease. Infection through contact with contaminated articles is very rare.

Fetal infection is most likely to occur if the mother is in primary, secondary, or early latent stage, but it can occur throughout the latent period. Infants can have infectious mucocutaneous lesions.

8. Risk groups—All people are considered susceptible to syphilis, though only approximately 30% of exposures result in infection. Untreated infection leads to gradual development of immunity against *T. pallidum* and, to some extent, against heterologous treponemes. Patients treated during the primary and secondary stages do not typically develop immunity and therefore remain susceptible to reinfection. Health professionals have developed primary lesions on the hands following unprotected clinical examination of infectious lesions.

9. Prevention—

1) Individuals can decrease their number of sex partners, establish mutually monogamous partnerships, and practice the correct and consistent use of condoms to decrease their risk of syphilis infection.

2) Health care providers should screen all patients with a confirmed or suspected sexually transmitted infection (STI), including HIV, for syphilis. High-risk groups according to local epidemiology, such as commercial sex workers and sexually active men who have sex with men, should be screened on a regular basis.

3) Pregnant women should be screened for syphilis at their first prenatal visit, and in high prevalence areas they should be screened again in the third trimester and at delivery.

4) Culturally appropriate prevention interventions should be available at low or no cost, including condoms, community-level education on the prevention of STIs, and health care for early diagnosis and treatment.

5) Through health care providers or public health organizations, cases should be interviewed to identify partners, and partners should be notified and treated.

10. Management of patient—All patients with syphilis should be tested for other STIs, particularly HIV. Universal precautions should be used when coming into contact with blood, lesion exudates, or other body fluids from patients with syphilis. Ideally, all patients should receive parenteral long-acting penicillin. The form and dose of penicillin depend on the stage and clinical manifestations of syphilis in the particular patient. Primary, secondary, and early latent (those known to be infected <1 year) syphilis are treated with 1 dose of intramuscular benzathine penicillin G, and late latent syphilis or those with unknown duration of latency are treated with 3 doses. Patients with CNS disease at any stage require intravenous aqueous crystalline penicillin G or procaine penicillin plus probenecid for 2 weeks.

There is limited data on the effectiveness of nonpenicillin regimens for syphilis. In nonpregnant, penicillin-allergic patients, regimens of doxycycline, tetracycline, or ceftriaxone can be tried with close follow-up.

Pregnant, penicillin-allergic patients should have their allergy verified with testing if possible, and then, if true allergy exists, they should be desensitized and treated with penicillin.

Patients should abstain from sexual contact until their treatment is completed and lesions disappear. To avoid reinfection, patients should not have sex with previous partners until the partners have also been treated.

Treatment failures might occur with any regimen. In patients who develop new clinical signs and symptoms of syphilis or a sustained 4-fold increase in nontreponemal titers, reinfection or treatment failure should be suspected. These patients should be evaluated and retreated. Most patients have a 4-fold decline in nontreponemal titers 6–12 months following appropriate therapy. Patients who do not have this expected titer drop should be tested for HIV, and evaluation for CNS disease with CSF testing should be considered; however, the ideal management of these patients is unclear. In HIV-infected patients, close follow-up with repeat serologic testing should be considered at 3, 6, 9, 12, and 24 months. Clinicians should examine the CSF of HIV-infected patients who do not respond appropriately to syphilis therapy.

11. Management of contacts and the immediate environment— Interviewing patients to identify sexual contacts is a fundamental part of syphilis control. The patient's stage of disease determines which partners should be notified and tested:

1) For primary syphilis, all sexual contacts during the 3 months preceding onset of symptoms.
2) For secondary syphilis, all contacts during the 6 months preceding onset of symptoms.
3) For early latent syphilis, those of the preceding year.
4) For late latent syphilis, long-standing partners and children if mothers are infected.
5) For congenital syphilis, all members of the immediate family.

Patients and their partners must be encouraged to obtain HIV counseling and testing. All infants born to seroreactive mothers should be treated unless it is documented that the mother had adequate penicillin-based treatment at least 30 days prior to delivery.

12. Special considerations—

1) Reporting: case report of early infectious syphilis and congenital syphilis is required in most countries; laboratories must report reactive serology and positive dark-field examinations in many areas. Confidentiality of the individual must be ensured.
2) Epidemic measures: intensification of measures outlined Prevention and Management of Contacts and the Immediate

Environment in this chapter. In protracted epidemics in selected populations (e.g., commercial sex workers) that remain refractory to standard interventions, mass treatment of the at-risk population might be considered.

3) International measures:

- Examine groups of adolescents and adults who emigrate from areas of high prevalence for treponemal infections.
- Adhere to international agreements concerning records, provision of diagnostic, and treatment facilities, and contact interviews at seaports for foreign merchant seamen (e.g., Brussels Agreement).
- Provide for rapid international exchange of information about contacts.

WHO Collaborating Centres provide support as required. Further information can be found at: http://www.who.int/collaboratingcentres/database/en.

[C. E. Introcaso, T. Peterman]

TAPEWORM

DISEASE	ICD-10 CODE
DWARF TAPEWORM	ICD-10 B71.0
RAT TAPEWORM	ICD-10 B71.0
DOG TAPEWORM	ICD-10 B71.1
BROAD OR FISH TAPEWORM	ICD-10 B70.0
TAENIASIS	ICD-10 B68
TAENIA SOLIUM TAENIASIS, INTESTINAL FORM	ICD-10 B68.0
TAENIA SAGINATA TAENIASIS	ICD-10 B68.1
TAENIASIS, UNSPECIFIED	ICD-10 B68.9
CYSTICERCOSIS	ICD-10 B69
Echinococcosis (see ''Echinococcosis'')	

I. DWARF TAPEWORM (hymenolepiasis due to *Hymenolepis nana*)

1. **Clinical features**—An intestinal infection with very small tapeworms; usually an infection of children. Light infections are usually

asymptomatic. Massive numbers of worms may cause enteritis with or without diarrhea, abdominal pain, and other nondescript symptoms such as pallor, loss of weight, and weakness.

2. Causative agent—*Hymenolepis nana* (dwarf tapeworm), the only human tapeworm without an obligatory intermediate host.

3. Diagnosis—Identification of eggs in feces; may require examination of multiple stool samples.

4. Occurrence—Cosmopolitan; more common in warm than cold and in dry than wet climates. Dwarf tapeworm is the most common human tapeworm in the USA and Latin America; it is also reported in Australia, Mediterranean countries, the Near East, and India.

5. Reservoir—Humans and rodents.

6. Incubation period—Onset of symptoms is variable; the development of mature worms requires about 2 weeks.

7. Transmission—Eggs of *H. nana* are infective when passed in feces, and therefore autoinfection or person-to-person transmission can occur. Infection is acquired through ingestion of eggs in contaminated food or water; directly from fecal-contaminated fingers; or through ingestion of insects such as mealworms, larval fleas, and beetles bearing larvae (cysticercoids) that have developed from eggs ingested by the insect. *H. nana* eggs, once ingested by humans, hatch in the intestine, liberating oncospheres that enter mucosal villi and develop into cysticercoids; these rupture into the lumen and grow into adult tapeworms. The infection is communicable for as long as eggs are passed in feces and may persist for years.

8. Risk groups—Children are more likely to be infected and susceptible to disease than adults; intensive infection occurs in immuno-deficient and malnourished children.

9. Prevention—

1) Educate the public in personal hygiene, especially handwashing, and safe disposal of feces.
2) Provide and maintain clean toilet facilities.
3) Protect food and water from contamination with human and rodent feces.
4) Treat those infected to remove sources of infection.
5) Eliminate rodents from home environment.

10. **Management of patient**—

1) Safe disposal of feces.
2) Treatment: drug of choice is praziquantel. Alternatively, niclosamide can be used but multiple doses are necessary for cure, and it is not available for human use in some countries. Nitazoxanide may be effective.

11. **Management of contacts and the immediate environment**— Fecal examination of family or institution members.

12. **Special considerations**—Outbreaks in schools and institutions can best be controlled through treatment of infected persons and special attention to personal and group hygiene.

II. RAT TAPEWORM (hymenolepiasis due to *Hymenolepis diminuta*)

Infection with the rat tapeworm, *Hymenolepis diminuta*, occurs accidentally in humans, usually in young children. Eggs passed in rodent feces are ingested by insects such as flea larvae, grain beetles, and cockroaches, in which cysticercoids develop in the hemocele. The mature tapeworm develops in rats, mice, or other rodents when the insect is ingested. People are rare accidental hosts, usually having a single or few tapeworms, and human infections are rarely symptomatic. Definitive diagnosis is based on finding characteristic eggs in the feces and treatment as for *H. nana*.

III. DOG TAPEWORM (dipylidiasis)

Toddler-age children are occasionally infected with the dog tapeworm (*Dipylidium caninum*), a parasite of dogs and cats worldwide. Infected children are usually asymptomatic, but parents may be alarmed by motile, seed-like proglottids (tapeworm segments) at the child's anus or on the surface of the stool. Infection is acquired when the child accidentally ingests adult fleas that, in their larval stage, have eaten eggs from proglottids. In 3–4 weeks the tapeworm becomes mature. Infection is prevented by keeping dogs and cats free of fleas and worms; treatment as for *H. nana*.

IV. BROAD OR FISH TAPEWORM (diphyllobothriasis)

1. **Clinical features**—An intestinal tapeworm infection of long duration. Symptoms are commonly trivial or absent; some patients, however, develop vitamin B12 deficiency anemia (*Diphyllobothrium latum* infections). Massive infections may be associated with diarrhea, obstruction of the bile duct or intestine, and toxic symptoms.

2. Causative agents—*D. latum* and 14 other primarily zoonotic species including *D. nihonkaiense*, *D. cordatum*, *D. lanceolatum*, *D. pacificum*, *D. dendriticum*, *D. ursi*, *D. dalliae,* and *D. klebanovskii*.

3. Diagnosis—Identification of eggs or segments (proglottids) of the worm in feces; may require examination of multiple stool samples.

4. Occurrence—The disease occurs in lake regions in the northern hemisphere and in subarctic, temperate, and tropical zones where eating raw or partly cooked freshwater fish is popular. Prevalence increases with age. In North America, endemic foci have been found among Eskimos in Alaska and Canada. Japan and Peru report cases of *D. nihonkaiense* infection among consumers of marine fish.

5. Reservoir—Primarily humans for *D. latum*; dogs, bears, and other fish-eating mammals and seagulls for the other *Diphyllobothrium* species.

6. Incubation period—3-6 weeks from ingestion of infected fish to passage of eggs in the stool.

7. Transmission—Humans acquire the infection by eating raw or inadequately cooked fish. Eggs in mature segments of the worm are discharged in feces into bodies of fresh or salt water where they mature and hatch; ciliated embryos (coracidium) infect the first intermediate host, usually copepods of the genera *Cyclops* and *Diaptomus*, and become procercoid larvae. Depending on the parasite species, freshwater, anadromous, or marine fish are second intermediate hosts when they ingest infected copepods; freshwater fish hosts include trout, pike, turbot, and perch; anadromous and salt water hosts include Pacific and Atlantic salmon and whitefish. The procercoid larvae transform into plerocercoids in the fish. This stage is infective for people, fish-eating mammals (e.g., foxes, mink, bears, cats, dogs, pigs, walruses, seals), and seagulls.

No direct person-to-person transmission. Humans and other definitive hosts disseminate eggs into the environment as long as worms remain in the intestine, sometimes for many years.

8. Risk groups—Those eating raw or undercooked fish that was harvested in geographic areas where transmission occurs..

9. Prevention—Cooking fish to an internal temperature of 63°C/ 145°F; freezing at −35°C/−31°F or below until solid and storing at that temperature or below for 15 hours or storing at −20°C/−4°F or below for 24 hours; freezing at −20°C/−4°F or below for 7 days; or applying radiation (irradiation).

10. **Management of patient—**

1) Sanitary disposal of feces.
2) Treatment: drug of choice is praziquantel; niclosamide is an alternative treatment but is not available for human use in some countries. Cobalamin injections and folic acid supplements may benefit patients with evidence of vitamin B_{12} deficiency.

11. **Management of contacts and the immediate environment—** No requirements.

12. **Special considerations—**Reporting: report indicated if a commercial source is implicated.

V. TAENIASIS AND CYSTICERCOSIS

1. **Clinical features—**Taeniasis is an intestinal infection with the adult stage of large tapeworms; cysticercosis is a potentially fatal tissue infection with the larval stage of one species, *Taenia solium*. Clinical manifestations of infection with the adult worm, if present, are variable and may include nervousness, insomnia, anorexia, weight loss, abdominal pain, and digestive disturbances. Except for the annoyance of having segments of worms emerging from the anus, many infections are asymptomatic.

Cysticercosis may produce serious somatic disease when larvae localize in the muscles, eye, or central nervous system (CNS). Clinical manifestations of cysticercosis depend on the number, location, and stage (viable, degenerating, or calcified) of the cysticerci and the intensity of the inflammatory response. The most important clinical manifestations occur when cysticerci are located in the brain. Seizures are the most common CNS manifestation; encephalitis, intracranial hypertension, hydrocephalus, chronic meningitis, and cranial nerve abnormalities are less frequent. CNS cysticercosis, or neurocysticercosis, may cause serious disability but with a relatively low case-fatality rate.

2. **Causative agents—***T. solium*, the pork tapeworm, causes both intestinal infection with the adult worm and extraintestinal infection with the larvae (cysticerci). *T. saginata*, the beef tapeworm, only causes intestinal infection with the adult worm in humans. *T. asiatica* is a recently classified organism that causes human infections similar to that caused by *T. saginata*.

3. **Diagnosis—**Infection with an adult tapeworm is diagnosed by identification of proglottids (segments), eggs, or antigens of the worm in the feces; examination of several samples may be necessary to detect eggs. Eggs of *T. solium* and *T. saginata* cannot be differentiated morphologically. Specific diagnosis is based on the morphology of the scolex (head) and/or

gravid proglottids. Specific serological tests should support the clinical diagnosis of cysticercosis. Subcutaneous cysticerci may be visible or palpable; microscopic examination of an excised cysticercus confirms the diagnosis. Cysticercosis in intracerebral and other tissues may be recognized by computerized axial tomography (CAT) scan or magnetic resonance imaging (MRI). Standard radiography is of limited use for detection of calcified cysticerci.

4. Occurrence—Worldwide; particularly frequent wherever beef or pork is eaten raw or insufficiently cooked and where sanitary conditions allow pigs and cattle to have access to human feces. Prevalence is highest in parts of Latin America, Africa, south and southeastern Asia, and eastern Europe. In Latin America, seroprevalence of cysticercosis in endemic villages has been reported to be 10%-25%. In some of the *T. solium*-endemic regions this tapeworm is considered responsible for more than 10% of acute case admission to neurological wards and one-third of late onset seizures. Transmission of *T. solium* is rare in Canada, the USA, western Europe, and most parts of Asia and the Pacific. Human infections with *T. asiatica* have been reported in Taiwan (China), Indonesia, the Republic of Korea, and Thailand.

5. Reservoir—Humans are the definitive host of all 3 species of *Taenia*; cattle are the intermediate hosts for *T. saginata* and pigs for *T. solium* and *T. asiatica*.

6. Incubation period—Symptoms of cysticercosis may appear from months to years after infection. For tapeworm infections, eggs appear in the stool 8-12 weeks after consumption of infected pork for *T. solium* and 10-14 weeks after consumption of infected beef for *T. saginata*.

7. Transmission—Eggs of *T. saginata* passed in the stool of an infected person are infectious only to cattle. The eggs develop into cysticerci in the muscle tissue of the cow. In humans, infection follows ingestion of raw or undercooked beef containing cysticerci; in the intestine, the adult worm develops attached to the jejunal mucosa.

Intestinal tapeworm infection due to *T. solium* in humans follows ingestion of raw or undercooked pork infected with cysticerci ("measly pork"), with subsequent development of the adult worm in the intestine. Human cysticercosis occurs when a person ingests *T. solium* eggs that are passed in the feces of a human tapeworm carrier. This can happen by drinking contaminated water or food or by putting contaminated fingers to the mouth. Importantly, a human tapeworm carrier can infect himself or herself with tapeworm eggs, resulting in cysticercosis (autoinfection), and can contaminate others in the household.

Ingested eggs hatch in the small intestine, and the larvae migrate hematogenously to the subcutaneous tissues, striated muscles, and other tissues and vital organs of the body where they form cysticerci.

T. asiatica infection is acquired by eating uncooked liver and other viscera of pigs infected with cysticerci of the parasite. In experimental studies this organism produced cysticerci only in the viscera of pigs, cattle, goats, and monkeys. It is unknown if human cysticercosis occurs with this species.

Eggs of both *T. solium* and *T. saginata* are disseminated into the environment as long as the worm remains in the intestine; the tapeworm lives about 3-5 years, while eggs may remain viable in the environment for months.

8. Risk groups—People who consume undercooked or raw pork or beef in areas with poor sanitation are at risk for adult tapeworm infection. People are at risk for cysticercosis if they live in areas where *T. solium* tapeworm infection is common. The greatest risk for cysticercosis is being a household member of a *T. solium* tapeworm carrier.

9. Prevention—

1) Cysticercosis can be prevented by improving public health education and sanitary measures.

2) Educate the public to prevent fecal contamination of soil, water, and human and animal food; to avoid use of sewage effluents for pasture irrigation; and to cook beef and pork thoroughly.

3) Identification and immediate treatment or institution of enteric precautions for people harboring adult *T. solium* is essential for prevention of human cysticercosis. *T. solium* eggs are infective immediately on leaving the host and may produce severe human illness.

4) Thoroughly cook meat to an internal temperature of 63°C/145°F and ground meat to at least 71°C/160°F. Freezing pork or beef at a temperature below −5°C (23°F) for more than 4 days kills the cysticerci effectively. Irradiation is very effective at 1 kGy.

5) Inspection of carcasses of cattle and swine will detect only a proportion of those that are infected; these should be condemned, irradiated, or processed into cooked products.

6) Prevent swine and cattle access to latrines and human feces.

10. Management of patient—

1) Dispose of feces in a sanitary manner; emphasize strict sanitation with handwashing after defecating and before eating, especially for *T. solium*.

2) Treatment: praziquantel is effective in the treatment of *T. saginata* and *T. solium* intestinal tapeworm infections. Niclosamide is an

effective alternative but is not widely available. Patients with neurocysticercosis require careful evaluation and tailored treatment based on their clinical manifestations and location and number and stage of cysticerci. The first goal of therapy is to control seizures, intracranial hypertension, edema, or hydrocephalus; in rare cases, emergency surgical intervention is indicated to prevent intracranial herniation. Treatment with praziquantel or albendazole may cause an inflammatory response to dying cysticerci, requiring administration of corticosteroids to help control cerebral edema. Where anthelminthic treatment is not indicated, symptomatic treatment, such as with antiepileptic drugs, may bring relief.

11. Management of contacts and the immediate environment— Investigation of contacts and source of infection. Evaluate symptomatic contacts. Ensure good sanitation and human waste disposal.

12. Special considerations—Reporting: reporting to local health authority may be required in some locations.

[S. Montgomery, P. Cantey]

TETANUS
(lockjaw)

DISEASE	ICD-10 CODE
TETANUS	ICD-10 A35
OBSTETRICAL TETANUS	ICD-10 A34
TETANUS NEONATORUM	ICD-10 A33

1. Clinical features—Tetanus is an acute disease that is caused by an exotoxin produced by the anaerobic bacterium *Clostridium tetani* at the site of an injury. However, history of an injury or an apparent portal of entry may be lacking. Four clinical types of disease are often described: generalized, localized, cephalic, and neonatal. Generalized tetanus is characterized by painful muscular contractions, primarily of the masseter and neck muscles (trismus), and secondarily of trunk muscles. Generalized spasms are frequently induced by sensory stimuli; typical features of the tetanic spasm are extreme hyperextension of the body, in which the head and heels are bent backward and the spine arches forward (opisthotonos), and the facial expression known as "risus sardonicus." A common first sign suggestive of tetanus in older children and adults is abdominal rigidity, though rigidity is sometimes confined to the region of injury (localized tetanus). Infected wounds of the head and neck area can lead to cranial nerve dysfunction or cephalic tetanus.

Tetanus neonatorum (neonatal tetanus) is typified by a newborn infant who sucks and cries well for the first few days after birth but who subsequently develops progressive difficulty and then inability to feed because of trismus—generalized stiffness with spasms or convulsions and opisthotonos.

The case-fatality rate of tetanus ranges from 10% to more than 80% depending on age, the quality of care available, and the length of the incubation period. Case-fatality rates for neonatal tetanus are highest, exceeding 80% among those with short incubation periods. Neurological sequelae including mild retardation occur in 5% to over 20% of those infants who survive. The case-fatality rate is also high in the elderly and varies inversely with the availability of experienced intensive care unit personnel and resources and with the length of the incubation period.

2. **Causative agent**—*C. tetani*, the tetanus bacillus.

3. **Diagnosis**—Attempts at laboratory confirmation are of little help. A negative culture does not rule out the diagnosis as the organism is rarely recovered from the site of infection, and usually antitetanus antibodies are undetectable in most cases.

4. **Occurrence**—Worldwide. The disease is sporadic and relatively uncommon in most industrialized countries but is more common in agricultural regions and in areas where contact with animal excreta is more likely and immunization is inadequate. Parenteral use of drugs, particularly intramuscular or subcutaneous injection, can result in individual cases and occasional circumscribed outbreaks. In 2006, an estimated 290,000 people worldwide died of tetanus, most of them in Asia, Africa, and South America. Populations in rural and tropical areas are especially at risk, and tetanus neonatorum is common.

Tetanus neonatorum is a serious health problem in many developing countries where maternity care services are limited and immunization against tetanus is inadequate. In the past 10 years the incidence of tetanus neonatorum has declined considerably in many developing countries as a result of improved training of birth attendants, hygienic deliveries, and immunization coverage with tetanus toxoid for women of childbearing age. Despite this decline, WHO estimated in 2011 that tetanus neonatorum still caused about 61,000 deaths, mainly in the developing world.

5. **Reservoir**—Spores of *C. tetani* are ubiquitous in the environment and are normal but harmless inhabitants of intestines of horses and other

animals. Tetanus spores in soil or fomites contaminated with animal and human feces can contaminate wounds of all types.

6. Incubation period—Usually 3-21 days, although it may range from 1 day to several months, depending on the character, extent, and location of the wound. Most cases occur within 14 days. In general, shorter incubation periods are associated with more heavily contaminated wounds, more severe disease, and a worse prognosis.

For tetanus neonatorum, the average incubation period is about 6 days, with a range from 3-28 days.

7. Transmission—No direct person-to-person transmission. Tetanus spores are usually introduced into the body through a puncture wound contaminated with soil, street dust, or animal or human feces; through a laceration, burns, and even a trivial or unnoticed wound; or by injected, contaminated drugs (e.g., street drugs). Tetanus occasionally follows surgical procedures, such as circumcision and abortions performed under unhygienic conditions. The presence of necrotic tissue and/or foreign bodies favors growth of the anaerobic pathogen. Cases have followed injuries considered too trivial for medical consultation.

Tetanus neonatorum usually occurs through introduction of tetanus spores via the umbilical cord during delivery through the use of an unclean instrument to cut the cord or after delivery by "dressing" the umbilical stump with substances heavily contaminated with tetanus spores, frequently as part of natal rituals.

Recovery from tetanus may not result in immunity; second attacks can occur and primary immunization is indicated after recovery.

8. Risk groups—Those with greater than usual risk of traumatic and puncture injury, especially workers in contact with soil, sewage, and domestic animals; members of the military forces; policemen, and others with greater than usual risk of traumatic injury; adults with diabetes mellitus; older adults who are currently at highest risk for tetanus and tetanus-related mortality; and unvaccinated women of reproductive age and their newborns. Most newborn infants with neonatal tetanus are born to nonimmunized mothers delivered by an untrained birth attendant outside a hospital.

9. Prevention—

1) Educate the public on the necessity for complete immunization with tetanus toxoid, the hazards of puncture wounds and closed injuries that are particularly liable to be complicated by tetanus, and the potential need after injury for active and/or passive prophylaxis.

2) Universal active immunization with adsorbed tetanus toxoid (TT), which gives durable protection for at least 10 years; after the initial basic series has been completed, single booster doses elicit high levels of immunity.

- For children younger than 7 years, tetanus toxoid is generally administered together with diphtheria toxoid and pertussis vaccine as a triple (diphtheria/tetanus and whole-cell pertussis vaccine [DTP] or diphtheria/tetanus and acellular pertussis vaccine [DTaP]) antigen or as double (diphtheria/tetanus vaccine [DT]) antigen when contraindications to pertussis vaccine exist. Immunization should be initiated in infancy with a formulation containing diphtheria toxoid, tetanus toxoid, and either acellular pertussis antigens (DTaP, preferred in many industrialized countries) or DTP. WHO recommends at least 3 primary DTP or DTaP doses given intramuscularly (IM) and starting as early as 6 months of age with a minimum interval of 4 weeks between doses, and a DTP booster given at 1-6 years. Some currently available formulations combine DTP or DTaP with one or more of the following: *Haemophilus influenzae* type b vaccine, poliomyelitis vaccine, or hepatitis B vaccine.

- For persons older than 7 years, tetanus and diphtheria (Td) vaccine is recommended for primary vaccination and boosters. For adolescents and adults and where available, combined tetanus, diphtheria, and acellular pertussis (Tdap) vaccine can be safely used as a single dose and for boosting as part of wound prophylaxis instead of Td. In countries with inadequate immunization coverage for children, all pregnant women should receive 2 doses of tetanus toxoid in the first pregnancy with an interval of at least 1 month and with the second dose at least 2 weeks prior to childbirth in order to prevent maternal and neonatal tetanus. Booster doses may be necessary to ensure ongoing protection (discussed later).

- Nonadsorbed ("plain") tetanus toxoid vaccines, as opposed to alum adjuvant tetanus toxoid preparations, are less immunogenic for primary immunization or booster shots. Minor local reactions following tetanus toxoid injections are relatively frequent but not clinically significant; severe local and systemic reactions are infrequent but do occur, particularly in persons who have received an excessive number of prior doses.

- Active immunity induced by tetanus toxoid persists for at least 10 years after full primary immunization and should be maintained by administering a dose of Td every 10 years thereafter. For added protection against pertussis, a one-time dose of Tdap may be substituted for the next Td dose in a person older than 18 years of age.

- Tetanus toxoid is recommended for universal use regardless of age; it is especially important for workers in contact with soil, sewage, and domestic animals; members of the military forces; policemen and others with greater than usual risk of traumatic injury; adults with diabetes mellitus; older adults who are currently at highest risk for tetanus and tetanus-related mortality; and women of reproductive age and newborns.

- For children and adults who are severely immunocompromised or infected with HIV, tetanus toxoid is indicated in the same schedule and dose as for immunocompetent persons, even though the immune response may be suboptimal.

- Transient passive immunity follows injection of tetanus immune globulin (TIG) or tetanus antitoxin (equine origin). Infants of actively immunized mothers acquire passive immunity that protects them from neonatal tetanus.

3) Prevention of tetanus neonatorum: improving maternity care, with emphasis on clean deliveries and increasing the tetanus toxoid immunization coverage of women of childbearing age (especially pregnant women).

- Nonimmunized pregnant women should receive at least 2 doses of tetanus toxoid, preferably as Td, with the first dose at initial contact or as early as possible during pregnancy and the second dose 4 weeks after the first and preferably at least 2 weeks before delivery. A third dose could be given 6–12 months after the second or during the next pregnancy. An additional 2 doses should be given at annual intervals or during subsequent pregnancies. In some industrialized countries including the USA, Tdap is recommended during pregnancy, preferably after the first trimester. A 5-dose series of tetanus toxoid protects the previously unimmunized woman throughout the entire child-bearing period. Women whose infants have a risk of neonatal tetanus, but who themselves have received 3 or 4 doses of DTP/DTaP as children, need only receive 2 doses of tetanus toxoid during each of their first 2 pregnancies.

- Increasing the proportion of deliveries attended by trained attendants. Important control measures include licensing of midwives, providing professional supervision and education as to methods, equipment, and techniques of asepsis in childbirth, and educating mothers, relatives, and attendants in the practice of strict asepsis of the umbilical stump. The latter is especially important in many areas where strips of bamboo are used to sever the umbilical cord or where ashes, cow dung poultices, or other contaminated substances are traditionally applied to the umbilicus. In those areas, any woman of childbearing age visiting a health facility should be screened and offered immunization, no matter what the reason for the visit.

4) Prophylaxis in wound management: tetanus prophylaxis in managing patients with wounds is based on careful assessment of whether the wound is clean or contaminated and the immunization status of the patient. It requires proper use of tetanus toxoid and/or TIG, wound cleaning, and—where required—surgical debridement and the proper use of antibiotics.

- Those who have been completely immunized and who sustain minor and uncontaminated wounds require a booster dose of toxoid only if more than 10 years have elapsed since the last dose was given. For major and/or contaminated wounds, a single booster injection of tetanus toxoid (preferably as Td or Tdap) should be administered promptly on the day of injury if the patient has not received tetanus toxoid within the preceding 5 years.

- Persons who have not completed a full primary series of tetanus toxoid require a dose of toxoid as soon as possible following the wound and may require passive immunization with human TIG if the wound is major and/or if it is contaminated with soil containing animal excreta. DTP/ DTaP, DT, or Td, as determined by the age of the patient and previous immunization history, should be used at the time of the wound and ultimately to complete the primary series. Passive immunization with at least 250 IU of human-derived TIG IM (or 1,500–5,000 IU of antitoxin of animal origin, if human TIG is not available), regardless of the patient's age, is indicated for patients with other than clean, minor wounds and a history of none, unknown, or fewer than 3 previous tetanus toxoid doses. When tetanus toxoid is given concurrently with human TIG (or equine antitoxin), separate syringes and separate sites must be used. When antitoxin of animal origin is given, it is essential to avoid anaphylaxis by first injecting 0.02 ml of a 1:100 dilution in physiologic saline intradermally with a syringe containing adrenaline on hand. Pretest with a 1:1000 dilution if there has been prior animal serum exposure, together with a similar injection of physiologic saline as a negative control. If after 15–20 minutes there is a wheal with surrounding erythema at least 3 mm larger than the negative control, it is necessary to desensitize the individual.

- Antibiotics may theoretically prevent the multiplication of *C. tetani* in the wound and thus reduce production of toxin, but this does not obviate the need for prompt treatment of the wound together with appropriate immunization. Metronidazole is the most appropriate antibiotic in terms of recovery time and case-fatality rate and should be given for 7–14 days in large doses; this also allows for a reduction in the amount of muscle relaxants and sedatives required.
- The wound should be debrided widely if possible. Wide debridement of the umbilical stump in neonates is not indicated.

10. **Management of patient—**

1) Case investigation to determine circumstances of injury.
2) Treatment: see Prophylaxis in Prevention in this chapter.
3) Maintain an adequate airway and employ sedation as indicated; muscle relaxant drugs, together with tracheotomy or nasotracheal intubation and mechanically assisted respiration, may be lifesaving.

11. **Management of contacts and the immediate environment—** Not applicable.

12. **Special considerations—**

1) Reporting: case report to local health authority required in most countries.
2) Epidemic measures: in the rare case of an outbreak, search for source, especially contaminated street drugs or other common-use injections.
3) Disaster implications: social upheaval (military conflicts, riots) and natural disasters (floods, hurricanes, earthquakes) that cause many traumatic injuries in nonimmunized populations may result in an increased need for TIG or tetanus antitoxin and toxoid for injured patients.
4) Up-to-date immunization against tetanus is advised for international travelers.

[T. S. P. Tiwari]

TOXOPLASMOSIS

DISEASE	ICD-10 CODE
TOXOPLASMOSIS	ICD-10 B58
CONGENITAL TOXOPLASMOSIS	ICD-10 P37.1

1. **Clinical features**—A systemic coccidian protozoan disease in which infections are frequently asymptomatic or present as acute disease with lymphadenopathy only, or resemble infectious mononucleosis, with fever, lymphadenopathy, and lymphocytosis persisting for days or weeks. Development of an immune response decreases parasitemia, but Toxoplasma cysts remaining in the tissues contain viable organisms. These cysts may reactivate if the immune system becomes compromised. Among immunodeficient individuals, including HIV-infected patients, primary or reactivated infection may cause a maculopapular rash, generalized skeletal muscle involvement, cerebritis, chorioretinitis, pneumonia, myocarditis, and/or death. Cerebral toxoplasmosis is a frequent component of AIDS.

Infections with genetically distinct subtypes have been described, predominantly in South America, with fatal outcome in otherwise immunocompetent patients. An increased occurrence of chronic chorioretinitis in acquired toxoplasmosis has also been described in this region.

A primary infection during early pregnancy may lead to fetal infection with death of the fetus or manifestations such as chorioretinitis, brain damage with intracerebral calcification, hydrocephaly, microcephaly, fever, jaundice, rash, hepatosplenomegaly, xanthochromic cerebrospinal fluid, and convulsions evident at birth or shortly thereafter. Later in pregnancy, maternal infection results in milder or subclinical fetal disease with delayed manifestations, such as recurrent or chronic chorioretinitis. In immunosuppressed pregnant women who are Toxoplasma-seropositive, a reactivation of latent infection may result in congenital toxoplasmosis, though this is thought to be a rare event.

2. **Causative agent**—*Toxoplasma gondii*, an intracellular coccidian protozoan that completes its sexual life cycle phase in cats and that belongs to the family *Sarcocystidae*, in the class *Sporozoa*.

3. **Diagnosis**—Based on clinical signs and supportive serological results, demonstration of the agent in body tissues or fluids by biopsy or necropsy, or isolation in animals or cell culture. Rising antibody titers are corroborative of active infection; the presence of specific immunoglobulin class M (IgM) and/or rising immunoglobulin class G (IgG) titers in sequential sera of newborns is conclusive evidence of congenital infection. The presence of immunoglobulin class A (IgA) is also helpful in determining infection in newborns. High IgG antibody levels may persist

for years with no relation to active disease. Reference laboratories may use the IgG avidity test, differential agglutination test, and IgA- and immunoglobulin class E (IgE)-specific antibody tests to help determine the timing of infection. In addition, polymerase chain reaction (PCR) assays of body fluids have been used to assist with the diagnosis.

4. Occurrence—Worldwide in mammals and birds. Infection in humans is common.

5. Reservoir—The definitive hosts of *T. gondii* are cats (felines), which acquire infection mainly from eating infected mammals (especially rodents) or birds, and probably also from oocysts in soil contaminated with cat feces, acquired during licking/grooming. Felines alone harbor parasites in the intestinal tract, where the sexual stage of the protozoan life cycle occurs, resulting in excretion of oocysts in feces for 10-20 days, and rarely longer. The intermediate hosts include sheep, goats, rodents, swine, cattle, chickens, and other birds; all may carry an infective stage encysted in tissue, especially muscle and brain. Tissue cysts remain viable for long periods, perhaps lifelong. Cattle seem to be only minimally affected by natural Toxoplasma infection.

6. Incubation period—From 10-23 days from ingestion of under-cooked meat in one common source outbreak; 5-20 days in another outbreak associated with cats.

7. Transmission—Transplacental infection occurs in humans when a pregnant woman has rapidly dividing cells (tachyzoites) circulating in the bloodstream, usually during primary infection. Children may become infected by ingesting infective oocystsin from sandboxes, playgrounds, and yards in which cats have defecated. Infections arise also from eating raw or undercooked infected meat containing tissue cysts (pork, mutton, or wild game, very rarely beef); ingesting infective oocysts on food such as raw vegetables; or ingesting water contaminated with feline feces. Presumed inhalation of sporulated oocysts was associated with one outbreak; another was associated epidemiologically with consumption of raw goat milk. Infection may occur through blood transfusion or organ transplantation from an infected donor. No direct person-to-person transmission except in utero. Oocysts shed by cats sporulate and become infective 1-5 days later and may remain infective in water or moist soil for over a year. Cysts in the flesh of infected animals remain infective throughout the period during which fresh meat is edible and uncooked; freezing meat, however, destroys infectivity.

Susceptibility to infection is general, but immunity is readily acquired and most infections are asymptomatic. Duration and degree of immunity are unknown but they are assumed to be long-lasting or permanent; antibodies persist for years, probably for life.

8. Risk groups—Risk for infection is primarily from cat feces or soil contaminated with cat feces and from ingestion of undercooked contaminated meat. In addition, infection can occur through blood transfusion or organ transplantation from an infected donor. Pregnant women who have not previously been infected with *T. gondii* are at risk for acute infection and congenital transmission to the fetus. Patients undergoing cytotoxic or immunosuppressive treatment and HIV-infected patients are at high risk of developing illness from reactivated infection.

9. **Prevention—**

1) Educate pregnant women about preventive measures:

   - Use irradiated meats or cook them to 66°C (150°F) before eating. Freezing meat down to −20°C (−4°F) for 24 hours is a good alternative. Carefully wash/clean raw vegetables before eating.
   - Unless they are known to have antibodies to *T. gondii*, pregnant women should avoid changing cat litter if possible. If no one else can perform the task, they should wear disposable gloves and wash their hands with soap and warm water afterwards. They should wear gloves during gardening and wash hands thoroughly afterward.
   - Raw fruits and vegetables should be peeled or thoroughly washed before eating.

2) Wash hands thoroughly before eating and after handling raw meat or after contact with soil possibly contaminated with cat feces. Cutting boards, dishes, counters, and utensils should be washed after contact with raw meat.

3) Cats should be fed dry, canned, or boiled food and discouraged from hunting (i.e., kept as indoor pets only).

4) Dispose of cat feces and litter daily (before sporocysts become infective). Feces can be disposed in trash destined for landfills, burned, or deeply buried. Disinfect litter pans by scalding; wear gloves or wash hands thoroughly after handling potentially infective material. Dispose of dried litter without shaking to avoid aerial dispersal of oocysts.

5) Control stray cats and prevent their access to sandboxes and sand piles used by children for play. Keep sandboxes covered when not in use.

6) Avoid drinking untreated water.

7) Toxoplasma-seropositive patients who have a cluster of differentiation 4 glycoprotein + (CD4+) T-lymphocyte count less than 100/μL should be administered prophylaxis against toxoplasmic encephalitis. A double-strength tablet daily dose of trimethoprim-sulfamethoxazole is the preferred regimen.

8) Patients with AIDS who have experienced symptomatic toxoplasmosis must receive prophylactic treatment throughout life with pyrimethamine, sulfadiazine, and folinic acid.

10. Management of patient—Treatment: not routinely indicated for a healthy immunocompetent host, except for confirmed initial infection during pregnancy or presence of active chorioretinitis, myocarditis, or other organ involvement. Pyrimethamine combined with sulfadiazine and folinic acid (to avoid bone marrow depression) for 4 weeks is the preferred treatment for those with severe symptomatic disease. Clindamycin has also been used in combination with pryimethamine and folinic acid as an alternative to treat ocular toxoplasmosis. In ocular disease, systemic corticosteroids are indicated when irreversible loss of vision can occur from lesions of the macula, papillomacular bundle, or optic nerve.

Treatment of pregnant women is problematic. Spiramycin is commonly used to prevent placental infection; pyrimethamine, sulfadiazine, and folinic acid should be considered if ultrasound, PCR of amniotic fluid, or other investigations indicate that fetal infection has occurred. Because of concerns about possible teratogenicity, pyrimethamine should not be given during the first 16 weeks of pregnancy; sulfadiazine may be administered alone in this case. Infants whose mothers had primary infections or were HIV positive during pregnancy should be treated with pyrimethamine-sulfadiazine-folinic acid during their first year of life or until congenital infection is ruled out in an attempt to prevent chorioretinitis and other sequelae. At time of writing, there is as yet no international consensus on the correct management of infants born to HIV-infected mothers who are seropositive for Toxoplasma.

11. Management of contacts and the immediate environment— In congenital cases, determine antibody titers in mother and child; in acquired cases, determine antibody titers in members of the household and common exposure to cat feces, soil, untreated water, raw meat, or unwashed vegetables.

12. Special considerations—

1) Reporting: reportable in some countries to facilitate further epidemiological understanding of the disease.
2) International measures: the EU zoonosis directive (92/117 EEG) mentions toxoplasmosis under category B (collection of data in Member States when available). WHO Collaborating Centres provide support as required. Further information can be found at: http://www.who.int/collaboratingcentres/database/en.

[J. Jones, F. Meslin, H. V. Nielsen]

❖

TRACHOMA

DISEASE	ICD-10 CODE
TRACHOMA	ICD-10 A71
Pneumonia due to *chlamydia trachomatis* (see "Pneumonia")	

1. **Clinical features**—A chlamydial conjunctivitis of insidious or abrupt onset; the infection may persist for a few weeks if untreated and tends to resolve with no consequence; in hyperendemic areas the characteristic lifetime duration of active disease is the result of frequent reinfections. Conjunctivitis ("active disease") is characterized by the presence of lymphoid follicles and diffuse conjunctival inflammation (papillary hypertrophy), particularly on the tarsal conjunctiva lining the upper eyelid. The inflammation can produce superficial vascularization of the cornea (pannus) and scarring of the conjunctiva, which increases with the severity and duration of inflammatory disease. The marked conjunctival scarring causes lid deformities and in-turning of eyelashes (entropion and trichiasis), which later in adult life cause chronic abrasion of the cornea and opacity in some individuals, resulting in visual impairment and blindness. Secondary bacterial infections frequently occur in populations with endemic trachoma and may contribute to the communicability and severity of the disease.

Active trachoma in some developing countries is an endemic early childhood disease. It may be clinically indistinguishable from conjunctivitis caused by other bacteria (including genital strains of *Chlamydia trachomatis*). Differential diagnosis includes molluscum contagiosum nodules of the eyelids, toxic reactions to chronically administered eye drops, and chronic staphylococcal lid-margin infection. An allergic reaction to contact lenses (giant papillary conjunctivitis) may produce a trachoma-like syndrome with tarsal nodules (giant papillae), conjunctival scarring, and corneal pannus.

2. **Causative agent**—*C. trachomatis* serovars A, B, Ba, and C; serovars B, Ba, and C have also been isolated from genital chlamydial infections.

3. **Diagnosis**—It is primarily made though clinical observation of the disease-specific signs. Confirmation of the causative organism can be made through polymerase chain reaction (PCR), Giemsa-stained smears for the detection of intracellular chlamydial elementary bodies in epithelial cells of conjunctival scrapings, immunofluorescence (IF) examination after methanol fixation of the smear, detection of chlamydial antigen by enzyme immunoassay (EIA) or deoxyribonucleic acid (DNA) by probe, or isolation of the agent in special cell culture.

4. Occurrence—Worldwide; as an endemic disease, most often of poor rural communities in developing countries. In endemic areas, trachoma presents in childhood, then subsides in adolescence, leaving varying degrees of potentially disabling scarring. Blinding trachoma is still widespread in sub-Saharan Africa. Pockets of blinding trachoma also occur in the Middle East, parts of the Indian subcontinent, southeastern Asia and China, Latin America, Australia (among Aboriginals), and the Pacific islands. The disease occurs among population groups with poor hygiene, poverty, and crowded living conditions, particularly in dry, dusty regions. The late complications of trachoma (trichiasis and corneal opacity) occur in older people who had active trachoma in childhood.

5. Reservoir—Humans.

6. Incubation period—From 5-12 days (based on volunteer studies).

7. Transmission—Through direct contact with infectious ocular or nasopharyngeal discharges on fingers or indirect contact with contaminated fomites such as towels, clothes, and nasopharyngeal discharges from infected people and materials soiled therewith. Flies, especially *Musca sorbens* in Africa and the Middle East, can contribute to the spread of the disease. In children with active trachoma, *Chlamydia* can be recovered from the nasopharynx and rectum, but the trachoma serovars do not appear to have a genital reservoir in endemic communities. The disease is probably communicable as long as active lesions are present in the conjunctivae and adnexal mucous membranes; communicability may continue for up to a few years. Concentration of the infectious agent in the tissues is greatly reduced with cicatrization but increases again with reactivation and recurrence of infective discharges. Infectivity ceases within 2-3 days of the start of antibiotic therapy, long before clinical improvement.

8. Risk groups—Susceptibility is general; while there is no absolute immunity conferred by infection, the severity of active disease due to reinfection gradually decreases over the childhood years, and active trachoma is no longer seen in older children or young adults. In endemic areas, children have active disease more frequently than adults. The severity of disease is often related to living conditions, particularly poor hygiene; exposure to dry winds, dust, and fine sand may also contribute.

9. Prevention—

1) Educate the public on the need for personal hygiene, especially to encourage face washing and avoid sharing towels.
2) Improve basic sanitation, including availability and use of soap and water.
3) Provide appropriate community-based (mass) treatment of meso- and hyperendemic populations with oral or topical

azithromycin to decrease the reservoir of infection and thereby reduce transmission.

4) Conduct epidemiological investigations to determine important factors in the occurrence of the disease for specific situations.

5) There is no available vaccine at present.

6) For those with trichiasis, surgery to reposition the eye lashes so that they no longer abrade the cornea.

10. **Management of patient—**

1) Treatment: in individuals with trichiasis, surgery to reposition the eye lashes so that they no longer abrade the cornea. In areas where the active trachoma is highly prevalent, community-based (mass) treatment of the whole population with oral or topical azithromycin.

2) Disinfection of contaminated fomites (hands, cloths, towels).

3) For hospitalized patients, drainage and secretion precautions.

11. Management of contacts and the immediate environment— Investigation of contacts and source of infection: members of family, playmates, and schoolmates.

12. **Special considerations—**

1) Reporting: case report to local health authority required in some countries of low endemicity.

2) Epidemic measures: in regions of hyperendemic prevalence, mass treatment campaigns have been successful in eliminating the disease as cause of visual impairment and blindness when associated with education in personal hygiene, especially cleanliness of the face and improvement of environmental hygiene (particularly increases in availability and use of water).

The WHO/Alliance for the Global Elimination of blinding Trachoma provides technical and coordination support. WHO Collaborating Centres can also provide support as required. Further information can be found at:

• http://www.who.int/blindness/causes/trachoma/en/index.html
• http://www.who.int/gho/neglected_diseases/en/index.html

[S. P. Mariotti, A. Solomon]

TRENCH FEVER
(quintana fever)

DISEASE	ICD-10 CODE
TRENCH FEVER	ICD-10 A79.0

1. Clinical features—A typically nonfatal, febrile bacterial septicemic disease varying in manifestations and severity, characterized by headache, malaise, shin pain, and dizziness. Onset is either sudden or gradual, and fever may be relapsing (usually with a 5-day periodicity), prolonged (typhoid-like), or limited to a single episode lasting several days. Splenomegaly, transient macular rash, and conjunctivitis may also be present. Symptoms may continue to recur many years after the primary infection; persistent bacteremia has been described. Bacteremia, osteomyelitis, lymphadenopathy, and bacillary angiomatosis can occur in immunocompromised patients, especially those with HIV infection. Endocarditis has been associated with trench fever infections, especially among homeless or alcoholic persons.

2. Causative agent—*Bartonella quintana* (formerly *Rochalimaea quintana*).

3. Diagnosis—Laboratory diagnosis is made by culture of patient blood on blood or chocolate agar under 5% CO_2. Microcolonies are visible after 8–21 days incubation at 37°C (98.6°F). Serologic testing may be performed using a commercially available immunofluorescence assay (IFA) test; this test may cross-react with other *Bartonella* spp., *Coxiella burnetii*, and *Chlamydia*. Polymerase chain reaction (PCR) of resected heart valve tissue may aid diagnosis of endocarditis.

4. Occurrence—Epidemics of trench fever occurred in Europe during World Wars I and II among those living in crowded, unhygienic conditions. Since then, *B. quintana* infections have been reported in every inhabited continent. Two forms of infection were documented during the 1990s in France and the USA: (1) an opportunistic febrile infection in patients with HIV infection (sometimes presenting as bacillary angiomatosis; see "Bartonellosis" and "Cat Scratch Disease"); and (2) a louse-borne febrile disease in homeless or alcoholic persons, so-called urban trench fever. Endocarditis has been reported in patients with and without typical risk factors for trench fever.

5. Reservoir—Humans. The intermediate host and vector is the body louse, *Pediculus humanus corporis*. The organism multiplies in the louse intestine for the duration of the insect's life, which is approximately 5 weeks after hatching; however, transovarial transmission does not occur.

Cat fleas may also carry the bacteria, but their role in transmission is undetermined.

6. Incubation period—Generally 3-30 days.

7. Transmission—Humans are infected by inoculation of louse feces through a break in the skin, usually when scratching bites. Infected lice begin to excrete infectious feces 5-12 days after ingesting infective blood; this continues for the remainder of their life span. The disease spreads when lice leave abnormally hot (febrile) or cold (dead) bodies in search of a normothermic host. Organisms may circulate in the host's blood (thus infecting lice) for weeks, months, or years and may recur with or without symptoms. A history of trench fever is a permanent contraindication to blood donation. Trench fever is not directly transmitted from person to person.

8. Risk groups—The disease is encountered especially among the homeless, refugees, and other persons infested with lice.

9. Prevention—Delousing procedures: clothing, bedding, and towels should be boiled or washed in hot water and machine dried at high heat. The patient's body should be cleaned thoroughly; however, insecticide treatment is generally not necessary since body lice reside in clothing and only visit the host's skin to feed. Mass treatments of body and clothing with appropriate pediculicides may be necessary in outbreak situations.

10. Management of patient—

1) Treatment: oral doxycycline for 4 weeks and gentamicin intravenous (IV) for 2 weeks for adults (consult an infectious disease specialist for treatment of children). Patients should first be evaluated carefully for endocarditis, as this will change the antibiotic therapy and duration. Relapse may occur, despite antibiotic treatment, in both immunocompromised and immunocompetent patients.
2) Treat louse-infested clothing to kill the lice.

11. Management of contacts and the immediate environment—Search bodies and clothing of people at risk for the presence of lice; delouse if indicated.

12. Special considerations—

1) Reporting: report to local health authority so that an evaluation of louse infestation in the population may be made and appropriate measures taken.
2) Epidemic measures: systematic application of residual insecticide to clothing of all people in affected population.

3) Disaster implications: risk is increased when louse-infested people are forced to live in crowded, unhygienic shelters.

[C. Nelson]

TRICHINELLOSIS
(trichiniasis, trichinosis)

DISEASE	ICD-10 CODE
TRICHINELLOSIS	ICD-10 B75

1. Clinical features—A roundworm disease in which clinical illness is highly variable and can range from inapparent infection to a fulminating, fatal disease, depending on the number of larvae ingested. Sudden appearance of muscle soreness and pain together with periorbital or facial edema and fever are early characteristic signs. These are sometimes followed by subconjunctival, subungual, and retinal hemorrhages, pain, and photophobia. Thirst, profuse sweating, chills, weakness, prostration, and rapidly increasing eosinophilia may follow shortly after the ocular signs.

Gastrointestinal symptoms, such as diarrhea due to the intra-intestinal activity of the adult worms, may precede the ocular manifestations. Remittent fever is usual, sometimes as high as 40°C (104°F); fever terminates after 1–6 weeks, depending on intensity of infection. Cardiac and neurological complications may appear in the third to sixth week; in the most severe cases, death due to myocardial failure may occur in either the first to second week or between the fourth and eighth weeks.

2. Causative agent—*Trichinella spiralis* and other *Trichinella* spp, intestinal nematodes. *T. spiralis* has a cosmopolitan distribution and broad host range in primarily temperate areas of the world. Separate taxonomic designations have been accepted for isolates found in carnivorous and omnivorous animals of the Arctic and subarctic (*Trichinella nativa*) and Palaearctic (*Trichinella britovi*), wild animals in temperate North America (*Trichinella murrelli*); in Africa (*Trichinella nelsoni*); in mammals and birds (*Trichinella pseudospiralis*); and in omnivorous and carnivorous animals (*Trichinella papuae*, *Trichinella zimbabwensis* and T6, T8, T9, T12 genotypes) in several specific regions of the world.

3. Diagnosis—Serological tests and marked eosinophilia may aid in diagnosis. Biopsy of skeletal muscle, taken more than 10 days after infection (most often positive after the fourth or fifth week of infection), frequently provides conclusive evidence of infection by demonstrating the uncalcified parasite cyst.

4. Occurrence—Worldwide, but variable in incidence, depending in part on practices of eating and preparing pork or wild animal meat, and the extent to which the disease is recognized and reported. Cases are usually sporadic and outbreaks localized, often resulting from eating sausage and other meat products containing pork or from sharing meat from Arctic mammals. Several outbreaks have been reported in France and Italy through infected horse meat. Ingestion of raw soft-shelled turtles was implicated in Taiwan.

5. Reservoir—Swine, dogs, cats, horses, rats, and many wild animals, including foxes, wolves, bears, moose, mountain lions, polar bears, wild boar, and marine mammals in the Arctic, and hyena, jackal, lion, and leopard in the tropics. Also found in farmed crocodiles; health risks from consuming crocodile meat are unknown.

6. Incubation period—Systemic symptoms usually appear about 8-15 days after ingestion of infected meat; this varies from 5-45 days depending on the number of parasites involved. Gastrointestinal (GI) symptoms may appear within a few days.

7. Transmission—Consumption of raw or insufficiently cooked flesh of animals containing viable encysted larvae, chiefly pork and pork products and wild game animals such as bear. Occasionally, beef products, such as hamburger that is adulterated intentionally or inadvertently with raw pork, are implicated. In the epithelium of the small intestine, larvae develop into adults. Gravid female worms then produce larvae, which penetrate the lymphatics or venules and are disseminated via the bloodstream throughout the body. The larvae become encapsulated in skeletal muscle (unless nonencapsulating type). Infection is not transmitted directly from person to person. Animal hosts remain infective for months, and their meat stays infective for appreciable periods unless cooked, frozen, or irradiated to kill the larvae. Infection results in partial immunity.

8. Risk groups—People who ingest raw or undercooked meat, especially pork and wild animal meat.

9. Prevention—

1) Educate the public on the need to cook all fresh pork, pork products, and meat from wild animals at a temperature and for a time sufficient to allow all parts to reach at least 71°C (160°F) or until meat changes from pink to grey, which allows a sufficient margin of safety. This should be done unless it has been

established that these meat products have been processed either by heating, curing, freezing, or irradiation adequate to kill trichinae.

2) Grind pork in a separate grinder, or clean the grinder thoroughly before and after processing other meats.

3) Adopt regulations to encourage commercial irradiation processing of pork products. Testing carcasses for infection with a digestion technique is useful, as is immunodiagnosis of pigs with an approved enzyme-linked immunosorbent assay (ELISA) test.

4) Adopt and enforce regulations that allow only certified trichinae-free pork to be used in raw pork products that have a cooked appearance or in products that are traditionally not heated sufficiently in final preparation to kill trichinae.

5) Adopt laws and regulations to require and enforce the cooking of garbage and offal before feeding to swine.

6) Educate hunters to cook the meat of bear, wild boar, walrus, seal, and other wild animals thoroughly.

7) Freezing temperatures maintained throughout the mass of the infected meat are effective in inactivating most *Trichinella* species; holding pieces of pork up to 15 cm thick at a temperature of −15°C (5°F) for 20 days or −25°C (−13°F) or lower for 10 days will effectively destroy most types of *Trichinella* cysts. Hold thicker pieces at the lower temperature for at least 20 days. These temperatures will not inactivate the freeze-resistant Arctic strains (*T. nativa* and possibly *T. britovi*) found in walrus and bear meat and—rarely—in swine.

8) Exposure of pork cuts or carcasses to low-level gamma irradiation effectively sterilizes and, at higher doses, kills encysted trichinae.

10. Management of patient—Treatment: albendazole or mebendazole should be given as early in the course of illness as possible and both are beneficial in the intestinal stage and in the muscular stage. In rare situations where infected meat is known to have been consumed, prompt administration of anthelminthic treatment may prevent development of symptoms. Corticosteroids are indicated only in severe cases to alleviate symptoms of inflammatory reaction when the central nervous system or heart is involved; however, they delay elimination of adult worms from the intestine.

11. Management of contacts and the immediate environment—Evaluate family members and persons who have eaten meat suspected as the source of infection. Dispose of any remaining suspected food.

12. **Special considerations—**

1) Reporting: case report required in most countries.
2) Epidemic measures: epidemiological study to determine the common food involved. Confiscate remainder of suspected food and correct faulty practices. Eliminate infected herds of swine.

WHO Collaborating Centres provide support as required. Further information can be found at: http://www.who.int/collaboratingcentres/database/en.

[J. Jones, S. Montgomery, R. Hall, M. Eberhard]

TRICHOMONIASIS

DISEASE	ICD-10 CODE
TRICHOMONIASIS	ICD-10 A59

1. **Clinical features**—Asymptomatic infection in about 70% of infected persons. Symptoms include mild-to-moderate genital inflammation, pruritus, vaginitis, urethritis, or prostatitis. Affected persons may notice pain during urination or sexual intercourse and malodorous genital discharge that can appear clear, white, yellow, or green. Infection can increase the risk of acquiring other sexually transmitted infections, including HIV.

2. **Causative agent**—*Trichomonas vaginalis*, a flagellated protozoan parasite.

3. **Diagnosis**—New point-of-care tests including a nucleic acid amplification test with high sensitivity and specificity can be used to test genital secretions or urine specimens. Although culture has been considered the gold standard, infection is most commonly diagnosed by identifying the motile parasite in genital secretions viewed on a microscope slide ("wet mount") within 20 minutes of collection. Wet mount testing is widely available and fairly inexpensive but has poor sensitivity (60%–70%).

4. **Occurrence**—The most common curable sexually transmitted infection worldwide, with an estimated 248 million new cases per year.

5. **Reservoir**—Humans only.

6. **Incubation period**—Symptoms may occur within 5-28 days after initial infection, but asymptomatic infections can last for years. Symptoms can recur.

7. **Transmission**—During sex. The parasite is transmitted by sexual contact with genital secretions from a penis or a vagina. It is not common for this parasite to infect fomites or other body parts, such as hands, mouth, or anus.

8. **Risk groups**—Prevalence increases with increasing age. Immuno-compromised persons may be at higher risk.

9. **Prevention**—Symptomatic women (i.e., with genital discharge) should be tested for trichomoniasis. Asymptomatic persons who are at high risk, such as those with HIV, may benefit from screening and treatment. Using latex condoms consistently and correctly can reduce the risk of acquiring or transmitting sexually transmitted infections including trichomoniasis.

10. **Management of patient**—Usually curable with a single oral dose of a nitroimidazole antimicrobial, such as metronidazole or tinidazole. Detailed treatment information can be found at: http://www.cdc.gov/std/treatment.

11. **Management of contacts and the immediate environment**—To reduce recurrence, sexual partner(s) should be treated concurrently. One option is to give patients medication to take to their partners.

12. **Special considerations**—None.

[E. Meites]

TRICHURIASIS
(trichocephaliasis, whipworm disease)

DISEASE	ICD-10 CODE
TRICHURIASIS	ICD-10 B79

1. **Clinical features**—A nematode infection of the large intestine, usually asymptomatic. Heavy infections may cause bloody, mucoid stools and diarrhea, and at times rectal prolapse, clubbing of fingers, hypoproteinemia, and anemia with growth retardation.

2. Causative agent—*Trichuris trichiura* (*Trichocephalus trichiurus*), or human whipworm, a nematode, soil-transmitted helminth.

3. Diagnosis—Made through demonstration of eggs in feces, or observation of worms attached to the wall of the lower colon during a sigmoidoscopic examination conducted for other reasons. Eggs must be differentiated from those of *Capillaria* species.

4. Occurrence—Worldwide, especially in warm, moist regions.

5. Reservoir—Humans. Animal whipworms do not infect humans.

6. Incubation period—Indefinite.

7. Transmission—Indirect, particularly through pica (eating of non-food items, in this context, especially soil contaminated with infective eggs) or ingestion of contaminated vegetables; no person-to-person transmission. Eggs passed in feces require a minimum of 10–14 days in warm moist soil to become infective. Hatching of larvae follows ingestion of infective eggs from contaminated soil, attachment to the mucosa of the cecum and proximal colon, and development into mature worms. Eggs appear in the feces 70–90 days after ingestion of embryonated eggs; symptoms may appear much earlier. Untreated carriers can communicate the disease for several years.

8. Risk groups—Susceptibility is universal. The highest prevalence and intensity of infection are found in school-age children.

9. Prevention—

1) Educate all members of the family, particularly children, in the use of toilet facilities and handwashing. Provide adequate facilities for feces disposal.
2) Encourage satisfactory hygienic habits, especially handwashing before food handling and before eating; avoid ingestion of soil by thorough washing of vegetables and other foods contaminated with soil.
3) WHO recommends a "preventive chemotherapy" strategy focused on mebendazole or albendazole treatment of high-risk groups at regular intervals for the control of morbidity due to the soil-transmitted helminths causing ascariasis, trichuriasis, and hookworm disease (http://www.who.int/neglected_diseases/preventive_chemotherapy/pct_manual/en). See "Ascariasis" for details.

10. Management of patient—

1) Sanitary disposal of feces.

2) Treatment: single-dose oral mebendazole or albendazole (half dose for children 12–24 months). For all drugs, longer treatment courses (≤3 days) are required in heavy infections. On theoretical grounds, pregnant women should not be treated in the first trimester unless there are specific medical or public health indications.

11. Management of contacts and the immediate environment— Examine feces of all symptomatic members of the family group, especially children and playmates.

12. Special considerations—Advise school health authorities of unusual frequency in school populations.

[M. Eberhard, A. Gabrielli, A. Montresor, L. Savioli]

TRYPANOSOMIASIS

DISEASE	ICD-10 CODE
AFRICAN TRYPANOSOMIASIS	ICD-10 B56, ICD-10 B56.1
AMERICAN TRYPANOSOMIASIS	ICD-10 B57

I. AFRICAN TRYPANOSOMIASIS (sleeping sickness)

1. Clinical features—A systemic protozoal disease that is generally fatal without treatment. There are 2 forms: the gambiense or chronic form, which may run a course of several years, and the rhodesiense or acute form, which is lethal within weeks or months.

In the early stage, a painful chancre, originating as a papule and evolving into a nodule, may be found at the primary tsetse fly bite site (more frequent in rhodesiense infection); there may also be fever, intense headache, painless enlarged lymph nodes, local edema, rash, and unspecific cardiac symptoms. In the late stage, after the parasite crosses the blood-brain barrier, neurological signs are added, such as disturbances of circadian rhythm, sensory disturbances, endocrine dysfunction, disorders of tonus and mobility, abnormal movements, mental changes, or psychiatric disorders. Neurological symptoms correlate with the damaged areas of central nervous system (CNS).

Occasional unapparent or asymptomatic infections have been documented. Spontaneous recovery in cases with the gambiense form without CNS involvement has been described.

2. Causative agents—Extracellular hemoflagellates subspecies of *Trypanosoma brucei*: *T. brucei gambiense* and *T. brucei rhodesiense*. There are no morphological criteria for subspecies differentiation. Clinically, acute cases contracted in eastern and southern Africa have been considered to be due to *T. brucei rhodesiense*, whereas chronic cases infected in western and central Africa have been considered to be due to *T. brucei gambiense*. It is now possible to differentiate both subspecies by molecular biology.

3. Diagnosis—Cannot be based on clinical symptoms. It relies on finding trypanosomes in blood, lymph, or eventually cerebrospinal fluid (CSF). Parasite concentration techniques are generally required in gambiense, and less often in rhodesiense disease; in blood, capillary tube centrifugation or minianion exchange centrifugation; and in CSF, single modified centrifugation or double centrifugation. Inoculation on laboratory rats or mice is sometimes useful in rhodesiense disease. The screening test of choice for *T. brucei gambiense* is the card agglutination test for trypanosomiasis, a simple 5-minute test based on the agglutination of whole, fixed, and stained trypanosomes in the presence of specific antibodies. The control programs in areas where *T. brucei gambiense* is endemic use it for seroscreening of at-risk populations. There is no seroscreening test available for *T. brucei rhodesiense*. New rapid serological tests (lateral flow) for *T. brucei gambiense* form have been recently developed and are under evaluation process. Diagnosis should be followed by CSF exams (white blood cells and parasites) to determine the involvement (late stage) or not (early stage) of the CNS. Molecular diagnostic tests are available using different targets, although these are not recommended to take therapeutic decisions.

4. Occurrence—The disease is confined to tropical Africa between 15°N and 20°S latitude, corresponding to the distribution of the tsetse fly. The annual incidence of cases reported to WHO is 6,000–10,000. WHO estimates some 20,000 people are currently infected per year, with up to 70 million people in 21 countries at risk of contracting the disease. The gambiense form of the disease represents 97% of the total cases reported. Sleeping sickness has a focal distribution and occurs at over 250 foci in the poorest rural areas of some of the least industrialized countries.

Outbreaks can occur when human-fly contact is intensified, when reservoir hosts introduce trypanosome human-infective strains into a tsetse-infested area, or when populations are displaced into endemic areas.

5. Reservoir—In *T. brucei gambiense* infection, humans are the major reservoir; however, the role of domestic and wild animals is not clear. Wild animals, cattle, and other domestic animals are the chief reservoirs for *T. brucei rhodesiense*.

6. Incubation period—Symptoms usually appear within 3 days to a few weeks after infection with *T. brucei rhodesiense*, but they may not be apparent or misdiagnosed for several months with *T. brucei gambiense* infection.

7. Transmission—Through the bite of infective Glossina, the tsetse fly. Six species are the main vectors in nature. The riverine species are vectors for *T. brucei gambiense*: *Glossina palpalis*, *Glossina fuscipes*, and *Glossina tachinoides*. The wooden savannah species are vectors of *T. brucei rhodesiense*: *Glossina morsitans*, *Glossina pallidipes*, and *Glossina swynnertoni*. The fly is infected by ingesting blood of a human or animal that carries trypanosomes. The parasite multiplies in the fly for 12-30 days, depending on temperature and other factors, until infective forms develop in the salivary glands. Once infected, a tsetse fly remains infective for life (average 3 months, but as long as 10 months); infection is not passed from generation to generation in flies. Congenital transmission can occur in humans. Transmission by blood transfusion is possible. Direct mechanical transmission by blood on the proboscis of Glossina and other biting insects, such as horseflies, or in laboratory accidents is possible.

The disease is communicable to the tsetse fly as long as the parasite is present in the blood of the infected person or animal. Parasitemia in humans occurs in waves of varying intensity in untreated cases, and occurs at all stages of the disease.

8. Risk groups—Susceptibility is general.

9. Prevention—Selection of appropriate prevention methods must be based on knowledge of the local ecology of vectors and infectious agents. In a given geographic area, priority must be given to one or more of the following:

1) Educate the public on personal protective measures against tsetse fly bites—this has limited impact because tsetse flies bite during the day at the workplace. Bednets are not useful.
2) Reduce the parasite population by screening and diagnosing exposed populations and treating those infected. This is effective for *T. brucei gambiense*, where humans are the main reservoir.
3) Reduce the parasite population by diagnosing and treating cattle. This is effective for *T. brucei rhodesiense*, where cattle are the main reservoir.
4) Destroy vector tsetse fly habitats if useful; indiscriminate destruction of vegetation is not recommended.
5) Reduce the tsetse fly population by appropriate use of traps and screens, impregnated with insecticide or otherwise; by local use of residual insecticide; or by sequential aerial spraying of

insecticide by helicopter or fixed-wing aircraft. Sterile insect technique has been successfully used to eradicate tsetse from Unguja island in Zanzibar.

6) Check for the disease in case of blood donation from those that have visited or lived in endemic areas in Africa.

10. **Management of patient—**

1) Systematic screening of exposed populations in each *T. brucei gambiense* focus aimed at identifying asymptomatic infections at an early stage. Early diagnosis reduces both the risk of sequelae and the late-stage drug-related risks and helps stop transmission. Regular surveillance in local health centers and villages for both rhodesiense and gambiense to identify areas at risk.

2) Prevent tsetse flies from feeding on patients with trypanosomes in their blood. Patient isolation is not recommended.

3) Treatment: differs according to form and phase of the disease. If diagnosis occurs early in the initial phase, chances of cure are high. Treatment of the neurological phase requires drugs that can cross the blood-brain barrier. If started too late, treatment cannot prevent irreversible neurological damage. Early diagnosis allows low-risk early-stage treatment, but the disease is notoriously difficult to treat in the neurological stage for which medicines are difficult to manufacture and complicated to administer. While some people tolerate drugs well, in others, fatal complications are common. Problems of drug resistance have increasingly been reported in several countries. Four drugs—suramin, pentamidine, melarsoprol, and eflornithine— are registered for treatment of African trypanosomiasis. Nifurtimox, a drug registered for American trypanosomiasis, is also used for African trypanosomiasis in combination regimens. All 5 drugs are available through WHO, the only provider, and are free of charge through donation programs. Pentamidine is used for early stages of *T. brucei gambiense* and suramin for early stages of *T. brucei rhodesiense* infections.

Late-stage disease, with CNS involvement, requires inpatient treatment with a drug that can cross the blood-brain barrier. Available medicines suffer from a range of difficulties, including substantial toxicity and lengthy or complicated parenteral administrations. Increasing rates of treatment failure have been observed in some foci of *T. brucei gambiense*. Melarsoprol is an arsenical derivate drug used to treat both forms at the neurological stage. Reactive encephalopathy, the main adverse effect of melarsoprol, occurs in 5%–10% of treatments and is often fatal. This drug must be administered on an inpatient basis, and in the intensive care unit if possible. Eflornithine is used for late-stage *T. brucei gambiense* infection. This drug is difficult to administer under field conditions. Although it can have fatal complications, it is safer than melarsoprol. The combination of nifurtimox and eflornithine has shown similar efficacy than eflornithine alone, but it is easier to administer and it is currently used for late-stage *T. brucei gambiense* infection. Patients must be followed up for at least 1 and preferably 2 years after treatment to assess drug efficacy.

11. Management of contacts and the immediate environment—If the case is a member of a tour group or a family, others in the group or family should be alerted and investigated.

12. Special considerations—

1) In some endemic areas, establish records of prevalence and encourage control measures.

2) Epidemic measures: mainly for *T. brucei rhodesiense*; mass surveys, urgent treatment for identified infections, cattle treatment, and tsetse fly control. If epidemics recur despite initial control measures, the measures recommended in "Infection Prevention and Control" must be pursued more vigorously.

3) International measures: the Pan-African Tsetse and Trypanosomosis Eradication Campaign is an Africa Union program to promote and coordinate antitrypanosomiasis efforts of governments in affected countries. WHO is leading a human African trypanosomiasis surveillance and control program, providing capacity building as well as technical and logistical support (diagnosis reagents and equipment, drugs, training) to countries where the disease is endemic and carrying out surveillance and control activities and improving reporting of the disease. WHO Collaborating Centres provide support as required. Further information can be found at: http://www.who.int/collaboratingcentres/database/en.

Further information on trypanosomiasis can be found at:

- http://www.who.int/trypanosomiasis_african/en
- http://www.who.int/mediacentre/factsheets/fs259/en

II. AMERICAN TRYPANOSOMIASIS (Chagas disease)

1. Clinical features—The acute disease, with variable fever, lymphadenopathy, malaise, and hepatosplenomegaly, generally occurs in children—although the majority of infections are asymptomatic or paucisymptomatic. In

20%-30% of infections, irreversible chronic manifestations generally appear later in life. An inflammatory response at the site of infection (chagoma) may last up to 8 weeks. Unilateral bipalpebral-edema (Romana's sign) occurs in a small percentage of acute cases. Life-threatening or fatal manifestations include myocarditis and meningoencephalitis. Chronic irreversible sequelae include myocardial damage with cardiac dilatation, arrhythmias and major conduction abnormalities, and intestinal tract involvement with megaesophagus and megacolon. Megavisceral manifestations occur mainly in central Brazil. The prevalence of megaviscera and cardiac involvement varies according to regions; the latter is not as common north of Ecuador as in southern areas. In AIDS patients, acute myocarditis and severe multifocal or diffuse meningoencephalitis with necrosis and hemorrhage occur as relapses of chronic infection. Reactivation of chronic Chagas disease may also occur with non-AIDS immunosuppression and is characterized by skin lesions, blood parasitemia, and, often, acute myocarditis. Central nervous system involvement is not usually seen.

Infection with *Trypanosoma rangeli* occurs in foci of endemic Chagas disease; prolonged parasitemia occurs, sometimes coexisting with *Trypanosoma cruzi* flagellates (with which *T. rangeli* shares reservoir hosts)—no clinical manifestations attributable to *T. rangeli* have been noted.

2. Causative agent—*T. cruzi* (*Schizotrypanum cruzi*), a protozoan that occurs in humans as a hemoflagellate (trypomastigote) and as an intracellular parasite (amastigote) without an external flagellum.

3. Diagnosis—In the acute phase (or in reactivation for immunosuppression) a blood wet smear or a blood concentration technique, such as microhaematocrit or Strout technique, must be used. Stained preparations, such as malaria films, detect parasites when parasitaemia is high (acute phase). Parasitemia is most intense during febrile episodes early in the course of infection. In the chronic phase serologic tests should be used, including anti-*T. cruzi* antibodies through a conventional or recombinant enzyme-linked immunosorbent assay (ELISA), indirect hemagglutination assay, indirect immunofluorescence assay, western blot, and rapid diagnostic tests such as immunochromatography. Special laboratory studies include blood culture, xenodiagnosis (faeces examination of uninfected triatomine bug fed with the patient's blood), and polymerase chain reaction (PCR). *T. cruzi* is best differentiated from *T. rangeli* by PCR, though it is distinctive by its shorter length (20 μm vs. 36 μm) and larger kinetoplast. Serologic tests are valuable for individual diagnosis as well as for screening purposes.

4. Occurrence—The disease is confined to the Western Hemisphere, with wide geographic distribution in rural Mexico and Central and South America. However, progress in reduction of vector-borne and bloodborne transmission in endemic countries, together with migration of chronically infected people to nonendemic countries, is changing the epidemiology of the disease. Based on limited data from seroprevalence studies among blood donors and other populations, it is estimated that at least 100,000 people in North America are infected with *T. cruzi*, mainly immigrants from endemic countries.

5. Reservoir—Humans and more than 150 domestic and wild mammals species, including dogs, cats, rats, mice, marsupials, edentates, rodents, chiroptera, carnivores, and primates.

6. Incubation period—About 5-14 days after bite of insect vector; 30-40 days if infected through blood transfusion.

7. Transmission—Infected vectors—that is, blood-sucking species of Reduviidae (cone-nosed or kissing bugs), especially various species from the genera *Triatoma, Rhodnius,* and *Panstrongylus*—have the trypanosomes in their feces. Defecation occurs during feeding; infection of humans and other mammals occurs when the freshly excreted bug feces contaminate conjunctivae, mucous membranes, abrasions, or skin wounds (including the bite wound). The bugs become infected when they feed on a parasitemic animal; the parasites multiply in the bugs' gut. Transmission may also occur by blood transfusion; there are increasing numbers of infected donors in cities because of migration from rural areas. Organisms may also cross the placenta to cause congenital infection (in 2%-8% of pregnancies for those infected); transmission through breastfeeding seems highly unlikely, so there is currently no reason to restrict breastfeeding by chagasic mothers. Transmission through ingestion of food or drink contaminated with triatomine feces has also been reported. Transplantation of organs from chagasic donors presents a growing risk of *T. cruzi* transmission.

Organisms are regularly present in the blood during the acute period and may persist in very small numbers throughout life in symptomatic and asymptomatic people. The vector becomes infective 10-30 days after biting an infected host; gut infection in the bug persists for life (as long as 2 years).

8. Risk groups—All ages are susceptible, but the acute disease is usually more severe in younger people. Immunosuppressed people, especially those with AIDS, are at risk of serious infections and complications.

9. Prevention—

1) Educate the public on mode of spread and methods of prevention.
2) Systematically attack vectors infesting poorly constructed houses and houses with thatched roofs, using effective insecticides with residual action (spraying, use of insecticidal paints, or fumigant canisters).
3) Construct or repair living areas to eliminate lodging places for insect vectors and shelter for domestic and wild reservoir

animals. In certain areas, palm trees close to houses often harbor infested bugs and can be considered a risk factor.

4) Use bed nets (preferably insecticide-impregnated) in houses infested by the vector.

5) Screen blood and organ donors living in or coming from endemic areas to prevent infection by transfusion or transplants as required by law in most countries in the Americas.

10. Management of patient—

1) Blood and body fluid precautions for hospitalized patients.

2) Treatment: benznidazole, a 2-nitroimidazole derivative, and nifurtimox, a nitrofurfurylidene derivative, have proven effective in acute cases. Clinical trials have shown that benznidazole modifies parasite-related outcomes among young persons with chronic, asymptomatic infection. Treatment is recommended for acute and congenital cases, for children with chronic asymptomatic infection, and for reactivated infection in immunocompromised patients. Many experts also offer treatment to asymptomatic adults; the potential of trypanocidal treatment in asymptomatic, chronically infected persons is under evaluation.

11. Management of contacts and the immediate environment—

1) Search thatched roofs, bedding, and rooms for vectors.

2) All family members of a case should be examined. Infants born to mothers with known seropositive status should be evaluated for congenital infection.

3) Serological tests and blood examinations on all blood and organ donors implicated as possible sources of transfusion- or transplant-acquired infection.

12. Special considerations—

1) Reporting: report to local health authority may be required in some endemic areas.

2) Epidemic measures: in areas of high incidence, field survey to determine distribution and density of vectors and animal hosts and implementation of measures described in "Infection Prevention and Control."

3) Although triatomine vectors are still responsible for most human infections, successful programs based on application of residual insecticides have substantially reduced transmission by this route in the "Southern Cone" of South America. Uruguay, Chile, and parts of Brazil have been certified free of vector-borne transmission. Further research and implementation efforts are necessary in the Amazon, Andean, and Central American regions, where

transmission occurs through both domiciliated and nondomiciliated vectors. Many Latin American countries have made considerable progress in improving blood safety. Further information can be found at: http://www.who.int/neglected_diseases/diseases/chagas/en.

[P. Simarro, J. R. Franco, D. L. Heymann]

TUBERCULOSIS AND OTHER MYCOBACTERIAL DISEASES
(TB, TB disease)

DISEASE	ICD-10 CODE
TUBERCULOSIS	ICD-10 A15-A19
DISEASES DUE TO OTHER MYCOBACTERIA	ICD-10 A31
Buruli ulcer (see "Buruli Ulcer")	

I. TUBERCULOSIS

1. Clinical features—There are 2 forms of TB, latent and active (pulmonary and/or extrapulmonary).

Latent TB infection can be established following exposure to an infectious patient expelling aerosolized particles containing viable bacilli. Initial infection generally causes no outward clinical manifestations and is called latent TB. It is characterized by microscopic lesions in the lungs that commonly heal, leaving no residual changes other than occasional small pulmonary or tracheobronchial lymph node calcifications.

Active TB disease can develop following infection and facilitated by certain risk factors. It can be pulmonary and/or extrapulmonary. Active pulmonary TB may arise from reactivation of a latent focus originating from the initial subclinical infection or from reinfection. Extrapulmonary TB occurs in 15%-30% of cases and may affect any organ or tissue as follows: lymph nodes (33%), pleura (20%), genitourinary tract (5%-10%), bones and joints (5%-10%), meninges (5%), gastrointestinal tract and peritoneum (3.5%), and pericardium (2%-3%).

Cough, fatigue, fever, night sweats, and weight loss are common symptoms associated with active pulmonary TB. In most cases, cough is initially nonproductive and later accompanied by purulent sputum.

Symptoms such as hemoptysis and hoarseness associated with laryngeal TB are sometimes prominent in advanced stages. Chest radiography reveals pulmonary infiltrates and cavitations in the upper segments of the lung lobes. In prolonged disease, fibrotic changes with volume loss are seen.

2. Causative agents—*Mycobacterium tuberculosis* (MTB) complex which includes *M. tuberculosis, Mycobacterium bovis* ("bovine tubercle bacillus," historically an important cause of TB transmitted through unpasteurized milk), *Mycobacterium africanum*, and *Mycobacterium canettii* are the causes of a small number of infections in Africa. Occasionally, *Mycobacterium microti, Mycobacterium caprae, Mycobacterium pinnipedii, Mycobacterium mungi,* and *Mycobacterium orygis* produce disease clinically indistinguishable from tuberculosis. *M. tuberculosis* is aerobic

3. Diagnosis—Latent TB can be detected by tuberculin skin testing (TST) and/or blood tests (interferon-gamma release assays [IGRAs], that is, QuantiFERON-TB Gold In-Tube, and T-SPOT.TB. These tests become positive 2–6 weeks after exposure.

The classification of active pulmonary TB has been traditionally based primarily on the presence or absence of acid-fast bacilli (AFB) in the microscopic examination of the sputum. At least 2 sputum specimens (1 early morning) should be obtained. Specimens should be transported using liquid media and undergo AFB smear microscopy; good quality microscopy of 2 consecutive sputum specimens identifies the vast majority (95%–98%) of smear-positive TB patients. Fluorescence microscopy using auramine staining is preferred over Ziehl-Neelsen staining.

Since 2010, a molecular method, such as Xpert MTB/RIF (diagnostic test for MTB/rifampicin), has been recommended by WHO for rapid diagnosis of pulmonary and extrapulmonary TB in adults and children, including in high HIV-prevalent settings and where multidrug-resistant TB (MDR-TB) is potentially present. This method also detects rifampicin resistance as a proxy of MDR-TB. In all instances, isolation of *M. tuberculosis* on culture confirms diagnosis and also permits determination of drug susceptibility. Persons suspected of having TB disease should have a full diagnostic evaluation, including a chest radiograph. In the absence of bacteriological confirmation, active disease can be presumed if clinical, histological, or radiological evidence is suggestive of TB and other likely diseases can be ruled out. Diagnosis of TB among HIV-positive persons may be complicated by the tendency to yield negative smears. Serological tests, TST, and IGRAs have no role in diagnosis of active TB.

Extrapulmonary TB is diagnosed by microscopy, culture, and histopathological examination on specimens from the involved sites. Ultrasound, computerized tomography (CT) scan, and magnetic resonance imaging (MRI) facilitate diagnosis.

All TB isolates, especially from previously treated patients, should be submitted for culture and drug susceptibility testing. Rapid molecular tests such as Xpert MTB-RIF and line-probe assays result in more rapid diagnosis and treatment of drug-resistant TB.

4. Occurrence—Worldwide. The prevalence of latent TB infection increases with age. It is estimated that one-third of the human population is infected today, mostly in the less-developed countries. Microepidemics of latent TB have been reported in high-income countries in confined populations within nursing homes, homeless shelters, hospitals, schools, and prisons.

The incidence of active pulmonary TB was estimated at 8.6 million persons in 2012 of which two-thirds were officially reported. Over 95% of active TB occurs in developing countries, where it remains a dominant cause of morbidity and mortality The highest rates of active pulmonary TB per capita are in sub-Saharan Africa, especially the eastern and southern regions (with rates ≤1,000/100,000 population), but approximately 60% of all cases are reported from Asia. Morbidity is highest among adult males. Incidence is increasing in many high-income countries due to poverty-related living conditions, immigration from high-incidence areas, HIV infection, alcohol abuse, smoking, and diabetes. Dismantling of well-resourced TB care services has facilitated this. Morbidity and mortality rates are higher among impoverished, disadvantaged, and minority populations, often living in urban areas.

It is estimated that 4%–5% of all active pulmonary TB is caused by MDR strains. In Eastern Europe and Central Asia up to 35% of newly diagnosed active pulmonary TB and 70% of that previously treated is MDR-TB. Five countries—India, China, Russia, Philippines, and Pakistan—account for 60% of all MDR-TB. Extensively drug resistant TB (XDR-TB) is defined as MDR-TB plus resistance to any fluoroquinolones and any of the 3 injectable drugs, amikacin, kanamycin, and capreomycin. It has emerged in settings where second-line drug use has been poorly managed. It is estimated that about 10% of all TB resistance is XDR-TB. In 2005–2006 a major outbreak of XDR-TB occurred in KwaZulu Natal, South Africa, where 52 of 53 (98%) patients died, and the median survival from date of diagnosis was 16 days.

HIV-associated active pulmonary TB (TB/HIV) is frequent in persons with untreated HIV infection, especially in Africa. Outbreaks of MDR-TB have occurred in hospitals, prisons, drug-treatment clinics, and residences where HIV-infected persons congregate. The mortality rates are high as are the rates of transmission to other patients and health care workers. Strict enforcement of infection control, proactive case-finding, intensive contact investigation, and ensuring completion of appropriate treatment regimens are effective in stopping and preventing MDR-TB outbreaks.

Human infection with *M. bovis* occurs where bovine TB in cattle is poorly controlled and unpasteurized milk or dairy products are consumed.

It is estimated that approximately 2% of active pulmonary TB and 9.4% of extrapulmonary TB worldwide is caused by *M. bovis.*

5. Reservoirs—Primarily humans; rarely other primates. *M. bovis,* is found in cattle and a variety of other wild mammals.

6. Incubation period—For latent TB, 2-10 weeks from infection to demonstrable primary lesion or significant TST reaction and positivity of IGRA. IGRAs are normally positive by 10 weeks from exposure, but the actual time from infection to IGRA conversion has not been adequately studied. Fewer than 10% of latently infected persons will develop active pulmonary TB disease in their lifetimes; half of those will develop active pulmonary TB within 18 months after initial infection. Latent TB infection can persist for a lifetime. It is not possible to identify those with latent TB who will progress to active pulmonary TB, nor the speed with which it will develop. Rapid clinical progression is more common among infants and in the immunosuppressed, such as the HIV-infected.

7. Transmission—Persons with active pulmonary tuberculosis transmit the tubercle bacilli during coughing, singing, or sneezing. The droplet nuclei are inhaled into the pulmonary alveoli of a vulnerable contact. The aerosolized particles containing *M. tuberculosis* are ingested by alveolar macrophages, initiating a new infection. Theoretically, the period of communicability lasts as long as viable tubercle bacilli are discharged in the sputum. Effective antimicrobial chemotherapy usually eliminates communicability within 2-4 weeks, although *M. tuberculosis* may still be cultured from sputum. Some untreated or inadequately treated patients with active pulmonary TB can be intermittently AFB sputum-positive and therefore contagious for years. Studies suggest that persons with smear-negative, culture-positive active pulmonary TB can also be contagious, although to a lesser extent. Younger children with latent TB generally are not contagious.

The degree of communicability depends on intimacy and duration of the exposure, the number of bacilli discharged, virulence of the bacilli, adequacy of ventilation, exposure of bacilli to sun or ultraviolet light, and opportunities for aerosolization through coughing, sneezing, or singing—or, for health care workers during aerosolizing procedures. The first 18 months after infection constitute the period of greatest risk for the development of active pulmonary TB. Laryngeal TB disease occurs rarely and is highly contagious.

Direct invasion of mycobacteria through mucous membranes or breaks in the skin can occur but are extremely rare. Bovine tuberculosis (caused by *M. bovis*) results from direct exposure to tuberculous cattle or the ingestion of unpasteurized contaminated milk or dairy products. Except for rare situations where there is a draining sinus, extrapulmonary tuberculosis (other than laryngeal) is not communicable.

8. Risk groups—The risk of infection is directly related to the degree of exposure to active pulmonary TB and less so to genetic or other host factors. However, the risk of active pulmonary TB once infected is highest in children younger than 3 years, adolescents, young adults, the very old, and the immunocompromised including those who are HIV-positive. Reactivation of latent infection accounts for a large proportion of active pulmonary TB in older people. Detection of latent TB infection through tuberculin skin testing or IGRA is used in child and adult contacts of pulmonary TB cases, people living with HIV, patients initiating antitumor necrosis factor treatment, patients receiving dialysis, patients preparing for organ or hematologic transplantation, patients with silicosis, immigrants from high-incidence countries, prisoners, and homeless to guide interventions that include preventive therapy.

In addition to a markedly increased risk of reactivation of latent infection among those with HIV infection and other forms of immunosuppression, there is also a risk among the underweight or undernourished, people with diabetes mellitus and a debilitating disorder (e.g., chronic renal failure, some forms of cancer, silicosis, gastrectomy), and illicit drug users. Tobacco smokers and alcoholics are also at increased risk of TB morbidity and mortality. For adults coinfected with HIV and latent TB, the lifetime risk of developing active pulmonary TB rises from an estimated 10% in a lifetime to up to 15% per year in the absence of antiretroviral treatment.

9. Prevention—

A. Primary prevention—

1) Prompt diagnosis and treatment: render smear-positive active pulmonary and extrapulmonary TB noninfectious within 2–4 weeks by using an effective management regimen. Active case finding by investigation of close contacts of infectious patients and among high-risk populations, and provision of adequate treatment for all cases are key to reducing transmission. This normally requires a well-functioning TB program at the lowest health authority level coordinated with primary care facilities and using national best practice, training, supervision, and performance monitoring. Required are clinical, laboratory, and radiology facilities; physical examination of patients and contacts; provision of a regimen based on 4 essential anti-TB drugs (discussed later); and support to patients through completion of treatment.

2) Public education: inform the public regarding mode of spread, symptoms, methods of control, and importance of early diagnosis and continued adherence to treatment.

3) Infection control measures: establish and maintain effective TB infection control measures in institutional settings where health care is provided and especially where immunocompromised

patients congregate, including hospitals, drug treatment programs, prisons, nursing homes, and homeless shelters.

4) Bacillus Calmette-Guérin (BCG) vaccination: BCG appears to be protective against extrapulmonary TB (TB meningitis and disseminated disease) in children younger than 5 years, but not against initial infection. Because the risk of infection is low in many industrialized countries, BCG is not used routinely in these settings. In countries with high TB prevalence, WHO recommends BCG vaccination for newborns as part of the routine immunization program. As it is a live-attenuated vaccine, BCG is contraindicated in persons with immunodeficiency disorders, including infants and children with symptomatic HIV infection, because of the risk of disseminated BCG disease. There are ongoing efforts to develop a vaccine more effective than BCG, and candidate vaccines are currently in human clinical trials for safety and immunogenicity.

5) Eliminate bovine tuberculosis among dairy cattle: tuberculin testing and slaughtering of positive reactors; pasteurize or boil milk and dairy products for human consumption.

6) Address social determinants: reduce or eliminate social and economic conditions that increase the risk of infection and progression to disease including poor living conditions, malnutrition, indoor air pollution, smoking, and alcohol abuse.

B. Secondary prevention—

1) Treatment of latent TB infections: treatment for latent TB may be warranted for persons with positive tuberculin skin tests or IGRA. Previously known as preventive chemotherapy or chemoprophylaxis, it consists, usually, in the administration of isoniazid (INH) for 6–9 months. This has been effective in preventing the progression of latent TB infection to TB disease in up to 70% of adherent individuals.

- It is essential to rule out active pulmonary and extrapulmonary TB before starting treatment for latent TB infection, especially in immunocompromised persons such as HIV-infected individuals, in order to avoid inadvertently treating active disease with a 1- or 2-drug regimen that would encourage the development of drug resistance.

- WHO recommends a preventive treatment with 6 months of daily INH for all HIV-infected individuals after careful exclusion of active disease. In high TB and HIV prevalence settings with high rate of transmission and reinfection risk, INH preventive therapy may need to be provided for life to maintain its efficacy.

- Other treatment options recommended include: 9-month INH, a 3-month regimen of weekly rifapentine plus INH, 3-4 months INH plus rifampicin, or 3-4 months rifampicin alone.
- Persons started on preventive treatment for latent TB must be informed of possible adverse effects and checked for symptoms monthly prior to prescription refills; they should be advised to discontinue treatment and seek medical advice if suggestive TB symptoms develop. Monitoring liver function tests is important in patients with signs, symptoms, or history of liver disease and in those who abuse alcohol.
- During pregnancy, it may be wise to postpone treatment for latent TB infection until after delivery, except in high-risk individuals, where it should be administered with caution. If INH treatment is prescribed for pregnant women or in the immediate postpartum period, monthly routine hepatic transaminases should be monitored. Breastfeeding is not contraindicated.
- Nontargeted treatment of latent TB is unsuitable in most communities unless there is a well-organized program to supervise and encourage adherence to treatment and unless a high rate of cure can at the same time be achieved among patients with symptomatic TB disease. However, vulnerable groups, such as the HIV-infected, may be targeted for selective, large-scale treatment.

2) Screening for active pulmonary and extrapulmonary TB: people living with HIV need to be screened for symptomatic TB at any clinical check-up using a simple symptom-based screening algorithm based on 4 symptoms (presence of cough of any duration, weight loss, fever, and night sweats). They should be investigated for active pulmonary or extrapulmonary TB disease if any one of the symptoms is reported through proper medical history and examination, including Xpert MTB/RIF and chest radiography. In the absence of symptoms and if they have tested positive with TST or IGRA, they should be offered treatment of latent TB as described earlier.

3) For treatment of latent TB in contacts infected from persons with known drug-resistant strains, treatment regimens have been based on in vitro data, extrapolation from treatment of known contacts, and expert opinion.

10. **Management of patient—**

1) Patients with active pulmonary TB should be taught to cover both mouth and nose when coughing or sneezing. Face masks,

such as the cloth or paper surgical masks, prevent spread of bacilli from the wearer to others by capturing the large wet particles expelled but do not protect the wearer from inhaling infectious droplets nuclei in the air.

2) All persons with evidence of active pulmonary or extrapulmonary TB should be counseled and tested for HIV infection, and offered the option of antiretroviral treatment and all other support measures for HIV-infected persons.

3) Where available, adult patients with sputum smear-positive active pulmonary TB who reside in congregate settings should be placed in an airborne-infection isolation room with negative pressure ventilation, with at least 6 air exchanges per hour. Patients whose sputum is bacteriologically negative, who do not cough, and who are known to be on adequate chemotherapy (known or probable drug susceptibility and clear clinical response to treatment) do not require isolation, nor do children with symptomatic active pulmonary TB with negative sputum smears and no cough, as they are not contagious. For patients with MDR-TB, sputum culture conversion to negative is likewise recommended for discontinuing isolation precautions.

4) If a patient willfully refuses treatment, especially if the infection is resistant, interference with freedom of movement when instituting quarantine or isolation may be necessary for the public good and could be implemented in a manner in which the isolation complies with applicable ethical and human rights principles. This must be viewed as a last resort and justified only after all voluntary measures to isolate such a patient have failed. A key factor in determining if the necessary protections exist when rights are restricted is that each one of the 5 criteria of the Siracusa Principles must be met (but these should be of a limited duration and subject to review and appeal).

5) Handwashing and good infection control practices must be maintained according to policy. Because active pulmonary TB has an airborne mode of transmission, no special precautions are necessary for handling fomites. Decontamination of air is achieved by ventilation; this may be supplemented by filtration and ultraviolet light.

6) Treatment: for all active pulmonary and extrapulmonary TB, WHO recommend short-course chemotherapy, that is, a treatment regimen of 2 months (intensive phase) of daily doses of INH, RIF, pyrazinamide (PZA), and ethambutol (EMB), followed by 4 months of daily administration of INH and RIF (continuation phase). All treatment should be supervised or directly observed to ensure the patient receives all prescribed drugs. Patients need

to be counseled and supported during the 6-month course of treatment. Community-based mechanisms should be put in place to ensure patients receive support within their own community. Directly observed therapy and other measures to facilitate adherence tailored to individual circumstances and mutually acceptable to patient and provider should especially be ensured for persons with suspected or proven MDR-TB, with a previous history of poor adherence to treatment linked to social factors, or who live in conditions where relapse would result in exposure of many other susceptible persons. The use of fixed-dose combinations including all 4 first-line drugs (or, in the continuation phase the 2 recommended drugs) is recommended to minimize the risk of inadvertent monotherapy. This may also facilitate adherence by reducing the number of tablets to be ingested.

Ideally, drug susceptibility testing should be available for all patients with active pulmonary and extrapulmonary TB (see Diagnosis under Tuberculosis section in this chapter). New rapid molecular tests (such as Xpert MTB/RIF and line-probe assays) allow selection of a specific drug regimen at the start of treatment if the test indicates the presence of RIF and/or INH resistance. Culture and phenotypic drug susceptibility testing should also be performed ideally in all cases to confirm molecular testing results.

All patients should be monitored throughout the course of treatment to ensure they respond to the regimen prescribed. If sputum smear microscopy fails to become negative after 2 months of treatment, it should be repeated a month later; if it is still positive, repeat culture and drug susceptibility testing should be performed. The clinical response should guide interventions as well. MDR-TB requires a different treatment approach. WHO recommends the use of pyrazinamide, plus a combination of 4 second-line drugs as follows: a later-generation fluoroquinolone, a parenteral agent (such as kanamycin, amikacin, or capreomycin), ethionamide or prothionamide, and either cycloserine and p-aminosalicylic acid. The intensive phase should last at least 8 months, and the recommended total treatment duration should be of at least 20 months.

WHO recommends children receive the same regimens as adults with minor modifications. Children with acute pulmonary or extrapulmonary TB can be treated with INH, RIF, PZA, and EMB for 2 months, followed by INH and RIF for 4 months. If treatment cannot be directly observed in the continuation phase, 6 months of INH and EMB can be substituted in place of 4 months of INH and RIF. Children with TB meningitis or HIV-coinfection should be treated for a minimum of 9 months.

- In HIV-infected patients, concomitant treatment for TB and antiretroviral therapy has several challenges, including adherence to multiple medications, overlapping medication side effects, immune reconstitution inflammatory syndrome, and drug–drug interactions. These patients should be treated by, or in close consultation with, a clinician with expertise in management of both TB and HIV.

- Thoracic surgery is rarely indicated but has been used successfully in certain MDR and XDR-TB cases with focal pulmonary disease and adequate pulmonary function. Patients in whom surgery is considered should have several months of adequate treatment before resection and should continue treatment for 12–24 months following surgery.

- Monitoring of treatment response necessitates symptom evaluation and sputum-smear microscopy and culture monthly, or at least after 1, 2, 5, and 6 months. In developing countries where smear microscopy is still the only readily available tool, the latter plan is most common. Radiological abnormalities may persist for months after a bacteriological response, often with permanent scarring, and monitoring by serial chest radiographs is thus neither useful nor recommended for evaluation of response. An end-of-treatment chest X-ray in patients with active pulmonary TB may help show new baseline anatomy and will document findings for future comparison.

- WHO strongly recommends that cohort analysis of treatment outcomes include all patients registered for treatment. The 6 mutually exclusive categories of treatment results are: bacteriologically proven cure, treatment completion (without bacteriological evidence of cure), failure (smear positive at month 5 after treatment start), default, death, and transfer to other administrative units. Cohort analysis allows proper evaluation of treatment program performance and prompts corrective measures when unacceptable levels of treatment failures, deaths, and defaulting occur.

  For WHO guidance on details of case management (including MDR and HIV-associated TB), see: http://whqlibdoc. who.int/publications/2010/9789241547833_eng.pdf. For WHO policy on collaborative TB/HIV activities, see: http:// whqlibdoc.who.int/publications/2012/9789241503006_eng. pdf. For WHO guidelines for the programmatic management of drug-resistant TB, see: http://whqlibdoc.who.int/ publications/2011/9789241501583_eng.pdf?ua=1. For further

details of case management in children, see: http://www.who.
int/entity/tb/publications/childtb_guidelines/en/index.html.

11. **Management of contacts and the immediate environment—**

1) Investigation of potentially exposed contacts is recommended, using TST or IGRA tests for all household members and other close contacts. If the initial result is negative, a repeat test should be performed at least 8–10 weeks after exposure to the person with active pulmonary TB has ended or they are no longer considered contagious. Clinical evaluation and a chest radiograph should be obtained for contacts with a positive test result to exclude active pulmonary TB.

2) Treatment of latent TB is indicated for contacts with positive TST or IGRA results. In addition, close contacts at high risk of developing active pulmonary or extrapulmonary TB (i.e., children <5 years and persons with HIV infection) should be started on presumptive treatment (i.e., "window prophylaxis") until the postexposure TST or IGRA result is available. In many developing countries, investigation of household contacts is limited to sputum microscopy of those contacts who have symptoms suggestive of TB disease.

3) Persons entering rooms where infectious TB patients reside should wear personal respiratory protective devices capable of filtering particles of less than a micron in diameter, such as N95 face respirators (surgical masks are not recommended).

12. **Special considerations—**

1) Reporting: report active pulmonary or extrapulmonary TB to local public health authorities when diagnosis is suspected; case reports are obligatory in most countries. They should state whether the case is bacteriologically confirmed (AFB smear positive, culture positive, or molecular detection) or if diagnosis was based on clinical and/or radiographic findings, and whether the case was previously treated. Public health authorities should maintain a register of cases requiring treatment and must be actively involved with planning and monitoring the course of treatment.

2) TB and air travel: several incidents of potential transmission of TB related to international air travel have been reported since the early 1990s. More recently, the emergence of MDR-TB and XDR-TB has raised the concern of air travel and TB transmission. The revision of the IHR, which provides a legal framework for a more effective and coordinated international response to public health emergencies and risks, including those caused by outbreaks of communicable diseases such as XDR-TB has important provisions for the detection

and control of TB during air travel. Available evidence indicates that the risk of transmission of *M. tuberculosis* on board aircraft is low and limited to persons in close proximity to an infectious case for 8 hours or longer. Passenger-to-passenger transmission of *M. tuberculosis* has been documented only among passengers seated in the same section as the index case. The risk of TB among cabin crew members is similar to that of the general population. Therefore, mandatory routine or periodic screening is not indicated for cabin crew. There is no evidence that recirculation of cabin air facilitates the transmission of infectious disease agents on board.

Further information can be found at:

● http://www.who.int/topics/tuberculosis/en.
● http://www.cdc.gov/tb/ http://www.who.int/gtb.
● http://www.stoptb.org.

II. DISEASES DUE TO OTHER MYCOBACTERIA (mycobacterioses, nontuberculous mycobacterial disease)

Nontuberculous mycobacteria (NTM, mycobacteria other than *Mycobacterium tuberculosis* complex organisms, and *Mycobacterium leprae*) are ubiquitous environmental microorganisms that can be recovered from soil, fresh water, and seawater (natural and treated). Until recently there was no evidence of human-to-human or animal-to-human transmission of NTM. However, 2 recent findings investigating outbreaks in cystic fibrosis patients by using thorough conventional epidemiologic and state-of-the-art molecular typing investigations such as whole genome sequencing suggest potential transmission of *Mycobacterium abscessus* subsp. *massiliense* and *M. abscessus* between these patients. Since NTM may be found in both natural and man-made reservoirs, human infections are suspected to be acquired from these environmental sources. However, the identification of the specific source of infection is usually not possible. NTM diseases are usually not mandatory to report since they are not generally communicable, and surveillance data is not only limited but also unreliable. The NTM are often classified based on their growth characteristics after subculture onto solid media. Some grow rapidly and within 7 days (*M. abscessus, Mycobacterium chelonae, Mycobacterium fortuitum, Mycobacterium peregrinum*). Others grow more slowly, requiring more than 7 days to form visible colonies (*Mycobacterium avium* complex [MAC], *Mycobacterium kansasii, Mycobacterium ulcerans, Mycobacterium marinum*). From 41 valid species in 1980, currently the genus *Mycobacterium* encompasses 169 recognized species and 13 subspecies. Clinical syndromes associated with the NTM can be classified broadly as follows:

1) Disseminated disease—often in the presence of severe immuno-deficiency such as that determined by HIV/AIDS—can be caused by MAC, *M. kansasii*, *Mycobacterium haemophilum*, and *Mycobacterium genavense*. *M. abscessus* and *M. fortuitum* can infect intravenous catheters and indwelling lines, causing disseminated disease. In the presence of disseminated NTM, symptoms include fever, weight loss, and fatigue. Diagnosis can be obtained through isolation in blood, liver, or bone marrow culture.

2) Pulmonary disease resembling tuberculosis—MAC, *M. kansasii*, *M. abscessus*, *Mycobacterium xenopi*, *Mycobacterium simiae*, and *Mycobacterium malmoense*. It should be suspected in cases of prolonged respiratory symptoms, especially in patients with underlying chronic pulmonary disease.

3) Lymphadenitis (primarily cervical)—MAC and *M. kansasii*.

4) Skin ulcers—*M. ulcerans* (see "Buruli Ulcer"), *M. fortuitum*, *M. chelonae*, *M. abscessus*, and *M. marinum*. These infections may appear as nodular or ulcerating; at times, they spread along the lymphatics.

5) Posttraumatic wound infections—*M. fortuitum*, *M. chelonae*, *M. abscessus*, *M. marinum*, and *M. avium* complex.

6) Nosocomial disease: surgical wound infections and catheter-related infections (bacteremia, peritonitis, postinjection abscesses)—*M. fortuitum*, *M. chelonae*, and *M. abscessus*.

A single isolation from sputum or gastric washings can occur in the absence of signs or symptoms of clinical disease. Multiple isolations of NTM from respiratory specimens, in the absence of illness or other specific pathology, may be evidence of colonization (e.g., with *Mycobacterium gordonae*), with no clinical significance. A single positive culture from a wound or tissue is generally considered diagnostic. In general, the diagnosis of disease requiring treatment is based on repeated isolations of many colonies from symptomatic patients with progressive illness. Where human infections with NTM are prevalent, cross-reactions may interfere with the interpretation of TST for *M. tuberculosis* infection, but less so if IGRAs are used.

Treatment is relatively effective against *M. kansasii* and *M. marinum* disease, but traditional antituberculosis drugs (especially PZA) may not be effective for NTM. Some cases of failure of TB treatment in settings with limited facilities for culture and drug susceptibility testing may in fact be cases of disease with NTM, which are commonly resistant in vitro to standard TB drugs. Drug susceptibility tests on the isolated organism will help select an effective drug combination. In general, pulmonary disease due to MAC can be treated with ethambutol, rifabutin plus a macrolide (clarithromycin or azithromycin), while that due to *M. kansasii* responds to clarithromycin, ethambutol, and rifampin. Cutaneous diseases caused by rapidly growing NTM can be treated with clarithromycin and/or amikacin, depending on the extent of skin disease. Skin infection caused by *M. marinum* is treated with a combination of clarithromycin, ethambutol, and a rifamycin (other active agents include tetracyclines and trimethoprim/sulphamethoxazole), usually for 3–4 months.

Further information can be found at: http://www.thoracic.org/sections/publications/statements/pages/mtpi/nontuberculous-mycobacterial-diseases.html.

[M. C. Raviglione, H. Getahun]

TULAREMIA
(rabbit fever, deer-fly fever, Ohara's disease, Francis disease)

DISEASE	ICD-10 CODE
TULAREMIA	ICD-10 A21

1. **Clinical features**—A bacterial zoonotic infection that causes 1 of 6 clinical syndromes depending on the site of inoculation and virulence of the infecting organism. The most common syndrome is ulceroglandular tularemia, characterized by a skin ulcer and regional lymphadenopathy. Glandular tularemia is similar but lacks an obvious skin ulcer. Oropharyngeal tularemia presents with painful pharyngitis (with or without ulceration) and marked cervical lymphadenopathy, which may be unilateral. Pneumonic tularemia may be primary, following inhalation of the organism, or secondary due to hematogenous spread to the lungs from other parts of the body. Although not readily distinguished from other forms of community-acquired pneumonia, pneumonic tularemia is often accompanied by a transudative pleural effusion that yields the organism if cultured. Purulent conjunctivitis, punctate palpebral ulcers, and periauricular lymphadenopathy characterize oculoglandular tularemia. The sixth syndrome, typhoidal tularemia, refers to patients who lack localizing symptoms. Sudden high fever, chills, fatigue, general body aches, headache, and nausea accompany all forms of tularemia. Pneumonic tularemia can be life threatening; however, the overall case fatality is less than 5% with proper treatment. Differential diagnosis includes anthrax, brucellosis, plague, staphylococcal and streptococcal infections, cat scratch fever, and tuberculosis.

2. Causative agent—*Francisella tularensis* is a highly infectious, small, faintly staining, pleomorphic Gram-negative coccobacillus. The majority of human infections are caused by 2 subspecies that differ in distribution and virulence: *F. tularensis* subsp. *tularensis* (Jellison type A, generally the more virulent) and *F. tularensis* subsp. *holarctica* (Jellison type B). A third subspecies, *F. tularensis* subsp. *mediasiatica*, has been isolated from animals in central Asia but has not been linked to human illness. Related species *Francisella novicida*, *Francisella philomiragia*, and *Francisella hispaniensis* are rare causes of human illness.

3. Diagnosis—The diagnosis of tularemia is generally established serologically by demonstrating a 4-fold rise in specific antibody titers between acute and convalescent sera using tube or microagglutination. Cross-reactions with *Brucella* species have been observed when using tube agglutination. In some instances a sufficiently high titer in a single specimen is considered positive. Enzyme-linked immunosorbent assay (ELISA) assays for tularemia have also been used. Culture can provide a conclusive diagnosis but must be attempted only with appropriate biosafety conditions. Appropriate specimens include swabs or scrapping of skin lesions, lymph node aspirates or biopsies, pharyngeal swabs, sputum, bronchial/tracheal washings, sputum, or pleural fluid, depending on the form of illness. Blood cultures should also be collected, although yield is low.

When tularemia is suspected, it should be communicated to laboratory personnel beforehand because of the need to select the most appropriate specimens and the requirement for using special isolation procedures. A presumptive diagnosis of tularemia may be made through the testing of suspected isolates using direct fluorescent antibody (DFA), immunohisto-chemical (IHC) staining, or polymerase chain reaction (PCR) assays. In some jurisdictions *F. tularensis* has been identified as a "select agent," and therefore only registered laboratories are allowed to work with the organism.

4. Occurrence—Tularemia occurs regionally throughout the northern hemisphere. It has been reported in Scandinavia, continental Europe, central Asia, Middle East, Russia, northern regions of China, and Japan, but not north of the Arctic or in the British Isles. In North America, *F. tularensis* has been found from northern Mexico to the Arctic Circle in Alaska. Whereas type B infections occur throughout the northern hemisphere, the more virulent type A infections are limited to North America. Seasonality depends on the predominant mode of transmission and can be bimodal, with arthropod-associated infections occurring in the warmer months and rabbit-associated infections occurring in the winter. Outbreaks of human tularemia usually occur in association with animal epizootics, although these may not be recognized without a careful environmental investigation. Epidemics among humans may also be triggered by war and social disruption.

5. Reservoir—Wild animals, especially rabbits, hares, voles, muskrats, water rats, beavers, and some domestic animals; also various hard ticks. A rodent-mosquito cycle has been described for *F. tularensis* subsp. *holarctica* in the Scandinavian countries and Russia. Recent studies have suggested a possible role for free-living amoeba as a reservoir for type B strains.

6. Incubation period—Related to size of inoculum; usually 3-5 days (range 1-14 days).

7. Transmission—Humans become infected through arthropod bites, handling infected animal tissues, ingestion of contaminated food or water, and inhalation of contaminated aerosols. Symptoms vary according to the route of exposure (see Clinical Features in this chapter). Principal tick vectors in North America include *Dermacentor variabilis*, *Dermacentor andersoni*, and *Amblyomma americanum*; Eurasian tick vectors include *Ixodes ricinus*, *Dermacentor reticulatus*, and *Dermacentor marginatus*. Tabanid flies (*Crysops* spp.) are mechanical vectors that can transmit infection to a wide a range of hosts. Mosquitoes have been implicated as vectors in Eurasia but not in North America. Hunting-associated cases are usually associated with rabbits, hares, muskrats, or voles; a small outbreak in Spain was linked to collecting freshwater crayfish. Waterborne transmission has been reported due to unchlorinated wells and municipal systems and to natural bodies of water. Inhalational exposures can occur during agricultural activities, including sorting contaminated hay and mowing. The average infectious dose for humans is estimated at 10 organisms by subcutaneous inoculation and 25 organisms by aerosol. All ages are susceptible, and long-term immunity follows recovery; reinfection is extremely rare but has been reported in laboratory staff. Person-to-person transmission has never been reported.

8. Risk groups—As with other zoonotic diseases, the risk of tularemia is closely linked to occupational and recreational activities. Hunters, trappers, sheep shearers, veterinarians, forest rangers, game wardens, hikers, campers, and others with frequent animal or arthropod exposure are at increased risk of infection. In some areas, farmers and landscapers appear to be at increased risk of pneumonic tularemia as a consequence of exposure to contaminated dust and aerosols. *F. tularensis* is highly infectious when grown in culture, and numerous cases have been documented among laboratory workers. A few recent cases have been linked to commercially traded pets, suggesting that persons in the pet industry may also be at increased risk.

9. Prevention—

1) Educate the public to avoid bites of ticks, flies, and mosquitoes, for example by using long sleeves and repellents, and to avoid

contact with untreated water where infection prevails among wild animals.

2) Use impervious gloves when skinning or handling animals, especially rabbits. Cook the meat of wild rabbits and rodents thoroughly. Avoid handling such meat together with vegetables.

3) Use universal precautions in direct handling of small animals (especially pets) that are exhibiting signs and symptoms of illness.

4) Live attenuated vaccines applied intradermally by scarification are used extensively in Russia and to a limited extent for occupational risk groups in some other countries such as Sweden.

5) Take appropriate precautions (using facemasks, gowns, and impervious gloves and carrying out work under Class II biosafety cabinets) when handling cultures of *F. tularensis.*

10. **Management of patient—**

1) Universal precautions during patient care; person-to-person transmission has not been reported.

2) Concurrent disinfection of discharges from ulcers, lymph nodes, or conjunctival sacs.

3) Treatment: aminoglycosides (gentamicin or streptomycin) are the drugs of choice in serious infections. Tetracyclines, also widely used effectively as prophylaxis and treatment, are associated with higher relapse rates. Recent experience of treatment with ciprofloxacin has shown excellent efficacy and is preferred if oral treatment is used. Many antibiotics, including all beta-lactam antibiotics and modern cephalosporins, are ineffective and many isolates show resistance to macrolides. Treatment with aminoglycosides or ciprofloxacin should last 10–14 days, and tetracyclines, for 21 days.

4) Most common complication is persistent lymphadenopathy with suppuration that may require surgical drainage.

11. **Management of contacts and the immediate environment—**
Investigation of the source of infection is important in each case.

12. **Special considerations—**

1) Reporting: report to local health authority may be required in some endemic areas.

2) Epidemic measures: search for sources of infection related to arthropods, animal hosts, water, and environments soiled by small mammals, including hay. Control measures as indicated in Prevention in this chapter.

3) Measures in the case of deliberate use: *Francisella* is considered to be a potential agent for deliberate use, particularly as an

aerosol. As with plague, cases acquired by inhalation present as primary pneumonia. Such cases require prompt identification and specific treatment to prevent a fatal outcome. All diagnosed cases, and especially clusters of pneumonia due to *F. tularensis*, must be reported immediately to the health department for appropriate investigation.

[P. Mead]

TYPHOID FEVER AND PARATYPHOID FEVERS

DISEASE	ICD-10 CODE
TYPHOID FEVER	ICD-10 A01.0
PARATYPHOID FEVER	ICD-10 A01.1-A01.4

1. Clinical features—A systemic bacterial disease characterized by the insidious onset of sustained fever, marked headache, and malaise. Other symptoms and signs that may be present in some patients include anorexia, relative bradycardia, splenomegaly, nonproductive cough in the early stage of the illness, rose spots on the trunk (visible in 25% of light-skinned patients), and constipation more often than diarrhea in adults. The clinical picture varies from mild illness with low-grade fever to severe clinical disease with abdominal discomfort and multiple complications. Severity is influenced by factors such as strain virulence, quantity of inoculum ingested, duration of illness before adequate treatment, age, and, for typhoid fever, previous exposure to typhoid vaccination. Inapparent or mild illnesses occur, especially in endemic areas; 60%-90% of patients with typhoid fever do not receive medical attention or are treated as outpatients. Mild cases show no systemic involvement; the clinical picture is that of gastroenteritis (see "Salmonellosis"). Nonsweating fevers, mental dullness, slight deafness, and parotitis may occur. Peyer patches in the ileum can ulcerate, with intestinal hemorrhage or perforation (~3% of cases in the developing world) occurring most commonly in the absence of timely, appropriate antimicrobial therapy. Severe forms with altered mental status and other neurologic complications have been associated with high case-fatality rates. The case-fatality rate of 10%-20% observed in the preantibiotic era can fall below 1% with prompt appropriate antimicrobial therapy. Depending on the antimicrobials used, 15%-20% of patients may experience relapses (generally milder than the initial clinical illness).

Paratyphoid fever presents a similar clinical picture. The ratio of typhoid fever to paratyphoid fever is estimated to be about 4 to 1. Relapses occur in approximately 3%-4% of cases.

2. Causative agents—*Salmonella enterica* serovar Typhi is the etiologic agent of typhoid fever. Paratyphoid fever may be caused by *S. enterica* serovars Paratyphi A, Paratyphi B, or Paratyphi C. The term "enteric fever" is sometimes used to describe invasive febrile infections caused by serovars Typhi, Paratyphi A, Paratyphi B, or Paratyphi C. Although nontyphoidal *Salmonella* serovars may also commonly cause invasive infections (e.g., Dublin), the term enteric fever is limited to disease caused by these 4 serovars.

3. Diagnosis—The causal organisms can be isolated from blood early in the disease and from urine and feces after the first week. Blood culture is the diagnostic mainstay for typhoid fever, but bone marrow culture provides the most sensitive method for bacteriological confirmation even in patients who have already received antimicrobials. Because of limited sensitivity and specificity, serological tests based on agglutinating antibodies (Widal) are generally of little diagnostic value. Although rapid serodiagnostic tests (such as TUBEX TF) based on the detection of specific antibodies have better sensitivity and specificity than the Widal test, these tests are still poorly suited for individual patient diagnosis; instead, they are most useful for rapid outbreak detection and confirmation.

4. Occurrence—Worldwide, the annual estimated incidence of typhoid fever is about 27 million cases with approximately 210,000 deaths. Most of the disease burden occurs in the developing world. The burden is sporadic in industrialized countries, where most cases are acquired during travel in endemic areas. Paratyphoid fever occurs sporadically or in limited outbreaks, probably more frequently than reports suggest. Of the 3 serovars, Paratyphi A is most common, Paratyphi B is less frequent, and Paratyphi C is extremely rare.

5. Reservoir—Exclusively humans for serovars Typhi and Paratyphi A; humans and possibly domestic animals for other serovars. A carrier state may follow acute or mild illness or even subclinical infections. Short-term fecal carriers are more common than urinary carriers. The chronic carrier state is most common (2%-5%) among persons infected during middle age, especially women; serovar Typhi colonizes the gallbladder, and carriers frequently have biliary tract abnormalities including gallstones. The chronic urinary carrier state may co-occur with schistosome infections or kidney stones.

6. Incubation period—Depends on inoculum size and on host factors; for typhoid fever, from 3 days to more than 60 days with a usual range of 8-14 days; for paratyphoid fever, the incubation period is 1-10 days.

7. Transmission—Through ingestion of food and water contaminated by feces or urine of patients and carriers. Important vehicles in some countries include shellfish (particularly oysters) from sewage-contaminated beds, raw fruit and vegetables, frozen fruit, contaminated milk/milk products (usually contaminated through hands of carriers), and untreated drinking water. Flies may contaminate foods in which the organism then multiplies to infective doses (those are reportedly lower for typhoid than for paratyphoid bacteria). Epidemiological data suggest that, while water-borne transmission of *S. enterica* serovar Typhi usually involves small inocula, foodborne transmission is associated with large inocula and high attack rates over short periods. Sexual transmission of typhoid fever from an asymptomatic carrier has been documented. Patients are infectious for as long as bacilli appear in excreta, usually from the first week throughout convalescence; variable thereafter (commonly 1-2 weeks for paratyphoid). About 10% of untreated typhoid fever patients discharge bacilli for 3 months after onset of symptoms. Both treated and untreated patients can become chronic carriers; fewer persons infected with paratyphoid organisms may become chronic carriers.

8. Risk groups—In endemic areas, typhoid fever is most common in preschool children and children 5-19 years; in epidemic areas, cases of typhoid fever have a broad age distribution. International travelers to endemic areas are also at risk, as are individuals with gastric achlorhydria. Relative specific immunity follows recovery from clinical disease, unapparent infection, and active immunization.

9. Prevention—Prevention is based on access to safe water and proper sanitation and on adherence to safe food-handling practices.

1) Instruct the community, patients, convalescents, and carriers in personal hygiene. Emphasize hand washing as a routine practice after defecation and before preparing, serving, or eating food. Provide suitable hand washing facilities, particularly for food handlers and attendants involved in the care of patients and children.

2) Dispose of human feces safely, and maintain fly-proof latrines. Where culturally appropriate, encourage use of sufficient toilet paper to minimize hand contamination. Under field conditions, dispose of feces by burial at a site distant and downstream from the source of drinking water. Discourage the use of human feces as fertilizer.

3) Protect, purify, and chlorinate public water supplies, provide safe private supplies, and avoid possible backflow connections between water and sewer systems. For individual and small

group protection and during travel or in the field, treat water chemically or by boiling.

4) Use scrupulous cleanliness in food preparation and handling; refrigerate as appropriate. Pay particular attention to the storage of salads and other foods served cold. These provisions apply to home and public eating places. If uncertain about sanitary practices, select foods that are cooked and served hot and fruit that is peeled by the consumer.

5) Pasteurize or boil all milk and dairy products. Supervise the sanitary aspects of commercial milk production, storage, and delivery.

6) Enforce suitable quality-control procedures in industries that prepare food and drink for human consumption. Use chlorinated water for cooling during canned food processing.

7) Limit the collection and marketing of shellfish to supplies from approved sources. Boil or steam ($\geq$10 minutes) before serving.

8) Encourage breastfeeding throughout infancy; boil all milk and water used for infant feeding in developing countries or where there may be breaches in pasteurization.

9) Typhoid carriers should be excluded from handling food and from providing patient care. Identify and supervise typhoid carriers. Chronic carriers should not be released from supervision and restriction of occupation until local or state regulations are met, often not until 3 consecutive negative cultures are obtained from authenticated fecal specimens (and urine in areas endemic for schistosomiasis) over the course of several days to 2 months and at least 48 hours after antimicrobial therapy has stopped. Fresh stool specimens are preferred to rectal swabs. It has been suggested that at least 1 of the 3 consecutive negative stool specimens should be obtained by purging, though this is rarely practical. Administration of ciprofloxacin or norfloxacin twice daily for 28 days provides successful treatment of chronic carriers in 80%-90% of cases. Several studies have suggested 14-21 days of treatment to be equally efficacious. Follow-up cultures are necessary to confirm cure.

10) Control flies by screening and use of insecticidal baits and traps or, where appropriate, spraying with insecticides. Control fly breeding through frequent garbage collection and disposal and through fly control measures in latrine construction and maintenance.

11) Immunization for typhoid fever is not routinely recommended in nonendemic areas except for those subject to unusual occupational exposure to enteric infections (e.g., clinical microbiology technicians) and household members of known carriers. WHO recommends vaccination for people who travel

to endemic high-risk areas and children living in endemic areas where typhoid fever control is a priority. Vaccination of high-risk populations is considered a promising strategy for the control of endemic typhoid fever; this approach has rarely been used as a control measure for ongoing outbreaks. An oral, live multidose vaccine using *S. enterica* ser. Typhi strain Ty21a and a single-dose parenteral vaccine containing the polysaccharide Vi antigen are widely available. However, Ty21a should not be used in patients receiving antibiotics until 24 hours or more after the last antibiotic dose. Booster doses every 2–5 years, according to vaccine type, are desirable for those at continuing risk of infection. Neither vaccine is licensed for children younger than 2 years; Ty21a is only licensed for children 6 years and older in the USA, but is licensed for younger children in other countries. Polysaccharide Vi conjugate vaccines in various stages of development have shown promise in stimulating a greater immune response of longer duration, even in children younger than 2 years. These are expected to be commercially available in the future. No vaccines for paratyphoid fever are currently available. Findings indicate that Ty21a offers limited cross-reacting humoral intestinal immune response against *S. enterica* ser. Paratyphi B antigens.

10. **Management of patient—**

1) Enteric precautions while ill; hospital care is desirable during acute illness. Release from supervision by local health authority based on not fewer than 3 consecutive negative cultures of feces (and urine in patients with schistosomiasis) at least 24 hours apart, at least 48 hours after any antimicrobials, and not earlier than 1 month after onset. If any of these are positive, repeat cultures at monthly intervals during the 12 months following onset until at least 3 consecutive negative cultures are obtained.

2) Concurrent disinfection of feces, urine, and soiled articles. In communities with adequate sewage disposal systems, feces and urine can be disposed of directly into sewers without preliminary disinfection.

3) Treatment: fluoroquinolones are the drugs of choice in adults, including pregnant women infected with amoxicillin-resistant strains. However, rapid emergence of decreased susceptibility and frank resistance to fluoroquinolones in both *S. enterica* ser. Typhi and *S. enterica* ser. Paratyphi A restricts widespread and indiscriminate use in primary care facilities and mandates antimicrobial testing of all isolates. If local strains are known to

be sensitive to traditional first-line antibiotics, oral chloramphenicol, amoxicillin, or trimethoprim-sulfoxazole (particularly in children) should be used in accordance with local antimicrobial sensitivity patterns. If strains are resistant to ciprofloxacin as well as traditional first-line antibiotics, azithromycin is an effective alternative treatment. Ceftriaxone, a parenteral once-daily antibiotic, is recommended in patients with dulled perceptions or those with complications such that oral antibiotics cannot be used. Short-term, high-dose corticosteroid treatment, combined with specific antibiotics and supportive care, reduces mortality in critically ill patients. Patients with concurrent schistosomiasis must also be treated with praziquantel to eliminate possible schistosome carriage of *S. enterica* ser. Typhi. Patients with confirmed intestinal perforation require immediate surgical intervention and intensive care. Early intervention is crucial, as morbidity rates increase with delayed surgery after perforation. Strains resistant to chloramphenicol and other recommended antimicrobials have become prevalent in several areas. Most isolates from southern and southeastern Asia, the Middle East, and northeastern Africa in the 1990s carry an R factor plasmid encoding resistance to those antimicrobial agents that were previously the mainstay of oral treatment, including chloramphenicol, ampicillin, and trimethoprim/sulfamethoxazole. Resistance to fluoroquinolones is now common in Asia and is emerging in sub-Saharan Africa. There have been limited reports of in vitro azithromycin resistance in isolates of *Salmonella* Typhi and Paratyphi A; in at least one patient with Paratyphi A infection, this was correlated with azithromycin treatment failure.

11. **Management of contacts and the immediate environment—**

1) Routine administration of typhoid vaccine is of limited value for family, household, and nursing contacts who have been or may be exposed to active cases; it should be considered for those who may be exposed to carriers on a prolonged basis. There is no effective immunization for paratyphoid fever.

2) Determine actual or probable source of infection of every case through search for unreported cases, carriers, or contaminated food, water, or milk. All members of travel groups in which a case has been identified should be followed. The presence of elevated antibody titers to purified Vi polysaccharide is highly suggestive of the typhoid carrier state, especially in the setting of an epidemiologically consistent history. Identification of the same phage type or molecular subtype in the carrier and in

organisms isolated from patients suggests a possible chain of transmission. Consideration should be given to obtaining 2 negative stool cultures, taken at least 24 hours apart, from household and close contacts before allowing them to be employed in sensitive occupations (e.g., as food handlers).

12. **Special considerations—**

1) Reporting: case report to local health authorities is obligatory in most countries.

2) Epidemic measures:

   - Search intensively for the case/carrier who is the source of infection, and for the vehicle (water or food) through which infection was transmitted.
   - Selectively eliminate suspected contaminated food. Pasteurize or boil milk, or exclude milk supplies and other foods suspected on epidemiological evidence, until safety is ensured.
   - Chlorinate suspected water supplies adequately under competent supervision, or avoid use. All drinking water must be chlorinated, treated with iodine, or boiled before use.
   - Preemptive vaccination before seasonal outbreaks or in areas at risk of an outbreak may be considered.

3) Disaster implications: with disruption of usual water supply and sewage disposal and of controls on food and water, transmission and large-scale outbreaks of typhoid fever may occur if there are active cases or carriers in a displaced population. Efforts should be made to restore safe drinking-water supplies and excreta disposal facilities. Selective immunization of stabilized groups such as schoolchildren, prisoners, and utility, municipal, or hospital personnel may be helpful.

4) International measures: for typhoid fever, immunization is advised for international travelers to endemic areas, especially if travel is likely to involve exposure to unsafe food and water or close contact in rural areas to indigenous populations. It is not a legal requirement for entry into any country.

WHO Collaborating Centers provide support as required. Further information can be found at: http://www.who.int/collaboratingcentres/database/en.

[E. Mintz, R. Slayton, M. Walters]

TYPHUS

DISEASE	ICD-10 CODE
EPIDEMIC LOUSE-BORNE TYPHUS FEVER	ICD-10 A75
BRILL-ZINSSER DISEASE	ICD-10 A75.1
ENDEMIC FLEA-BORNE TYPHUS FEVER	ICD-10 A75.2
SCRUB TYPHUS	ICD-10 A75.3
Queensland tick typhus (see "Rickettsioses")	

I. EPIDEMIC LOUSE-BORNE TYPHUS FEVER
(louse-borne typhus, typhus exanthematicus, classic typhus fever)

1. Clinical features—A rickettsial disease with variable onset; often with sudden onset of headache, chills, malaise, fever, and general pains. A macular eruption appears on the fifth or sixth day, initially on the upper trunk, followed by spread to the entire body, but usually not to the face, palms, or soles. The eruption is often difficult to observe on patients with darkly pigmented skin and/or absent in up to 40% of patients. Cough and tachypnea may be present and neurological signs are common, including confusion, drowsiness, coma, seizures, and hearing loss. The case-fatality rate increases with age and varies from 10%–40% in the absence of treatment. Mild infections may occur without eruption, especially in children. The disease may recrudesce years after the primary attack (Brill-Zinsser disease); this form of disease is milder, has fewer complications, and has a lower case-fatality rate.

2. Causative agent—*Rickettsia prowazekii*.

3. Diagnosis—As with many rickettsial diseases, thrombocytopenia and elevated serum liver enzymes are common and may aid in making a diagnosis. Laboratory confirmation of a diagnosis typically occurs late in the disease process and is therefore not useful for making treatment decisions. The immunofluorescence assay (IFA) is the most accurate method for laboratory confirmation and requires a 4-fold increase in antibody titers when comparing a patient's acute and convalescent sera. An acute serum sample should be obtained in the first week of symptoms and a convalescent serum sample obtained 3–4 weeks later. Antibody tests usually become positive in the second to third week of illness. Therefore, an acute titer taken in the first week of illness should be used as a baseline for comparison to the convalescent sample and a negative acute result does not rule out active infection, nor does a positive acute result confirm the diagnosis. Common serologic tests cannot discriminate between louse-borne and murine typhus unless the sera are differentially absorbed with the respective rickettsial antigen prior to testing. Other diagnostic methods with varying degrees of sensitivity and specificity are enzyme immunoassay (EIA), polymerase chain reaction (PCR), immunohistochemical (IHC) staining of tissues, complement fixation with group specific or washed type-specific rickettsial antigens, and the toxin neutralization test. The Weil-Felix agglutination test is commonly used and available worldwide but is notoriously unreliable and not recommended. Skin biopsy samples of rash sites can be tested by IHC or PCR, but only PCR and sequence analysis provides definitive agent identification. Sending lice to a reference laboratory for PCR testing may help detect an outbreak.

4. Occurrence—Worldwide distribution where people live under unhygienic conditions and are infested with lice. Explosive epidemics may occur during war and famine. Endemic foci exist in the mountainous regions of Mexico, in Central and South America, in central and eastern Africa, and numerous countries in Asia. Recent outbreaks have been observed in Burundi and Rwanda. In the eastern USA, cases of epidemic typhus associated with contact with flying squirrels and their ectoparasites have been reported sporadically.

5. Reservoir—Humans are the reservoir for louse-associated epidemic typhus and are responsible for maintaining the infection during interepidemic periods. Although not a major source of human disease, sporadic cases may be associated with flying squirrels, possibly via the squirrel flea.

6. Incubation period—From 1-2 weeks, commonly 12 days.

7. Transmission—The body louse, *Pediculus humanus corporis*, is infected by feeding on the blood of a patient with acute typhus fever. Patients with Brill-Zinsser disease can infect lice and may serve as foci for new outbreaks in louse-infested communities. Infected lice excrete rickettsiae in their feces and usually defecate at the time of feeding. People are infected by rubbing feces or crushed lice into the bite or into superficial abrasions. Inhalation of infective louse feces in dust may account for some infections. Transmission from the flying squirrel is presumed to be through the bite of the squirrel flea, but flea feces may also be infectious. One attack usually confers long-lasting immunity.

The disease is not directly transmitted from person to person. Patients are infective for lice during the febrile illness, and possibly for 2-3 days after the temperature returns to normal. Infected lice pass rickettsiae in their feces within 2-6 days after the blood meal; they are infective earlier if crushed. The louse invariably dies within 2 weeks after infection; rickettsiae may remain viable in the dead louse for weeks.

8. Risk groups—Susceptibility is general.

9. **Prevention—**

   1) Apply an effective residual insecticide powder at appropriate intervals by hand or power blower to clothes and skin of persons of populations living under conditions favoring louse infestation. The insecticide used should be effective on local lice and used according to safety labeling and instructions.

   2) Improve living conditions with provisions for bathing and washing clothes.

   3) Treat prophylactically those who are subject to risk by application of residual insecticide to clothing (dusting or impregnation), and in the case of an epidemic, directly to the skin as well (see Appropriate Insecticide under Management of Patient).

10. **Management of patient—**

    1) Appropriate insecticide powder applied to clothing and bedding of patient and contacts; launder clothing and bedclothes. Lice tend to leave abnormally hot or cold bodies in search of a normothermic clothed body. If death from louse-borne typhus occurs before delousing, delouse the body and clothing by thorough application of an insecticide.

    2) Isolation is not required after proper delousing of patient, clothing, living quarters, and household contacts.

    3) Treatment: treatment should be initiated empirically as soon as typhus is suspected based on clinical signs, symptoms, and epidemiology, because early treatment is more likely to prevent adverse outcomes. Doxycycline is the drug of choice for adults and children of all ages. The pediatric dose is 2.2 mg/kg twice a day for 3 days after resolution of fever (usually a 5- to 10-day course); the adult dose is 100 mg twice a day for 5-10 days. Chloramphenicol is an acceptable alternative drug. Ciprofloxacin is not recommended because treatment failures have occurred. In epidemic situations in which antimicrobial agents may be limited, a single dose of doxycycline may provide effective treatment (100 mg for children; 200 mg for adults).

11. **Management of contacts and the immediate environment—**

    1) All immediate contacts should be kept under surveillance for 2 weeks.

    2) Appropriate insecticide powder applied to clothing and bedding of contacts; launder clothing and bedclothes.

    3) Every effort should be made to trace the infection to the immediate source.

12. **Special considerations—**

1) Reporting: report of louse-borne typhus fever required as a Disease under Surveillance by WHO. Further information can be found at: http://www.who.int/collaboratingcentres/database/en.

2) Epidemic measures: the best measure for rapid control of typhus is application of an insecticide with residual effect to all contacts. Where louse infestation is known to be widespread, systematic application of residual insecticide to all people in the community is indicated. Treatment of cases in an epidemic may also decrease the spread of disease. In epidemics, individuals may protect themselves by wearing silk or plastic clothing tightly fastened around wrists, ankles, and neck and impregnating clothes with repellents or permethrin.

3) Disaster implications: typhus can be expected to be a significant problem in louse-infested populations in endemic areas if social upheavals and crowding occur.

4) International measures: notification by governments to WHO and to adjacent countries of the occurrence of a case or an outbreak of louse-borne typhus fever in an area previously free of the disease.

5) Measures in case of deliberate use: *R. prowazekii* has been produced as a possible bioweapon and was used before World War II. It is infectious by aerosol, with a high case-fatality rate. The initial reference treatment of any suspected case is a single dose of 200 mg of doxycycline in situations where doxycycline is limited in supply.

II. ENDEMIC FLEA-BORNE TYPHUS FEVER (murine typhus, shop typhus, flea-borne rickettsiosis)

1. **Clinical features**—The course of flea-borne rickettsial diseases resemble that of louse-borne typhus but are frequently milder, with abrupt onset of fever, headache, and myalgias. Rash occurs in 50%-80% of patients, however, it typically is not present at initial presentation. Abdominal symptoms such as nausea, vomiting, and abdominal pain may occur and are more common in children. Complications such as acute renal failure and respiratory failure can occur but are not common. The case-fatality rate for all ages is less than 5% but increases with age. Presence of fleas and absence of louse infestation, geographic and seasonal distribution, and sporadic occurrence of the disease help differentiate it from louse-borne typhus.

2. **Causative agents**—*Rickettsia typhi, Rickettsia felis*.

3. **Diagnosis**—See Epidemic Louse-Borne Typhus Fever section in this chapter.

4. Occurrence—Worldwide. Found in areas where people and rats occupy the same buildings. Multiple cases may occur in the same household.

5. Reservoir—Rats, mice, and possibly other small and medium sized mammals. Infection is maintained in nature by a host-flea-host cycle (commonly *Xenopsylla cheopis* on *Rattus rattus* and *Rattus norvegicus*). A related organism, *R. felis*, is found worldwide in diverse flea species, particularly *Ctenocephalides felis*, and maintained transovarially.

6. Incubation period—From 1-2 weeks, commonly 12 days.

7. Transmission—Infective fleas defecate rickettsiae while taking a blood meal; this contaminates the bite site and other fresh skin wounds. Occasionally, a case may follow inhalation of dried infective flea feces. Not directly transmitted from person to person. Once infected, fleas remain so for life (up to 1 year) and transfer infection to their progeny. One attack confers immunity.

8. Risk groups—Susceptibility is general.

9. Prevention—

1) To avoid increased exposure of humans, wait until flea populations have first been reduced by insecticides before instituting rodent control measures (see "Plague").
2) Apply insecticide powders with residual action to rat runs, burrows, and harborages.

10. Management of patient—Treatment: treatment should be initiated empirically as soon as typhus is suspected based on clinical signs, symptoms, and epidemiology, because early treatment is more likely to prevent adverse outcomes. Doxycycline is the treatment of choice for flea-borne rickettsioses, regardless of patient age. The pediatric dose is 2.2 mg/kg twice a day for 3 days after resolution of fever (usually a 5- to 10-day course); the adult dose is 100 mg twice a day for 5-10 days. Chloramphenicol may be used as an alternative; however, relapses after treatment with this medication have been documented.

11. Management of contacts and the immediate environment—Control rodents or opossums (North America) around premises or home of patient.

12. Special considerations—

1) Reporting: case report to local health authority obligatory in most countries.

2) Epidemic measures: in endemic areas with numerous cases, use of a residual insecticide effective against rat or cat fleas will reduce the flea index and the incidence of infection in humans.

3) Disaster implications: cases can be expected when people, rats, and fleas are forced to coexist in close proximity, but murine typhus has not been a major contributor to elevated disease rates in such situations.

WHO Collaborating Centres provide support as required. Further information can be found at: http://www.who.int/collaboratingcentres/database/en.

III. SCRUB TYPHUS (Tsutsugamushi disease, mite-borne typhus fever)

1. Clinical features—A rickettsial disease often characterized by a primary "punched out" skin ulcer (eschar) corresponding to the site of attachment of an infected mite (chigger). Not all patients with scrub typhus have an eschar and the frequency of this symptom varies by region. An acute febrile onset follows within several days, along with headache, profuse sweating, conjunctival injection, and lymphadenopathy. A transient maculopapular rash appears on the trunk in about half of patients around day 7 of fever. Cough and X-ray evidence of pneumonitis are common and may progress to acute respiratory distress syndrome (ARDS) and respiratory failure. Neurological findings such as confusion or hearing loss may occur. This disease may cause spontaneous abortions in pregnant women. Without antibiotic therapy, fever lasts for about 14 days. The case-fatality rate in untreated cases varies from 1%–60% according to area, strain of infectious agent, and previous exposure to disease; it is consistently higher among older people.

2. Causative agent—*Orientia tsutsugamushi* with multiple, serologically distinct strains.

3. Diagnosis—See Epidemic Louse-Borne Typhus Fever section in this chapter. While IFA detection of a 4-fold rise in titer and/or an immunoglobulin class M (IgM) titer greater than 1:32 remain the gold standard, complement fixation tests are available that detect either antibodies or antigen in a patient's serum. Reinfections with different strains may occur and serologic diagnosis may need to include testing for multiple *O. tsutsugamushi* strains to improve assay sensitivity and specificity. Five major serotypes have been identified (Kato, Karp, Boryon, Kawazaki, and Gilliam) and country-specific antigenic pools may also be available and assessed. Commercial rapid diagnostic kits are available that provide results within 1 hour although the cost of these kits may be prohibitive in some areas. PCR of eschar and swabs of subeschar lesions are often diagnostic.

4. Occurrence—Central, eastern, and southeastern Asia; from southeastern Siberia and northern Japan to northern Australia and Vanuatu, as far west as Pakistan, to as high as 3,000 m (10,000 ft) above sea level in the Himalaya Mountains, and particularly prevalent in northern Thailand. Acquired by humans in one of innumerable small, sharply delimited typhus islands (some covering an area of only a few square feet) where causative agent, vectors, and suitable rodents exist simultaneously. Epidemics occur when susceptibles are brought into endemic areas, especially in military operations in which 20%–50% of troops have been infected within weeks or months.

5. Reservoir—Infected larval stage of trombiculid mites (chigger); *Leptotrombidium deliensis* and related species (varying with area) are the most common vectors for humans. Infection is maintained by transovarial passage in mites.

6. Incubation period—From 6–21 days, usually 10–12 days.

7. Transmission—Through the bite of infected larval mites; nymphs and adults do not feed on vertebrate hosts. No direct person-to-person transmission.

8. Risk groups—Military troops brought into endemic areas. Occupational infection is restricted mainly to adult workers (males more than females) who frequent overgrown terrain or other mite-infested areas, such as forest clearings, reforested areas, new settlements, or even newly irrigated desert regions.

Susceptibility is general. An attack confers prolonged immunity against the homologous strain of *O. tsutsugamushi* but only transient immunity against heterologous strains. Heterologous infection results in mild disease within a few months but produces typical illness after a year or so. Second and even third attacks of naturally acquired scrub typhus (usually benign or inapparent) occur among people who spend their lives in endemic areas or who have not been completely treated.

9. Prevention—

1) Prevent contact with infected mites through personal prophylaxis by impregnating clothes and blankets with miticidal chemicals (permethrin and benzyl benzoate) and application of mite repellents (diethyltoluamide) to exposed skin surfaces.

2) Eliminate mites from the specific sites through application of chlorinated hydrocarbons, such as lindane, dieldrin, or chlordane,

to ground and vegetation in environs of camps, mine buildings, and other populated zones in endemic areas.

3) In a small group of volunteers in Malaysia, the administration of 7 weekly doses of doxycycline was an effective prophylactic regimen.

10. Management of patient—Treatment: treatment should be initiated empirically as soon as typhus is suspected based on clinical signs, symptoms, and epidemiology, because early treatment is more likely to prevent adverse outcomes. Doxycycline is the drug of choice for adults and children of all ages. The pediatric dose is 2.2 mg/kg twice a day for 3 days after resolution of fever (usually a 5- to 10-day course); the adult dose is 100 mg twice a day for 5–10 days. Chloramphenicol is an acceptable alternative drug. Combination therapy with doxycycline and rifampin may be needed in regions where strains with reduced susceptibility to tetracyclines have been identified. Azithromycin may be a suitable alternative in some cases.

11. Management of contacts and the immediate environment—

1) Every effort should be made to trace the infection to the environmental source.

2) Persons with similar exposures should be monitored for fever and treatment initiated quickly when needed.

12. Special considerations—

1) Reporting: report to local health authority may be required in some endemic areas.

2) Epidemic measures: rigorously employ procedures described in Prevention in this chapter in the affected area; daily observation of all people at risk for fever and appearance of primary lesions; institute treatment on first indication of illness.

3) Disaster implications: only if refugee centers are sited in or near a "typhus island."

WHO Collaborating Centres provide support as required. Further information can be found at: http://www.who.int/collaboratingcentres/database/en.

[J. Regan, G. Dasch]

VARICELLA/HERPES ZOSTER

DISEASE	ICD-10 CODE
VARICELLA	ICD-10 B01
HERPES ZOSTER	ICD-10 B02

1. Clinical features—Varicella/herpes zoster (VZV) causes 2 distinct diseases: varicella, or chickenpox, is the primary infection, and later, if VZV reactivates, herpes zoster, or shingles. Varicella is characterized by fever and generalized, pruritic, maculopapulovesicular rash typically consisting of 250-500 lesions in varying stages of development. The lesions are maculopapular for a few hours, vesicular and pustular for 3-4 days, then crust, leaving granular scabs. The vesicles are superficial, unilocular, and collapse on puncture. Lesions commonly occur in successive crops for 3-7 days with several stages of maturity present at the same time; they tend to have central distribution and are more abundant on the trunk and proximal extremities. Lesions may appear on the scalp, high in the axilla, on mucous membranes of the mouth and upper respiratory tract, and on the conjunctivae; lesions tend to be more severe and can become confluent in areas of irritation, such as sunburn or diaper rash.

Breakthrough varicella is defined as varicella that develops more than 42 days after vaccination; most (~70%) breakthrough disease is mild with mildly elevated or no fever, fewer than 50 lesions, and with papules that do not generally progress to vesicles and may be so few in numbers as to escape observation.

Occasionally, especially in adults and in persons with cellular immune deficiencies, such as malignancies and HIV/AIDS, fever and constitutional manifestations of varicella may be severe.

Serious complications of varicella include pneumonia, secondary bacterial infections, hemorrhagic complications, and encephalitis. Secondary bacterial infections of the vesicles may leave disfiguring scars or result in necrotizing fasciitis or septicemia. Rarely, complications may result in death; the case-fatality rate is lower for children (1:100,000 varicella cases in the 5-9 age group) than for adults (1:5,000).

Herpes zoster is a local manifestation of reactivation of latent VZV in the dorsal root ganglia. Vesicles with an erythematous base are restricted to skin areas supplied by sensory nerves of a single or associated group of dorsal root ganglia. Rash is typically unilateral, and most commonly affects thoracic, cervical, and ophthalmic dermatomes. Small numbers of lesions may appear outside the primary dermatome. In the immunosuppressed and those with malignancies, but sometimes in otherwise healthy individuals, extensive varicella-like lesions may appear outside the dermatome. Lesions are histologically identical to those of varicella, but are deeper seated and more closely aggregated. The rash lasts about 7–10 days and heals within 2–4 weeks. The most common complication of herpes zoster is chronic severe pain, also called postherpetic neuralgia, that can last for months, or even years; about 10%–15% of shingles patients have pain for at least 90 days after shingles onset. Nonpain complications may occur in about 10% of cases. Herpes zoster occasionally results in permanent neurological damage, such as cranial nerve palsy and contralateral hemiplegia, or visual impairment following herpes zoster ophthalmicus.

2. Causative agent—Human (alpha) herpesvirus 3 (VZV), a member of the *Herpesvirus* group.

3. Diagnosis—Laboratory tests are not routinely required for diagnosis, but are useful in complicated cases. Viral strain identification may be needed (e.g., to document whether rash in a vaccine recipient is due to vaccine or wild virus). Several antibody assays are now commercially available, but they are not sensitive enough to be used for post-immunization testing of immunity.

4. Occurrence—Worldwide. Infection is nearly universal. In temperate climates, at least 90% of the population has had varicella by age 15, and at least 95%, by young adulthood. In temperate zones, varicella occurs most frequently in winter and early spring. In tropical countries, a higher proportion of cases occur among adults. In developed countries, herpes zoster occurs in up to 30% of the population, mostly in adults older than 50 years.

5. Reservoir—Humans.

6. Incubation period—10–21 days; commonly 14–16 days; may be prolonged to 28 days after passive immunization against varicella and may be shorter in the immunodeficient.

7. Transmission—Person-to-person by direct contact, airborne spread of vesicle fluid of skin lesions of acute varicella and herpes zoster, or infected secretions of the respiratory tract of varicella cases that also might be aerosolized; indirectly through articles freshly soiled by discharges from vesicles and mucous membranes of infected people. In contrast to vaccinia and variola, scabs from varicella lesions are not infective.

Varicella is communicable from 1–2 days before onset of rash until all lesions are crusted (usually about 5 days) after rash onset. Infectiousness may be prolonged in patients with altered immunity. Herpes zoster patients are infectious while they have active (vesiculopustular) lesions (usually 7–10 days). Susceptible exposed individuals should be considered potentially infectious for 8–21 days following exposure (or 28 days if they received passive immunization).

Varicella in unvaccinated persons is one of the most readily communicable diseases; secondary attack rates in susceptible household contacts range from 61% to 100%. Herpes zoster has a lower rate of transmission: data from a household study showed that approximately 20% of those who were varicella susceptible developed varicella when they were in contact with persons who had herpes zoster.

8. Risk groups—Infants, adolescents, adults, immunocompromised persons, and pregnant women are at higher risk for severe varicella and complications. Neonates whose mothers are not immune and patients with leukemia may suffer severe, prolonged, or fatal varicella. Among neonates whose mothers develop varicella 5 days prior to, or within 2 days after delivery, and who do not receive varicella-zoster immune globulin (discussed later) or antiviral therapy, the case-fatality rate can reach 30%.

Infection during the first trimester of pregnancy may lead to congenital varicella syndrome in 1% of cases; at 13-20 weeks gestation the risk for congenital varicella syndrome is 2%. Few cases consistent with congenital varicella syndrome have been reported after 20 weeks gestation. Intrauterine infection and varicella in the first year of life are associated with herpes zoster in childhood.

Deficiencies in cell-mediated immunity are risk factors for both herpes zoster and its severe manifestations. The incidence of both herpes zoster and postherpetic neuralgia increases with age. Cancer and HIV patients have a higher risk of herpes zoster, with highest rates among children. Herpes zoster is also more common following hematopoietic stem cell and solid organ transplants, especially in the first year and among patients on immunosuppressive medications. Additionally, persons with cancer, especially of lymphoid tissue, immunodeficient patients, and those on immunosuppressive therapy have an increased frequency of severe herpes zoster.

Varicella infection usually confers immunity for life; second attacks of varicella are rare in immunocompetent persons but have been documented; subclinical reinfection is common.

9. Prevention—

1) Varicella vaccination: live attenuated varicella vaccines are available throughout the world. They are licensed for use in healthy persons aged 12 months and older, except for the GSK vaccine, which can be administered as early as 9 months of age in some countries. A quadrivalent vaccine (measles, mumps, rubella, and varicella) has been licensed for use in healthy children aged 9-12 months to 12 years. One dose of varicella vaccine has an effectiveness estimated at 70%-90% (median 84%) for prevention of all varicella and at greater than 95% for prevention of combined moderate and severe disease in children

followed for up to 10 years. Two doses of varicella vaccine produce an improved immune response that correlates with improved protection against disease. Routine varicella vaccination programs for children have been introduced primarily in industrialized countries. Countries that adopted varicella vaccination programs have recommended either 1 or 2 doses among children; while the first dose is usually recommended at the minimum age, the age for the second dose is variable with some countries recommending it at 4-6 years of age and others at 4-6 weeks after the first dose. In the USA, for example, the recommendations are for the first dose at 12-15 months of age, the second dose at 4-6 years of age, and second dose catch-up vaccination for persons who previously received only one dose. Routine childhood immunization may be considered in countries where the disease is a public health and socioeconomic problem, where immunization is affordable, and where sustained high vaccine coverage (85%-90%) can be achieved.

For persons aged 13 years and older, 2 doses of vaccine 4-8 weeks apart are recommended for susceptible persons. Vaccination is generally offered based on a negative history of varicella and without confirmation of seronegativity. Some countries have vaccination programs targeted for population considered at high risk. Priority groups for adult immunization include close contacts (e.g., health care workers and household contacts of immunocompromised persons of persons at high risk for serious complications); persons who live or work in environments where transmission of varicella is likely (e.g., teachers of young children, day care employees, residents, staff in institutional settings) or can occur (e.g., college students, inmates, staff members of correctional institutions, military personnel); nonpregnant women of childbearing age; adolescents and adults; and international travelers.

Duration of immunity after one dose is unknown, but antibody persistance for more than 10 years has been documented in settings in which wild virus continues to circulate. Large-scale vaccination of children with varicella vaccine and older adults with herpes zoster vaccine may have an important impact on the incidence of herpes zoster and postherpetic neuralgia. Postlicensure data indicate that children (both immunocompetent and immunocompromised) immunized against varicella have a lower risk for herpes zoster, and the clinical presentations of herpes zoster seem to be milder varicella. Rare occasions of herpes zoster following varicella vaccination and confirmed to be due to vaccine strain VZV show that the currently used vaccine strains may induce latency with the subsequent risk of reactivation, although in children the rate is lower than after natural disease.

A mild varicella-like rash at the site of vaccine injection or at distant sites has been observed in 2%–4% of children and about 5% of adults.

Contraindications to varicella vaccination:

- Immunocompromised persons, including those with:

  o Blood discrasias, leukemia, lymphoma of any type, or malignant neoplasms affecting the bone marrow or lymphatic systems;
  o HIV infection; single antigen varicella vaccine can be considered, however, for HIV-infected children with cluster of differentiation 4 glycoprotein + (CD4+) T-lymphocyte counts greater than or equal to 200 cells/μL ($\geq$15%) and for HIV-infected adolescents and adults with CD4+ counts greater than or equal to 200 cells/μL;
  o Immunosuppressive therapy (including systemic steroids within the previous month).

- History of anaphylactic reactions to any component of the vaccine (including neomycin).
- Pregnancy (theoretical risk to the fetus—pregnancy should be avoided for 4 weeks following vaccination).
- Acute severe illness.
- History of congenital immune disorders in first-degree relatives unless the immune competence of potential vaccine recipient has been demonstrated.

2) A herpes zoster vaccine for older adults has been approved and recommended for use in some countries for healthy persons aged 50 years and older (in the USA the vaccine is recommended for persons $\geq$60 years). The herpes zoster vaccine contains the same VZV strain used in the varicella vaccine, but with a higher potency.

10. **Management of patient**—

1) Infectious patients should be isolated and excluded from school, work, or other public places until all lesions are crusted (usually after 5 days in nonimmunized persons). Vaccinated persons with varicella may develop lesions that do not crust (macules and papules only); these persons should be isolated until no new lesions appear within a 24-hour period. In hospital, observe

strict isolation because of the risk to immunocompromised patients.

2) Concurrent disinfection of articles soiled by discharges from the nose and throat.

3) Treatment: antiviral therapy is moderately effective in treating varicella and herpes zoster infections: acyclovir, valacyclovir, or famciclovir are considered the agents of choice. Some authorities do not recommend routine use of oral antivirals in uncomplicated cases of varicella in healthy children but endorse their use for groups of people at risk for severe disease. In addition to these drugs, for herpes zoster, brivudin can be used. These drugs may shorten the duration of symptoms and reduce acute and chronic pain, especially if administered within 48–72 hours of rash onset. In case of resistance, foscarnet is considered the second-line drug. For the treatment of postherpetic neuralgia, amitriptylin, gabapentin, pregabalin, or carbamazepine are recommended.

11. **Management of contacts and the immediate environment—**

1) All contacts should be evaluated promptly to determine the need for postexposure prophylaxis.

2) Exposed susceptibles eligible for immunization should receive vaccine as soon as possible after exposure to prevent disease and transmission with potential occurrence of an outbreak. Varicella vaccine is effective in preventing illness or modifying severity if used within 3 days, and possibly up to 5 days, of exposure.

3) For exposed susceptibles ineligible for vaccination, passive immunization with varicella-zoster immune globulin prepared from the plasma of normal blood donors with high VZV antibody is available in several countries and recommended. Varicella-zoster immune globulin effectively modifies or prevents disease if given as soon as possible after exposure, but it may be efficacious if administered up to 10 days postexposure. Several formulations are available and recommendations for use vary, but they usually include exposed susceptible immunocompromised patients, neonates whose mothers develop varicella within 5 days prior to or 2 days after delivery, premature infants, and pregnant women. Antiviral drugs such as acyclovir appear useful in preventing or modifying varicella in exposed individuals if given for 7 days starting 7–10 days after exposure. Most studies have been carried out in healthy children. However, in some countries there is experience with

administration of acyclovir as postexposure prophylaxis to immunocompromised children.

4) Quarantine: in places where susceptible, children with known recent exposure must remain for medical reasons, the risk of spread to steroid-treated or immunodeficient patients may justify quarantine of known susceptible contacts for at least 8–21 days after exposure (≤28 days if varicella-zoster immune globulin was given).

12. Special considerations—

1) Reporting: deaths may be reportable to health authorities.
2) Epidemic measures: outbreaks of varicella are common in schools and other institutional settings, such as emergency housing situations; they may be protracted, disruptive, and associated with complications. Infectious cases should be isolated, and susceptible contacts immunized promptly. Persons ineligible for immunization should be evaluated immediately for administration of varicella-zoster immune globulin.

[M. Marin, S. R. Bialek]

WEST NILE VIRUS DISEASE

DISEASE	ICD-10 CODE
WEST NILE FEVER	ICD-10 A92.3
WEST NILE VIRUS ENCEPHALITIS	ICD-10 A83.8
WEST NILE VIRUS MENINGITIS	ICD-10 A87.8
WEST NILE VIRUS ACUTE FLACCID PARALYSIS	ICD-10 A88.8
KUNJIN	ICD-10 A83.4

1. Clinical features—Approximately 70%–80% of human West Nile virus (WNV) infections are asymptomatic. Most symptomatic people experience an acute systemic febrile illness that often includes headache, myalgia, or arthralgia; gastrointestinal tract symptoms and a transient maculopapular rash also are commonly reported. Less than 1% of infected people develop neuroinvasive disease, which typically manifests as meningitis, encephalitis, or acute flaccid paralysis. WNV meningitis is indistinguishable clinically from aseptic meningitis caused by most other viruses. Patients with WNV encephalitis usually present with seizures, mental status changes, focal neurologic deficits, or movement disorders. WNV acute flaccid paralysis often is clinically and pathologically identical to poliovirus-associated acute flaccid paralysis, with damage of anterior horn cells, and may progress to respiratory paralysis requiring mechanical ventilation. WNV-associated Guillain-Barré syndrome has also been reported and can be distinguished from WNV acute flaccid paralysis by clinical manifestations and electrophysiologic testing. Cardiac dysrhythmias, myocarditis, rhabdomyolysis, optic neuritis, uveitis, chorioretinitis, orchitis, pancreatitis, and hepatitis have been described rarely after WNV infection.

Most patients with WNV nonneuroinvasive disease (i.e., West Nile fever) or meningitis recover completely, but fatigue, malaise, and weakness can linger for weeks or months. Patients who recover from WNV encephalitis or acute flaccid paralysis often have residual neurologic deficits. Among patients with neuroinvasive disease, the overall case-fatality rate is approximately 10% but significantly is higher in WNV encephalitis and acute flaccid paralysis than in WNV meningitis.

WNV disease should be considered in the differential diagnosis of acute neurologic or febrile illnesses associated with recent exposure to mosquitoes, blood transfusion, or organ transplantation and of illnesses in neonates whose mothers were infected with WNV during pregnancy or while breastfeeding. In addition to other more common causes of aseptic meningitis and encephalitis (e.g., herpes simplex virus and enteroviruses), other arboviruses should also be considered in the differential diagnosis (see "Arboviral Encephalitides").

2. Causative agent—WNV, of the family *Flaviviridae* and genus *Flavivirus*.

3. Diagnosis—Identifying anti-WNV immunoglobulin class M (IgM) antibodies in serum or cerebrospinal fluid (CSF) is the most common way to diagnose WNV infection. The presence of anti-WNV IgM usually is good evidence of recent WNV infection but may indicate infection with another closely related flavivirus. Because anti-WNV IgM can persist in some patients for longer than 1 year, a positive test result occasionally may reflect past infection. IgM antibody to WNV develops in a majority of WNV-infected patients by the fourth day of symptom onset; 95% of infected patients develop IgM antibody within 7 days of symptom onset. Detection of WNV IgM in CSF is diagnostic of neuroinvasive disease. For patients in whom serum collected within 10 days of illness lacks detectable IgM, testing should be repeated on a convalescent-phase sample. Immunoglobulin class G (IgG) antibody generally is detectable shortly after IgM and can persist for years.

Plaque-reduction neutralization tests can be performed to measure virus-specific neutralizing antibodies and to discriminate between cross-reacting antibodies in primary flavivirus infections. A 4-fold or greater increase in virus-specific neutralizing antibodies between acute- and convalescent-phase serum specimens collected 2–3 weeks apart may be used to confirm recent WNV infection. In patients who have been immunized against or infected with another flavivirus in the past (i.e., who have secondary flavivirus infections), cross-reactive antibodies in IgM, IgG, and neutralization assays may make it difficult to identify which flavivirus is causing the patient's illness. Immunization history, date of symptom onset, and information regarding other flaviviruses known to circulate in the geographic area that may cross-react in serologic assays should be considered when interpreting results.

Viral culture and WNV nucleic acid amplification tests (including reverse transcription polymerase chain reaction [RT-PCR]) can be performed on acute-phase serum, CSF, or tissue specimens. However, by the time most immunocompetent patients present with clinical symptoms, WNV ribonucleic acid (RNA) is usually no longer detectable, thus RT-PCR is not recommended for diagnosis in immunocompetent patients. The sensitivity of these tests is likely higher in immunocompromised patients. Immunohistochemical staining can detect WNV antigens in fixed tissue, but negative results are not definitive.

4. Occurrence—WNV disease has been documented on every continent except Antarctica. In temperate and subtropical regions, most human WNV infections occur in summer or early fall. Seasonal outbreaks often occur in local areas with the location of outbreaks often varying from year to year.

Since the 1990s, the largest outbreaks of WNV neuroinvasive disease have occurred in the Middle East, Europe, and North America. WNV was first detected in the Western Hemisphere in New York City in 1999 and subsequently spread across the continental United States and Canada and into Central and South America. In recent years, several countries in Southern Europe (e.g., Italy, Greece, and Spain) have reported outbreaks of WNV neuroinvasive disease.

5. Reservoir—WNV is transmitted in an enzootic cycle between mosquitoes and amplifying vertebrate hosts, primarily birds. Birds infect feeding vector mosquitoes that then transmit the virus to humans and other mammals during subsequent feeding. Some birds (e.g., corvids) will become sick and may die due to WNV infection, while others (e.g., chickens) develop viremia but do not become unwell. Viremia in humans usually lasts fewer than 7 days in immunocompetent persons, and concentrations of the virus in blood are generally too low to infect mosquitoes, making humans incidental or "dead-end" hosts. Several other mammals can be infected by WNV but most are incidental hosts. Some mammals, like horses, can become symptomatic following WNV infection.

6. Incubation period—Usually 2–6 days but ranges from 2–14 days and can be as long as 21 days in immunocompromised people.

7. Transmission—WNV is transmitted to humans primarily through the bite of infected mosquitoes, predominantly *Culex* mosquitoes. These mosquitoes feed most avidly from dusk to dawn and breed mostly in peridomestic standing water with high organic content or pools created by irrigation or rainfall.

Humans usually do not develop a level or duration of viremia sufficient to infect mosquitoes. However, person-to-person WNV transmission can occur through blood transfusion and solid organ transplantation. Intrauterine transmission and probable transmission via human milk also have been described but appear to be uncommon. Transmission through percutaneous and mucosal exposure have occurred in laboratory workers and occupational settings.

8. Risk groups—Risk of WNV infection is generally determined by exposure to infected vectors and is dependent on many factors including environmental conditions, season, and human activities. Once infected, older age, chronic renal disease, immune suppression, history of alcohol abuse, diabetes, and hypertension have been associated with higher risk of neuroinvasive or severe disease (e.g., hospitalization or death). Infection generally results in lifelong immunity.

9. Prevention—

1) Vector prevention measures (see "Arboviral Encephalitides").
2) Vaccine: WNV vaccines for horses are available in several countries. Human WNV vaccines are not yet available, but several candidate vaccines have been evaluated in preclinical and clinical trials.
3) Other prevention measures:

   - Screening of blood and organ donations is useful in certain settings. Since 2003, blood products have been routinely screened for WNV in the USA and Canada leading to thousands of infected products being removed from the blood supply.
   - To prevent laboratory infections, precautions should be taken when handling viruses in the laboratory at the appropriate biosafety level (http://www.cdc.gov/biosafety/publications/bmbl5/BMBL5_sect_VIII_f.pdf).
   - WNV also may be transmitted through human milk, but transmission appears rare. Because the benefits of breastfeeding likely outweigh the risk of illness in breastfeeding infants, mothers should be encouraged to breastfeed even in areas of ongoing WNV transmission.

10. Management of patient—The primary treatment of WNV disease is supportive. Although various therapies have been evaluated or used for WNV disease, none has shown specific benefit thus far. Standard blood and body substance precautions are sufficient. Virus is not usually found in blood, secretions, or discharges during clinical disease.

11. Management of contacts and the immediate environment—A search for unreported or undiagnosed cases in areas where the patient may have been exposed during the 2 weeks prior to onset should be considered for sporadic or travel-associated cases in unexpected locations.

12. Special considerations—

1) Reporting: local health authority may be required to report cases in selected endemic areas or in areas where WNV previously has not been reported.
2) Epidemic measures: use personal protective measures, including mosquito repellents. Eliminate or treat all potential mosquito breeding places. Consider adult mosquito control measures.

[E. Staples, M. Fischer]

YAWS
(framboesia tropica)

DISEASE	ICD-10 CODE
YAWS	ICD-10 A66

1. Clinical features—Yaws is a chronic relapsing nonvenereal treponematosis. It is characterized by highly contagious primary and secondary cutaneous lesions (early yaws) and noncontagious tertiary destructive lesions (late yaws).

The typical initial lesion (mother yaw) is a papilloma on the face or extremities (usually the leg) that persists for weeks or months and is painless unless secondarily infected. This proliferates slowly and may form a framboesial (raspberry) lesion or ulcerate (ulcero papilloma).

Secondary disseminated or satellite papillomata and/or papules and squamous macules appear before, or shortly after, healing of the initial lesion. These appear in successive crops, often accompanied by periostitis of the long bones (saber shin) and fingers (polydactylitis), with mild constitutional symptoms. In the dry season, papillomatous crops are usually restricted to the moist skinfolds, and papules or macular lesions predominate. Painful, and usually disabling, papillomata and hyperkeratosis on palms and soles may appear in early and in late stages. Lesions heal spontaneously; relapses may occur after periods of latency. Early yaws can last up to 5 years after initial infection.

The late stage, with destructive lesions of skin and bone, occurs in about 10%-20% of untreated patients, usually 5 or more years after infection. Unlike in syphilis, the brain, eyes, heart, aorta, and abdominal organs are not involved. The infection is rarely, if ever, fatal but can be very disfiguring and disabling, resulting in social stigma and economic impact.

Almost all cases of yaws occur in children younger than 5 years, with the peak incidence in children aged 6-10 years. The incidence is about the same in males and females.

2. **Causative agent**—*Treponema pallidum* subsp. *pertenue*, a spirochete.

3. **Diagnosis**—Based on clinico-epidemiological findings in the field. Confirmed through dark-field or direct fluorescent antibody (DFA) microscopic examination of exudates from primary or secondary lesions. Molecular methods using polymerase chain reaction (PCR) and deoxyribonucleic acid (DNA) sequencing have been developed to detect *T. pallidum* subsp. *pertenue*-specific sequences in lesion exudate. Nontreponemal serological tests for syphilis (e.g., Venereal Disease Research Laboratory and rapid plasma reagin) become reactive during the initial stage, remain so during the early infection, and tend to become nonreactive after many years of latency, even in the absence of specific treatment; in some patients, they remain reactive at a low titer for life. Treponemal serological tests (e.g., fluorescent treponemal antibody absorption and microhemagglutination assay for *T. pallidum* antibodies) usually remain reactive for life despite adequate treatment. A nontreponemal test should be confirmed by treponemal testing. Yaws, bejel, and venereal syphilis cannot be distinguished on the basis of serological testing.

4. **Occurrence**—Predominantly a disease of children living under lower socioeconomic conditions in rural humid tropical areas. Mass penicillin treatment campaigns in the 1950s and 1960s dramatically decreased worldwide prevalence, but yaws has reemerged in parts of equatorial and western Africa, with scattered foci of infection persisting in Latin America, the Caribbean islands, south eastern Asia, and some South Pacific islands. In September 2006, India declared yaws eliminated with no cases reported since 2004. WHO has commenced a global program to eradicate yaws, initially focusing on selected endemic districts in seven countries (Cameroon, Ghana, Indonesia, Papua New Guinea, the Solomon Islands, Timor Leste, and Vanuatu). Yaws should be considered in the evaluation of a reactive syphilis serology in any person who has emigrated from an endemic area.

5. Reservoir—Humans and possibly higher primates.

6. Incubation period—From 10-90 days (average 21 days).

7. Transmission—Principally transmitted via person to person through direct physical contact with exudate of primary and secondary skin lesions of infected people. Indirect transmission through contamination from scratching, skin-piercing articles, and flies on open wounds is probable but of unknown importance. The morphology, distribution, and infectiousness of the early lesions are greater in warm and humid regions. Unlike syphilis, congenital transmission does not occur. The period of communicability varies and may extend intermittently over several years when moist lesions are present. The infectious agent is not usually found in late destructive lesions.

8. Risk groups—No evidence of natural resistance. Infection produces immunity to reinfection and may offer some protection against infection by other pathogenic treponemes. Yaws is promoted by overcrowding and poor hygiene.

9. Prevention—The following apply to yaws and other nonvenereal treponematoses.

1) Educate the public about the value of better sanitation, including liberal use of soap and water, and the importance of improving social and economic conditions over a period of years to reduce incidence. Improve access to health services.

2) Organize intensive control activities on a community level suitable to the local problem. Examine entire populations and treat patients with active or latent disease. Treatment of asymptomatic contacts is beneficial. WHO recommends treating the entire population when the prevalence rate for active disease is above 10%; if prevalence is 5%-10%, treat patients, contacts, and all children younger than 15 years; if 5%, treat active cases plus household and other contacts. Periodic clinical resurveys and continuous surveillance are essential for success.

3) Conduct serological surveys for latent cases, particularly in children. This is to prevent relapses and development of infective lesions that maintain the disease in the community, and to detect ongoing community transmission, if any.

4) Provide facilities for early diagnosis and treatment as part of a plan in which mass control campaigns are eventually consolidated into permanent local health services.

10. Management of patient—

1) Treatment: for patients with active disease and their contacts, treat with a single intramuscular (IM) injection of benzathine

penicillin G or single dose oral treatment with azithromycin. There are no reports of azithromycin treatment failures for the nonvenereal treponematoses. Surgery for disfiguring and incapacitating late manifestations may be required.

2) Until lesions are healed, patients should be advised to avoid intimate contact with others and contamination of the environment.

3) Care in disposal of contaminated discharges and articles.

11. Management of contacts and the immediate environment—

1) Treat all family contacts. Those with no active disease should be regarded as latent cases. In low-prevalence areas, treat all active cases, all children, and close contacts of infectious cases.

2) Epidemic measures:

   - Active mass treatment programs in areas of high prevalence.
   - Examine a high percentage of the population through field surveys.
   - Extend treatment of active cases to family and community contacts, based on the demonstrated prevalence of active yaws as described earlier.
   - Survey at yearly intervals for 1–3 years as part of the established rural public health activities of the country.

12. Special considerations—

1) Reporting: in some endemic areas, yaws must be reported to the local health authority. Differentiation of venereal and non-venereal treponematoses, with proper reporting of each, has particular importance in the evaluation and consolidation of mass campaigns.

2) Disaster implications have not been observed, but potentially there is a risk in refugee or displaced populations in endemic areas without hygienic facilities.

3) International measures: to protect countries from reinfection where active mass treatment programs are in progress, adjacent countries in the endemic area should institute measures against yaws. Movement of infected people across frontiers may require supervision (see "Syphilis").

[A. Pillay]

❖

YELLOW FEVER

DISEASE	ICD-10 CODE
YELLOW FEVER	ICD-10 A95

1. Clinical features—Majority of infected persons are asymptomatic. Clinical disease varies from mild febrile illness to severe disease with jaundice and hemorrhage. Initial symptoms include sudden onset of fever, chills, headache, backache, general muscle pain, prostration, nausea, and vomiting. The pulse may be slow and weak, out of proportion to the elevated temperature (Faget sign). Leukopenia appears early and is most pronounced about the fifth day; however, leukocytosis is often seen in the second week of the disease. Most symptoms resolve at this stage.

In approximately 15% of cases, there is a brief remission of hours to a day, followed by recurrence of initial symptoms with progression to jaundice and hemorrhagic symptoms, including epistaxis, gingival bleeding, hematemesis, or melena. Elevated liver enzymes, abnormal clotting factors, albuminuria, and anuria may occur as a result of liver and renal failure. The overall case-fatality rate for severe cases is 20%–50%. Recovery from yellow fever results in life-long immunity.

2. Causative agent—Yellow fever virus, of the family *Flaviviridae* and genus *Flavivirus*.

3. Diagnosis—In acute disease, laboratory diagnosis often can be made through: (a) isolation of virus from blood by inoculation into suckling mice, mosquitoes, or cell cultures; (b) demonstration of viral antigen in tissues, especially liver, by use of labeled specific antibodies; or (c) demonstration of viral ribonucleic acid (RNA) in blood or tissue by reverse transcription polymerase chain reaction (RT-PCR). RT-PCR can also be used to distinguish acute infections with yellow fever virus from recent vaccination. Serological diagnosis includes demonstrating virus-specific IgM in early sera or a 4-fold or greater rise in titer of virus-specific antibodies in paired acute and convalescent sera. Serological cross-reactions occur with other flaviviruses. In natural infections, antibodies appear in the blood within the first week.

4. Occurrence—Disease occurrence is influenced by the specific transmission cycle present in an area, including a sylvatic or jungle cycle that involves *Aedes* or *Haemagogus* mosquitoes and nonhuman primates; an intermediate cycle involving various *Aedes* spp., humans, and nonhuman primates in savannah regions of Africa; and an urban cycle involving mainly *Aedes aegypti* mosquitoes and humans. Sylvatic transmission is restricted to tropical regions of Africa and Latin America, where a few

684 / YELLOW FEVER

hundred cases occur annually, most often among occupationally exposed young adult males in forested or transitional areas. The intermediate cycle involves humans in humid or semihumid areas of Africa where infected mosquitoes feed on both monkeys and humans, resulting in small-scale epidemics. Urban outbreaks are often reported in Africa, particularly West Africa. In the Americas, urban outbreaks are relatively uncommon, although one occurred as recently as 2008 in Asunción, Paraguay.

According to WHO, yellow fever is endemic in 45 countries, including 32 in Africa and 13 in Central and South America. Although disease occurs most frequently in sub-Saharan West Africa, recent outbreaks have been documented in Central and East African countries, including Central African Republic, Chad, Democratic Republic of Congo, Ethiopia, Sudan (Darfur), and Uganda. From 2007–2009 in the Americas, human and epizootic disease due to yellow fever virus was documented in many areas and countries that had not seen activity for several decades, such as Argentina, southern Brazil, Paraguay, and Trinidad and Tobago.

Yellow fever disease and transmission has been documented previously in Europe and North America, but no recent cases have been identified. There is no evidence that yellow fever has ever been present in Asia.

5. Reservoir—In urban areas, humans and *Aedes* mosquitoes; in forest areas, vertebrates other than humans, mainly nonhuman primates and possibly marsupials and forest mosquitoes. Transovarian transmission of the infection in mosquitoes has been documented, but its contribution to maintenance of infection is unknown. Humans have no essential role in transmission of jungle yellow fever but are the primary amplifying host in the urban cycle.

6. Incubation period—From 3–6 days.

7. Transmission—In urban and certain rural areas, through the bite of infective *Aedes* spp. mosquitoes. In South American forests, through the bite of several species of forest mosquitoes, *Haemagogus* spp. and *Sabethes* spp. In Africa, *Aedes africanus* is the principal vector in sylvatic transmission, while semidomestic *Aedes* spp., such as *Aedes furcifer*, *Aedes luteocephalus*, and *Aedes simpsoni* complex, are involved in intermediate transmission. *Aedes simpsoni* was also believed to be the person-to-person vector during large epidemics in Ethiopia. While *Aedes albopictus* is a relatively inefficient vector for yellow fever virus transmission, its recent territorial expansion raises concern about this species as a potential bridging vector for sylvatic and urban cycles of yellow fever.

Blood of patients is infective for mosquitoes shortly before onset of fever and for the first 3–5 days of illness. However, the virus has been found in the blood up to 17 days after illness onset. The extrinsic incubation period in *A. aegypti* is 9–12 days at the usual tropical temperatures. Once infected, mosquitoes remain so for life.

The disease is not communicable through contact or fomites. Since yellow fever vaccine virus has been documented to be transmitted through breastfeeding and blood transfusions, it is likely that natural yellow fever virus is also transmitted through breastfeeding or exposure to infected blood or organs.

8. Risk groups—Risk groups include unvaccinated travelers to endemic areas, forest workers in endemic areas, and those living near forest areas or in *A. aegypti*-infested areas who have not been vaccinated against yellow fever. The disease is highly communicable where many susceptible people and abundant vector mosquitoes coexist. Transient passive immunity in infants born to immune mothers may persist for up to 6 months.

9. Prevention—Mechanisms to prevent yellow fever disease include maintaining human and nonhuman primate disease surveillance, vaccinating persons at risk, and implementing mosquito surveillance and control.

1) Vaccination: all people aged 9 months or older who are at risk of becoming infected due to residence, occupation, or travel should be immunized. A single subcutaneous injection of attenuated yellow fever 17D vaccine is effective in more than 95% of recipients with antibodies appearing 7–10 days after immunization. Although some countries may require reimmunization within 10 years as stipulated by the International Health Regulations (IHR) for travel from endemic areas, a booster dose is no longer recommended by WHO as a single dose is considered sufficient to provide life-long immunity.

Many endemic countries have incorporated yellow fever vaccine into their routine childhood immunization programs (Expanded Program on Immunization). Beginning in 2007, WHO and public health partners under the Yellow Fever Initiative have conducted mass vaccination campaigns in 12 African countries with the highest risk of yellow fever (i.e., Benin, Burkina Faso, Cameroon, Central African Republic, Côte d'Ivoire, Ghana, Guinea, Liberia, Mali, Senegal, Sierra Leone, and Togo). Due to the large number of doses needed, a preventive campaign has not yet been conducted in Nigeria, but the first phase of a Nigerian campaign is scheduled for late 2013. Several South American countries, such as Bolivia, Peru, and Brazil, have also conducted recent preventive campaigns to improve the vaccination coverage in their populations at risk.

Yellow fever vaccine can be given any time after 9 months of age and can be administered simultaneously with other vaccines such as measles vaccine. The vaccine is contraindicated in children younger than 6 months and should be considered for those aged 6–8 months only if the risk of exposure is judged to exceed the risk of vaccine-associated encephalitis, the main complication in this age group.

The vaccine is not recommended during pregnancy or breastfeeding unless the risk of disease is believed to be higher than the theoretical risk to the fetus or infant. There is no evidence of major malformations occurring in the fetus secondary to the vaccine. However, one study observed lower rates of maternal seroconversion; checking antibody titers or reimmunizing women after the end of the pregnancy may therefore be warranted. At least 3 cases of breastfeeding-associated transmission of vaccine virus to infants, resulting in neurotropic disease in the child, have been documented. All infants were younger than 1 month at the time of exposure suggesting that age of the infant may impact whether or not an adverse event might occur.

There is insufficient evidence as to whether yellow fever vaccination poses a risk for people infected with HIV. Limited data suggest the vaccine may be tolerated in individuals with asymptomatic infection, but immunity wanes more rapidly than in persons without HIV. The vaccine is not currently recommended for individuals with symptomatic HIV, and a waiver therefore applies.

Serious adverse events have been observed following yellow fever vaccination, including anaphylaxis, neurologic disease, and viscerotropic disease. With the latter 2 conditions, the vaccine virus replicates either in the brain or other organs, such as the liver, to cause disease or incite an autoimmune event (e.g., Guillain-Barré syndrome or acute disseminating encephalomyelitis). Two possible risk factors for developing a serious reaction, in particularly viscerotropic disease, are advanced age and diseases of the thymus gland. Proper surveillance and support for adverse events following immunization should be part of any standard vaccine program or large vaccination campaign.

A list of yellow fever vaccination requirements and recommendations by country can be found at: http://www.who.int/ith/chapters/ith2012en_countrylist.pdf.

2) Mosquito prevention measures:

- For urban yellow fever, eliminate or control the vector through disposal of standing water-holding containers (reducing breeding sites) and the use of larvicides and insecticides.

- For sylvan or jungle yellow fever, vector control measures are typically not successful. Protective clothing, bed nets, and repellents are advised for those not immunized.
- For travelers who cannot be immunized and travel is unavoidable, using protective clothing, staying in locations with air-conditioning, screens, or bed nets, and using repellents may help lower the risk of disease.

10. Management of patient—No specific antiviral therapies available; treatment is supportive.

Blood and body fluid precautions should be used. Prevent access of mosquitoes to the patient for at least 5 days after onset by screening the sick room, spraying quarters with residual insecticide, and using insecticide-treated bed nets. The homes of patients and all houses in the vicinity should be sprayed promptly with an effective insecticide.

11. Management of contacts and the immediate environment—In endemic areas, family and other contacts and neighbors not previously immunized should be immunized promptly.

Inquire about all contacts and all places, including forested areas, visited by the patient 3-6 days before onset to locate focus of yellow fever; observe all people visiting that focus. Search patient's premises and places of work or visits over the preceding several days for mosquitoes capable of transmitting infection; apply effective insecticide. Investigate mild febrile illnesses and unexplained deaths suggesting yellow fever.

12. Special considerations—

1) Reporting: IHR require events involving yellow fever cases to be assessed at the national level for potential notification to WHO.
2) Epidemic measures:

- Urban or *A. aegypti*-transmitted yellow fever: mass immunization, beginning with people most exposed and those living in *A. aegypti*-infested areas who have not been vaccinated against yellow fever in the last 10 years. Eliminate or treat all potential breeding places. Spraying the inside of all houses in the community with insecticides has shown promise for controlling urban epidemics.
- Jungle or sylvan yellow fever: immediately immunize all people living in or near forested areas or entering such areas. Ensure that nonimmunized individuals avoid those tracts of forest where infection has been localized and that those just immunized avoid those areas for 7-10 days after immunization.

- In regions where yellow fever may occur, a diagnostic post-mortem examination service should be organized to collect small specimens of tissues, especially liver, from fatal febrile illnesses, provided biological safety can be ensured. Facilities for viral isolation or serological confirmation are necessary to establish diagnosis, since histopathological changes in the liver are not pathognomonic.

- In Central and South America, confirmed deaths of howler and spider monkeys in the forest are presumptive evidence of the presence of yellow fever. Confirmation by the histopathological examination of livers of moribund or recently dead monkeys, or by virus isolation, is highly desirable. In Africa, monkeys are rarely symptomatic and rarely die from infections with yellow fever virus and thus cannot be used to indicate the presence of yellow fever.

- Serosurveys through neutralization tests of wild primates captured in forested areas are useful in defining enzootic areas. Serological surveys of human populations are not useful where yellow fever vaccine has been widely used and can be difficult to interpret in places with other endemic flaviviruses.

3) Disaster implications: consider mass vaccination if an epidemic is feared.

4) International measures:

- Measures applicable to ships, aircraft, and land transport arriving from areas with ongoing yellow fever transmission are no longer specified in the IHR. There are, however, applicable guidelines listed in the IHR for any areas with ongoing disease transmission.

- Animal quarantine: Due to the risk of nonhuman primates carrying zoonotic pathogens such as yellow fever, the World Organisation of Animal Health (OIE) recommends in the Terrestrial Animal Health Code (2010) that captive-bred nonhuman primates be held in quarantine for 30 days and nonhuman primates captured from the wild be held in quarantine for 12 weeks.

- International travel: a valid International Certificate of Vaccination or Prophylaxis (yellow card) against yellow fever is required by many countries for entry of travelers coming from or going to recognized yellow fever zones of Africa and South America; otherwise, quarantine measures are applicable for up to 6 days. Immunizing practitioners and travelers should consult country-specific requirements and recommendations for yellow fever vaccination to determine if vaccine administration should be considered (see http://www.who.int/ith/chapters/ith2012en_countrylist.pdf). The International Certificate of Vaccination against yellow fever is valid for 10 years from 10 days after date of immunization. If reimmunization occurs within that period, it is valid 10 years from date of reimmunization.

[E. Staples, I. Rabe]

YERSINIOSIS

DISEASE	ICD-10 CODE
INTESTINAL YERSINIOSIS	ICD-10 A04.6
EXTRAINTESTINAL YERSINIOSIS	ICD-10 A28.2

1. **Clinical features**—Typically manifested by acute febrile diarrhea with abdominal pain (especially in young children). Other manifestations include acute mesenteric lymphadenitis mimicking appendicitis (especially in older children and adults), exudative pharyngitis, and systemic infection. The most common postinfectious complications are erythema nodosum and reactive arthritis. Bloody diarrhea can also occur in patients with *Yersinia* enteritis; diarrhea may be absent in up to a third of *Yersinia enterocolitica* infections. Ileitis is the characteristic lesion induced by *Y. enterocolitica*. *Yersinia pseudotuberculosis* causes acute mesenteric lymphadenitis, characterized by an appendicitis-like syndrome, sometimes with diarrhea. Because infections in older children and adolescents can mimic acute appendicitis, outbreaks can sometimes be recognized by a local increase in appendectomies.

2. **Causative agents**—Gram-negative bacilli. Globally, *Y. enterocolitica* is the species most commonly associated with human infection, causing up to 1%–3% of acute enteritis in some areas. *Y. enterocolitica* has more than 60 serotypes and 6 biotypes, many nonpathogenic. *Y. pseudotuberculosis* has 6 serotypes with 4 subtypes. Most human and animal infections are caused by O-group I.

3. **Diagnosis**—Usually made through stool culture. Cefsulodin irgasan novobiocin medium is highly selective and should be used if infection with *Yersinia* is suspected; at 28°C (78.4°F), it permits identification in 24 hours. The organisms may be recovered on usual enteric media if precautions are taken to prevent overgrowth of fecal flora. Cold enrichment in buffered

saline at 4°C (39°F) for 2–3 weeks can be used, but this procedure usually enhances the isolation of nonpathogenic species. *Yersinia* can be isolated from blood with standard commercial blood culture media. Serological diagnosis is possible (agglutination test or enzyme-linked immunosorbent assay [ELISA]), but availability is generally limited to research settings.

4. Occurrence—The distribution of pathogenic *Y. enterocolitica* varies by geographic region. Serotypes O:3 and O:9 account for most cases in Europe. In the USA and Canada, most isolates are serotypes O:3 and O:8. The highest isolation rates have been reported during the cold season in temperate climates, including northern Europe (especially Scandinavia), North America, and temperate regions of South America. Approximately two-thirds of *Y. enterocolitica* illness occurs among infants and children. Three-quarters of those with *Y. pseudotuberculosis* illness are aged 5–20 years.

Humans are primarily incidental hosts of *Y. pseudotuberculosis*, but in some countries, such as Japan and the Russian Federation, it is the main cause of human yersiniosis. Specific *Y. pseudotuberculosis* syndromes (Izumi fever, Far East scarlet-like fever) have been reported in Japan and the Russian Federation.

5. Reservoir—Animals. The pig is the main reservoir for *Y. enterocolitica* (serotype O:3). Asymptomatic pharyngeal carriage is common in swine, especially in winter, and serotype O:9 has been isolated from ovine, bovine, and caprine origins. *Y. pseudotuberculosis* is widespread among many avian and mammalian hosts, particularly rodents and other small mammals.

6. Incubation period—Probably 3–7 days, generally under 10 days.

7. Transmission—Fecal-oral transmission through consumption of contaminated food or water or through contact with infected people or animals. *Y. enterocolitica* has been isolated from many foods, and pathogenic strains, most commonly from raw pork or pork products. Vehicles implicated in outbreaks attributed to *Y. enterocolitica* include soybean cake (tofu), pork chitterlings (large intestines), and milk. *Y. enterocolitica* can multiply under refrigeration and microaerophilic conditions. Nosocomial transmission has occurred, as has transmission by transfusion of stored blood from donors who were asymptomatic or had mild gastrointestinal (GI) illness.

Human illness with *Y. pseudotuberculosis* has been reported in association with infections in household pets, particularly puppies and kittens. Outbreaks of *Y. pseudotuberculosis* have been reported from northern Europe, Japan, and Canada; vehicles implicated include produce, pasteurized milk, and vegetable juice.

Secondary transmission appears rare. There is fecal shedding at least as long as symptoms exist, usually for 2–3 weeks. Untreated cases may excrete the organism for 2–3 months. Prolonged asymptomatic carriage has been reported in both children and adults.

8. Risk groups—Gastroenterocolitis diarrhea is more severe in children. Postinfectious arthritis is more severe in adolescents and older adults. *Y. enterocolitica* equally affects men and women. Reactive arthritis and Reiter syndrome occur more often in people with the HLA-B27 genetic type. Septicemia occurs most often among people with iron overload (hemochromatosis) or immunosuppression.

9. Prevention—

1) Prepare meat and other foods in a sanitary manner. Avoid eating raw pork, and pasteurize milk. Irradiation of meat is effective.
2) Wash hands before food handling and eating, after handling raw pork, and after contact with animals.
3) Protect water supplies from animal and human feces; purify appropriately.
4) Control rodents and birds (for *Y. pseudotuberculosis*).
5) Dispose of human, dog, and cat feces in a sanitary manner.
6) During the slaughtering of pigs, the head and neck should be removed from the body to avoid contaminating meat from the pharynx, which may be heavily colonized.

10. Management of patient—

1) Enteric precautions for patients in hospitals. Remove anyone with diarrhea from food handling, patient care, and occupations involving care of young children.
2) Concurrent disinfection of feces. In communities with modern and adequate sewage disposal systems, feces can be discharged directly into sewers without preliminary disinfection.
3) Treatment: organisms are sensitive to many antibiotics but are generally resistant to penicillin, ampicillin, and third-generation cephalosporins. The benefit of antibiotic treatment for uncomplicated gastrointestinal infection is unclear, but treatment is definitely indicated for septicemia and other invasive disease. Agents of choice against *Y. enterocolitica* are the aminoglycosides (septicemia only), trimethoprim/sulfamethoxazole, doxycycline, and ciprofloxacin. *Y. pseudotuberculosis* infection can be treated with ampicillin, tetracycline, chloramphenicol, cephalosporins, and aminoglycosides.

11. Management of contacts and the immediate environment—

1) Searching for unrecognized cases and convalescent carriers among contacts is indicated only when a common-source exposure is suspected.

2) Investigate general sanitation and search for common source vehicle. Pay attention to consumption of, or possible cross-contamination with, raw or undercooked pork. Look for evidence of close contacts with pet dogs, cats, and other domestic animals.

12. Special considerations—Reporting: any group of cases of acute gastroenteritis or a cluster of suspected appendicitis should be reported at once to the local health authority, even in the absence of specific causal identification.

[L. H. Gould, P. M. Griffin]

EXPLANATION OF TERMS

Technical meaning of certain terms used in *CCDM20*
(not binding definitions)

1. **Carrier**—A person or animal that harbors a specific infectious agent without discernible clinical disease and that serves as a potential source of infection. The carrier state may exist in an individual with an infection that is unapparent throughout its course (such an individual is commonly known as **healthy** or **asymptomatic carrier**) or during the incubation period, convalescence, and post-convalescence of a person with a clinically recognizable disease (commonly known as an **incubatory** or **convalescent carrier**). Under either circumstance the carrier state may be of short or long duration (**temporary** or **transient carrier**, or **chronic carrier**).

2. **Case-fatality rate** (fatality rate, fatality percentage, case-fatality ratio)—Usually expressed as the proportion of persons diagnosed as having a specified disease who die within a given period as a result of acquiring that disease. In communicable disease epidemiology, this term is most frequently applied to a specific outbreak of acute disease in which all patients have been followed for a period of time sufficient to include all deaths attributable to the given disease. The case-fatality rate—where the numerator is "deaths from a given disease in a given period" and the denominator is "number of diagnosed cases of the disease during that period"—must be differentiated from the **disease-specific mortality rate**, where the denominator is "total population."

3. **Chemoprophylaxis**—The administration of a chemical, including antibiotics, to prevent the development of an infection or the progression of an infection to active manifest disease or to eliminate the carriage of a specific infectious agent in order to prevent transmission and disease in others. **Chemotherapy** refers to use of a chemical to treat a clinically manifest disease or to limit its further progress.

4. **Cleaning**—The removal by scrubbing and washing, as with water, soap, antiseptic, or suitable detergent, or by vacuum cleaning, of infectious agents and of organic matter from surfaces on which and in which infectious agents may find favorable conditions for surviving or multiplying.

   Terminal cleaning is the cleaning after the patient has been removed by death or transfer or has ceased to be a source of infection, or after hospital isolation or other practices have been discontinued (see **Terminal disinfection**).

5. **Communicable disease** (infectious disease)—An illness due to a specific infectious agent or its toxic products that arises through transmission of that agent or its products from an infected person, animal, or inanimate source to a susceptible host, either directly or indirectly through an intermediate plant or animal host, vector, or the inanimate environment.

6. **Contact**—In the context of communicable disease, a person or animal that has been in such association with an infected person or animal or a contaminated environment and thus has had an opportunity to acquire the infection.

7. **Contamination**—The presence of an infectious agent on a body surface, in or on clothes, bedding, toys, surgical instruments or dressings, or in other inanimate articles or substances including water, milk, and food. Contamination of a body surface does not imply a carrier state. **Pollution** is distinct from contamination and implies the presence of offensive, but not necessarily infectious, matter in the environment.

8. **Disinfection**—Killing of infectious agents outside the body by direct exposure to chemical or physical agents. **High-level disinfection** may kill all microorganisms with the exception of high numbers of bacterial spores; extended exposure is required to ensure killing of most bacterial spores. High-level disinfection is achieved after thorough detergent cleaning through exposure to specific concentrations of certain disinfectants (e.g., 2% glutaraldehyde, 6% stabilized hydrogen peroxide, ≤1% peracetic acid) for at least 20 minutes. **Intermediate-level disinfection** does not kill spores; it can be achieved through pasteurization (75°C [167°F] for 30 minutes) or appropriate treatment with approved disinfectants.

    Concurrent disinfection is the application of disinfective measures as soon as possible after the discharge of infectious material from the body of an infected person or after the soiling of articles with such infectious discharges; all personal contact with such discharges or articles should be minimized prior to concurrent disinfection.

    Terminal disinfection is the application of disinfective measures after the patient has been removed by death or transfer or has ceased to be a source of infection, or after hospital isolation or other practices have been discontinued. Terminal disinfection is rarely practiced; terminal cleaning generally suffices (see **Cleaning**), along with airing and sunning of rooms, furniture, and bedding. Steam sterilization or incineration of bedding and other items is sometimes recommended after a disease such as Lassa fever or another highly infectious disease.

Sterilization involves destruction of all forms of microbial life by physical heat, irradiation, gas, or chemical treatment.

9. **Disinfestation**—Any physical or chemical process serving to destroy or remove undesired small animal forms, particularly arthropods or rodents, present upon the person or clothing or in the environment of an individual, or on domestic animals (see **Insecticide** and **Rodenticide**). Disinfestation includes delousing for infestation with *Pediculus humanus*, the human body louse. Synonyms include the terms **disinsection** and **disinsectization** when only insects are involved.

10. **Endemic**—A term denoting the habitual presence of a disease or infectious agent within a given geographic area or a population group; may also refer to the usual prevalence of a given disease within such an area. **Hyperendemic** expresses a habitual presence at all ages at a high level of incidence, and **holoendemic** (a term applied mainly to malaria) expresses a high level of prevalence with high spleen rates in children and lower rates in adults. (See also **Zoonosis**.)

11. **Epidemic**—The occurrence, in a defined community or region, of cases of an illness (or an outbreak) with a frequency clearly in excess of normal expectancy. The number of cases indicating the presence of an epidemic varies according to the infectious agent, size and type of population exposed, previous experience or lack of exposure to the disease, and time and place of occurrence; epidemicity is thus relative to usual frequency of the disease in the same area, among the specified population, and at the same season of the year. A single case of a communicable disease long absent from a population or the first invasion by a disease not previously recognized in that area requires immediate reporting and full field epidemiological investigation; two cases of such a disease associated in time and place are sufficient evidence of transmission to be considered an epidemic (see **Report of a disease** and **Zoonosis**).

12. **Food irradiation**—A technique that provides a specific dose of ionizing radiation from a source such as a radioisotope (e.g., cobalt 60) or from machines that produce accelerated electron beams or X-rays. Doses for irradiation of food and material are **low**—1 or less kiloGrays (kGy), used for disinfestation of insects from fruit, spices, and grain and for parasite disinfection in fish and meat; **medium**—1–10 kGy (commonly 1–4 kGy), used for pasteurization and the destruction of bacteria and fungi; and **high**—10–50 kGy, used for sterilization of food as well as medical supplies (including intravenous (IV) fluids, implants, syringes, needles, thread, clips, and gowns).

13. **Fumigation**—A process by which the killing of animal forms, especially arthropods and rodents, is accomplished by the use of gaseous agents (see **Insecticide** and **Rodenticide**).

14. **Health education** (patient education, education for health, education of the public, public health education)—The process by which individuals and groups of people learn to behave in a manner conducive to the promotion, maintenance, or restoration of health. Education for health begins with people as they are, with whatever interests they may have in improving their living conditions. Its aim is to develop their sense of their own responsibility for health conditions as individuals and as members of families and communities. In communicable disease control, health education commonly includes an appraisal of what is known by a population about a disease, an assessment of habits and attitudes of the people as they relate to spread and frequency of the disease, and the presentation of specific means to remedy observed deficiencies.

15. **Herd immunity**—The immunity of a group or community. The resistance of a group to invasion and spread of an infectious agent, based on the resistance to infection of a high proportion of individual members of the group.

16. **Host**—A person or other living animal, including birds and arthropods, that affords subsistence or lodgment to an infectious agent under natural (as opposed to experimental) conditions. Some protozoa and helminths pass successive stages in alternate hosts of different species. Hosts in which a parasite attains maturity or passes its sexual stage are **primary** or **definitive** hosts; those in which a parasite is in a larval or asexual state are **secondary** or **intermediate** hosts. A **transport host** is a carrier in which the organism remains alive but does not undergo development.

17. **Immune individual**—A person or animal that has specific protective antibodies and/or cellular immunity as a result of previous infection or immunization or is so conditioned by such previous specific experience as to respond in a way that prevents the development of infection and/or clinical illness following reexposure to the specific infectious agent. Immunity is relative: a level of protection that could be adequate under ordinary conditions may be overwhelmed by an excessive dose of the infectious agent or by exposure through an unusual portal of entry; protection may also be impaired by immunosuppressive drug therapy, concurrent disease, or the ageing process.

18. **Immunity**—A status usually associated with the presence of antibodies or cells having a specific action on the microorganism concerned with a particular infectious disease or on its toxin. Effective immunity includes both **cellular immunity**, conferred by T-lymphocyte sensitization, and **humoral immunity**, based on B-lymphocyte response. **Passive immunity** is attained either naturally through transplacental transfer from the mother or artificially by inoculation of specific protective antibodies (from immunized animals or from convalescent hyperimmune serum or immune serum globulin [human]). Passive immunity is of short duration (days to months). **Active humoral immunity**, which usually lasts for years, is attained either naturally through infection with or without clinical manifestations or artificially through inoculation of the agent itself in killed, modified, or variant form or of fractions or products of the agent.

19. **Inapparent infection** (synonyms: asymptomatic, subclinical, occult, unapparent infection)—See **Unapparent infection**.

20. **Incidence**—The number of instances of illness commencing, or of persons falling ill, during a given period in a specified population. The **incidence rate** is the ratio of new cases of a specified disease diagnosed or reported during a defined period of time to the number of persons at risk in a stated population in which the cases occurred during the same period of time (if the period is 1 year, the rate is the **annual incidence rate**). This rate is expressed, usually as cases per 1,000 or 100,000 per annum, for the whole population or specifically for any population characteristic or subdivision such as age or ethnic group (see **Prevalence rate**). **Attack rate**, or **case rate**, is a proportion measuring cumulative incidence for a particular group, over limited periods, and under special circumstances, as in an epidemic; it is usually expressed as a percentage (cases/100 in the group). The numerator can be determined through the identification of clinical cases or through seroepidemiology. The **secondary attack rate** is the ratio of the number of cases among contacts occurring within the accepted incubation period following exposure to a primary case to the total number of exposed contacts; the denominator may be restricted to the numbers of susceptible contacts when this can be determined. The **infection rate** is a proportion that expresses the incidence of all identified infections, manifest or unapparent (the latter identified by seroepidemiology).

21. **Incubation period**—The time interval between initial contact with an infectious agent and the first appearance of symptoms associated with the infection. In a vector, it is the time between entrance of an organism into the vector and the time when that vector can transmit

the infection (**extrinsic incubation period**). The period between the time of exposure to an infectious agent and the time when the agent can be detected in blood or stool is called the prepatent period.

22. **Infected individual**—A person or animal that harbors an infectious agent and who has either manifest disease or unapparent infection (see **Carrier**). An **infectious** person or animal is one from whom the infectious agent can be naturally acquired.

23. **Infection**—The entry and development or multiplication of an infectious agent in the body of persons or animals. Infection is not synonymous with infectious disease; the result may be unapparent (see **Unapparent infection**) or manifest (see **Infectious disease**). The presence of living infectious agents on exterior surfaces of the body, or on articles of apparel or soiled articles, is not infection but represents contamination of such surfaces and articles (see **Infestation** and **Contamination**).

24. **Infectious agent**—An organism (virus, rickettsia, bacteria, fungus, protozoan, or helminth) that is capable of producing infection or infectious disease. **Infectivity** expresses the ability of the infectious agent to enter, survive, and multiply in the host. **Infectiousness** indicates the relative ease with which an infectious agent is transmitted to other hosts.

25. **Infectious disease**—A clinically manifest disease of humans or animals resulting from an infection (see **Infection**).

26. **Infestation**—For persons or animals, the lodgment, development and reproduction of arthropods on the surface of the body or in the clothing. Infested articles or premises are those that harbor or give shelter to animal forms, especially arthropods and rodents.

27. **Insecticide**—Any chemical substance used for the destruction of insects; can be applied as powder, liquid, atomized liquid, aerosol, or "paint" spray; an insecticide may or may not have residual action. The term **larvicide** is generally used to designate insecticides applied specifically for the destruction of immature stages of arthropods; **adulticide** or **imagocide**, to those destroying mature or adult forms. The term insecticide is used broadly to encompass substances for the destruction of all arthropods; **acaricide** is more properly used for agents against ticks and mites. Specific terms such as **lousicide** and **miticide** are sometimes used.

28. **Isolation**—As applied to patients, isolation represents separation, for a period at least equal to the **period of communicability**, of infected persons or animals from others in such places and under such conditions as to prevent or limit the direct or indirect transmission of the infectious agent from those infected to those who are susceptible to infection or who may spread the agent to others.

   Universal precautions should be used consistently for all patients (in hospital settings as well as outpatient settings), regardless of their bloodborne infection status. This practice is based on the possibility that blood and certain body fluids (any body secretion that is obviously bloody, semen, vaginal secretions, tissue, cerebrospinal fluid [CSF], and synovial, pleural, peritoneal, pericardial, and amniotic fluids) of all patients are potentially infectious for agents such as HIV, hepatitis B virus (HBV), and other bloodborne pathogens. Universal precautions are intended to prevent parenteral, mucous membrane, and nonintact skin exposures of health care workers to bloodborne pathogens. Protective barriers include gloves, gowns, masks, and protective eyewear or face shields. A private room is indicated if patient hygiene is poor. Local and state authorities control waste management. Two basic requirements are common for the care of all potentially infectious cases:

   1) Hands must be washed after contact with the patient or potentially contaminated articles and before taking care of another patient.
   2) Articles contaminated with infectious material must be appropriately discarded or bagged and labeled before being sent for decontamination and reprocessing.

   Recommendations made for isolation of cases in Management of Contacts and the Immediate Environment sections in disease chapters may allude to the methods that have been recommended as category-specific isolation precautions based on the mode of transmission of the specific disease, in addition to universal precautions. These categories are as follows:

   Strict isolation: to prevent transmission of highly contagious or virulent infections that may be spread by both air and contact. The specifications, in addition to those discussed earlier, include a private room and the use of masks, gowns, and gloves for all persons entering the room. Special ventilation requirements with the room at negative pressure to surrounding areas are desirable.

   Contact isolation: for less highly transmissible or less serious infections; for diseases or conditions that are spread primarily by close or direct contact. In addition to the 2 basic requirements, a private room is indicated, but patients infected with the same pathogen may share a room. Masks are indicated for those who come close to the patient, gowns if soiling is likely, and gloves for touching infectious material.

Respiratory isolation: to prevent transmission of infectious diseases over short distances through the air, a private room is indicated, but patients infected with the same organism may share a room. In addition to the basic requirements, masks are indicated for those who come in close contact with the patient; gowns and gloves are not indicated.

Tuberculosis isolation (acid-fast bacilli [AFB] isolation): for patients with pulmonary tuberculosis who have a positive sputum smear or a chest X-ray that strongly suggests active tuberculosis. Specifications include use of a private room with special ventilation and closed doors. In addition to the basic requirements, those entering the room must use respirator-type masks. The use of gowns will prevent gross contamination of clothing. Gloves are not indicated.

Enteric precautions: for infections transmitted by direct or indirect contact with feces. In addition to the basic requirements, specifications include use of a private room if patient hygiene is poor. Masks are not indicated; gowns should be used if soiling is likely and gloves should be used when touching contaminated materials.

Drainage/secretion precautions: to prevent infections transmitted by direct or indirect contact with purulent material or drainage from an infected body site. A private room and masking are not indicated. In addition to the basic requirements, gowns should be used if soiling is likely and gloves used when touching contaminated materials.

29. **Molluskicide**—A chemical substance used for the destruction of snails and other mollusks.

30. **Mortality rate** (death rate)—A rate calculated in the same way as an **incidence rate** by dividing the number of deaths occurring in the population during the stated period of time, usually a year, by the number of persons at risk of dying during the period or by the mid-period population. A **total** or **crude mortality rate** refers to deaths from all causes and is usually expressed as deaths per 1,000. A **disease-specific mortality rate** refers to deaths due to a single disease and is often reported for a denominator of 100,000 persons. Age, ethnicity, or other characteristics may define the population base. The mortality rate must not be confused with the **case-fatality rate**.

31. **Nosocomial infection** (hospital-acquired infection)—An infection occurring in a patient in a hospital or other health care facility in

whom the infection was not present or incubating at the time of admission, or the residual of an infection acquired during a previous admission. This includes infections acquired in the hospital but appearing after discharge and also such infections among the staff of the facility.

32. **Pandemic**— A communicable disease epidemic that rapidly spreads to affect susceptible populations over much of the world. A pandemic can be of variable mortality and can in some cases lead to endemicity.

33. **Pathogenicity**—The property of an infectious agent that determines the extent to which overt disease is produced in an infected population, or the power of an organism to produce disease. Measured by the ratio of the number of persons developing clinical illness to the number of persons exposed to infection.

34. **Period of communicability/communicable period**—The time during which an infectious agent may be transferred directly or indirectly from an infected person to another person, from an infected animal to humans, or from an infected person to animals, including arthropods. In diseases (e.g., diphtheria and streptococcal infection) in which mucous membranes are involved from the initial entry of the infectious agent, the period of communicability starts at the date of first exposure to a source of infection and lasts until the infecting microorganism is no longer disseminated from the mucous membranes, that is, from the period before the prodromata until the termination of a carrier state, if the latter develops. Some diseases (e.g., hepatitis A, measles) are more easily communicable during the incubation period than during the actual illness. In diseases such as tuberculosis, leprosy, syphilis, gonorrhea, and some of the salmonelloses, the communicable state may persist—sometimes intermittently—over a long period, with discharge of infectious agents from the surface of the skin or through the body orifices. For diseases transmitted by arthropods, such as malaria and yellow fever, the periods of communicability (or infectivity) are those during which the infectious agent occurs in the blood or other tissues of the infected person in sufficient numbers to permit infection of the vector. For the arthropod vector, a period of communicability (transmissibility) is also to be noted, during which the agent is present in the tissues of the arthropod in such form and locus as to be transmissible (infective state).

35. **Personal hygiene**—In the field of infectious disease control, those protective measures, primarily within the responsibility of the

individual, that promote health and limit the spread of infectious diseases, chiefly those transmitted by direct contact. Such measures encompass:

1) Washing hands in soap and water immediately after evacuating bowel or bladder and always before handling food or eating
2) Keeping hands and unclean articles, or articles that have been used for toilet purposes by others, away from the mouth, nose, eyes, ears, genitalia, and wounds
3) Avoiding the use of common or unclean eating utensils, drinking cups, towels, handkerchiefs, combs, hairbrushes, and pipes
4) Avoiding exposure of other persons to droplets from the nose and mouth expelled when coughing, sneezing, laughing, or talking
5) Washing hands thoroughly after handling a patient, or a patient's belongings, and keeping the body clean by frequent soap and water washing.

36. **Prevalence**—The total number of instances of illness or of persons ill in a specified population at a particular time (**point prevalence**), or during a stated period of time (**period prevalence**), without distinction between old and new cases. A **prevalence rate** (not to be confused with prevalence) is the ratio of prevalence to the population at risk of having the disease or condition at the stated point in time or midway through the period considered; it is usually expressed per 1,000, per 10,000, or per 100,000 population.

37. **Quarantine**—Restriction of activities for well persons or animals who have been exposed (or are considered to be at high risk of exposure) to a case of communicable disease during its period of communicability (i.e., **contacts**) to prevent disease transmission during the incubation period if infection should occur. The 2 main types of quarantine are

Absolute or complete quarantine: The limitation of freedom of movement of those exposed to a communicable disease for a period of time not longer than the longest usual incubation period of that disease, in such manner as to prevent effective contact with those not so exposed (see **Isolation**).

Modified quarantine: A selective, partial limitation of freedom of movement of contacts, commonly on the basis of known or presumed differences in susceptibility and related to the assessed risk of disease transmission. It may be designed to accommodate particular situations. Examples are exclusion of children from school, exemption of immune persons from provisions applicable to susceptible persons, or restriction of military populations to post or to quarters.

Modified quarantine includes **personal surveillance**, the practice of close medical or other supervision of contacts to permit prompt recognition of infection or illness but without restricting their movements, and **segregation**, the separation of some part of a group of persons or domestic animals from the others for special consideration, control, or observation; removal of susceptible children to homes of immune persons; or establishment of a sanitary boundary to protect uninfected from infected portions of a population.

38. **Repellent**—A chemical applied to the skin or clothing or other places to discourage arthropods from alighting on and biting a person or to discourage other agents, such as helminth larvae, from penetrating the skin.

39. **Report of a disease**—An official report notifying an appropriate authority of the occurrence of a specified communicable or other disease in humans or in animals. Diseases in humans are reported to the local health authority; those in animals, to the livestock, sanitary, veterinary, or agriculture authority. Some few diseases in animals, also transmissible to humans, are reportable to both authorities. Each health jurisdiction declares a list of reportable diseases appropriate to its particular needs. Reports should also list suspected cases of diseases of particular public health importance, ordinarily those requiring epidemiological investigation or initiation of special control measures. When a person is infected in one health jurisdiction and the case is reported from another, the health authority receiving the report should notify the jurisdiction where infection presumably occurred, especially when the disease requires examination of contacts for infection, or if food, water or other common vehicles of infection may be involved. In addition to routine reports of cases of specified diseases, special notification is required of most epidemics or outbreaks of disease, including diseases not listed as reportable (see **Epidemic**). Special reporting requirements are specified in "Reporting of Communicable Diseases under the International Health Regulations."

   Zero reporting (null reporting) consists in the explicit reporting of "zero cases" when no cases have been detected by the reporting unit. This is a way of checking that the relevant data have not been forgotten or lost.

40. **Reservoir** of infectious agents—Any person, animal, arthropod, plant, soil, or substance (or combination of these) in which an infectious agent normally lives and multiplies, on which it depends primarily for survival, and where it reproduces itself in such manner that it can be transmitted to a susceptible host.

41. **Rodenticide**—A substance used for the destruction of rodents, generally but not always through ingestion (see also **Fumigation**).

42. **Source of infection**—The person, animal, object or substance from which an infectious agent passes to a host. **Source of infection** should be clearly distinguished from **source of contamination**, such as overflow of a septic tank contaminating a water supply (see **Reservoir**).

43. **Surveillance of disease**—In communicable disease control, surveillance consists in the process of systematic collection, orderly consolidation, analysis, and evaluation of pertinent data, with prompt dissemination of the results to those who need to know, particularly those who are in a position to take action. It includes the systematic collection and evaluation of

    1) Morbidity and mortality reports.
    2) Special reports of field investigations of epidemics and of individual cases.
    3) Isolation and identification of infectious agents by laboratories.
    4) Data concerning the availability, use, and untoward effects of vaccines and toxoids, immune globulins, insecticides, and other substances used in control.
    5) Information regarding immunity levels in segments of the population.
    6) Other relevant epidemiological data.

    A report summarizing this data should be prepared and distributed to all cooperating persons and others with a need to know the results of the surveillance activities. The procedure applies to all jurisdictional levels of public health, from local to international.

    Serological surveillance identifies patterns of current and past infection using serological tests for antibody detection.

44. **Susceptible**—A person or animal not possessing sufficient resistance to a particular infectious agent to prevent contracting infection or disease when exposed to that agent.

45. **Suspect**—In the context of infectious disease control, illness in a person whose history and symptoms suggest that he or she may have, or be developing, a communicable disease.

46. **Terminal cleaning**—See **Cleaning**.

47. **Terminal disinfection**—See **Disinfection**.

48. **Transmission of infectious agents**—Any mechanism by which an infectious agent is spread from a source or reservoir to a person. These mechanisms are as follows:

Direct transmission: Direct and essentially immediate transfer of infectious agents to a receptive portal of entry through which human or animal infection may take place. This may be by direct contact, such as touching, biting, kissing, or sexual intercourse, or through direct projections (droplet spread) of droplet spray onto the conjunctiva or onto the mucous membranes of the eye, nose, or mouth during sneezing, coughing, spitting, singing, or talking (risk of transmission in this manner is usually limited to a distance of about ≤ 1 m from the source of infection). Direct transmission may also occur through direct exposure of susceptible tissue to an agent in soil, through the bite of a rabid animal, or transplacentally.

Indirect transmission:

- **Vehicle-borne**: Contaminated inanimate materials or objects (fomites) such as toys, handkerchiefs, soiled clothes, bedding, cooking or eating utensils, and surgical instruments or dressings; water, food, milk, and biological products including blood, serum, plasma, tissues, or organs; or any substance serving as an intermediate means by which an infectious agent is transported and introduced into a susceptible host through a suitable portal of entry. The agent may or may not have multiplied or developed in or on the vehicle before being transmitted.

- **Vector-borne**:

  - **Mechanical:** Includes simple mechanical carriage by a crawling or flying insect through soiling of its feet or proboscis or by passage of organisms through its gastrointestinal tract. This does not require multiplication or development of the organism.
  - **Biological:** Propagation (multiplication), cyclic development, or a combination of these (cyclopropagative) is required before the arthropod can transmit the infective form of the agent to humans. An incubation period (extrinsic) is required following infection before the arthropod becomes infective. The infectious agent may be passed vertically to succeeding generations (**transovarian transmission**); **transstadial transmission** indicates its passage from one stage of life cycle to another, as from nymph to adult. Transmission may be by injection of salivary gland fluid during biting or by regurgitation or deposition

on the skin of feces or other material capable of penetrating through the bite wound or through an area of trauma, often created by scratching or rubbing. This transmission is by an infected nonvertebrate host and not simple mechanical carriage by a vector as a vehicle. An arthropod in either role is termed a vector.

Airborne transmission: The dissemination of microbial aerosols to a suitable portal of entry, usually the respiratory tract. Microbial aerosols are suspensions of particles in the air consisting partially or wholly of microorganisms. They may remain suspended in the air for long periods of time, some retaining and others losing infectivity or virulence. Particles in the 1-5 μm range are easily drawn into the alveoli of the lungs and may be retained there. Not considered as airborne are droplets and other large particles that promptly settle out (see **Direct transmission**).

- **Droplet nuclei**: Usually the small residues that result from evaporation of fluid from droplets emitted by an infected host. They may also be created purposely by a variety of atomizing devices or accidentally as in microbiology laboratories or in abattoirs, rendering plants, or autopsy rooms. They usually remain suspended in the air for long periods.
- **Dust**: The small particles of widely varying size that may arise from soil (e.g., fungus spores), clothes, bedding, or contaminated floors.

49. **Unapparent infection** (asymptomatic, inapparent, subclinical, occult infection)—The presence of infection in a host without recognizable clinical signs or symptoms. Unapparent infections are identifiable only through laboratory means such as a blood test or through the development of positive reactivity to specific skin tests.

50. **Universal precautions**—See **Isolation**.

51. **Virulence**—The ability of an infectious agent to invade and damage tissues of the host; the degree of pathogenicity of an infectious agent, often indicated by case-fatality rates.

52. **Zoonosis**—An infection or infectious agent transmissible under natural conditions from vertebrate animals to humans. May be **enzootic** or **epizootic** (see **Endemic** and **Epidemic**).

INDEX